Central Pain Syndrome

Pathophysiology, Diagnosis, and Management

Second Edition

Central Pain Syndrome

Pathophysiology, Diagnosis, and Management

Second Edition

Sergio Canavero
Turin Advanced Neuromodulation Group, Turin, Italy

Vincenzo Bonicalzi
Turin Advanced Neuromodulation Group, Turin, Italy

CAMBRIDGE
UNIVERSITY PRESS

CAMBRIDGE UNIVERSITY PRESS
Cambridge, New York, Melbourne, Madrid, Cape Town,
Singapore, São Paulo, Delhi, Tokyo, Mexico City

Cambridge University Press
The Edinburgh Building, Cambridge CB2 8RU, UK

Published in the United States of America by Cambridge University Press, New York

www.cambridge.org
Information on this title: www.cambridge.org/9781107010215

First edition published by Cambridge University Press 2007

Second edition published 2011

Printed in the United Kingdom at the University Press, Cambridge

A catalog record for this publication is available from the British Library

Library of Congress Cataloging in Publication data

Canavero, Sergio, 1964–
Central pain syndrome : pathophysiology, diagnosis, and management / Sergio Canavero, Vincenzo Bonicalzi. – 2nd ed.
p. ; cm.
Includes bibliographical references and index.
ISBN 978-1-107-01021-5 (hardback)
1. Central pain. I. Bonicalzi, Vincenzo, 1956– II. Title.
[DNLM: 1. Pain – drug therapy. 2. Pain – physiopathology. 3. Central Nervous System – physiopathology.
4. Central Nervous System Diseases – drug therapy. WL 704]
RC368.C36 2011
616′.0472–dc22

2011011286

ISBN 978-1-107-01021-5 Hardback

To
Marco and Serena
Per aspera ad astra
and
Francesca

To Cecilia
with love

Contents

Preface to the second edition

Ever since the publication of the first edition of this book, we have been flooded with emails from patients who bought the book asking for therapeutic advice. Patient after patient, file after file, what we found left us dumbstruck. Not only did pain therapists from the most celebrated centers in the world sometimes get the diagnosis wrong, but when they got it right the therapeutic program they laid out was outlandish, to say the least – wrong drugs, wrong doses, wrong surgeries. Amazingly, we found that some therapists combine gabapentin with pregabalin at the same time in the same patient! Patients are still being subjected to deep brain stimulation as the first-line surgical option or, worse, sympathetic blocks. The medical literature too is a source of ludicrous statements, such as "SCS has not to our knowledge been used to treat central pain" or "combination of opioids and promonoaminergic drugs . . . a new strategy for central pain."

At the same time, theories have been advanced, even by people without direct experience of central pain, which are totally flawed, and these have been published by the most prestigious journals.

What accounts for this state of affairs? According to Dr. Smith, former editor of the *BMJ*, and author of *The Trouble with Medical Journals* (2006), several reasons can be adduced:

(1) low scientific quality and relevance of most published articles;
(2) manipulation of or downright fraudulent trial data, poor reporting, duplicate/redundant publications, ghost writing (i.e., articles written by compliant contract firms instead of actual researchers), and highly deficient peer review;
(3) all-pervasive conflicts of interest, with academia/industry entanglement, suppression of "undesired" negative data, economic dependency of many journals from advertisers ("medical journals are an extension of the marketing arm of pharmaceutical companies");
(4) naiveté of doctors and inability to muddle through misinformation.

As an aside, "there is evidence that patients in trials do better than patients receiving routine treatment, even if they receive a placebo."

There are also profound reasons for the failure of science to advance itself, including in the field of chronic pain. As beautifully synthesized by Prof. Montgomery (2010):

> It is human nature to discount observations that are counter to current theories, but these new observations are the source of new and better theories . . . it is important to recognize what is the basis of disagreement and the problem is that many times it appears to be based on habits and uncritical imitations of others. These do not represent knowledge . . . attacking the paradoxes is most likely to truly advance the field . . . some conservative scientists will continue to promote a theory even in the face of accumulating paradoxes and crumbling support for the theory (Kuhn 1996). Their reasons for hanging on range from polemical (Kuhn 1996) to psychological . . . science has its own "denial" mechanisms for preventing paradoxes from becoming too uncomfortable. These mechanisms include ignoring the paradoxes by not allowing their publication in peer-reviewed journals, by not funding research to explore them, by not inviting scientists who unearth them to present at conferences, and by not addressing them in articles that do get published. Another mechanism for discounting paradoxes is to attribute them to some unseen error in methods and interpretation. This discounting is easy to do because of the Quine–Duhem theorem, which holds that if the inferences from an observation are in fact wrong, it is impossible to know which of the underlying assumptions is at fault. Consequently, any underlying assumption may be at fault. Thus the paradoxical finding can be discounted by indicting an assumption, any

> assumption. And there are always assumptions. On the other hand, some radical scientists are willing to throw out any theory in the face of any paradox and redirect their research. This mechanism is supported by the concept of pessimistic induction, or the belief that because every theory in history has proven wrong, every theory in the future will also be proven wrong. Solipsism aside, such radicals, although rare, are necessary and need to be supported, if only to prevent conservatism from becoming dogma.

In a brutal, but to-the-point, remark, Dr. Sonnenberg (2007) wrote:

> Why is academic medicine run by former C-students? ... Physicians with few talents and lots of time to spare will accumulate in administration and politics, whereas those with talents and little time will remain committed to biomedical research or clinical practice.

We would add another peccadillo to the list: reliance on "glitzy" technology with imposing names (our favorite: "neuromagnetic resonance spectroscopy using wavelet decomposition and statistical testing"), but no guiding hypothesis behind.

Thus, reviewing paper after paper published in "prestigious" journals, we flushed out incongruities between reported data, poor referencing, poor analysis, etc. Witness to this, different publications labeled as below-level pain (i.e., cord central pain) pain one, two, three, four, or five levels below injury! So much for exact science. The result is that we had a real hard time wading through the morass of incomprehensible data behind central pain studies. Not surprisingly, many patients seek alternative treatments instead of the usual "old hat," as the chasm between society and science has grown ever more.

That said, the first edition of this book has met with success and good reviews, and we are fortunate that Cambridge University Press accepted to press on with a second edition.

A few highlights:

(1) Revised treatment guidelines after critical, conflict-of-interest-free assessment of the latest literature. In the chapter summarizing the options for treatment, a flow chart guides the reader through the interventions step by step. Neuromodulation (including non-invasive cortical stimulation, which is new to this edition) is one of the strong points. Useless or dangerous drugs are black-boxed.
(2) The text has been completely reorganized into 26 chapters plus an appendix. Highly specialized material has been confined to boxes and tables. While Section 4 is for the researcher only, Sections 2 and 3 are for all, including busy clinicians and patients, who can easily refer to the primary text for clear information. Pharmacologic discussion of mechanisms of action and their relevance to our understanding of the neurochemistry of central pain is left to a separate chapter in Section 4. Older material covered in the first edition and no longer felt of immediate interest has been deleted.
(3) Conditions such as multiple sclerosis, Parkinson's disease (which is not central pain), epilepsy, and other conditions are now covered in depth in a separate chapter.
(4) Extensive discussion of diagnostic methods.
(5) A new chapter on alternative and complementary therapies used by patients.
(6) Many more figures and new-to-this-edition pictures, emphasizing the corticothalamic generator.
(7) Erroneous theories of central pain (including those based on animal studies) have been confined to the appendix.
(8) Discussion of the "attractor dynamic reverberation theory" of central pain, which evidence strongly suggests to be The Theory of central pain. It offers a definitive cure and does away with all competing theories.
(9) Epidemiological data now cover Asian countries, where the bulk of the patients is found.

We have also included a few (mostly irrelevant) publications we missed in our all-out search for the first edition.

We have no qualms in saying that this new edition of *Central Pain Syndrome* sets the standard in the field and does away with the multitude of authors that pack current books with no single "clear view" and no clear conclusions. Hopefully, statements such as "the pathophysiology of central pain is poorly understood," "treatment is unsatisfactory," or "central pain remains a mysterious syndrome" (Fishman *et al.* 2010: *Bonica's Management of Pain*, 4th edition, p. 370) will be relegated to the dustbin of history.

Special thanks go to Deborah Russell, medical editor at Cambridge University Press, who spurred us in our endeavor, Nisha Doshi for providing effective editorial assistance, and Charlotte homus for bringing the whole ball of wax to fruition. Thanks girls! And equally hearty thanks to Hugh "Hawk Eye" Brazier, without whom this written endeavor would have been a few cuts below excellent. Thanks lad!

Sergio Canavero, Vincenzo Bonicalzi
Turin, April 2011

Preface to the first edition (or, the story of an idea)

"The man with a new idea is a crank – until the idea succeeds"
(Mark Twain)

The story of this book goes back 15 enthusiastic years. At the end of 1991, S.C., at the time 26, was asked by C. A. Pagni, one of the past mavens of the field, to take up central pain. S. C. was back from a semester as an intern at Lyon (France) neurosurgical hospital. A dedicated bookworm, he often skipped the operating theater in favor of the local well-stocked library. In that year a paper was published by two US neurobiologists, espousing the idea of consciousness arising from corticothalamic reverberation: this paper drew his attention, as he was entertaining a different opinion as to how consciousness arises. At the beginning of 1992 he came across a paper written by two US neurologists, describing a case of central post-stroke pain abolished by a further stroke: the authors were at a loss to explain the reason.

Discoveries sometimes happen when two apparently distant facts suddenly fit together to explain a previously puzzling observation. And so it was. During a "girl-hunting" bike trip at Turin's best-known park, a sunny springtime afternoon, the realization came thundering in. Within a short time, a name was found and so the dynamic reverberation theory of central pain was born. It was first announced in a paper published in the February 1993 issue of *Neurosurgery* and then in *Medical Hypotheses* in 1994.

In May 1992 Pagni introduced Dr. Bonicalzi, a neuroanesthesiologist and pain therapist, to S.C. Over the following years, the combined effort led to further evidence in favor of the theory, in particular a neurochemical foundation based on the discovery that propofol, a recently introduced intravenous anesthetic, could quench central pain at nonanesthetic doses (September 1992). The idea of using propofol at such dosage came from reading a paper by Swiss authors describing its use in central pruritus. The similitude between central pain and pruritus, at the time not clearly delineated in the literature, was the driving reason. In 1988 Tsubokawa in Japan introduced cortical stimulation for central pain: it was truly ad hoc, as cortex plays a major role in the theory. Happily, since 1991, the cortex has gone through a renaissance in pain research, although neurosurgical work already pointed in that direction. We soon combined three lines of research – drug dissection, neuroimaging and cortical stimulation data – in our effort to tease out the mechanism subserving central pain.

Central pain as a scientific concept was the product of an inquisitive mind, that of Dr. L. Edinger, a neurologist working in Frankfurt-am-Main, Germany, at the end of the 1800s. Despite being recognized by early-twentieth-century neurologists as the initiator of the idea of "centrally arising pains," this recognition soon faded, shadowed by Dejerine and Roussy and their thalamic syndrome. At the beginning of the twenty-first century, due credit must go to the physician who deserved it in the first place, namely Dr. Edinger.

For a century, central pain has remained neglected among pain syndromes, both for a lack of pathophysiological understanding and a purported rarity thereof. Far from it! Recent estimates make it no rarer than Parkinson's disease, which, however, commands a huge literature. Worse yet, the treatment of central pain has only progressed over the past 15 years or so and much of the new acquisitions have not yet reached the pain therapist in a rational fashion.

As we set out to write this book, we decided to review the entire field and not only expound the dynamic reverberation theory, which, as we hope to show, may truly represent "the end of central pain." It has truly been a "sweatshop work" as we perused hundreds of papers and dusted off local medical libraries in search of obscure and less obscure papers in many languages, as true detectives. We drew out single cases lost in a *mare magnum* of unrelated data and in the process gave new meaning to long-overlooked reports. We also realized that some bad science mars the field, and this is properly addressed.

The result is – hopefully – the most complete reference source on central pain over the past 70 years or so. The reader should finish the book with a sound understanding of what central pain is and how it should be treated. The majority of all descriptive material has been tabulated, so that reading will flow easily. We hope this will be of help to the millions who suffer from central pain.

Special thanks go to the "unsung heroes" at the National Library of Medicine in Washington, DC, whose monumental efforts made our toil (and those of thousands of researchers around the world) less defatiguing. Thanks also to the guys behind Microsoft Word, which made the tabulations easy as pie. Also, due recognition must go to the Cambridge staff who have been supervising this project over the past two years, especially Nat Russo, Cathy Felgar, and Jennifer Percy and the people at Keyword, above all Andy Baxter and Andrew Bacon for the excellent editorial work.

Sergio Canavero, Vincenzo Bonicalzi
Turin, May 2006

Abbreviations

ACC	anterior cingulate cortex
AD	antidepressant
AED	antiepileptic drug
AIDS	acquired immune deficiency syndrome
AMPA	alpha-amino-3-hydroxy-5-methyl-4-isoxazolepropionic acid
ASAS	anterior spinal artery syndrome
ASIA	American Spinal Injury Association
AVM	arteriovenous malformation
BCP	brain central pain
BOLD	blood-oxygen-level dependent
BPA	brachial plexus avulsion
BPI	Brief Pain Inventory
BS	brainstem
CAM	complementary and alternative medicine
CBF	cerebral blood flow
CBT	cognitive behavioral therapy
CC	cingulate cortex
CCP	cord central pain
CD	central dysesthesia
CDT	cold detection threshold
CES	cranial electrotherapy stimulation
CESD-SF	Center for Epidemiologic Studies Depression Scale – Short Form
CGIC	Clinical Global Impression of Change
CGRP	calcitonin gene-related peptide
CHEP	contact heat evoked potential
CK	creatine kinase
CL	central lateral nucleus
CM	centromedian nucleus (centrum medianum)
CNP	central neurogenic pruritus
CNS	central nervous system
CP	central pain
CPAC	central pain-allied conditions
CPSP	central post-stroke pain
CPT	cold pain threshold
CRPS	complex regional pain syndrome
CS	cortical stimulation
CSF	cerebrospinal fluid
CT	computed tomography
CT	corticothalamic
CVS	caloric vestibular stimulation
DBS	deep brain stimulation
DC	dorsal column
DLPFC	dorsolateral prefrontal cortex
DM	dorsomedian
DMN	default mode network
DPN	diprenorphine
DREZ	dorsal root entry zone
DRG	dorsal root ganglion
DSIS	Daily Sleep Interference Scale
DTI	diffusion tensor imaging
ECD	ethylene cysteine dimer
ECG	electrocardiography
ECoG	electrocorticography
ECS	extradural cortical stimulation
ECT	electroconvulsive therapy
EDSS	Expanded Disability Status Scale
EEG	electroencephalography
EMA	European Medicines Agency
EP	evoked potential
EPSP	excitatory postsynaptic potential
EQ-5D	Euro Quality of Life 5 dimensions
FBSS	failed back surgery syndrome
FDA	Food and Drug Administration
FDG	fluorodeoxyglucose
fMRI	functional magnetic resonance imaging
FPS	Faces Pain Scale
FWHM	full width at half-maximum
GABA	gamma-aminobutyric acid
HADS	Hospital Anxiety and Depression Scale
HMPAO	hexamethylpropyleneamineoxime
HPC	heat-pinch-cold
HPT	heat pain threshold
IASP	International Association for the Study of Pain
IC	internal capsule

IPG	implanted pulse generator
ITT	intention to treat
LANSS	Leeds Assessment of Neuropathic Symptoms and Signs
LDH	lactate dehydrogenase
LEP	laser evoked potential
LFP	local field potential
LMI	lateral medullary infarction
LOI	level of injury
LORETA	low-resolution tomography
LTMP	long-term microcircuit plasticity
LTS	low-threshold spike
MCA	middle cerebral artery
MCC	mid cingulate cortex
MCS	motor cortex stimulation
MD	mediodorsal
MEG	magnetoencephalography
MEP	motor evoked potential
MI	primary motor cortex
ML	medial lemniscus
MMPI	Minnesota Multiphasic Personality Inventory
MMSE	Mini Mental State Examination
MOS	Medical Outcome Study
MPI	multidimensional pain inventory
MPQ	McGill Pain Questionnaire
MRI	magnetic resonance imaging
MRS	magnetic resonance spectroscopy
MT	mirror therapy
NAA	*N*-acetyl-aspartic acid
NMDA	*N*-methyl-D-aspartic acid
NNT	number needed to treat
NP	neuropathic pain
NPS	Neuropathic Pain Scale
NPSI	Neuropathic Pain Symptom Inventory
NRS	numerical rating scale
NSAID	non-steroidal anti-inflammatory drug
NVS	numerical verbal scale
NWC	number of words chosen
OFC	orbitofrontal cortex
OGMUR	oxygen–glucose molar utilization ratio
OR	opioid receptor
OXCBZ	oxcarbazepine
PAG	periaqueductal gray
PCA	patient-controlled analgesia
PCP	primary central pain
PD	Parkinson's disease
PDI	Pain Disability Index
PET	positron emission tomography
Pf	parafascicular nucleus
PF	projected field
PFC	prefrontal cortex
PGIC	Patient's Global Impression of Change
PHN	postherpetic neuralgia
PICA	posteroinferior cerebellar artery
PNP	peripheral neuropathic pain
Pom	posterior medial nucleus
PPC	posterior parietal cortex
PPI	patient pain intensity
PRI	Pain Rating Index
PRI(R)	Pain Rating Index (rank)
PS	parasylvian
PSS	pure sensory stroke
PVG	periventricular gray
PW	pulse width
QANeP	Quantitative Assessment of Neuropathic Pain
QoL	quality of life
QST	quantitative sensory testing
QTT	quintothalamic tract
rCBF	regional cerebral blood flow
rCMRGlu	regional cerebral glucose metabolic rate
$rCMRO_2$	regional cerebral oxygen metabolism rate
RCT	randomized controlled trial
RF	receptive field
RMT	resting motor threshold
rOEF	regional oxygen extraction fraction
rTMS	repetitive transcranial magnetic stimulation
SAH	subarachnoid hemorrhage
SF-36	Short Form-36
SF-MPQ	Short Form McGill Pain Questionnaire
SCI	spinal cord injury
SCS	spinal cord stimulation
SI	primary somatosensory cortex
SII	secondary somatosensory cortex
SMA	supplementary motor area
SNRI	serotonin–norepinephrine reuptake inhibitor
SPECT	single photon emission computed tomography
SRPC	subparietal radiatotomy/posterior capsulotomy
SRT	spinoreticulothalamic tract
SSEP	somatosensory evoked potential

SSRI	selective serotonin reuptake inhibitor
STP	spinothalamoparietal
STrT	spinotrigeminothalamic tract
STT	spinothalamic tract
TANG	Turin Advanced Neuromodulation Group
TC	thalamocortical
TCD	thalamocortical dysrhythmia
tDCS	transcranial direct current stimulation
TENS	transcutaneous electrical nerve stimulation
TMS	transcranial magnetic stimulation
TN	trigeminal neuralgia
TOPS	Treatment Outcomes of Pain Survey
TRN	thalamic reticular nucleus
TSL	thermal sensory limen
UPDRS	United Parkinson Disease Rating Scale
VAS	visual analog scale
Vc	ventrocaudalis (ventrocaudal nucleus)
Vim	ventralis intermedius
VM	ventral medial nucleus
VMpo	ventral medial nucleus, posterior part
VPI	ventral posterior inferior nucleus
VPL	ventral posterolateral nucleus
WBPQ	Wisconsin Brief Pain Questionnaire
WDT	warm detection threshold

Section 1 Introduction

Those who cannot remember the past are condemned to repeat it.
G. Santayana

Chapter 1

Introducing central pain

Definition

Ever since Dejerine and Roussy's description of central pain (CP) after thalamic stroke in 1906, *thalamic pain* (itself part of the *thalamic syndrome*) has remained the best-known form of CP and it has often – misleadingly – been used for all kinds of CP. Since CP is due to extrathalamic lesions in the majority of patients, this term should be discarded in favor of the terms central pain of brain–brainstem or cord origin (BCP and CCP). Unacceptable terms include *pseudothalamic pain*, *parainsular pain*, *central deafferentation pain*, *neural injury pain*, *anesthesia dolorosa* (if it refers to central nervous system [CNS] lesions). If a stroke is the cause of CP, the term central post-stroke pain (CPSP) is used. Even though some clinical features are similar, peripheral neuropathic pain (PNP), e.g., brachial plexus avulsion pain, postherpetic neuralgia, and complex regional pain disorder, is not CP, although in some cases the dorsal horn may be involved.

CP is akin to central dysesthesias/paresthesias (CD) and central neurogenic pruritus (CNP): actually, these are facets of the same disturbance of sensory processing following CNS lesions. Dysesthesias and paresthesias differ from pain in being abnormal unpleasant and non-unpleasant sensations with a non-painful quality. Virtually all kinds of slowly or rapidly developing disease processes affecting the spinothalamic and quintothalamic tracts (STT/QTT), i.e., the pathways that are most important for the sensations of pain and temperature, at any level from the dorsal horn/sensory trigeminal nucleus to the parietal cortex, can lead to CP/CD/CNP. These do not depend on continuous receptor activation.

CP/CD/CNP is defined as:

Spontaneous and/or evoked, anomalous, painful or non-painful, sensations projected in a body area congruent with a clearly imaged lesion impairing – transitorily or permanently – the function of the spinothalamoparietal thermoalgesic pathway.

For simplicity, we will refer to CP *tout court* throughout the text. Parkinson's disease (PD), epileptic pains, and perhaps other diseases with a painful CP-like component should be classified as *central pain-allied conditions* (CPAC). In PD there is no impairment of the spinothalamoparietal (STP) path, but an anomalous modulation of the acute pain networks (no thermoalgesic deficit), and in epilepsy there is an over-recruitment of pain-coded neurons.

History

Cases of CP following brain or cord damage have most certainly been observed since antiquity, but never understood as such. We have to wait until the nineteenth century for published descriptions of what we now understand to be CP (Table 1.1) in Western medicine (there appear to be reports of what is most likely CP in ancient Chinese medicine, this being the result of a "deficiency of the Qi and attendant blood stasis, in turn depriving the nourishing of meridians and tendons"; see Kuong 1984). However, the possibility of *centrally arising* pains was simply dismissed by most authorities.

It was not until 1891 that Edinger, a German neurologist, challenging the prevailing opinion of the day, and "*avec une rare sagacité*" (with rare sagacity; Garcin 1937), introduced the concept of *centrally arising pains*. In his landmark paper "Are there centrally arising pains? Description of a case of bleeding in the nucleus externus thalami optici and in the pulvinar, whose essential symptom consisted in hyperesthesia and terrible pains in the contralateral side, besides hemiathetosis and hemianopsia" (Fig. 1.1), he remarked how only a few cases of pains associated with damage of the brain, brainstem, and spinal cord were on record ("*Die Durchsicht der Literatur nach aehnlichen Beobachtungen hat nur wenig ergeben*" – a literature review of similar cases has borne little

Table 1.1. Historic highlights of central pain (CP), from De Ajuriaguerra (1937), Garcin (1937)

Viesseux (1810)	Presented his own experience of dissociated sensory loss after brainstem stroke
Marcet (1811)	Describes pain after bulbar lesions
Fodera (1822)	Describes pain after spinal hemisection
D'Angers (1824)	First describes syringomyelia
Brown-Séquard (1850)	Describes the syndrome named after him; confirms previous description of hyperesthesia below lesion level on the plegic side
1860–70s	Descriptions of pain after spinal trauma during the US Civil War
Charcot (1872) [pp. 239–40]	Description of multiple sclerosis and the associated pains
Marot (1875)	Further describes pain after bulbar lesions
Nothnagel (1879)	First precise description of constant pain following tumors of the pons (mentioned by other authors) and other sites
Page (1883)	Describes pain in spinal cord injury patients
Edinger (1891)	Birth of the concept of CP
Hardford (1891)	Describes pain of cortical origin
Mann (1892)	Matches CP to infarctions of medulla at nucleus ambiguus level
Gilles de la Tourette (1889)	Describes syringomyelic pain
Wallenberg (1895)	(Re)describes the syndrome named after him; insists on facial pains; ascribes it to PICA embolism (verified autoptically in 1901)
Reichenberg (1897)	Describes CP as resulting from parietal stroke (autopsy confirmed)
Link (1899)	Describes CP as resulting from pontobulbar lesions
Dejerine and Roussy (1906)	Describe the syndrome named after them
Head and Holmes (1911)	First quantitative assessment of sensory deficits in CP
Holmes (1919)	"Typical thalamic pain" observed in spinal cord injured patients (World War I soldiers)
Souques (1910), Guillain and Bertrand, Davison and Schick, Schuster, Wilson, Parker (1920s–30s)	Autoptic confirmation that CP may arise without thalamic involvement
Cassinari and Pagni (1969)	Pinpoint the anatomic basis of CP

Also of note: Elsberg (cordonal pain), Förster (dorsal horn pain), Gerhardt (recognized CP in multiple sclerosis), Anton. See Canavero and Bonicalzi (2007a) for other authors.

fruit), but that other reasons were adduced to explain them (generally peripheral nerve causes or muscle spasms).

One of the few "well investigated" cases was that of Greiff (1883), concerning a 74-year-old woman who developed "*Hyperaesthesie und reissenden Schmerzen im linkem Arm, geringgradiger im linkem Beine*" (hyperesthesia and tearing pains in the left arm and of lesser intensity in the left leg) as a consequence of several strokes, which lasted for two months until death. At autopsy, two areas of thalamic softening were found, one of which was in what appears to be ventrocaudalis (Vc). Greiff commented on vasomotor disturbances as a possible cause of pain. According to Edinger, "*Vielleicht giebt es auch corticale Schmerzen*" (perhaps there are also cortical pains), and he cited as evidence "*schmerzhaften Aura bei epileptischen, abnorme Sensationen bei Rindenherden und*

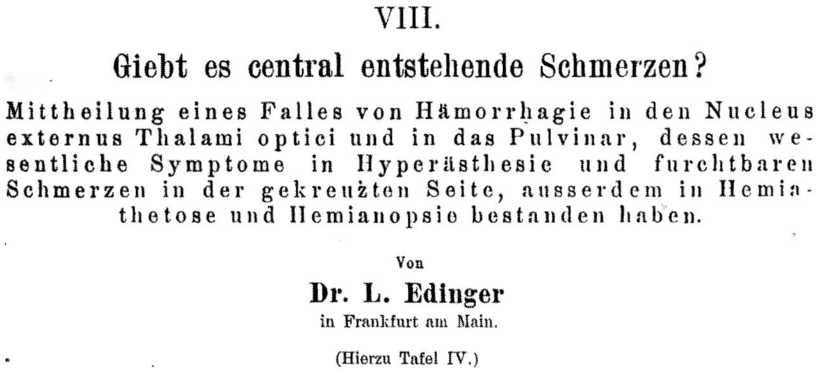

VIII.

Giebt es central entstehende Schmerzen?

Mittheilung eines Falles von Hämorrhagie in den Nucleus externus Thalami optici und in das Pulvinar, dessen wesentliche Symptome in Hyperästhesie und furchtbaren Schmerzen in der gekreuzten Seite, ausserdem in Hemiathetose und Hemianopsie bestanden haben.

Von

Dr. L. Edinger

in Frankfurt am Main.

(Hierzu Tafel IV.)

Figure 1.1. Title page of Edinger's 1891 paper marking the birth of the concept of central pain.

Reizerscheinungen im Bereich des Opticus bei Affectionen des Hinterhaupts-lappens" (painful aura in epileptics, abnormal sensations in cortical foci, and signs of excitation in the territory of the opticus following diseases of the occipital lobe). Edinger reported on "*einen Krankheitsfall … in dem als Ursache ganz furchtbaren Schmerzen post mortem ein Herd gefunden wurde, der dicht an die sensorische Faserung grenzend im Thalamus lag. Der Fall erscheint dadurch besonders beweiskraftig fuer die Existenz 'centraler Schmerzen', weil die Hyperaesthesie und die Schmerzen sofort nach dem Insulte und monatelang vor einer spaeter auftretenden Hemichorea sich zeigten*" (a patient … in whom the origin of truly terrible pains was at autopsy a lesion that impinged on the fibers abutting the thalamus. This case is thus especially convincing evidence for the existence of "central pains," as the hyperesthesia and the pains showed immediately after the insult and months before a later arising hemichorea). The patient was "*Frau R*" (Mrs. R), aged 48, who developed "*heftige Schmerzen und deutliche Hyperaesthesie in den gelaehmten Gliedern*" (violent pains and clear-cut hyperesthesia in the paretic limbs: right arm and leg), "*Wegen der furchtbaren Schmerzen Suicidium 1888*" (due to the terrible pains, suicide 1888). This woman developed an intense tactile allodynia for all stimuli bar minimal, which hindered all home and personal activities (e.g., dressing) and made her cry; also "*Laues Wasser wurde als sehr heiss, kaltes als unertraeglich schmerzend*" (lukewarm water was felt as very hot, and cold water as intolerably painful) in both limbs. Very high doses of "*Morphium*" were basically ineffective. This patient's pain reached intolerable peaks, but sometimes could be tolerated for a few hours or at most half a day before shooting up again. In this patient, "*Vasomotorische Stoerungen, wie sie in dem Lauenstein (D.Arch.f.klin.Med. Bd.XX.u.A.)'schen … Falle bestanden haben, sind nicht zur Beobachtung gekommen*" (vasomotor disturbances, as present in Lauenstein's case, were nowhere to be observed). At autopsy, "*Der Herd im Gehirn nimmt also den dorsalen Theil des Nucleus externus thalami und einen Theil des Pulvinar ein, er erstreckt sich lateral vom Pulvinar fuer 1 mm in den hintersten Theil der inneren Kapsel hinein. Der Faserausfall, der dort in Betracht kommt, ist sehr gering*" (the brain lesion involved the dorsal portion of the nucleus externus thalami and a portion of the pulvinar, extending laterally from the pulvinar for 1 mm into the most posterior part of the inner capsule. The loss of fibers, which can be observed at this point, is minimal). Thus, in Greiff's and Edinger's patients, lesions were respectively found at autopsy in right thalamic nucleus internus and ventral thalamus, and in thalamic nucleus externus and pulvinar.

Edinger should be given the credit for introducing the concept of CP to neurology, as he wrote: "*Man kommt zum Schlusse, dass hier wahrscheinlich durch directen Contact der sensorischen Kapselbahn mit erkranktem Gewebe die Hyperaesthesie und die Schmerzen in der gekreuzten Koerperhaelfte erzeugt worden sind*" (one concludes that here both the hyperesthesia and the pains in the crossed half of the body have been likely caused by direct contact of injured tissue with the sensory path coursing in the internal capsule).

One year later, Mann (1892), another German neurologist, concluded, in Edinger's wake, that CP can be also observed outside the thalamus, namely in the medulla oblongata, thus antedating Wallenberg's classic description (autopsy of this patient performed

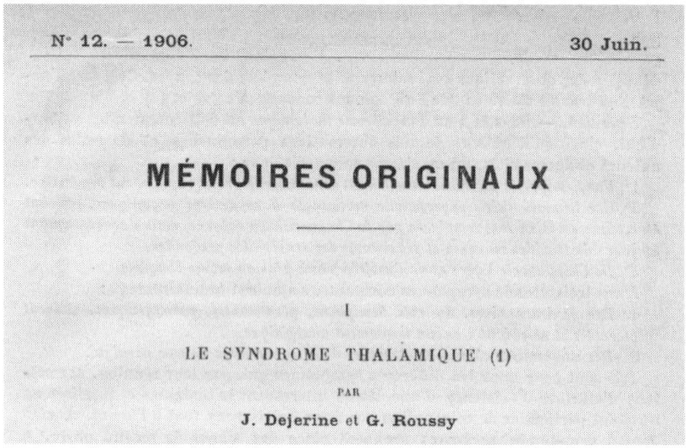
N° 12. — 1906. 30 Juin.

MÉMOIRES ORIGINAUX

I

LE SYNDROME THALAMIQUE (1)

PAR

J. Dejerine et G. Roussy

Figure 1.2. Title page of Dejerine and Roussy's 1906 paper introducing the "thalamic syndrome."

in 1912 confirmed Mann's clinical diagnosis and the involvement of the spinothalamic tract). Thereafter, an explosion of reports ensued.

In the first decade of the twentieth century, Dejerine and Egger (1903) and Dejerine and Roussy (1906) described six cases of what they called "*syndrome thalamique,*" (Fig. 1.2), whose signs and symptoms were defined thus (Roussy 1907):

> *Définition – Sous le nom de syndrome thalamique on doit comprendre aujourd'hui, ainsi qu'il ressort de nos observations personnelles et de celles des auteurs ci-dessus cités, un syndrome caractérisé par:*
> 1° *Une hémiplégie légère habituellement sans contracture et rapidement regressive.*
> 2° *Une hémianestésie superficielle persistante à caractères organiques, pouvant être, dans certains cas, remplacée par de l'hyperesthésie cutanée, mais s'accompagnant toujours de troubles marqués et persistants des sensibilités profondes.*
> 3° *De l'hémiataxie légère et de l'astéréognosie plus ou moins complete.*
> *A ces trois grands symptômes constants, s'ajoutent ordinairement:*
> 4° *Des douleurs vives, du côté hèmiplégié, persistantes, paroxystiques, souvent intolérables et ne cédant à aucun traitement analgésique.*
> 5° *Des mouvements choréo-athétosiques dans les membres du côté paralysé.*
>
> [(1) slight hemiparesis usually without contracture and rapidly regressive; (2) persistent superficial hemianesthesia of an organic character which can in some cases be replaced by cutaneous hyperesthesia, but always accompanied by marked and persistent disturbances of deep sensations; (3) mild hemiataxia and more or less complete astereognosis. To these principal and constant symptoms are ordinarily added: (4) severe, persistent, paroxysmal, often intolerable pain on the hemiparetic side unyielding to any analgesic treatment; (5) choreoathetotic movements in the limbs on the paralyzed side.]

Dejerine and Roussy wrote:

> *Les douleurs ... Nous les retrouvons ... dans la plupart des cas de syndrome thalamique ... avec assez de fréquence, pour nous autoriser à admettre que ces douleurs sont sous la dépendence de la lésion thalamique, ou mieux de la destruction et de l'irritation des fibres qui viennent s'arboriser dans sa portion ventrale.*
>
> [The pains ... We find them ... in most cases of the thalamic syndrome ... with enough frequency to warrant the conclusion that these pains are due to the thalamic lesion, or better to the destruction and irritation of the fibers branching throughout its ventral portion.]

Thereafter, on the basis of an autopsy study of three cases (Joss ..., Hud ..., Thal ...), they concluded that:

> *Une lesion de la couche optique intéressant le noyau externe dans sa partie postéro-externe et prenant en outre une partie des noyeaux médian et interne ainsi que le fragment correspondant de la capsule interne, donne en clinique un tableau symptomatique toujours semblable à lui-meme ... Ce tableau symptomatique constitue ... un nouveau syndrome qui doit prendre rang dans la nosologie: le syndrome thalamique.*
>
> [A lesion of the optic bed involving the postero-exterior side of the external nucleus and also a portion of the median and internal nuclei plus a corresponding fragment of the internal capsule leads to a consistent clinical picture ... this collection of symptoms adds up to ... a new, nosologically separate syndrome: the thalamic syndrome.]

A few years later, Head and Holmes (1911), on the basis of personal and literature autoptic evidence, concluded that thalamic pain depends on the destruction of the posterior part of the external thalamic nucleus. In their book-size article, they provided the best and first quantitative description ever of somatosensory alterations in CP patients.

During World War I several observations on "thalamic pains" associated with spinal cord war lesions were published, as had previously been done – but only descriptively – during the American Civil War in the 1860s. The term *central pain* was first used in the English literature by Behan (1914). In 1933 Hoffman reported a tiny lesion in the most basal part of the Vc, where spinothalamic fibers end (Hassler's Vcpc), the smallest reported lesion causing CP at the time. Interestingly, he commented that *"Der Fall spricht gegen die Schmerztheorie von Head und legt den Gedanken nahe, dass die Spontanschmerzen durch eine funktionwandelung im Bereiche des Schmerzleitungsystem selbst entstehen"* (the report speaks against Head's theory and suggests that the spontaneous pain is self-generated through a functional change of the pain conducting system).

In the 1930s three major reviews on CP were published (De Ajuriaguerra 1937, Garcin 1937, Riddoch 1938). Here, the interested reader will find an unparalleled review of the literature of the nineteenth and early twentieth centuries, plus unsurpassed descriptions of CP, whose ignorant neglect (admittedly also due to language barriers) on the part of modern investigators is responsible for several "rediscoveries." Nothing new has basically been added to the clinical literature since then. Riddoch (1938) gave this definition:

> By central pain is meant spontaneous pain and painful overreaction to objective stimulation resulting from lesions confined to the substance of the central nervous system including dysesthesiae of a disagreeable kind.

It was clear how "thalamic pains" could follow a lesion of the lateral thalamic area, in the territories of the lenticulo-optic, thalamo-geniculate, and thalamo-perforating arteries, but also of the cortex (rarely), internal capsule, medulla oblongata, and less frequently the pons (no mesencephalic lesions were on record) and the spinal cord (not infrequently; particularly following injury and syringomyelia). Thermoalgesic sensory loss and somatotopographical constraints were clearly delineated.

The most frequent cause of CP appeared to be vascular at all levels, except the brainstem, where tumors, tuberculomas, multiple sclerosis, syringobulbia, and hematobulbia contributed. Epileptic pains were also considered CP.

Unfortunately, over the years, despite ample evidence that other lesions can cause CP as well, the term *thalamic syndrome* became synonymous with CP, despite it being clear to many that it was not so.

In 1969 Cassinari and Pagni, in their monograph *Central Pain: a Neurosurgical Survey*, wrote:

> The conclusions of the various workers who have tried . . . to identify the structure in which lesions are responsible for the onset of central pain sometimes conflict. The divergence of opinion is fairly easily explained by the fact that spontaneous lesions are usually extensive, difficult to define, often plurifocal, and affect several systems with different functions.

By studying iatrogenic "pure" lesions (which they equated to "*experimental lesions*") giving rise to CP, they reached the conclusion that the essential lesion was damage to the pain-conveying spinothalamoparietal tract. Also, they observed how operations that interrupt the central pain pathways in order to allay pain may themselves lead to CP (sometimes more severe than the pain that led to the operation), an occurrence practically impossible to foresee. However, the genesis of CP remained an enigma. Thereafter, the subject received little additional attention (the "*hidden disorder*": Schott 1996), with most physicians in practice having little appreciation of the subject. In 1994, Canavero put forth the *dynamic reverberation* theory of central pain (Fig. 1.3), which, as this book will show, is the only one that can explain the genesis of this syndrome and provide what biomedical theories should strive for: a definitive cure.

Medical Hypotheses

Medical Hypotheses (1994) 42, 203–207
© Longman Group Ltd 1994

Dynamic Reverberation. A Unified Mechanism for Central and Phantom Pain

S. CANAVERO

Figure 1.3. Title page of Canavero's 1994 paper introducing the dynamic reverberation theory of central pain. Reproduced with permission from Elsevier.

Section 2

Clinical features and diagnosis

Per me si va nella città dolente,
Per me si va nell'eterno dolore,
Per me si va tra la perduta gente.

[Through me you pass into the city of woe,
Through me you pass into eternal pain,
Through me among the people lost for aye]

Written above Hell's Gate
Dante Alighieri, Inferno, *Canto III, 1–3*
(early fourteenth century)

Chapter 2

Epidemiology

Brain central pain

Close to 10% of all strokes (brain and brainstem, ischemic and hemorrhagic), regardless of the presence of sensory deficits, lead to central pain as defined in Chapter 1. This is a much higher figure than previously accepted (*c.* 1%). The presence of sensory deficits increases the risk, but it is not yet clear whether certain brain sites actually carry a higher risk of brain central pain (BCP). In the USA there are 6.5 million people who have suffered a stroke, while each year *c.* 600 000 suffer a first stroke and another 200 000 or so a recurrence. In Europe, 6 million survivors are currently recorded, with 1.1 million new strokes yearly (113/100 000/year). In China, the incidence ranges between 135/100 000 in Beijing and 70/100 000 in Shanghai (Jiang *et al.* 2006); in the 1980s the prevalence was about 900/100 000. In India, surveys found a 105–262/100 000 stroke incidence (Banerjee and Kumar 2006; see also Table 2.1). In Singapore, people of Chinese ethnicity are more affected than Indians or Malays. In Brazil a city survey found a 80/100 000 yearly incidence (Cabral *et al.* 2009). Estimates based on WHO data suggest that the current global burden of stroke is 16 million first-ever strokes and 62 million stroke survivors. Yearly, 2 million people suffer spontaneous non-traumatic intracerebral hemorrhages, which make up 10–15% of all strokes in Western countries and 20–30% in the East. Thus, **stroke alone should account for several (*c.* 6) million BCP patients globally**. Given current projections of stroke prevalence, this figure is destined to increase (Strong *et al.* 2007).

No prospective study exists on the prevalence and incidence of CP following brain injury. Its supposed rarity must therefore be called into question.

Central pain is rarely due to brain tumors. For instance, in a series of 123 cases of BCP, only two were due to tumors (Amancio *et al.* 2002).

An under-recognized cause of CP is surgery (and particularly neurosurgery), either via direct brain (and cord) damage or postoperative strokes. Unfortunately, no epidemiological data are available.

There do not appear to be clear-cut differences in age distribution between the general stroke population and CPSP (Table 2.3 in Canavero and Bonicalzi 2007a). In a recent series, median age of patients with CPSP was 62.5 years (Klit *et al.* 2011). The suggestion that CP may depend in some way on the maturity of the nervous system is refuted by reports of CP in children (Ameri 1967: infant; Zaki *et al.* 2010: 10-year-old male) and cases of central pruritus in children are on record (Chapter 5).

A majority of studies find men more affected than women, with some exceptions (e.g., Andersen *et al.* 1995: male/female 0.77; Lampl *et al.* 2002: male/female 0.69; Klit *et al.* 2011: male/female 0.86; see Table 2.4 in Canavero and Bonicalzi 2007a). Moreover, after age 80, females are more affected by stroke than males (USA).

Cord central pain (below-level pain)

Literature series are often inconsistent and contradictory, because pain terms used are not homogeneous, research methods vary widely (e.g., cross-sectional, retrospective, by questionnaire or postal survey), and cord central pain (CCP) can be "simulated" by other concurrent pains, which are often not well differentiated (Cardenas and Felix 2009, Dijkers *et al.* 2009). Most importantly, there is no agreement on the definition of at-level versus below-level neuropathic pain, with authors classifying as CCP pain found one, two, three, four, or five levels below injury. Thus, it is not surprising that quoted estimates range from *c.* 5% to *c.* 95% of all patients with spinal cord injury (SCI). The lack of prospective longitudinal studies also means that no significant determining or predictive factor can be validated. Burke (1973) reported different incidences of pain among paraplegics in different societies.

Table 2.1. Incidence and prevalence of brain central pain (BCP)

Reference	Pathology	No. of patients	Patients with CP
Kameyama (1976–77)	Ventrocaudalis (Vc) vascular lesions	87	Clinicopathological study. Cases selected at random from a routine autopsy series Thalamic spontaneous pain present in 12 patients (**14%**) "Dysesthesia" in 25 patients (**29%**)
Graff-Radford *et al.* (1985)	Non-hemorrhagic thalamic infarction	25	"Dysesthesia" in 4 patients (**16%**) Dysesthesias present only in a subgroup of patients with posterolateral (geniculothalamic) infarction, in whom the incidence was raised to **44.4%** (4/9 patients)
Kawahara *et al.* (1986)	Small thalamic hemorrhage	37	"Paresthesia and/or dysesthesia" in 6 patients (**16.2%**). Symptoms present only in patients with posterolateral thalamic lesions: 6/28 patients (**21.4%**)
Bogousslavsky *et al.* (1988)	Thalamic infarct	40	**Prospective study** (all patients with a thalamic infarct admitted to the neurology department between 1978 and 1986) reporting clinical findings and long-term follow-up of 40 patients with a CT-proven "pure" thalamic infarct. Delayed-onset (1 week, 2 months, and 3 months) severe (2 cases) or moderate (1 case) CP in 2 women and 1 man out of 27 patients with sensory dysfunctions Pain incidence: • whole group: 3/40 patients (**7.5%**) • patients with sensory impairment: 3/27 (**11%**) • patients with inferolateral territory infarct and lesion of the thalamic Vc region: 3/18–19 (**c. 17%**) patients with infarcts outside the Vc region: no CP observed
Samuelsson *et al.* (1994)	Lacunar infarct syndromes	39	Patients collected from a series of 100 **consecutive** patients. Pure sensory stroke (thalamic) in 10 cases Pain incidence: • whole group: 3/39 (**7.7%**) (severe in 2 [5.1%]) • pure sensory stroke: 3/10 (**30%**) (severe in 2 [20%])
Kumral *et al.* (1995)	Thalamic hemorrhage	100	**Consecutive** patients affected by thalamic hemorrhage and admitted to a single neurology department between 1988 and 1993 Sensory deficits: 66/100 patients Acute thalamic pain: 0/100 patients Delayed (1 month) thalamic pain: 3 patients (large anterolateral, posterolateral, and dorsal thalamic hemorrhage, respectively) Delayed (1 month) thalamic pain plus chorea plus ataxia (thalamic syndrome): 6 patients: small posterolateral hemorrhage (1 case), large posterolateral hemorrhage (4 cases), large medial hemorrhage (1 case) CPSP incidence in the whole group: **9%** (not reported if CPSP arose only in patients with somatosensory deficits)
Andersen *et al.* (1995)	Unselected stroke population	267	Study evaluating the incidence of CPSP in 207 (out of 267) patients (age < 81 years) surviving at least 6 months after a stroke and who were able to communicate reliably. Sampling bias reduced by also examining 1/3 of the 10% non-hospitalized patients. 60 patients (23%) died in the first 6 months after stroke and were not examined. Exclusion criteria: patients with subarachnoid hemorrhage, Binswanger's disease, degenerative or expansive neurological diseases. Characterization of the site and

Table 2.1. (cont.)

<table>
<tr><th>Reference</th><th>Pathology</th><th>No. of patients</th><th>Patients with CP</th></tr>
<tr><td></td><td></td><td></td><td>extension of the lesions by means of a CT scan. Neuropsychiatric examinations and detailed sensory test made in the first week, at 1, 6, and 12 months after the stroke. Patients lost to follow-up: < 5%
Incidence of CPSP at follow-up (% of patients):
• 1 month: 4.8%; 6 months: 6.5%; 1 year: 8.4% (16/191 patients) (moderate or severe in 5%)
Evoked dysesthesia or allodynia in all but 1 patient. One further patient had persistent evoked non-painful dysesthesia. In 2 additional patients pain disappeared spontaneously; 1 patient had evoked dysethesia and shoulder pain at 1 month and another (lower brainstem infarction), complained of ocular pain with a Horner syndrome
Incidence of CPSP in patients with some somatosensory deficits: 18%
Authors' conclusion: 8% CPSP incidence may be a minimum figure. CP is not associated with age, sex, or previous stroke</td></tr>
<tr><td>Naver et al. (1995)</td><td>Stroke</td><td>37</td><td>Consecutive patients with acute monofocal stroke. Hemispheric lesion in 26 patients, brainstem stroke in 11 patients. Pain contralateral to the lesion side in 6 patients (16.2%), most of them with impaired temperature sensibility</td></tr>
<tr><td>Mori et al. (1995)</td><td>Thalamic hematoma</td><td>104</td><td>104 patients with thalamic hematoma. 86 survivors at 6 months (52/63 men, 34/41 women)
<table>
<tr><th>Extent of hematoma</th><th></th><th>Thalamic pain</th></tr>
<tr><td>Localized within the thalamus</td><td>21 (20.2%)</td><td>2 (9.5%)</td></tr>
<tr><td>Extending to the internal capsule</td><td>52 (50%)</td><td>3 (5.7%)</td></tr>
<tr><td>Extending to the midbrain or putamen</td><td>31 (29.8%)</td><td>1 (3.2%)</td></tr>
<tr><td>Total</td><td>104</td><td>6 (5.7%)</td></tr>
</table></td></tr>
<tr><td>Chung et al. (1996)</td><td>Thalamic hemorrhage</td><td>175</td><td>Retrospective survey of 175 consecutive patients with thalamic hemorrhage
Paresthesia and decreased touch and pain sensation at onset in 31/77 patients (40%) with posterolateral lesions. "About one-third of them developed Dejerine–Roussy thalamic syndrome between 3 and 15 days after the onset"
Paresthesia at onset also noted in 34% of patients with dorsal thalamic lesions
Incidence of thalamic syndrome:
• 25% of patients with posteromedial hemorrhage (6 cases)
• 32% of patients with posterolateral hemorrhage (25 cases?)
• 25% of patients with dorsal hemorrhage (8 cases)
Data from text and figure (Fig. 8) are not in agreement as far as posterolateral lesions are concerned. The presence of pain in thalamic syndrome is not specifically noted. No follow-up reported</td></tr>
<tr><td>Kim and Bae (1997)</td><td>Brainstem stroke</td><td>17</td><td>Pure or predominant sensory stroke. MRI or CT confirmed lesions. Follow-up: 1 month – 3 years</td></tr>
</table>

Table 2.1. (cont.)

Reference	Pathology	No. of patients	Patients with CP
			Paresthesia was the initial and main complaint in all patients. Sensory symptoms (almost) completely resolved in 5 patients. Paresthesia usually persisted in the others **CPSP:** in 2 patients (12%) paresthesia worsened, became painful, and was often exacerbated by cold weather or fatigue, mimicking the so-called "thalamic pain syndrome" (follow-up: 18 months, 3 years)
Nasreddine and Saver (1997)	Thalamic stroke	180	Systematic review on pain after thalamic stroke. Frequency of CP after any thalamic stroke: **11%** (range 8–16%). Frequency of CP after geniculothalamic artery stroke: **24%** (range 13–59%).
McGowan *et al.* (1997)	Lateral medullary infarction (LMI) (Wallenberg's syndrome)	63	Mainly retrospective analysis. LMI diagnosis confirmed by MRI. Frequency of CP: 16/63 patients (25.4%). Loss of some patients to follow-up Rare (less than twice-monthly) non-painful dysesthesias in a limb or cheek in 11 additional patients. **Two patients with crossed sensory deficits without pain suffered from a compulsive urge to scratch and pick their painless cheek** and developed excoriated ulcers No CP after medial medullary stroke in Bassetti *et al.* (1997)
Paciaroni and Bogousslasky (1998)	Pure thalamic sensory stroke	3628	Isolated sensory dysfunction with confirmed thalamic lesion in 25 patients among 3628 included in the Lausanne Stroke Registry. Clinical symptoms strongly suggestive of pure thalamic sensory stroke with normal findings on CT or MRI scans in other 34 patients Symptoms during the stroke: • pain and/or dysesthesias in 4/25 patients (transient in all 4) • contralateral paresthesia in 18/25 • delayed pain and/or dysesthesias in 4/25 patients (**16%**)
Kim and Choi-Kwon (1999)	Lateral medullary infarction (LMI) (Wallenberg's syndrome)	41	Group of 55 (out of 64 consecutive patients) with a single episode of MRI-identified medullary infarction Subjective residual sensory symptom 6–40 months (mean 21 months) after stroke onset: • on the face: LMI: 56% of patients; MMI: 7% of patients • on the body/limbs: LMI: 83% of patients; MMI 71% of patients CPSP incidence: **about 25%** (according to the authors' statement that "pain" was defined as sensory symptoms more severe than grade 5 or 6 on a 10-point visual analog scale)
	Medial medullary infarction (MMI)	14	Symptoms were not described as "pain" by the majority of these patients, so the term *central post-stroke paresthesia* is a more appropriate description of their sensory sequelae **LMI**: predominantly burning or cold sensations (visual analog scale ≥ 5) on the face in 6 patients (14.6%) and/or on the body/limbs in 10 (24.3%). Severe lancinating sensations on the face in 1 patient. Severe paresthesias in 14 patients (**34.1%**) **MMI**: Severe burning or cold body/limb sensations in 1 patient (7.1%) and severe squeezing/numbness sensations in 4 patients (**28.5%**)
Mukherjee *et al.* (1999)	Stroke	17 000	Door-to-door survey of 4600 families in Calcutta. 37/17 000 people suffered a stroke (prevalence 217/100 000). CPSP in 17/37 patients (12 F, 5 M) (**46%; prevalence: 0.1%**)

Table 2.1. (cont.)

Reference	Pathology	No. of patients	Patients with CP
Kumral *et al.* (2001)	Bilateral thalamic infarction	16	1/16 patients (**6.25%**) developed CPSP with burning pain. Another patient reported Dejerine–Roussy syndrome. CPSP among thalamogeniculate infarct patients: 1/3 patients (**33.3%**)
Bowsher (2001)	Stroke	1071	Elderly post-stroke population. Survey of stroke in 1071 elderly people (median age 80 years, range 69–102 years). Completed stroke in 72/1071 (6.7%) CPSP observed in 8/72 patients (5 men) (**11%**). Shoulder pain excluded
Lampl *et al.* (2002)	Ventrocaudalis (Vc) thalamic stroke	39	**Prospective** study aimed at investigating the incidence of CPSP in thalamic stroke patients either under prophylactic treatment (1 year) with amitriptyline or assuming placebo CPSP incidence: whole group: 18%; amitriptyline group: 17%; placebo group: **21%**
Weimar *et al.* (2002)	Ischemic/ hemorrhagic stroke	119	11 (**9.2%**). CPSP probable in 6 patients, confirmed in 5 patients. 1 patient with recurrent pain in the right extremities from recurrent focal seizures Frequency of (assumed) CPSP after hemorrhagic stroke: 4/13 patients (31%)
Widar *et al.* (2002)	Ischemic/ hemorrhagic stroke	43	Neurological clinic inpatients with CT-confirmed stroke and long-term pain CPSP (2 years after stroke) in 15/43 patients (**35%**). Nociceptive (shoulder) pain in 18/43
Kim (2003)	Lenticulocapsular hemorrhage (LCH)	20	20 patients with CPSP or paresthesia after LCH Not all patients were evaluated so no data on general prevalence of CPSP among patients with LCH can be extrapolated
Gonzales *et al.* (2003)	Cancer-associated CP		Retrospective review of medical records of patients evaluated by 2 different services: the Pain Service and the Neurology Service at Memorial Sloan-Kettering Cancer Center CP prevalence: **4%** and **2%**, respectively. Primary and metastatic tumors and their therapy, including surgery, radiation, and chemotherapy, were all potential causes of CP CP in patients with primary CNS tumors higher in patients with spinal cord tumors compared to patients with brain tumors ($p < 0.0001$)
Kameda *et al.* (2004)	MRI-confirmed medullary infarction (LMI and MMI)	214	157 LMI patients with information on sensory function. CP (thermal hypoesthesia with touch and thermal allodynia) in 40 patients (**25%**). No correlation with a specific topographical subgroup
Kong *et al.* (2004)	Ischemic/ hemorrhagic stroke	107	107/475 patients attending the outpatient clinic of a rehabilitation center, without significant cognitive and/or language deficits, post-stroke duration more than 6 months. CPSP in 13 patients (**12.1%**)
Nakazato *et al.* (2004)	Wallenberg's syndrome	32	CPSP in 14/32 patients (**44%**)
Widar *et al.* (2004)	Stroke	356 (?)	Patients with cerebral infarct or hemorrhage registered in an inpatient register at a neurological clinic in a university hospital, Sweden. 356 people contacted, 65 non-responders, 245 no pain or other pain conditions. 15 CPSP patients. CPSP incidence in the whole group: **4.2–5.1%** (15/356 or 15/291 patients)

Table 2.1. (cont.)

Reference	Pathology	No. of patients	Patients with CP
Jönsson *et al.* (2006)	Stroke	416	416 consecutive, unselected patients in Lund, Sweden. Prospective, 1 year. Visual analog scale in 297 patients (98% of all survivors); 84 dead, 35 patients too old or incapacitated for assessment. At 16 months, 4 patients (**1.3%**) diagnosed as CPSP. Diagnosis of CPSP not performed by neurologist.
Appelros (2006)	Stroke	377	Patients with first-ever stroke ($n = 377$) were examined at baseline and after 1 year in Stockholm, Sweden. After 1 year survivors ($n = 253$) were examined. 28 patients (11%) had stroke-associated pain (several of these may have been CPSP, but the number was not specifically ascertained)
Lundstrom *et al.* (2009)	Stroke	140	Cross-sectional survey in Uppsala, Sweden. At 1 year, 4 CPSP patients (**2.85%**). No detailed sensory assessment
Kuptniratsaikul *et al.* (2009)	Stroke	327	Multicenter, prospective, cohort study of patients in rehabilitation in Thailand. Neuropathic pain in 14 (**4.3%**) patients (**6.5%** after hemorrhage, **3.4%** after ischemia)
Zvan and Zaletel *et al.* (2010) (duplicate of Zaletel *et al.* 2007)	Stroke	297	Random investigation (duration 1 year) of 297 patients (mean age 72 ± 5.4 years) with first-time stroke. Patients evaluated at 6 and 12 months after stroke. 27 patients (**9.2%**) developed CPSP. Factors significantly associated with having CP with visual analog score > 4 were younger age and higher depression scores ($p < 0.01$). Constantly present in 37%; sleep disturbed in 67%
Klit *et al.* (2011)	Stroke	964	Stroke patients identified through a Danish stroke database. Questionnaire mailed to all (2006). 644 questionnaires returned. 608 patients included in study. 67 had suspected CPSP (11%). 12 deceased at study end. 51 examined directly. 21 patients with definite CPSP, 14 with probable CPSP, 6 with dysesthesias. In sum: minimum prevalence of definite CPSP 4.4%, definite and probable **7.3%**, CPSP dysesthesias **8.6%**
Bugnicourt *et al.* (2011)	Cerebral venous (and sinus) thrombosis	43	Observational study (2002–7). 7/43 developed CP within 12 months of stroke, 8 by study end (**19%**). Initial motor deficit (87% vs. 17%, $p < 0.001$), initial sensory deficit (62% vs. 20%, $p = 0.03$), cerebral infarction (75% vs. 23%, $p = 0.009$), right-sided lesion on initial MRI (62% vs. 17%, $p = 0.017$), thalamic (37% vs. 0%, $p = 0.005$) and basal ganglia involvement (25% vs. 0%, $p = 0.03$) and vein of Galen occlusion (25 vs. 0%) significantly associated with CP

It can be estimated that *c.* 3.5 million SCI patients are alive globally (223–755 per million inhabitants), 1.3 million in the USA, with an incidence of between 10.4 and 83 per million inhabitants per year. One-third of patients with SCI are tetraplegic and half have a complete lesion. The mean age of patients is 33 years and the sex distribution (men/women) is 3.8/1, reflecting younger males' susceptibility to trauma (Wyndaele and Wyndaele 2006). **Around 1 million people may suffer CCP worldwide.**

Multiple sclerosis (MS) likely affects far more than the commonly quoted figure of 1.3 million people globally, perhaps 3 million (Multiple Sclerosis Society UK, 2008). The largest and most reliable of all surveys (1672 MS patients from 26 Italian centers) found dysesthetic pain in 303 patients (18.1%; 71.6% female, mean age 43.6 years, mean Expanded Disability Status Scale [EDSS] 3.8, mean disease duration 11.9 years): 60% were relapsing/remitting (RR), 30% of the secondary progressive (SP) type, and only 10%

primary progressive. The vast majority of those affected by trigeminal neuralgia (2.2%) were female (> 80%; mean age 48.5, mean EDSS 4.4, mean disease duration 15.3 years), with almost similar proportions between RR and SP (Solaro *et al.* 2004). **Worldwide, *c.* 300 000–400 000 MS patients may suffer CP.**

It has been estimated that 2–4% of cancer patients suffer CP from both primary and metastatic tumors. CP is more prevalent in patients with spinal cord rather than brain masses (Gonzales *et al.* 2003; see also Beatty 1970). In 2002, of the 11 million new cancer cases estimated worldwide, *c.* 45% were in Asia, 26% in Europe, and *c.* 15% in the USA. Metastatic tumors are the most common CNS neoplasms: the true incidence is probably underestimated but the literature reports up to 11/100 000 per year. **Tens or even hundreds of thousands could suffer CP.**

Dieleman *et al.* (2008) found an incidence rate of neuropathic pain following spinal cord injury (including metastatic compression) of 1.1/100 000 person-years (12 incident cases; 95% CI 0.6–1.8), and 0.5/100 000 person-years (6 cases; 95% CI 0.2–1.1) for syringomyelia in the Dutch general population (1996–2004).

Chapter 3

Clinical features

Lesions associated with CP

Brain central pain (BCP) has been caused by all kinds of lesions at any level along the spinothalamoparietal path, from brainstem to cortex (Table 3.1). These include rapidly or slowly developing processes, compressive or disruptive/distractive. Stroke, either hemorrhagic or ischemic, is the commonest cause of BCP; dismayingly, iatrogenic CP is not rare. In agreement with their known incidence, in all studies, infarcts are more common than hemorrhages, although in Asian countries hemorrhages are more frequent than in the West.

Cord central pain (CCP, also known as below-level or remote pain) has been reported with virtually every type of disease or lesion affecting the spinal cord substance, be it a complete or an incomplete lesion (Table 3.2). Trauma/concussion (e.g., civilian gunshot wounds and road accidents) is the leading cause of CCP worldwide; again, iatrogenic lesions are not rare. CP, although only one of the many chronic pains observed after spinal cord injury (SCI), is by far the most severe and disabling, and in many patients may limit their functional ability and daily activities. Traumatic central cord syndrome (TCCS, Schneider's syndrome) is the most frequent type of incomplete SCI. Patients may immediately experience quadriplegia, but recover gradually in more than 50% of cases; they may also complain of a burning sensation of the upper limbs and severe touch allodynia (Harrop *et al.* 2006, Aarabi *et al.* 2008). Surgery does not generally relieve this pain (Chen *et al.* 2009). CCP is also common in patients with spina bifida (62% of 10% suffering neuropathic cord pains: Werhagen *et al.* 2010).

Location of lesions causing CP

When the lesion is thalamic, the nucleus ventrocaudalis (Vc) is always involved. Pure thalamic lesions account for a minority of all CPSP cases. In all other cases, lesions are cortico-subcortical, capsulothalamic, or lenticulocapsular, in the brainstem or diffuse. Most CPSP is supratentorial. All cortical lesions responsible for BCP involve, exclusively or in combination, the parietal lobe, i.e., SI and/or SII/insula (Table 3.3). Thalamic tumors or tumors restricted to the parietal lobe associated with CP are on record (e.g., Lozano *et al.* 1992, Amancio *et al.* 2002).

It has been emphasized that up to half of all insular lesions may release CP (see Appendix), but this contention is not backed up by prospective data. There are many insular strokes that do not release CPSP. Birklein *et al.* (2005) reported on an isolated insular infarction eliminating contralateral cold, cold pain, and pinprick sensation. CPSP was not seen. Cattaneo *et al.* (2007) reported on a patient with a right posterior dorsal insula infarction, not crossing the putative border with SII. There was a stable (1 year) deficit of contralateral non-painful thermal sensations, non-overlapping with other somatic painful/non-painful sensations (including hot/cold pain), with partial somatotopy. CPSP did not arise over a period of 18 months, with moderate recovery of thermal sensations in the arm. A man developed analgesia and thermoanesthesia in the right half of his body, with deep sensation preservation following a stroke affecting the thalamocortical sensory pathways to the secondary somatosensory cortex (SII), but not to SI: no CP arose (Hiraga *et al.* 2005).

The most common site of brainstem lesions (either stroke or hematobulbia, syringobulbia, tumors, and multiple sclerosis [MS]) is the medulla oblongata, with few cases of pontine and no pure midbrain spontaneous CP having been reported. However, this may actually be an underestimation. CP of bulbar origin is generally due to thrombosis of the posteroinferior cerebellar artery (PICA) giving rise to Wallenberg's syndrome, in which a lesion impinges on the spinothalamic tract and on the nucleus and/or the descending root of the trigeminal nerve on the same side (see below).

Table 3.1. Lesions associated with brain central pain (BCP)

(1) Vascular lesion: ischemia/infarct,[a] hemorrhage, including intracerebral,[b] and subarachnoid (independent of surgery, due to spasm and infarction or direct brain injury), vascular malformations (arteriovenous malformation through compression, ischemia by steal, or hemorrhage, cavernomas through hemorrhage and perhaps compression, compressing non-hemorrhagic saccular aneurysm, venous angioma), migraine-induced vasospasm [est. 85%]
(2) Penetrating trauma [est. 1–2%]
(3) Inflammation: MS, etc.
(4) Infection: abscess (e.g., toxoplasma), gumma, tuberculoma, encephalitis, etc. [est. 4%]
(5) Tumor: glioma, meningioma, etc., including intratumoral hemorrhage [est. 1–2%]
(6) Epilepsy
(7) Iatrogenic[c]

[a] There appears to be no difference between hemorrhages and infarcts as regards the tendency to induce CP, but infarcts, being more frequent (85% vs. 15%), are more commonly the cause of CPSP. Likewise, about 80% of all infarcts occur in the carotid territory and engage the thalamus (thalamogeniculate and thalamostriate arteries), while posteroinferior cerebellar artery (PICA) strokes engage the lower brainstem. Ischemic lesions may be multiple, often small infarcts, especially in the corona radiata and brainstem.
[b] Intracerebral hemorrhages may act like tumors and provoke CP by compression.
[c] Also includes one patient with a thalamic deep brain stimulation (DBS) apparatus for motor control who developed CP after cardioversion, and patients with resected vestibular schwannomas and cerebellar tumors.

Table 3.2. Lesions associated with cord central pain (CCP)

(1) Spinal trauma with fracture and/or dislocations producing complete or partial transection or concussion of the spinal cord (Schneider's syndrome)
(2) Ischemic/hemorrhagic: e.g., aortic dissection, systemic hypotension, atherosclerosis/thromboembolism/infarcts, hematomyelia[a]/subarachnoid hemorrhage due to arteriovenous malformations,[b] cavernomas, dural fistula, traumatic/non-traumatic/iatrogenic cervical anterior spinal cord syndrome, spontaneous abdominal compartment syndrome, etc.
(3) Rheumatological and degenerative disorders: e.g., myelopathy due to cervical spinal stenosis–spondylosis and cervical discal hernia, ankylosing spondylitis with conus lesions, Paget's disease, rheumatoid arthritis, posterior longitudinal ligament ossification
(4) Intra- and extramedullary tumors[c]
(5) Congenital and developmental: non-tumoral cysts, syringomyelia, dysraphism, diastematomyelia, spina bifida, myelomeningocele, etc.
(6) Inflammatory/infective: multiple sclerosis, transverse myelitis, viral (e.g., herpes zoster, cytomegalovirus, HIV, poliovirus), bacterial (e.g., mycobacteria/Pott's disease, luetic gumma[d]), fungal (e.g., cryptococcus), or parasitic infections/abscesses (e.g., toxoplasma, schistosoma), infective transverse myelitis
(7) Degenerative CNS disorders
(8) Toxic: antiblastic agents, radiation, etc.
(9) Genetic and metabolic
(10) Iatrogenic: cordotomy, aortic repair surgery, surgery for spinal angiomas/fistulas/hernias/spondylosis/intra- and extramedullary tumors, spinal fusion surgery, myelography, anticoagulant therapy with epidural/subdural hematomas

[a] Sudden at-level pain, sometimes followed by below-level pain.
[b] Initially produce at-level pain, then commonly below-level pain.
[c] Cervical–thoracic extramedullary tumors generally produce long-lasting at-level pain and shorter-lasting below-level pain more often involving the lower limbs. Pain or dysesthesias can be the only (or initial) symptom for a long time. Intramedullary tumors generate less frequent, below-level (short-lived) pain/(long-lived) dysesthesias, often in both legs and at-level ("armor-like" constrictive band).
[d] The pathological process in tabes dorsalis, which can cause CP, is known not to be confined to the posterior columns (Vierck 1973).

Table 3.3. Cortical central post-storke pain (CPSP) (selected series)

Biemond (1956)

Small subinsular infarct (thalamus and SI spared). Dramatic loss of pain perception. CPSP

Michel *et al.* (1990)

12 cases of cortical CP due to ischemia (11) or hemorrhage (1) sparing the thalamus (on MRI or CT), but involving SI or extending to the thalamoparietal radiations. In 3 cases SI was spared and the cortex involved was prerolandic or posterior parietal. In this series, painful paroxysms resembled painful fits with a jacksonian march in 3 cases (patients 7, 8, 11)

Case	Hand	Pain site	Sensibility			Cortical lesion site and type (CT scan)	Notes
			Pin	Ther	Tact		
1	R	L Hemibody (+ head)	I	I	Lo	R parietal (postcentral gyrus, supramarginalis gyrus) ischemic infarct	Cigarette smoking induced severe pain over the trunk. Spontaneous very slow (years) pain improvement (dysesthesia with smoke). No allodynia. Max. pain site: face
2	R	L Hand	I	N	I	R parietal (postcentral gyrus, gyrus angularis) – occipital ischemic infarct	Pain disappearance after a 2nd infarct. No allodynia
3	R	L Hemibody	Lo	Lo	Lo	R perisylvian (postcentral gyrus, SII, supramarginalis gyrus) ischemic infarct	Hemianesthesia (all modalities). Mechanical allodynia. Hyperpathia. Max. pain site: lower limb
4	R	L Hemibody (+ head)	I	I	I	Massive R sylvian (MCA) ischemic infarct sparing the thalamus (MRI-confirmed)	Hemihypoesthesia (all modalities). No allodynia. Patchy max. pain (more intense over joints)
5	R	R Hemibody (+ head)	I	I	I	L fronto-insular (prerolandic) ischemic infarct. Postcentral gyrus spared (?)	No allodynia. Max. pain: calf/ankle
6	R	L Hand/wrist	I	I	I	R parietal (postcentral gyrus, supramarginalis gyrus, gyrus angularis) ischemic infarct	Hypoesthesia (all modalities). Allodynia (mechanical, cold). Hyperalgesia
7	R	L Hemibody	I	I	I	Massive R sylvian (MCA) ischemic infarct sparing the thalamus (MRI-confirmed)	No allodynia. Patchy max. pain (joints). CPSP appearance 2 years after the infarct. Lancinating radiating pains. 50% pain improvement with TENS
8	R	L Face and forearm/ hand	I	I	I	R rolandic-parietal (postcentral gyrus, SII, supramarginalis gyrus) ischemic infarct (MRI-confirmed)	Lancinating radiating pains. No allodynia

Table 3.3. (cont.)

Case	Hand	Pain site	Sensibility			Cortical lesion site and type (CT scan)	Notes
			Pin	Ther	Tact		
9	R	L Leg (distal half)/foot	I	I	I	R MRI-confirmed small infarct of the ascending frontal convolution (precentral gyrus) (not showed by CT scan). Postcentral gyrus spared (?)	Allodynia
10	R	L Leg/foot	I	I	N	R parietal prerolandic ischemic infarct (or hematoma?). Postcentral gyrus spared (?)	Tactile allodynia. Lesion described as ischemic in Table 1, but as hematoma in text
11	R	L Face, hand, stump	N	(Lo)	N	R frontal-rolandic (postcentral gyrus) hematoma	Previous (3 years) L leg amputation (ischemic disease). Phantom limb without phantom pain. Patchy pain. No allodynia. Warm hypoesthesia over the L hand, with **cold and pinprick sensibility spared**. **Epileptic painful fits** (showing a jacksonian march from hand to face and involving the phantom foot), phenytoin-responsive (disappearance of fits and pain). Pain relief from **cold** bath
12	R	L Forearm/ hand	N	I	N	R sylvian (postcentral gyrus, SII, supramarginalis gyrus) ischemic infarct	Tactile (and cold?) allodynia

Hand, handedness; R, right; L, left; Pin, pinprick; Ther, thermal; Tact, tactile; I, impaired (reduced); Lo, lost; N, normal.

Authors' conclusion: Cortical areas generally involved in cortical CP: postcentral gyrus (particularly operculus parietalis, SII, and insula) with extension to gyrus supramarginalis; Brodmann's area 7 and SI. If parietal areas are spared, the thalamoparietal radiations are involved.

Masson *et al*. (1991)

One patient with a pseudothalamic cortical syndrome, associated with pain asymbolia; MRI confirmed right infarction restricted to the posterior insula, superior margin of T1, the parietal operculum, and the supramarginal gyrus (SI, thalamus, posterior parietal cortex, and MI [primary motor cortex] were spared)

Left hemibody (head included): complete hemianalgesia, no response to pinprick and pressure pain. Impaired thermal, tactile, vibratory, and position sensibilities. Right hemibody: pain sensibility completely lost. Normal pinprick, tactile, thermal, vibratory, and position sensibilities

Asymbolia was imputed to a disconnection between SII at insula level and the limbic system

Schmahmann and Leifer (1992)

Parietal CP: 6 patients

Table 3.3. (cont.)

Cortical lesion site and type (CT scan)	Notes
White matter deep to the inferior aspect of the postcentral and supramarginal gyri; cortex and white matter of the superior aspect of the L postcentral gyrus and posterior parietal region; caudal superior temporal gyrus	Resection of L-sided parietal meningioma. Discomfort in the R hand 4 months later. Traumatic hemorrhage in the inferior aspect of the L postcentral gyrus and rostral part of the L posterior parietal cortex (within the surgical scar) 7 years later. Max. pain: R hand
White matter deep to the L postcentral and supramarginal gyri; some involvement of the cortex of the postcentral gyrus; white matter deep to the middle and inferior frontal gyri (small lesion)	Embolic L stroke. CPSP 1 year later
White matter deep to the postcentral and supramarginal gyri; posterior aspect of the insular cortex	L postraumatic temporoparietal hematoma. CP 1 week later
Caudal part of the insula; cortex and underlying white matter of the R angular and supramarginal gyri and superior temporal gyrus	R temporoparietal infarct (recurrent). Carotid endarterectomy. CP 4 years later. Pain exacerbated by cold and damp weather
Pericentral regions, posterior parietal cortex, superior temporal gyrus; caudate nucleus and basal ganglia atrophy	Carotid occlusive disease. Incomplete L MCA territory infarction
L sylvian fissure, extending upward into the white matter beneath the postcentral gyrus and the rostral inferior parietal lobule	Embolic cerebral infarction. Acute hemianesthesia and hemiparesthesias. Touch-provoked dysesthesias. Max. pain: distal arm and hand (overlapping max. sensory impairment area)

Authors' conclusion: In all cases the thalamus was spared and a common lesioned area was identified in the parietal lobe, located in the white matter deep to the caudal insula and deep to the opercular region of the rostral posterior parietal cortex. Cerebral cortex lesions were also noted, but the area of overlap was in the white matter. The cortex overlying this common white-matter injury zone includes the rostral inferior parietal lobule and SII.

Bassetti *et al.* (1993)

20 consecutive patients with acute CT/MRI-confirmed parietal stroke without thalamic involvement (1% of over 2000 patients of the Lausanne Stroke Registry). 6 women, 14 men, mean age 53 years (range 26–74 years). Infarct side: R, 5 patients; L, 14 patients, R ICH, 1 patient (stroke localization on CT templates). Hemisensory disturbances, no visual deficit, no or only slight motor weakness.

Sensory examination: light touch, superficial pain (pinprick), position sense, vibration, stereognosis, graphesthesia. Not systematically tested: temperature, deep pain, two-point discrimination, baresthesia, and topesthesia. Long-term follow-up (mean, 6 months; range 3–12 months) in 8 patients (with significant sensory loss at discharge)

Main sensory syndromes

Syndrome	Stroke topography	Patients and symptoms	Sensibility impairment
Pseudothalamic	Inferior-anterior parietal infarct (parietal operculum, anterior part of the supramarginal gyrus, posterior insula) in 10/10 patients Extension to the underlying white matter in 9/10 patients (patient VIII: almost no subcortical involvement)	10 patients: 4 F, 6 M, mean age 45.5 years Lesion side: R 2, L 8 Numbness or paresthesia (contralateral hemibody) in 7 patients. **Transient pain sensation (arm) in 1 patient** Patient VIII: hemihypoesthesia (all modalities) then arm's	Hemibody (including face): 8 patients; face + upper limb: 1 patient; upper limb: 1 patient Faciobrachiocrural elementary sensory loss (touch, pain, temperature, vibration). All elementary modalities of sensation impaired in 5 patients.

Table 3.3. (cont.)

Main sensory syndromes			
Syndrome	**Stroke topography**	**Patients and symptoms**	**Sensibility impairment**
	Medial-superior part of the postcentral gyrus additionally involved in 4 patients (discriminative sensory loss in all)	isolated sensory loss (touch, pain, temperature) Long-term disabling sensory loss in patients VI and X	Touch and superficial pain sensation impaired in 10/10 patients Pain: diminished in 9, abolished in 1 (deep pain sensibility preserved in most patients) Temperature (5 patients tested): diminished in 4, abolished in 1
Cortical	Superior-posterior parietal infarct in 7/7 patients. Medial-superior part of postcentral gyrus involvement in 4 patients. Mainly subcortical lesion in 2 patients	7 patients: 7 M, mean age 66.8 years Lesion side: R 3, L 4 Some numbness in the upper limb in all patients; left perioral numbness + sensory loss in the hand in 1 patient	Upper + lower limbs: 3 patients; upper limb: 1 patient; cheiro-oral: 1 patient Isolated loss of discriminative sensory loss (stereognosis, graphesthesia, position sense) in one or two body parts
Atypical (probably a minor variant of the two previously described syndromes)	Heterogeneous parietal stroke topography: posterior insula and supramarginal gyrus (patient XVIII); medial-superior part of the postcentral gyrus (patient XIX). Subcortical hemorrhage underneath the superior part of the postcentral gyrus (patient XX)	3 patients: 2 F, 1 M, mean age 46 years Lesion side: R 1, L 2 Patient XVIII: paresthesias (R arm) + hand numbness (same distribution for the sensory loss, demarcation line over the wrist) Patient XIX: cheiro-oral paresthesias + sudden feeling of disappearance of R arm + sensory loss in the ulnar side of the hand (C8-like lesion) Patient XX: cold sensation in L leg + "pins and needles" in the L side of the body (L pseudospinal sensory loss below T3)	Complete sensory loss (all modalities of sensation) with partial (pseudoperipheral) distribution

No delayed pain in any patients

Authors' conclusion: parietal stroke can cause different sensory syndromes depending on the topography of the underlying lesion. Clinical differentiation between thalamic and pseudothalamic parietal stroke cannot be made on the basis of sensory deficits alone. Only constant association: conduction aphasia and R-sided pseudothalamic sensory deficit.

Cereda *et al.* (2002)

MRI-confirmed acute insular strokes (according to published templates). 4 consecutive patients among 4800 cases (< 1/1000) of first-ever acute stroke (Lausanne Stroke Registry); mean age 65 years

Table 3.3. (cont.)

Case 1. 73-year-old R-handed woman. MRI: cerebral infarct restricted to the posterior portion of the R insula. Marked improvement within 3 days, discharged asymptomatic
Case 2. 69-year-old R-handed man. Diffusion-weighted MRI (7 h after onset of symptoms): infarct restricted to the L posterior insula. Numb sensation (R arm) at onset. R-sided sensory deficits (light touch, superficial pain, temperature, vibration [dramatic in the R leg], and position sense). Mild deficit of stereognosia and graphesthesia. Deficit in recognizing saline and acidic solutions bilaterally. Marked improvement within a week (minimal residual hypoesthesia of the R upper limb + taste discrimination deficit)
Case 3. 48-year-old R-handed woman. MRI (T2-weighted): infarct restricted to the L posterior insula. Sense of heaviness (R hemibody) R hemisensory deficit (touch, pain, temperature, vibration, and postural sense + two-point discrimination, graphesthesia, stereognosia). Normalization in the following 48 h
Case 4. 75-year-old R-handed hypertensive woman. MRI (diffusion-weighted): R posterior insular stroke. Hypoesthesia (touch and pain) of L upper limb, alteration of graphesthesia, and stereognosis. Favorable clinical evolution within 2 weeks
Authors' conclusion: Strokes restricted to the posterior insula may present with pseudothalamic sensory syndrome. Isolated posterior insular damage can also produce transient painful syndromes.
Bowsher *et al.* (1998, 2004), Bowsher (2006a, 2006b)
Parietal cortex: 13 patients (4 controls)
5 patients with small restricted cerebral cortical infarcts, in all cases sparing SI (postcentral gyrus)
• Patient 1 (CP+): lesion confined to the parietal operculum (SII)
• Patient 2 (CP+): SII lesion also encroaching on the posterior insula
• Patient 3 (CP–): lesion involving both banks of the sylvian fissure and the dorsal insula
• Patient 4 (CP–): lesion involving the upper bank of the sylvian fissure
• Patient 5 (CP+): lesion involving the left parietal operculum and posterior insula, and a little of the inferior part of the postcentral gyrus
Case report. Visceral CPSP. MRI (14 months after pain onset): increased density in the R anterior superior insular region + slightly suspicious appearance in the contralateral symmetrical region.
R-handed man. Appearance of burning sensation (R shoulder), lasting only for a few weeks, 6 months after a stroke. 3 months later appearance of a burning, scalding superficial (lower chest), and internal (upper abdomen, occasionally radiating to the L groin) sensation. Constant pain aggravated by contact with the bedclothes and partially relieved by hot bath. 18 months after the stroke complaint of internal ("like a stomachache") bilateral viscerosomatic abdominal pain (burning and tingling: L > R, best visual analog score 45, worst 100), rarely radiating to the L thigh, associated with occasional superficial and separate girdle pains (lower thorax). On examination (T7–T8): normal touch, sharpness, and heat sensibility. Pain thresholds unaffected. Warmth threshold raised (8 °); skinfold pinch and cold not tested. Tactile allodynia (T8). 2.5 years after the stroke no more pain (only numbness) on amitriptyline. Reappearance of pain after stopping tricyclic antidepressants. **Author's note**: *reservations are necessary because the patient lacks reliability as a witness*, but it would seem that this may be a genuine case of visceral pain following infarction in the anterior insula.
Kim (2007a)
24 patients who had prominent sensory symptoms without definitive motor dysfunction, divided into:
(1) dominant impairment of primitive sensation (DIPS) group: 6 patients, 4 developed CPSP. On longer follow-up, CPSP gradually diminished in intensity (?); lesions were generally located in the lower part of the parietal and frontal area, and parietal opercular area and insular cortex were always involved
(2) dominant impairment of cortical sensation (DICS) group: 12 patients. No frank CPSP, although 7 patients had mild residual numb or tight sensation in the affected body parts: **not CP** (but he says in *methods* that CPSP also included "numb" and "tight" sensations); responsible lesions generally located in the upper part of the parietal lobe, with SI always lesioned, with posterior insula involved in 2 patients

Table 3.3. (cont.)

(3) paresthesia-only without objective sensory impairment group (5 patients)

(4) both sensations impaired to a similar degree (1 patient: CPSP!!!)

DIPS was related to lesions involving the parietal operculum and the insular cortex, whereas DICS was related to the lesions affecting the postcentral gyrus. Patients with paresthesia only had smaller lesions located in the postcentral gyrus. DIPS-group patients were more often women ($p = 0.013$), more often had dysarthria ($p = 0.043$), and more often developed central post-stroke pain or paresthesia ($p = 0.005$) than the DICS group patients. Restricted sensory changes were common, predominantly involving the perioral or finger areas.

Author's note: *"the lesion-sensory symptoms correlation was **not perfect**; there was impaired positional sensation in most DIPS group patients and impaired primitive sensation in most DICS group patients"*

Peskine *et al.* (2008)

Female, 28 years, with aneurysmal clot in left sylvian fissure extending into the left frontal lobe. Global pansensory deficits of right hemibody and disagreeable sensations of right hemibody. MRI: left insular hypointensity.

Garcia-Larrea *et al.* (2010)

Overall population (2002–09): 22 patients with **cortico-subcortical lesions** (thalamus and brainstem spared). CP and dissociated loss of thermoalgesic sensations in 5 patients. MRI confirmed lesion; extension determined on published atlases.

(1) CP with dissociated loss of thermoalgesic sensations: 5 patients (insula/operculum ischemic stroke in all). R-sided 3, L-sided 2 cases (*data disagreement between text, tables, and figures in the original paper*). **Lesion site**: (1) L posterior insula + innermost parietal operculum; (2) L (*R in Table 2 and Fig. 1*) posterior insula + medial operculum; (3) R (*Tables 1 & 2 and Fig 1; L in text*) posterior and mid-insula (*4/5th; 3/4th in text*) + antero-inferior parietal operculum; (4) R insula (2/3rd) + lower parietal lobe (subcortical extension to the IC); (5) R posterior insula + medial and lateral operculum

(2) CP with lemniscal and pain/temperature deficit: 13 patients (cortical stroke, ischemic in 6 cases, hemorrhagic in 6 cases, post-surgical in 1 case). R-sided 4, L-sided 2; not reported: 7 cases. **Lesion site**: parietal + frontal: 3 patients (extended in 2, in 1 patient site of a further lesion not reported); parietal: 1 patient (R+L lesion); parietal-frontal + insula/operculum/temporal/basal ganglia/internal capsule: 4 patients; fronto-temporal + operculum + insula: 1 patient; temporal/insular-basal ganglia: 1 patient; opercular ablation: 1 patient; basal ganglia: 2 patients (extended in 1, capsulolenticular in 1). In 4 patients cortical lesions without CP.

(3) Patients with cortical lesion without central pain: 4 patients (cortical lesion, 2 tumor, 1 surgical, 1 ischemic). R-sided 1, L-sided 3

CP patients with pure dissociated loss of thermoalgesic sensations (ischemic stroke in all cases)

Patient /lesion site	Pain site/features	Notes
(1) M, 55 years. L posterior insula + innermost parietal operculum	R side of body + face. Continuous, burning; allodynia + [C, Br (R face)]	9-month follow-up: R-sided burning pain (face, arm, foot, genitalia). Face allodynia. Drug-resistant pain (2 years therapy). MCS effective (NRS from 8 to 5 after 1 year)
(2) F, 36 years. L (*R in Table 2 and Fig. 1*) posterior insula + medial operculum	R (*L in Table 2*) UL and trunk. Continuous, burning and freezing cold; allodynia + (C, Br)	50% pain relief by amitriptyline, pregabalin, duloxetine, escitalopram. Development of painting abilities after stroke (pain reduction by warm colors)
(3) M, 33 years. R (*Tables 1 & 2 and Fig 1; L in text*) posterior and mid-insula (*4/5th; 3/4th in text*) + antero-inferior parietal operculum	L (*in text*) UL and trunk . Continuous, burning, aching; allodynia + [C (L face)]	Summation hyperpathia. Partial pain relief by pregabalin, opioids, ketamine (TCA ineffective). Scheduled for TMS/MCS

Table 3.3. (cont.)

CP patients with pure dissociated loss of thermoalgesic sensations (ischemic stroke in all cases)		
Patient /lesion site	**Pain site/features**	**Notes**
(4) F, 52 years. R insula (2/3rd) + lower parietal lobe (subcortical extension to the internal capsule)	L hand and trunk. Continuous, burning; allodynia + [M (UL and trunk)]	Drug resistant pain (2 years therapy). Pain relief by TMS (30%) and MCS (80% pain relief at 6 months)
(5) M, 59 years. R posterior insula + medial and lateral operculum	L UL/LL (dyesthesiae, 1 d long, during the acute phase only)	No analgesic therapy at discharge

R, right; L, left; UL, upper limb; LL, lower limb; C, cold; Br, brushing; P, prick; W, warmth; HP, heat pain; M, mechanical; Abn, abnormal; Abs, absent; TCA, tricyclic antidepressants; TMS, transcranial magnetic stimulation; MCS, motor cortex stimulation. *Data disagreement in text, tables, and figure for patients 2 and 3.*

Sensory examination: Tactile thresholds: von Frey hairs; cotton (patient 2). Vibration: 100 Hz tuning fork. Pinprick (pain) thresholds: laser stimuli. Warm thresholds: contact thermode (patients 1–3); laser (patients 3–5). Contact heat and cold thresholds: thermode (patients 1–3); cold tubes and a metal fork (patients 4–5). Heat pain thresholds: laser. Pain assessment: NRS. **Neuroimaging**: MRI; lesion extension determined on published atlases

Patient	Allodynia	Spinothalamic tract sensibility (abnormal thresholds)	Laser evoked potentials
1	C, Br (R face)	P,W,C,HP	Abnormal (depressed and delayed)
2	C, Br	P,W,C,HP	Abnormal (reduced and delayed)
3	C (L face)	P,W,C,HP	Abnormal (delayed and depressed)
4	M (UL and trunk)	P, C, HP	Absent
5	–	–	Abnormal (attenuated and delayed)

Veldhuijzen *et al.* (2010)

7 patients. Cold and heat hypoalgesia were found only in the patient with the most extensive parietal and insular lesion. Cold allodynia occurred clinically and by thresholds in 2 patients with isolated ischemic lesions of the posterior insular/retroinsular cortex, and by thresholds in 2 patients with a lesion of parietal cortex with little or no insular involvement. Central pain occurred in the 2 patients with clinical allodynia secondary to isolated lesions of the posterior insular/retroinsular cortex, which spared the anterior and posterior parietal cortex.

Conclusion: **non-painful cold and heat sensations are jointly mediated by parietal and insular cortical structures** so that lesions anywhere in this system may diminish sensitivity. In contrast, **thermal pain requires larger cortical lesions of these same structures** to produce hypoalgesia. In addition, cold allodynia can result from restricted lesions that also produce thermal hypoesthesia, but not from all such lesions. Thus, anterior and posterior parietal lobe necessary for CP to arise.

- In this study physiologic abnormalities of cold sensation were independent of the occurrence of CPSP.
- Posterior insular/retroinsular lesions in isolation can lead to robust cold allodynia.
- CP was found in cases with substantial lesions of posterior insular/retroinsular cortex in the absence of involvement of the anterior/posterior parietal cortex BUT NOT with any case that included lesions of parietal cortex, with or without insular cortex.

Table 3.3. (cont.)

• [NB: authors say that allodynia alone is not enough to diagnose CPSP: wrong! One patient with parietal damage plus retroinsula (E1003) had cold allodynia.]
• 1 patient had an SII cavernoma that produced painful epileptic fits, but no ongoing pain. Resection: fits improved but not abolished.
• 1 patient with a relatively small lesion restricted to the posterior insula and retroinsula showed marked cool and warm hypoesthesia **bilaterally**. Bilateral thermal hypoesthesia for cold in 2 patients and for warm for 3 (also in Vestergaard *et al.* 1995).
• 1 patient had **bilateral** cold allodynia from unilateral lesion.
Thomas-Anterion *et al.* (2010)
Stroke of left posterior insula and adjacent SII. Right hemianesthesia to warm, heat and pinprick. CPSP. Migraines abated but anxiety and phobia increased. MR: small portion of posterior insula and a deep part of left SII. Intense pleasure from creative activity and she did not intend to get medication for pain relief. Manipulating cold colors gray and blue activated the pain but not passive viewing (polymodal insula-SII: synesthesia). (Garcia-Larrea *et al.* 2010.)

In two representative series (A: Tasker *et al.* 1992; B: Rogano *et al.* 2003) for a total of 208 patients, CCP was caused by cervical lesions in 42% (A) and 28.4% (B) of the cases, thoracic in 21% (A: down to T9) and 44.4% (B: up to T11?), and conocaudal in 37% (A: T10–L2) and 27.2% (B). In sum (Table 3.4), conocaudal lesions are not the most frequent lesions causing CCP, and that is also our experience (Canavero and Bonicalzi 2004a) and that of others (Beric 1999). Injuries that result in severe damage or disruption of the spinal cord and its adjacent tissues (e.g., gunshot wounds), as well as those with large intraspinal hemorrhages, are more prone to produce pain than a compression lesion produced by simple fracture dislocation (Nashold 1991, Tasker 2001a). CCP is equally represented at cervical, thoracic, and lumbar levels and with similar intensity; superimposed paroxysms are more frequently reported in conocaudal injury. Quadriplegics may suffer more pain than paraplegics. Neither vertebral level nor completeness of lesion affect the incidence of steady CCP, although steady (usually burning) perineal pain may occur more frequently with complete lesions. Intermittent pain occurs equally in complete and incomplete lesions at all spinal levels, but most frequently with lesions at the T10–L2 level (57%) (Tasker *et al.* 1992).

Pain onset

Acute onset (within a day) is frequent (15–75%: ≈ 30%) – often immediate (!) or within hours – and 43–100% of all patients develop BCP within 3 months. Pain onset delayed for more than 1 year is rare (8 years in Silver 1957; 10 years in a patient of Schott *et al.* 1986; 8 years in Kumral and Celebisoy 1996; 6 years in Bowsher 1996; 2 years in Garcia-Larrea *et al.* 2010): in such cases, the pain may sometimes commence after an infection, a trivial accident, or surgery (Tasker and Dostrovsky 1989). In some patients, the onset coincides with improvement of the sensory loss. The time of onset does not appear to depend on lesion level, and early- and late-onset pains appear to be clinically identical. CP may precede other neurological signs.

CCP can start immediately or even years after injury. Many patients develop it immediately, and practically all within a year (most within 6 months), but 6–8 years have also been reported (Nashold 1991, Defrin *et al.* 2001). About one-third of patients with a delay of up to 1 year and more than half with a delay of more than 1 year harbored a post-traumatic syrinx in the series of Tasker *et al.* (1992). In these cases, the syrinx rather than the original injury seems responsible for the pain. Thus, late onset of pain (and always facial pain) must raise suspicions of a syrinx. Like CPSP, CCP usually appears with some functional recovery in more severe cases.

Side of the lesions

In most, but not all (e.g. Misra *et al.* 2008: 7 right extrathalamic cases out of 15, Goto *et al.* 2008: R/L

Table 3.4. Frequency of lesions causing cord central pain (CCP)

Etiology	Series A (%)[a]	Series B (%)[b]	Notes
Trauma	65	75.3	Gunshot – closed trauma
Tumors	6	6.2	Ependymoma, meningioma, schwannoma, etc.
Inflammatory	9	5	Multiple sclerosis, etc.
Infective	–	3.6	
Skeletal	2	2.5	Cervical stenosis, etc.
Vascular/ischemic	2	1.2	
Congenital (or uncertain: A)	4	1.2	Syrinx, etc.
Iatrogenic	12	10	Surgery for cervical disk (2.5% in B), radiotherapy, etc.

[a] Tasker *et al.* (1992): 127 CCP patients seen between 1961 and 1989, Canada.
[b] Rogano *et al.* (2003): 81 patients seen prospectively, Brazil.

0.3, M/F 0.89) series, right-sided lesions predominate among CPSP patients at both thalamic and cortical levels (Table 2.6 in Canavero and Bonicalzi 2007a; Garcia-Larrea *et al.* 2010: R/L 1.5, M/F 1.5). This does not appear to be due simply to the higher prevalence of right strokes, since men show CPSP laterality much more commonly than women. Studies also find that pain processing is associated with a predominant right-hemisphere involvement.

Size of the lesions causing CPSP

Data are available only for thalamic vascular strokes (Table 2.7 in Canavero and Bonicalzi 2007a; Tong *et al.* 2010: volume of thalamic hemorrhage 0.3–6.3 mL, mean 2.3 ± 1.9 mL). The volume of the lesion in patients with thalamic CPSP does not seem to differ from the expected volume in thalamic hemorrhage, nor between patients with somatosensory deficits with and without CPSP. However, other data strongly suggest that total destruction of the thalamus is incompatible with a CP generator on that side (Chapter 22). Goto *et al.* (2008) suggested that a small thalamic or putaminal lesion is associated with pain in a limited area of the body, whereas a large lesion (extending to the medial side or to the wall of the lateral ventricle) is associated with pain in the hemisoma. In their diffusion tensor imaging (DTI) study, they concluded that the kind of sensory disturbance is unrelated to the volume of fiber tracking or lesion location.

Pain distribution

Refer to Tables 3.5 and 3.6. Contrary to the notion that CP is diffuse and difficult to localize, most patients can describe the location of their pain. Its distribution corresponds somatotopically to the site of the lesion, less frequently in a dermatomal pattern, but more commonly in terms of body parts, supporting a role of somatotopically organized structures. Roughly 40% of all BCP patients complain of hemibody pain (hemipain), with or without the hemiface, patchily or totally. In all other cases, CP is restricted to one or more body parts, e.g., the hemiface (*c.* 5%), one hand, one foot, a quadrant of the body, or the mouth and hand (the cheiro-oral syndrome, generally following thalamic lesions), without a transition zone. The face and arm are most affected, with the leg somewhat less so, reflecting greater cortical representation. The pain may vary in site ("wander"), disappearing from one limb only to arise in another, and intense pains in the limbs may be found simultaneously with only paresthesias in the face, or vice versa (Garcin 1937, Riddoch 1938). Langworthy and Fox (1937) emphasized how CP may appear to be localized in the abdominal viscera: one of their patients was misdiagnosed as gastric ulcer!

The area of pain (spontaneous and evoked, and rarely evoked only) may match the sensory and/or motor deficit, but may also be patchy, i.e., confined to a fraction of the disabled region, even after lesions causing extensive loss of somatic sensibility. In contrast, CP is never localized to an unaffected area. CP is

Table 3.5. General features of CP (representative series)

Attal *et al.* (2008)

Evaluation of associations between NP-positive symptoms (assessed with NPSI) and etiologies, types of nerve lesion, pain localizations. Statistical analysis: multiple correspondence analyses (MCA)

482 patients (53% men); quantitative sensory tests (QST) in 90 patients matched to the entire group. NP: peripheral (349 patients) or central (133 patients, 27.6%)

CP: Lesion site: spinal cord 78 patients (16.1%), brain 55 patients (11.4%). Etiologies: **syringomyelia** 40 patients (8.3%); **multiple sclerosis (MS) 32 patients** (6.5%); **CPSP 31 patients** (6.4%). Stroke type: ischemic (18 patients), hemorrhagic (12 patients), lacunar infarct (1 patient). Stroke site: rolandic or parietal areas (17 patients), thalamus (8 patients), brainstem (6 patients). **CCP**: SCI (25 patients); spinal tumor (ependymoma, schwannoma, cavernoma, neurinoma, or angioma: 6 patients)

Note: the number of reported cases adds up to 134 patients

Frequency of dimensions of the NPSI (%)

	Spinal lesion (25 patients)	MS (32 patients)	Syrinx (40 patients)	Stroke (31 patients)
Burning pain	76	56.2	75	74.2
Deep pain	74	62.5	60	64.5
Paroxysmal pain	72	65.6	65	58
Evoked pain	70	75	62.5	74
Paresthesia/ dysesthesia	80	84.4	87.5	83.9

Reported pain symptoms (whole population): tingling (69%), pins and needles (66%), burning (65%), electric shocks (57%), squeezing (50%), pressure (47%), stabbing (36%). Evoked pain: brush-evoked (55%), pressure-evoked (52%), cold-evoked (31%).

Mean pain intensity: 64 ± 19 (similar across all the neuropathic entities).

Association indicated by MCA: (1) idiopathic TN and electric shocks; (2) PHN and burning pain + allodynia without deep pain and paresthesia/dysesthesia; (3) plexus avulsion and amputation pain and pain paroxysms (electric shocks, stabbing). **No associations** between neuropathic symptoms (or dimensions) and other etiologies, types, or locations of lesions or pain localizations (exception: localization "face/neck in PHN and TN"), duration of pain, sex, or age.

Authors' conclusion: NP clinical expression is "trans-etiological". There are more similarities than differences in the neuropathic symptoms associated with peripheral and central lesions. Symptoms alone are not discriminant enough to indicate specific etiologies.

Lesion topography does not influence neuropathic characteristics of pain and should not determine the response to therapy.

This is different from the conclusions of Maier *et al.* (2010).

experienced as superficial (projected to the skin), deep (originating in muscle and bone), or both in varying proportions.

Sensory findings in brainstem lesions do not always correspond well with their anatomical site. Following lateral medullary infarction (LMI or Wallenberg's syndrome), four patterns of thermoalgesic sensory symptoms are described: type I (hypoalgesia in ipsilateral face and contralateral trunk and limbs), type II (both hemifaces plus contralateral hypalgesia, due to involvement of the crossed trigeminothalamic tract), type III (contralateral hemisoma), type IV (hypoalgesia in ipsilateral hemiface and contralateral trunk and leg, but not arm), and type V (contralateral hemiface, arm, and upper trunk) (Zhang *et al.* 2008). CP, when present, affects, diffusely or sectorially, the hemiface and contralateral hemisoma, the contralateral arm and leg, the hemiface, or

Table 3.6. Clinical findings in cord central pain (CCP) (selected recent series)

Finnerup *et al.* (2001)	
Assessment of the prevalence and characteristics of (neuropathic) pain and dysesthesia (P/D) in a community-based sample of spinal cord injury (SCI) patients. Postal survey (self-reported pain, drawn on a body chart, sub-classified as superficial, deep and/or abdominal, diffuse or patchy). P/D classification: above-level P/D and at- or below-level P/D.	
330 answers (76% of mailed questionnaires, 230 men). Median age: 42.6 years (range 19–80 years). Traumatic SCI in > 75% of patients. Complete lesion in 48% of responders. Median time since injury: 9.3 years (range 0.5–39 years).	
Demographic and clinical findings in 221 CP patients reporting P/D at or below lesion (67% of responders)	
Time to pain onset (% of patients)	Immediate: 31; ≤ 6 months: 36; delayed (> 6 months): 29
Change in pain intensity over time since onset (% of patients)	Decreased: 21; no change: 43; increased: 37
Temporal quality of pain (% of patients)	Constant: 38; intermittent shooting or electric shock-like: 56
Pain distribution (% of patients)	diffuse: 63; patchy: 35
Allodynia (% of patients)	48
Paresthesias (% of patients)	54 (34 in patients without P/D)
Abnormal unpleasant sensations (% of patients)	93
Median visual analog scale (mm)	47
Most frequently used words to describe P/D	Pricking, tingling, shooting, tiring, taut, annoying, burning
Interference with daily life (% of patients)	93 (in 19 interference ≥70 on a VAS)
Aggravating factors (% of patients)	Stress or anxiety (49), tiredness (38), weather change (30), cold (29)
Alleviating factors (% of patients)	Rest (51), physical activity (37), alcohol (18)
Increased risk for P/D	Incomplete lesions, sex (male)
Ducreux *et al.* (2006)	
MRI-confirmed spinal syringomyelia. 46 patients. Etiology of the syrinx: Chiari malformation (I) 27 patients, trauma 15 patients, primitive 4 patients. CP (= pain in an area of sensory deficit directly related to the SCI, not attributable to other condition, with specific characteristic descriptors) in 31 cases.	
Demographic and clinical findings in 31 CP patients	
Sex distribution (F/M)	16/15
Mean age	50 ± 14 years
Mean dermatomal extension of pain (painful area always located within the area of maximal thermal deficit, but more restricted)	5.8 ± 2.7 (unilateral: 24 patients)
Spontaneous ongoing pain (without evoked pain)	11 patients
Allodynia (brush, pressure, cold, heat) and/or hyperalgesia	20 patients (64%) (brush 12 patients; cold 11 patients; pressure 7 patients; heat 5 patients). (Allodynia to cold, pressure, or heat always associated with hyperalgesia to the same stimuli)
Pain location	**Upper limb**: 27 patients (+ neck: 7 patients); **thorax**: 5 patients; **thorax and lower limb**: 4 patients

Table 3.6. (cont.)

Demographic and clinical findings in 31 CP patients	
Mean pain duration	10.4 ± 8.3 years
Mean pain intensity (visual analog scale, mm)	56 ± 76
Pain quality (NPSI)	**Paresthesia/dysesthesia** (tingling, pins and needles): 24 patients (77%); **burning**: 23 patients (74%); **paroxysmal** (electric shocks, stabbing): 19 patients (63%); **deep** (pressure/squeezing): 14 patients (45%)

No relationship between pain intensity, duration, quality, and magnitude or extent of thermal deficits. No significant difference in thermal and mechanical deficits, graphesthesia, detection of movement direction impairment between maximal spontaneous pain area and adjacent lesioned but painless area.

Finnerup *et al.* (2007)

10 SCI (7 complete, 6 traumatic) patients with diffuse below-level NP (below-level pain only in 2 patients, + at-level pain in 4 patients, + at-level pain distinguished from the below-level pain in 4 patients); 10 SCI (9 complete, 0 traumatic) patients without NP at any level (paresthesias +). NP: chronic pain in an area of sensory abnormality, onset < 6 months after the SCI (traumatic or disease-based, border zone at the thoracic level).

Quality of pain (NPSI)/NRS (0–10, mean ± SD): **burning** (5.9 ± 3.8); **pressing/squeezing** (3.8 ± 3.2); **paroxysmal** (1.2 ± 2.8); **evoked** (1.9 ± 0.5); **tingling/pins and needles** (6.8 ± 7.0).

Felix *et al.* (2007)

194 SCI patients. 81% of patients with > 1 pain (87% men). Study aimed at determining most disturbing and less disturbing pain characteristics in SCI patients. Results: most disturbing pains: pain located at the level of injury, labeled "sharp" and "stabbing," with a high intensity rating, with a high interference score, with a high aggravating factors score, and with a high constancy of pain score.

Finnerup *et al.* (2008)

Study on hypothetical neuropathic origin of visceral pain in SCI patients. Questionnaire survey. No relation between the report of abdominal pain/discomfort and the report of burning, pricking, or shooting pain. Authors' conclusion: no suggested correlation between abdominal and NP. Still, a role of peripheral or central neuropathic mechanisms for the development of abdominal pain in some patients with SCI cannot be excluded.

Cruz-Almeida *et al.* (2009)

156 patients (135 men, 86.5%) with traumatic SCI and chronic pain (pain duration > 6 months, injury occurrence >2 years, average pain intensity > 3 on NRS). Mean age: 40.5 ± 12.8 years. Mean time since injury: 9.2 ± 8.8 years.

330 pains reported (on average 2.11 different pains/patient). Pain classification (% of cases): at (27.9%), **below (59.4%)**, **at and below (12.7%)** the neurological level of injury. Most common pain locations: back (30.0%), legs/feet (26.7%), thighs (23.0%).

Most common pain descriptors: burning (43.6%), aching (34.8%), sharp (30.6%), throbbing (22.4%), stabbing (19.4%), electric (19.1%), penetrating (18.2%), stinging (17.9%).

Soler MD *et al.* (2010a)

Investigation of the referred sensation (RS) phenomenon and its correlation with neuropathic pain (NP).

48 SCI patients with complete lesion. Chronic NP in 24 patients; no pain/paresthesias in 24 patients.

Assessment tools: NPSI, NRS. Examination of patient's perceptions (quality and location) in response to light touch and pinprick stimulation (repeated after 2 and 10 weeks if RS present). Random stimulation of 10–80 R/L, standardized, above-level key points. Stimulation carried out twice (patient's eyes closed and eyes open). Tactile self-stimulation in patients able to do it. Neurophysiological evaluation: MEPs, SSEPs (absent in all patients).

RS in 7/24 patients (29%) with below-level NP. No RS in any patients without NP.

Table 3.6. (cont.)

Demographic and clinical findings in 221 CP patients reporting P/D at or below lesion (67% of responders)]			
NP present more than 3 dermatomes below the neurological level of injury (LOI), complete lesion in all . Pain description: burning (4/7), pressing (3/7), paroxysmal (1/7), dysesthesia (2/7).			
Patient	**Levels/stimuli eliciting RS**	**CCP and RS description/site**	**Notes**
M, 50 years, T9 lesion, NRS (pain): 9	T5–T10; light touch, pinprick	Stabbing pain; R leg; 20 episodes/day; unrelated to position/movement, worsened by urinary tract infections Non-painful electric currents in the ipsilateral thigh (PA) + contralateral toes NPA)	RS evoked by light-touch self-stimulation. Unchanged EO/EC
M, 41 years, T5 lesion, NRS (pain): 5	Above but close to the lesion level + head and upper limbs; light touch, pinprick	Pressure and burning sensation; legs, toes and the perineal region; continuous, unrelated to position and movement, worsened by fatigue Non-painful tingling sensations in multiple areas below the lesion, predominantly in the PA and ipsilateral to the stimulated side (contralateral or bilateral RSs after stimulation of few points)	Upon stimulation, patient's awareness of the body areas experiencing RSs (patient's self-stimulation to produce sensations from anesthetic parts of the body). Stable RSs eliciting sites
M, 43 years, T10 lesion, NRS (pain): 8	R chest; light touch, pinprick	Constant pressure in R leg and groin, affected by mood, attention and weather changes Vivid, non-painful electric current sensations, ipsilateral to the stimulated side, located in the same area	RS evoked by light-touch self-stimulation. Unchanged EO/EC
M, 59 years, T12 lesion, NRS (pain): 10	Chest and back (T5–T12); light touch, pinprick	Burning, oppressive pain in the genital area (+ constant desire to defecate), worsened by trunk or fast wheelchair movements. NRS (pain): 10 **Painful sensations** (similar to the usual NP)	RS evoked by light touch self-stimulation **Only patient with painful** (similar to the usual NP) **referred sensations**
M, 35 years, C6 lesion, NRS (pain): 10	Head, shoulders, arms; light touch, pinprick	Burning, "pins and needles," tingling sensations on both soles Tingling, non-painful sensations in the PA + L thigh (ipsilateral to head and forearm stimulation)	
M, 45 years, C6 lesion (hemorrhage), NRS (pain): 8	Transition area; light touch, pinprick	Constant burning sensation in the thoracic area and in both legs, worsened with bowel function problems	Stable RS-eliciting sites. RS unchanged EO/EC

Table 3.6. (cont.)

Patient	Levels/stimuli eliciting RS	CCP and RS description/site	Notes
		Tingling, non-painful sensations in multiple areas, predominantly in the L leg (PA)	
M, 30 years, T4 lesion, NRS (pain): 5	Above the lesion area; light touch, pinprick	Constant, moderately intense pins and needles (dysesthetic pain) in the R foot. Tingling, non-painful sensation in the right foot (PA) + ipsilateral R chest (NPA)	RS evoked by self-stimulation

Below-level pain = NP present more than 3 dermatomes below the neurological level of injury (LOI); U, upper; L, lower; PA, painful area(s); NPA, non-painful area(s); L, left; R, right; NP, neuropathic pain; EO/EC, eyes open/eyes closed.

RSs well located and consistently evoked on repetition, elicited by both touch and pinprick stimulation, unchanged by visual feedback.

Authors' conclusion: RSs located in the same area as NP are relatively frequent in patients with complete SCI and NP. Pain and RSs could share common pathophysiological mechanisms.

the contralateral arm only, simultaneously or at different intervals. Rarely, LMI can lead to isolated contralateral spinothalamic sensory impairment (Kueper *et al.* 2008).

CCP may involve the entire body region below the level of injury (diffuse pain), but is usually more intense in the sacral dermatomes, buttocks and genitalia, and the feet, never following a dermatomal distribution. Pain is usually diffusely and symmetrically (although not at all times during follow-up) referred to the parts of the body whose sensation is affected by the cord lesion. However, a quarter complain of localized pain within a much larger area of sensory alteration, some having a pain sharply localized to a small body part, usually the saddle area. Tasker *et al.* (1992) found, in patients with complete lesions, that steady pain occurred as a band at the upper level of cord damage in about 7% of cases, diffusely below that level in less than 20%, patchily below that level in about 60%, and in the perineum in 15%. In those with incomplete lesions, the pain occurred diffusely below the level of cord dysfunction in two-thirds of cases, patchily in three-quarters, and as a band at the upper level in less than 20%. Patients with facial pain (about 4%) all had incomplete lesions and a syrinx. Intermittent pain tended to run around the trunk at the level of the cord lesion in complete cases, and shoot up and down the body and/or the legs in incomplete lesions. While pain generally starts from the level of injury and caudad, there may be a free area from the zone of injury to the area of dysesthesias. In a series, the most common locations included the legs (84%), posterior trunk (63%), anterior trunk (42%), and arms (16%; 100% in quadriplegics) (Beric 1999). In another series (Defrin *et al.* 2001), pain was described as deep by most patients (superficial only by 7%). The bizarre distribution of CCP is demonstrated by Jefferson (1983), who broke down his paraplegia pain patients into three groups:

(1) Six patients had an area of pain on the front of, or just above, the knees (a "blob" of about the same size as, or marginally bigger than, the patella), symmetrically or with side prevalence. Invariably there were also pains occupying the front of the thighs or else the front of the shins. One had pain on the tops of his feet and some (very localized) pain on the back of his calves (the only patient with a significant proportion of the pain occupying the posterior aspect of the leg in the first two groups). Only one patient complained of pain involving the pelvis (rectum and vagina).
(2) Three patients described pain occupying the anterior aspect of the thighs. In two of them the pain was symmetrical and there was no pain felt in any other part of the body. In the third patient, the pain occupied a large part of the front of the right thigh, extending upwards almost to the groin and

downwards to the middle of the patella. There was less severe pain in a similar distribution on the left, together with an area of pronounced hyperesthesia in the skin overlying the medial aspect of the left knee. Additionally, there was slight pain behind the right knee.

(3) The third group (6 patients) had fairly widespread pain, extending from the groin to the feet. Unlike groups 1 and 2, the pain spread downwards from iliac crests or groins and in half the patients it also involved the backs of the legs. Two patients had diffuse pain down the fronts of the thighs, knees, and shins, and in one of them the pain extended round the hips symmetrically into the lateral part of the buttocks. Three of the patients felt pain as extensively on the back of the legs as on the front, in two with involvement of the feet. One of these patients additionally described an episodic sensation which was likened to "an explosion" in the rectum. One patient had leg pains and pain involving the lower abdomen, the genitalia, and the buttocks. Two patients with no involvement of mid-thighs, knees, or shins had pains in areas that would be covered by bathing trunks (i.e., top of thighs, lower abdomen, buttocks plus anus and rectum either on the anterior or the posterior aspect). One of these patients also had isolated pains around the heels and ankles. Of the three patients who had lesions involving T10 vertebra the pains were distributed either throughout the leg or legs or else in a "bathing trunks" distribution.

Like BCP, CCP can be felt superficially or – perhaps more frequently – deeply. In Brown-Séquard's syndrome, below-level CP is observed in the contralateral hemisoma with respect to the lesion (end-zone pain is observed ipsilateral to hemisection). In some cases, pain is felt contralaterally after stimulation of the affected hypoesthetic areas (allochiria).

Quality of pain

Most patients experience one or more pain qualities (Table 3.7), simultaneously (two to four), in the same or different body regions (e.g., burning in leg and aching in face or, for example, in Wallenberg's syndrome dysesthesias to the hemiface and shooting pains to the limbs and trunk or vice versa), and seemingly identical lesions may cause different combinations of pain qualities in different patients. CP can have any quality, although some qualities are commoner; bizarre qualities are the exception rather than the rule. Variation in pain qualities is highest in CPSP and SCI-CP. Attempts to correlate various pain descriptors with some pathophysiology have failed. Dysesthetic pain is common in MS and incomplete SCI (including post-cordotomy), but, upon close questioning, may turn out to consist of a number of specific pain qualities. A burning quality is not a hallmark of CP, and in some series is not the most common descriptor. It is suggested that burning is commoner after brainstem lesions and following lesions confined to the white matter, but this remains moot. The more introspective point out that their symptoms bear no relation to anything they have experienced in the past. Whereas the majority have pain that can be described, several have no pain at all, but an unpleasant and difficult-to-describe sensation that drastically reduces their quality of life; moreover, there may be no sharp transition from non-painful to painful dysesthesias. Some patients complain of pruritus, singly or in combination with some of the other qualities mentioned above (Chapter 5). Paresthesias may also be the main complaint. Numbness is experienced by many; it can occur with total loss of tactile sensibility, but also with normal thresholds to touch, and sometimes it describes patients' paresthesias or dysesthesias.

According to Dr. McHenry, himself a CP patient (www.painonline.org), patients when asked to describe their pain quality sound like pain imbeciles and will only tell of the components if they "listen" very carefully, and then only with cues from the examiner. The result is that clinicians receive the false impression that CP is singular when it is plural, especially in symptoms other than dysesthetic burning. The patient of necessity borrows verbal descriptors from nociceptive pain, but these may mislead the examiner, leading to conflicts that the patient cannot explain and decreased credibility. Burning dysesthesia is an amalgam of pain sensations, but most closely corresponds to the second pain that follows, for example, touching a hot stove. There is nearly always a cold component, and frequently there is a metallic quality, as well as a sensation of wetness.

CCP is rather bizarre. There are different pains present in different patients, and also different pains present in the same patient at different times or simultaneously. Sometimes, characteristics change as they appear or disappear. As with BCP, there is no one quality prevailing in all studies, and patients may use many terms

Table 3.7. Pain quality

Muscle spindle pain	A cramp or contraction, with burning. There are sometimes areas of constant cramping sensation, usually in a single muscle belly, as well as diffuse burning when the muscle takes on a load. Weight-bearing while sleeping or resting on a surface also causes great soreness, so that patients feels as if they have been sleeping on rocks. (This, plus the burning dysesthesia from touching bedclothes, can make sleeping a torment.) Patients may describe muscle spindle pain as "drawing" or "pulling" or "crushing"
Burning	A chemical, not a purely physical, burn. Terms used: • mentholated burning • *like the skin of my legs has been destroyed and the charred flesh turned up at the edges* • *like in a dry lake bed* • *a sick burn, like that inflicted by a toxic chemical* • *a scalding, scathing torment, like in hell*
Cold	• *like touching dry ice so that it burns* • *my hand tells me the skin of my legs is cold but it feels like burning* • *like I am touching an incredibly cold pipe in a freezing night, so that it drains the flesh and burns me* • *like a dentist is touching the nerve in my tooth, only very cold*
Metallic	• *like tinfoil under my skin* • *creepy, like chewing tinfoil*
Wetness	• *When I am wet and sweaty, my skin is really sensitized and the burning lights up and I feel wet and uncomfortable underneath the burning*
Dysesthesia in the aggregate	• *I feel like I am being put on ice and then put into a fire with a million ice picks plunged into my body* (Bette Hamilton, one of Dr. Kevorkian's clients): this includes the burn, the cold, the metallic, and adds the lancinating component of CP • *often intolerable . . . crushed feeling, scalding sensation, as if boiling water was being poured down the arm, cramping, aching, soreness, as if the leg was bursting, something crawling under the skin, pain pumping up and down the side, as if the painful region was covered with ulcers, as if pulling a dressing from a wound, as if a log of wood was hanging down from the shoulder, as if little pins were sticking into the fingers, like a wheel running over the arm, cold stinging feeling* (Head and Holmes 1911) • *boiling hot, deep as though in the bones, showers of pain like electric shocks or red-hot needles evoked by touch, as though the arm and leg were being twisted, continuous sensation of pins and needles, a strange sensation of the limbs being abnormally full* (Loh *et al.* 1981) • *as if knives heated in Hell's hottest corner were tearing me to pieces* (Holmes 1919)
Circulatory	Pins and needles, tingling
Visceral (peristaltic)	Burning in the bladder, fullness or nausea in the gut ("like my bowels will explode"), heightened sense of distension and urgency with flatus or stool
Pruritus	This may occur singly or combined with other qualities
Other descriptors	Aching, lancinating, pricking, lacerating, pressing, shooting, stabbing, squeezing, throbbing, tearing, bruising, grabbing, pinching, cutting, crushing, sore, splitting, stinging, swollen, tiring, taut, numb, "like a tight armor," "sitting heavily on a ball," "like a flash of lightning"

to describe CCP. Intermittent pain is generally described as shooting or coming in electric shocks. As for the steady component, the most common qualities reported in a series by Widerström-Noga *et al.* (2001) were burning (59.9%) and aching (54.4%): burning was significantly associated with pain in frontal parts of the torso and genitals, buttocks, and lower extremities, whereas aching was associated with neck, shoulders, and back. In another series (Defrin *et al.* 2001), most frequent were burning (73%) and electric shock-like

(53%). Other descriptors include cutting, sharp/stabbing, piercing, cramping/pressing, stinging/pricking/pins and needles, electrical/shooting, throbbing/aching, cold/freezing, vibrating, radiating, tight, cruel, nagging, and others. No quality seems to prevail if series are pooled, but some authors emphasize how SCI and syringomyelia pain may have a prominent dysesthetic element, e.g., "pins and needles," stretching or pressure of the skin, and cold. Dysesthesias may be particularly common in incomplete spinal lesions (Davidoff *et al.* 1987a, Beric *et al.* 1988). Cruz-Almeida *et al.* (2009) identified three distinct symptom profiles: (1) aching, throbbing pain, aggravated by cold weather and constipation; (2) stabbing, penetrating, and constant pain of high intensity; and (3) burning, electric, and stinging pain aggravated by touch and muscle spasms. The patients of Davis and Martin (1947) complained of hot burning suddenly turning into "streams of fire" or pressure of a knife being burned in the tissue, twisted around rapidly and finally withdrawn.

Intensity of pain

Intensity varies widely between individuals, and severe pain is commoner among paretics than plegics (the suicidal people are usually paretic). After lenticulocapsular stroke, intensity tends to be maximal in the leg rather than in the arm or face (Kim 2003). Generally speaking, CP tends to be worst in areas of most severe initial sensory loss, while its evoked components are usually worst in areas of retained or only mildly impaired sensibility. The mean intensity of CP as reported in the literature varies: visual analog scale (VAS) 3 (Vestergaard *et al.* 1995); VAS 3.8 (median) for aching pain and VAS 5 (median) for burning pain (Bowsher *et al.* 1998); VAS 5 (Klit *et al.* 2011, Misra *et al.* 2008, median); VAS 5.6 (Kim 2003); and VAS 6 (Widar *et al.* 2002). While some reports found higher intensities for brainstem or thalamic lesions, Misra *et al.* (2008) found no differences between thalamic and other lesions. Among 18 CP patients, Yanagida *et al.* (2003) found intensity to be mild (81.6%) to moderate (13.3%); in only 4% was it severe. Exacerbations were due to specific factors (77.3%): stress, somatic stimuli, weather, fatigue, visceral activity. Their conclusion was that "to state that the intensity of central pain continues to be intolerable and severe throughout the day is an exaggeration ... the strategy to manage central pain should primarily focus ... on prevention of the exacerbating factors of central pain."

In the series of Andersen *et al.* (1995), most pain was mild to moderate, and severe in *c.* 19% of the patients. Sadosky and Dukes (2007), in their study of 38 CPSP and 32 SCI patients, found that, despite high adherence to drug therapy (91%), 63% still reported moderate pain and 22% severe pain. Anyway, even when low or moderate, CP may be assessed as severe because it causes much suffering and burden due to its irritating character and constant presence. For most patients, the intensity of CP is sufficient to interfere with daily activities and is a potential or active factor in the development of anxiety and depression, along with neurologic disabilities, themselves a risk factor. Depression may, in turn, increase the perceived intensity and affective quality of the pain. Pain can be assessed as a worse handicap than, for example, severe motor impairment. Sleep (both slow-wave and REM) is disturbed in up to two-thirds of the patients. In general, its intensity increases in the mid-afternoon to evening (Bruguerolle and Labrecque 2007), probably due to changes in central monoamine levels. There appears to be no meaningful difference among suprathalmic, thalamic, brainstem, or cord lesions. Intensity can be constant or more often may fluctuate spontaneously, even paroxysmally, or following aggravating or mitigating stimuli. Interestingly, variation in intensity may differ between pain qualities in the same patient. In its more extreme, intractable form, the patient is motivated to commit suicide.

The intensity of the CCP varies from mild, unpleasant tingling to one of the most agonizing torments known to humans. When more components of pain are present, the intermittent will be the more severe. The steady component generally fluctuates during the day and from day to day, also in bursts of activity and cyclically (e.g., every other day or even every other week) and is not always so harassing as to induce the patient to ask for medical help. Pain may be more intense in the legs (Widerström-Noga *et al.* 2001). Generally speaking, CCP is always very intense: for instance, in the series described by Rogano *et al.* (2003), mean VAS score was 9.4, with pain more severe with gunshot injuries ($p < 0.001$). Pain located in the frontal aspects of the torso (including genitals), "burning," or "electric" pain are especially intense (Widerström-Noga and Turk 2004). A higher level of education may be reflected in more perceived pain. SCI-CP may or may not be perceived as worse than motor deficits (Nepomuceno *et al.* 1979, Davidoff *et al.* 1987a).

Components

Patients with BCP demonstrate three types of pain: (1) a constant spontaneous component (85–100%); (2) an intermittent (every day, with pain-free intervals lasting a few hours at most), brief (seconds to minutes), intense, spontaneous component (*c.* 15%), generally shooting, shock-like or lancinating and with a similar distribution to that of steady pain; when present, it can be the major complaint, more common in brainstem; and (3) evoked pain (see below), that is, hyperesthesia, hyperpathia, hyperalgesia, and/or allodynia. Any single patient may, however, complain of only one of these three components. Only a minority of CPSP patients have their spontaneous CP absent for up to a few hours each day.

Shooting (lancinating) pain is the most distinct, most severe, and most startling, but it does not cause the most suffering, because the pain is limited to the surface area affected and can often be eliminated by shifting position or rubbing the area. This pain shoots from distal to proximal sites. The phenomenon is most dramatic early in the disease and tends to diminish with time, leading to false notions of drug benefit. It is indistinguishable clinically from the "lightning pains" of tabes dorsalis. Lancinating pain is said to originate where mini-fasciculations occur (Dr. McHenry, www.painonline.org).

Paretics display the greatest number of CP components, unlike plegics and MS patients (although the ones they have can be severe). Gradients can be observed: spontaneous pain tends to be distal (i.e., where sensory loss becomes greatest) and evoked pains proximal (i.e., where sensory loss is present but least marked).

CCP consists of three components (Tasker *et al.* 1992): a steady, spontaneous pain (almost all), an intermittent, spontaneous pain (about one-third, found singly in 1% of patients), and evoked pain (about one-half, singly in 3%). So, for instance, a single patient may complain of episodic lightning pains down a leg, superimposed on a continuous background of burning pain. Intermittent pain is particularly common in patients with T10–L1 injuries, whether complete or incomplete (57%), and often shooting down one or both legs: 69% of Tasker's CCP patients with intermittent pain had thoracolumbar lesions. The steady, intermittent, and evoked components are often associated in a single patient. The type of pain has no rapport with the causative lesion (Tasker *et al.* 1992).

At-level pain (also known as transitional-zone, radicular/root, girdle, segmental, end-zone, junctional, or boundary-zone pain) is not the same as below-level pain, i.e., it is not CCP. This pain occurs at or just above the level of the sensory loss, in the cutaneous transition zone from the area of analgesia to areas of normal sensation (i.e., hypoesthetic) and extends for 1–2 dermatomes into the anesthetic zone. Often it is not strictly dermatomal (radiculometameric), it may be unilateral or bilateral (more often than not asymmetrical), and it may be observed at all levels, perhaps with some preponderance, often in clinically complete injuries. It is generally described as dull, aching (sometimes burning) with superimposed paroxysms of throbbing, stabbing, electric shock-like, or cramping pain lasting from one to several minutes. Allodynia and hyperalgesia are frequent: touching/stroking the skin in the painful dermatomes, which may also present as a very narrow band of hyperalgesia, often activates the pain itself, causing it to radiate into the lower parts of the body, especially the legs. At-level pain is usually due to direct injury to the dorsal roots at or near the site of trauma, but also Lissauer's tract and posterior horns, or even local arachnoiditis/scarring with entrapment (occasional worsening by arm/leg movement suggests traction on these roots). One-third of SCI patients have it, making it the most common type of pain in association with paraplegia (Nashold 1991, Beric 1999). A subset of these pains is cauda equina pain (damage from T12 caudad), involving the legs, feet, perineum, genitals, buttocks, and rectum. It is generally very severe; usually burning, it may often be seen with dysesthesias and neuralgic pain in the thighs, calves, or feet.

Evoked pains

The spontaneous discomfort of CP is often (*c.* 70%: 50–90%) accompanied by unpleasant (dysesthesias, paresthesias) or painful sensations induced by somatosensory stimuli applied to areas of complete somatosensory interruption. It is unusual in the complete absence of clinically detectable sensory loss. Infrequently, these can be the only symptoms, i.e., in the absence of constant pain: 2/12 in the series of Michel *et al.* (1990), 3/27 in Shieff (1991), 7% in Tasker (2001a). They may first be noticed after several years with the disease. Evoked sensations may be unbearable and evoke violent emotional and defensive reactions (but only 6/31 patients of Misra *et al.* 2008 rated them as more intense than spontaneous pain), generally being referred to as the worst component of CP. Often poorly localized to the hemisoma (*c.* 90% in Tasker's series), patchily or diffusely, they may be elicited either by normally non-painful stimuli, namely touch (including caresses) – but not, at least initially, deep pressure – vibration, moderate cold and heat (***allodynia***), or by mildly to moderately painful stimuli, particularly sharp objects plus noxious cold and heat (***hyperesthesia***: ***hyperalgesia*** and ***hyperpathia***) delivered to an area of nearly (but not) always elevated threshold to stimuli of one or more somatosensory modalities (thermal, mechanical, either static or dynamic). Hyperalgesia may be less frequent in brainstem CP. These evoked pains are elicited most prominently by a single sensory modality, a little more often than by several (Tasker 2001a). Riddoch (1938) and others noted how pain can be evoked by simple pressure in areas of analgesia to pinprick. Also, even in the presence of nearly abolished pinprick sensibility, firm pinching or repeated pinpricks may be felt as painful. Head and Holmes (1911) also noted how pressure (deep tissue pain) with an algometer could evoke discomfort in cases with complete analgesia to pinprick (rediscovered by Mailis and Bennett 2002). In patients with complete thermoanesthesia, extremes of heat and cold may evoke disagreeable nonthermal sensations (Riddoch 1938). Hyperpathia (a term first introduced by Förster) refers to an abnormally painful reaction to a stimulus, especially a repetitive stimulus: the painful sensation develops explosively. There is usually little relation between the strength of the stimulus and the amount of sensation excited: it is nearly all or nothing. Moreover, there is no refractory period for hyperpathic responses. The effective stimulus may include all somatosensory stimuli or only a specific type of input (such as cold or draft, the light touch of clothing or pinprick, even smoke). These grossly unpleasant sensations may demonstrate temporal or spatial spread.

Simple neurologic sensory tests characterize (1) ***radiation of pain*** or ***dysesthesia*** (to body areas not directly in contact with the pain-evoking stimulus: "in a hot room . . . if one rubs the whiskers of the face with the palm of the hand, burning is felt in the ulnar forearm. Sitting on a chair until the burning is prominent on points of contact, burning is also felt in the lateral thigh which is not in contact with the fabric of the chair"), present in half the cases; (2) ***after-sensations*** (the persistence of pain long after the stimulus and the arrival of primary afferent impulses that evoke pain), seen in about 40% of cases; and (3) prolonged ***temporal summation*** (the gradual build-up of pain with repeated stimulation) (Garcin 1937, Riddoch 1938). Radiation of sensations from the stimulus site and spatial and temporal summation appear to be more common in CP than in peripheral neuropathic pain (PNP).

Although response latencies can be normal, anomalous ***summations*** may be seen: (1) ***slow temporal*** (pain or dysesthesias start after a delay, and, during the daytime, the patient can anticipate and avoid them: "if occlusive touch is applied to the skin, within minutes, evocation of the spontaneous dysesthetic burning occurs. The stimulus may be roughness, but the patient perceives it as heat. The search for ever 'cooler' shoes may be launched when what is needed is smooth leather, not the sueded tongue which is common"); (2) ***very slow temporal*** (starting after hours: "as to confinement or weight-bearing it renders a night's recumbency as feeling like the bed was hard as rocks. As to exercise, it means the muscle soreness the day after exertion is overwhelming"); (3) ***delayed with overshoot*** (this is not a temporal delay; rather it is a heightened threshold for pain, which, when reached, overshoots wildly; most easily seen in the response to sharp objects – a person with normal responses will note graded sharpness as painful before a CP patient will, but, because the pin in pinprick testing is so sharp, this delay is often missed at examination); and (4) ***spatial*** (an unexpected increase in pain as the area of stimulus is increased: it appears never to have been tested in CP).

Wind-up pain (increasing pain with increasing numbers of pinpricks, i.e., temporal summation) has been reported by 16.3% of CP cases in a large series (Maier *et al.* 2010). Parenthetically, dynamical mechanical allodynia, which is painful, is suggested to be the "hyperbole" of dynamical mechanical dysesthesia (non-painful), the difference being the number of Aβ fibers having access to the nociceptive system (Landerholm and Hannson 2011).

In sum, evoked pains are characterized by late onset and poor localization, they generally radiate from the stimulated point to the entire half of the body or lesser body areas, and they may persist for an unusually long time after stimulation has ceased. Evoked pains have a distribution which is less widespread than that of steady or intermittent pain. As a rule, somatic stimuli can cause or aggravate pain only when applied to the affected side, but sometimes even the stimulation of the normal side gives rise to exacerbation of pain (***synesthesalgia***).

Patients may wear as little clothing as possible over affected areas and seek a narrow window of room temperature, or alternatively wear gloves to avoid contact with the painful hand.

Cold allodynia is observed in *c.* 20–50% of the patients, heat allodynia/hyperalgesia in *c.* 10–19% (Nurmikko and Hietaharju 1992, Attal *et al.* 2000, Maier *et al.* 2010). Paradoxical burning on cold stimulation was reported by 26% in the series of Maier *et al.* (2010) (see also Hansen *et al.* 1996 for MS).

Hair sensation is usually unaffected and has never been reported to cause burning. Tactile allodynia is reported by *c.* 40% (with differences among series) of the patients.

In a large series (Klit *et al.* 2011), 66% of CPSP patients had allodynia or hyperalgesia, in particular cold allodynia (40%), pinprick hyperalgesia (57%), and dysesthesias in response to cold (66%), brush (51%), and touch (40%). Spreading and after-sensations were found in 29% and 34% of the patients respectively.

In cord lesions, evoked pain does not depend on the vertebral level or on the completeness of the spinal lesion, and exclusively occurs in areas of incomplete or clinically undetectable sensory loss or as a band at the upper margin of complete sensory loss. It can be elicited throughout the entire area of hypoesthesia or only in part of it, by one or several modalities of sensory stimulation. Trigger points can be identified even distant from areas of sensory deficit. In rare instances, evoked pain affects skin with clinically normal sensation (hyperesthesia). Different series report different frequencies of evoked pains (7–60%), which may (or may not) be lower than in BCP.

CP can be exacerbated by environmental changes (wind, weather changes, low atmospheric pressure, altitude, cold or warm temperatures), emotional stress (sudden fear, joy, anxiety, depression, others: *mental/cognitive allodynia*), tiredness, smell, loud noises, sad or distasteful music, (sudden) bright light, movements (including vibrations and changing – or maintaining for a long time – position), physical activity (e.g., walking, non-strenuous activity, isotonic/isometric muscle contraction of one or more muscles together, with ensuing activation of muscle stretch receptor afferents – so-called *movement/kinesthetic/proprioceptive/muscle (myo)allodynia*, seen in about 10–20% of patients, which can hinder rehabilitation and virtually paralyze some patients), visceral stimuli (e.g., a full urinary bladder or rectum, drinking cold and warm water, passing urine, cough, Valsalva maneuver), the thermal grill, smoking (and even the curling of cigar smoke along the fingers), intellectual concentration, inactivity (such as attempts to sleep), merely blowing on the skin and combing the hair. Less commonly, similar stimuli may reduce the pain. Dyskinesias and other anomalous motor reactions can also worsen CP. Rarely, an over-response to pleasant stimuli or relief by pleasant stimuli (e.g., warmth or orgasm) may also be found (Riddoch 1938): for instance, Biemond (1956) described a patient who drew a passing sensation of pleasure with cold drinks and ice creams. Bowsher *et al.* (1998) found orgasm as triggering the pain in 8.7% of their cases. Bowsher *et al.* (2004) also reported on a pontine CPSP patient who displayed allodynia to mechanical and acoustic startle, but not to mechanical stimulation when she knew it was coming. Widerström-Noga and Turk (2004) found that > 50% of SCI patients indicated that prolonged sitting, infections, fatigue, muscle spasms, cold weather, and sudden movements exacerbated their pain. A principal components analysis detected five sets of factors that were reported to magnify pain: negative mood, prolonged afferent activity (bowel, bladder, somatic), weather, voluntary physical activity, and transient somatic afferent activity. Other aggravating factors include pressure ulcers and a poor fit in a brace or wheelchair. Factors such as secondary gain or drug-seeking behavior will significantly affect the severity and chronicity of CP.

Sympathetic and other signs and symptoms

Signs of abnormal sympathetic nervous system activity within the region of disability (i.e., focal distribution) may sometimes be present: cooler and vasoconstricted skin in the painful area, edema, hypo/hyperhydrosis (rare), altered skin texture and color (mottled skin or livedo) (Garcin 1937, Riddoch 1938). However, these signs are equally present in non-CP patients with CNS injury; decreased movement alone can cause autonomic changes. A cerebral lesion can cause trophic disturbances in contralateral limbs (Arseni and Boetz 1971), particularly the shoulder–hand syndrome, even paroxysmally (Montgomery and King 1962). A common (30–40% of the cases) source of pain after stroke is

pain localized to the shoulder resulting from paresis and changed muscular tone/posture and sensory loss, but also painful spasticity and tension-type headache. Musculoskeletal pain is often reported in the back and lower limbs, particularly in the knees and hips. Post-stroke shoulder pain has been suggested to be central more than peripheral (Roosink *et al.* 2011). Heterotopic ossification (seen after brain/cord injury and rarely after stroke) may amplify CPSP (Chari and Tunks 2010).

Lance (1996) described the complaint of a ***painful, burning, red ear*** in a CP patient with a right sylvian infarction (female, 42 years old, case 10). Some 6 weeks later she developed sharp pains "like a hot needle" in the left side of her head, which recurred with increasing frequency until it became a diffuse burning ache in the left side of her head and face, similar to the pain she experienced in her left shoulder and upper limb. When the burning pain was exacerbated, onlookers commented that her left ear became red and sometimes stayed red all day. Sensory loss and weakness of her left arm persisted. Her pain was diminished to about half of the previous severity by imipramine 125 mg daily. Three years after the accident, she developed left-sided migraine-like headaches associated with increased intensity of the burning pain.

Eames (1997) reported on 13 patients who suffered severe head injury and a ***cold feeling***: all felt slightly cool to the touch, but not cold. Eleven stopped feeling cold, completely and permanently, after 1 month's treatment with vasopressin.

Often, following total spinal cord transection, after the phase of spinal shock, the patient complains of ***phantom sensations*** referred to the legs, and these are very similar to amputees' sensations, being painful, uncomfortable, and unpleasant, but not disabling. They appear early, almost immediately after SCI, and vanish soon after SCI (rarely, they linger on for months). Unlike amputees, telescoping or shrinkage of the involved body parts occurs only rarely in paraplegics, and the length and posture of the phantom do not change; in addition, they are less vivid. Paraplegics describe sensations projected from the surface, but few postural sensations, with both voluntary and involuntary movements of the phantoms. Phantom sensations must be distinguished from phantom pain. CP appears when phantom sensations fade.

Bilateral painful gynecomastia arising some time after dorsal level SCI has been described (Biju *et al.* 2005).

Following both brain lesions and spinal cord injury, the patient sometimes perceives pain and temperature (but also non-painful) stimuli applied to analgesic or hypalgesic regions in a part of the affected or contralateral side of the body in which the sensibility is normal (variously defined as ***referred/reference of pain, allo(ch)esthesia, mirror pain, allochiria***), a phenomenon first described by Obersteiner (1881). Referred sensations are seen after both stroke and SCI and may be experienced as mild electric-current and tingling (but also painful) sensations (Turton and Butler 2001, Soler MD *et al.* 2010a). Kawamura *et al.* (1987) observed alloesthesia in 20/123 patients with hypertensive cerebral hemorrhage in the acute stage (within 20 days), all but one in the right hemisphere. This phenomenon was observed in 17/35 patients with right putaminal hemorrhage and only 1/30 patients with right thalamic hemorrhage. Three patients, with cervical tumor, cervical disc herniation, and MS, all with anterolateral lesions of the spinal cord, also showed the phenomenon. The cerebral and spinal cord lesions presented similar symptomatic characteristics of alloesthesia. In cases of unilateral cord lesions, pain is usually referred to the symmetrical contralateral part of the body; in cases of bilateral cord lesions, giving rise to bilateral analgesia, it is referred to the ipsilateral or contralateral side above the analgesic zone. The patient reports that the pain slowly spreads, as stimulation is maintained, and arises from the interior, unlike the stimulus to the skin, which is felt as external (Nagaro *et al.* 1993). However, referred pain is not CP, as, in spinal cord cases, a cordotomy on the opposite side abolishes it. In two syringomyelia pain patients, brush-evoked allodynia with the patients watching the reflected image of their corresponding but opposite skin region being brushed in a mirror (dysynchiria) did not evoke any sensation at the affected area (Kraemer *et al.* 2008a).

Chapter 4

Somatosensory findings

A wide spectrum of sensory abnormalities can be found among patients with CP (Tables 4.1–4.4). They range from a slightly raised threshold for one of the submodalities, to complete loss of all somatic sensibility in the painful region, or a very painful hyperesthesia. In some patients the abnormalities are subtle, but they can often be detected by quantitative sensory tests (QST), as demonstrated by Head and Holmes (1911). A survey of the literature shows that the common feature of more than 90% of all CP patients is impaired temperature and pain (i.e., spinothalamic) sensibility at clinical or electrophysiological examination. Appreciation of pinprick and temperature is nearly always impaired, and there is almost always a raised threshold to innocuous thermal (heat and cold) detection, and to a lesser extent also to painful heat and cold pain. Some patients who have lost the ability to perceive heat and cold due to CNS lesions can nonetheless distinguish warm or cool objects by the distinctly different feelings they evoke (e.g., Kinnier Wilson 1927, Davison and Schick 1935). Impairment of the spinothalamocortical pathway has also been confirmed by diffusion tensor imaging (DTI) (Hong *et al.* 2010). No unequivocal report of CP arising from lesions restricted to the lemniscal pathways has been published, and several patients (particularly in Wallenberg's syndrome) have normal thresholds for touch, vibration, and kinesthesis (in such cases, the posterior columns may mediate evoked pains); instead, many cases of lesions restricted to the spinothalamic tract (STT) are on record (cordotomy, anterior spinal artery syndrome, medullary stroke).

CP is independent of other neurological symptoms, including paresis, tremor, dystonia, speech disturbances, and hemianopsia; only somatosensory abnormalities are always present, although these are far from uniform among patients.

Pain distribution is usually well correlated with sensory abnormalities.

The pain may also occur in patients with brain lesions who have recovered from clinically detectable sensory loss, and it may persist in time; in this case, a crude sensory examination, weeks or months after the lesion, reveals no sensory deficit. Nonetheless, a lesion affecting the STT system "is a necessary but not sufficient condition" for the development of CP, as many patients who diplay this loss have no CP. The question whether there is any significant association between thermoalgesic thresholds and severity of CP is unresolved, with conflicting results (e.g. Defrin *et al.* 2001, Felix and Widerström-Noga 2009).

It is the experience of all groups doing research with CP that some patients do not display thermoalgesic abnormalities either clinically or electrophysiologically (e.g. Schott *et al.* 1986: 5/43; Michel *et al.* 1990: thermal 8.3%, pinprick 16.7%; Tasker *et al.* 1991: 5.5%; Andersen *et al.* 1995: 6%). However, in all those cases where no sensory loss was seen in the first place, imaging techniques generally suggest a central lesion appropriately located to damage the somatosensory system.

Table 4.1. Somatosensory troubles in Head and Holmes' (1911) cases of central pain

Case no.	5	6	7	8	9	10	11	12	13
Sex	F	M	F	M	M	F	F	M	M
Age (years)	51	49	60	64	59	65	52	65	43
Side of pain	L	R	L	L	L	L	R	L	R
Tactile sensibility (von Frey)	–	0	=	=	–	– –	– –	0/– – (head)	– –
2-point discrimination	0	nt	=	=	– –	nt	– –	nt	nt
Localization of stimuli	– –	nt	=	=	=	nt	=/–	0	nt
Threshold for prick	=	++	=	=	=	+	+	++ = (sole)	++
Unpleasant response to prick	+	++	+	+	+	++	+	++	++
Threshold for painful pressure	=/+	++	=/– (sole)	– –	=	– (palm, sole) = (hand) + (shin)	– –	++	++ – – (sole)
Unpleasant response to pressure	+	++	++	++	+	++	++	++	++
Sensibility to heat	–	0	=	= (shifting)	-	0	=	0	0
Sensibility to cold	–	0	=	= (shifting)	–	0	=	0	0
Unpleasant response to extreme heat	+	++	+	+ +	+	+ +	=	nr	++
Unpleasant response to extreme cold	+	++	+	++	+	+ +	=	++	++
Pleasant response to mild warmth	nr	nr	nr	++	++	++	nr	nr	nr
Unpleasant response to visceral stimulation	+	nr	nr	nr	nr	nr	nr	+	++
Unpleasant response to tickling/scraping	nr	nr	0	= / +	+	+ +	++	+	++
Appreciation of vibration	nr	nr	–	=	–	– –/0	–	0	– –/0

0, lost; =, unchanged (no difference between affected and unaffected side); –, diminished; – –, strongly diminished; +, increased; ++, strongly increased; nt, not tested; nr, not reported.

Head and Holmes objectively analyzed sensory loss and dissociation of sensibility in patients with lesions of the CNS at spinal, mid-brain, thalamic, and cortical level by means of instrumentation that in some cases was designed expressly for this purpose. Results on the affected part were always compared with results obtained in the unaffected similar part of the body. Data were recorded as accurately and objectively as possible. Light touch was examined first by applying a *wisp of fine cotton wool*, avoiding any deformation of structure. For determining the threshold for light touch the authors employed *von Frey graduated hairs* ranging from 8 to 110 g/mm^2. They always performed 16 contacts in 1 minute, avoiding rhythmicity. The series of tests were performed without word exchange; hallucinatory responses were also recorded. Pressure-touch was tested by *contact with the observer's finger* provided that its surface temperature was similar to that of the part to be examined. The threshold for pressure-touch was determined by a *pressure-esthesiometer*. Specific methods, as accurate as possible, were used to test the faculty of localization, the threshold for the appreciation of roughness, the ability to discriminate two simultaneous contacts, the ability to recognize the posture of any part of the body, the ability to appreciate passive movements and the weight, size, bi-dimensional shape, three-dimensional form, texture, and consistency of objects. The ability to recognize vibration was tested by means of *a tuning-fork*, beating at 128 Hz, also noting the duration of the sensation. Tickling and scraping were employed to evaluate the affective component of sensation.

Superficial sensibility to pain was tested first by pricking with a *sharp steel pin or needle*, and a comparison between normal and affected parts was always performed. Being well aware that this test was subject to a source of error due to the reduction of the power of recognizing the size (sharpness) of the stimulating object, in cases with slight disturbances of pain sensation they determined the threshold for pain by means of an esthesiometer (algesimeter). They also noted that if a pain-spot was not directly stimulated, the same pressure was reported as touch. Finally, pressure-pain was tested by means of a *Cattell algometer*, measuring the amount of pressure (kg) on a standard area necessary to evoke pain. Results of the test on the affected part were always compared with results in the similar unaffected part of the body.

The **thermal sensibility** was examined by means of *silver tubes filled with hot or cold water*. The temperature of the water at the moment of testing was read on a *thermometer*. The authors determined the threshold for heat and cold on similar parts of the two halves of the body, as well as the ability to distinguish the relative warmth or coldness of two tubes. Moreover, the sensation evoked by neutral temperature was compared with that of a distinctly cold or warm tube. They also observed the effect of extreme heat (≥ 50 °C) and cold (≤ 15 °C) and compared the sensation evoked on normal and abnormal parts of the body. To study the affective component of thermal stimuli, they used large glass tubes (4 cm in diameter) filled with water at various temperatures. They also noted that the temperature tests were liable to lead to erroneous conclusions because of the tendency to call all sensations evoked during the testing either hot or cold. Patients with thalamic lesions and capable of no thermal appreciation were more liable to call every thermal stimulus, and even repeated pricking, "hot." This confusion was more likely to occur in patients with over-response to affective stimuli. In many patients it was also difficult to determine the extent of the neutral zone between heat and cold threshold, as patients possessed no word which expressed this neutral sensation ("nothing but a touch").

They reported data on one patient with SCI (Brown–Séquard paralysis) without CP, three cases of brainstem lesion (one of them with CP following Wallenberg's syndrome), nine cases of thalamic lesion (thalamic syndrome), and five patients with cortical lesions (one of them reporting pain during sensory epileptic attacks). Their conclusions on neurological features in thalamic syndrome were however based on data on 24 patients. In their opinion, the essential feature of thalamic syndrome is the tendency to react excessively to unpleasant stimuli (over-reaction).

In the patient with CP following *Wallenberg's syndrome* the sensibility to light touch (cotton-wool, von Frey hairs), the appreciation of roughness (Graham–Brown esthesiometer) or of two simultaneous contacts, and the ability to recognize vibration were not different between the two sides of the face, even if the patient complained that all forms of touch were less vivid over the affected (right) side. The affected side of the face was insensitive to superficial pain (prick), but pressure-pain was not lost (the Cattell algometer gave approximately equal readings on the two sides). Both heat and cold were appreciated on the two halves of the face and the thresholds were the same, but heat seemed hotter over the affected side while cold seemed less cold. On the body there was no difference in appreciation of touch, roughness, and vibration, but sensations were more vivid on the normal (right) half of the body. Heat and cold could be appreciated, but heat seemed hotter on the affected (left) half of the body and cold seemed less cold. The left half of the body, except an area in the left perineum, penis, and scrotum, was insensitive to prick. The pressure of the algometer necessary to evoke pain was considerably higher on the affected hemibody than in the normal half. The left testicle was insensitive to the pressure.

Somatosensory troubles in their patients suffering from "*thalamic syndrome*" (central pain) are summarized in Tables 4.1 and 4.2.

Concerning loss of *superficial and "deep" sensibility*, "in some patients with thalamic syndrome this loss is so insignificant that it can be discovered by measurement only, so we can imagine the existence of the over-reaction without it." Even if all patients with over-reaction had a more or less recognizable sensory loss, the excessive response bears no relation to the extent of the accompanying loss of sensation.

They noted that the *appreciation of posture and recognition of passive movements* was impaired more frequently than any other sensory quality. The amount of this loss varied from a scarcely measurable defect to a complete loss of these sensibilities.

Tactile sensibility was frequently diminished and in some cases totally lost, but generally a threshold could be obtained, especially by increasing the strength of the stimulus. Tactile threshold, measured with von Frey hairs, was unchanged between the two halves of the body in five cases, but in the majority of cases it was raised on the affected side. Only in a few cases were the affected parts totally insensitive to the tactile hairs and also to pressure-esthesiometer. In some patients, the consecutive contacts (especially with increasing strength) caused widespread tingling that made conclusive demonstration of the threshold impossible. Determination of tactile threshold was also prevented by the occurrence of involuntary (induced) movements, with accessory sensations misinterpreted as stimulation.

Many patients (50% of cases) could not recognize the *position* of a stimulated spot. In many cases where tactile sensibility was diminished, the inability was maintained even with pricks or painful pressure, to which the patient was sensitive. Patients could be at a loss to know where they were touched, or could refer touch to wrong areas. When the posture was not recognized and the power of localization was lost, patients recognized the stimulus as a change within the part of themselves and did not refer the discomfort to the action of an external agent. Moreover, when localization was affected, unpleasant sensations could spread widely over the affected part: for instance, they noted that a prick on the hand could cause a painful sensation in the cheek or side.

In no instance among 22 patients was the threshold for pinprick pain lower on the affected body side; it was identical on both sides in 13 cases and raised in nine cases, in whom a stronger stimulus was needed to produce a sensation of prick. Yet most patients (20/22) showed an over-response to prick.

They also attempted to measure the amount of pressure evoking pain, comparing the two sides of the body. They noted that the same pressure produced more disagreeable discomfort and increased reaction on the affected side in every one of 24 patients tested. Moreover, the pain developed explosively, as the pressure increased above a certain point. They noted that the threshold for pressure pain was frequently lower on the affected side of the body (15 cases), but it was higher in three cases and unchanged in six cases. No patient showing a lowered threshold for painful pressure showed a lower threshold for pinprick pain. Yet the response on the affected half of the body was excessive in all 24 patients. They also stated that excessive pressure (especially on a bone) normally caused discomfort rather than pain, and that the distressing sensation differed profoundly from the pain produced by a prick, even if both stimuli were perceived as painful. They concluded that pressure pain contained some sensory factors to which the affected half of the body was peculiarly susceptible, and that the over-reaction was due to this increased susceptibility, rather than increased sensibility to pain (as demonstrated by the fact that threshold to pinprick might be raised in patients with lowered threshold to pressure). A reduced sensibility to pain delays the appearance of the over-reaction, but, as the stimulus is strong enough to cause pain, the discomfort greatly exceeds that produced over the unaffected part.

Table 4.1 (cont.)

Concerning heat and cold sensibility, they wrote: "Twenty-two out of twenty-four patients who showed signs of a thalamic lesion responded excessively to the unpleasant aspect of heat and cold. In nine of these cases the threshold for thermal stimuli was the same on the two sides, and but for the over-response sensibility to heat and cold appeared to be normal; the range of discrimination was identical on the two halves of the body. This class is peculiarly interesting, for in them may appear the remarkable over-response to pleasurable heat we have described on p. 134. But, not infrequently, all appreciation of heat and cold is abolished and ice and water at over 50 °C evoke nothing but discomfort. This sensation is the same, whichever of the two extremes is used; the patient cannot tell the difference and may not recognize the cause of the unpleasant sensation. Occasionally, the insensibility is less profound and temperatures below 26 °C and above about 40 °C may evoke a response from the affected half of the body. But this response may be the same for heat and cold; water above 40 °C and below 26 °C produces the same sensation and may therefore be called indiscriminately hot or cold. For, if the patient knows from the experience on his normal side that thermal sensibility is under examination, he concludes that this vivid sensation is caused by 'something hot' or 'something cold.' No such confusion between the extreme degrees of heat and cold ever occurs when the patient is able to distinguish intermediate degrees. We have seen no reason so far to think that at this level of the nervous system the power of appreciating either heat or cold can be lost alone. The few apparent exceptions were due to the adoption by the patient of the same thermal nomenclature for the unpleasant reaction produced by certain temperatures towards the two ends of the scale, a confusion rendered possible by the absence of thermal appreciation. Sometimes the disturbance of sensibility to heat and cold is less severe; temperatures above 38–40 °C are recognized as warm and those below about 26–28 °C as cold. Under such conditions any temperature that can be appreciated is thought to be respectively 'hotter' or 'colder' on the affected side, and yet there is no evidence that the supposed greater heat or cold is due to anything but the increased affective reaction. Throughout all these cases, where the loss of thermal sensibility was not absolute, a threshold could always be determined. It might be the same on the two sides, or it might be more or less raised on that half of the body which showed an excessive response. But never did we find that remarkable loss of threshold and inability to discriminate between two temperatures, both of which were recognized to be hot or to be cold, so characteristic a feature with cortical lesions."

In other words, heat and cold are not dissociated: if one form of sensation is lost, the other will be gravely disturbed.

The loss of thermal sensibility generally affected intermediate temperatures, yielding a sensation of pleasant warmth. However, in several patients able to appreciate mild heat (34 °C), the application of water at 38 °C on the affected part evoked a higher degree of pleasure than the same application over the unaffected part. In one case, excessive pleasure could be converted into excessive discomfort as soon as water temperature exceeded 46 °C. In a few patients, when thermal sensibility was abolished, warmth applied over a sufficiently large surface evoked a feeling of pleasure, even if the patient did not recognize it was warm, and extreme hot or cold evoked great discomfort.

Head and Holmes analyzed the effects of visceral stimulation in patients suffering from thalamic syndrome by comparing the effect elicited by squeezing testicles (without pinching the scrotum). They noted that in many patients the discomfort was more intense and the cremasteric movements were more brisk after squeezing the testicle of the affected side. They also noted that even when pinprick pain threshold on the glans penis was the same on both sides, the discomfort described by the patients was greater after pricking of the affected half.

Patients complaining of thalamic pain could complain of unpleasant sensations after scraping the palm or the sole of the foot, or moving a rough object over the skin or even rubbing the hairs over the affected part of the body. Sometimes, these sensations were not painful, but very unpleasant, and frequently they spread from the stimulated area to the entire limb or half of the body. Examination with a *Graham–Brown esthesiometer* (to estimate the appreciation of roughness) frequently induced this anomalous response. Nevertheless, the threshold of appreciation of roughness was never lowered. It was always unchanged or increased, but in the large majority of the patients the esthesiometer induced greater discomfort on the affected side. Occasionally even the vibration of the tuning fork was able to give rise to similar spreading sensations. In patients characterized by an over-response to painful stimuli tickling was also unpleasant and induced greater reaction.

The vibrations of a tuning fork were generally appreciated on both halves of the body, but in almost every case for a shorter time on the affected side. In many cases, the patient complained that vibrations were "not so plain" or that the tuning fork vibrated less rapidly on the affected side. Only in a few cases (in whom most other sensations were gravely affected) was the affected half of the body insensitive to this stimulus. They noted that a shortened appreciation of the vibration of a tuning fork was associated with the over-response to painful stimuli, independently of the unpleasant feeling-tone evoked by vibration.

Response to pleasurable stimuli (p. 133):

"We were anxious to discover if sensations, normally accompanied by a pleasurable feeling-tone, also produced a similar over-reaction. Unfortunately, the greater number of methods . . . either produce discomfort or . . . an entirely indifferent sensation. But in the milder degrees of heat we possess a **measurable stimulus** [!!] endowed with a pleasant feeling-tone . . . In a few cases when thermal sensibility was abolished, warmth applied over a sufficient large surface evoked a feeling of pleasure . . . One of our patients found a hot-water bottle pleasant and soothing to the affected foot, but did not recognize that it was warm until he touched it with some normal part . . . Many patients found the warm hand of the observer unusually pleasant on the abnormal side, although no such manifestations of pleasure were produced when it was applied to the normal part of the body. In one case . . . the patient could not recognize any thermal stimulus as such, and yet over the affected half of the chest . . . water at from 38 °C to 48 °C evoked intense pleasure. Temperature of 50 °C and above, or of 18 °C and below, caused great discomfort . . . [three cases are described and "several patients" referred to]. So far we have been unable to find any temperature which produces a sensation of pleasurable cold."

Behavior of the affected half of the body in states of emotion (p. 135):

"A highly educated patient confessed that he had become more amorous since the attack, which had rendered the right half of his body more responsive to pleasant and unpleasant stimuli. 'I crave to place my right hand on the soft skin of a woman. It's my right hand that wants the consolation. I seem to crave for sympathy on my right side.' Finally he added, 'My right hand seems to be more artistic.' "

Table 4.2. Synopsis of the findings of Head and Holmes (1911)

24 CP patients.
As far as the loss of superficial and "deep" sensibility is concerned, "in some patients with thalamic syndrome this loss is so insignificant that it can be discovered **by measurement only**, so we can imagine the existence of the over-reaction without it." Even if **all patients with over-reaction had a more or less recognizable sensory loss**, the excessive response bears **no relation** to the extent of the accompanying loss of sensation.
Tactile threshold (von Frey hairs):
• **identical** on both sides: 5/24 patients (20.8%)
• **raised** or **lost** or **undetermined** on the affected side: 19/24 patients (79.2%) [a]
Tactile sensibility was frequently diminished and in some cases totally lost, but generally a threshold could be obtained, especially by increasing the strength of the stimulus. In a few cases only the affected parts were totally insensitive to the tactile hairs and also to pressure-esthesiometer
Threshold for pinprick pain:
• **identical** on both sides: 13/22 patients (59.1%)
• **raised** on the affected side (a stronger stimulus was needed to produce a sensation of prick): 9/22 patients (40.9%)
• **lower** on the affected side: 0/22 patients (0%)
Over-response to prick: 20/22 patients (90.9%)
Threshold for thermal stimuli and range of discrimination:
• **raised** on the affected side: 15/24 patients (62.5%)
• **normal** and **identical** on both sides: 9/24 patients (37.5%)
• **lower** on the affected side: 0/24 patients (0%)
Sensibility to heat and cold could show all degrees of change from total loss to a slight increase of the neutral zone. Thermal appreciation could be unaltered, even though, in the majority of cases, it was diminished or lost. The loss of thermal sensibility generally affected intermediate temperatures.
Patients with normal threshold could show an over-response to pleasurable heat. In patients with abolished appreciation of heat and cold, ice and water over 50 °C evoked only discomfort on the affected side. In patients suffering from thalamic lesions, the ability to appreciate either heat or cold could not be lost singly. In other words, **heat and cold are not dissociated**; if one form of sensation is lost, the other will be gravely disturbed.
Threshold for heat-induced over-reaction:
c. 40–45 °C in most patients (55–60 °C in some cases)
Threshold for cold-induced over-reaction:
• generally below 15 °C
The evoked sensation was the same whichever of the two extremes was used, and the patient could not recognize the cause of the unpleasant sensation.
Threshold for pressure pain:
• **lower** on the affected side: 15/24 patients (62.5%)
• **identical** on both sides: 6/24 patients (25%)
• **raised** on the affected side: 3/24 patients (12.5%)
Visceral stimulation (comparison of the effects elicited by squeezing testicles without pinching the scrotum):

Table 4.2. (cont.)

In many patients the discomfort was more intense and the cremasteric movements were more brisk after squeezing the testicle of the affected side. Even when pinprick pain threshold on the glans penis was the same on both sides, the discomfort described by the patients was greater after pricking of the affected half.
Vibrations of a tuning fork (128 Hz):
Generally appreciated on both halves of the body, but in almost every case for a shorter time on the affected side; vibrations "not so plain" or tuning fork vibrating less rapidly on the affected side. Only in a few cases (in whom most other sensations were gravely affected) was the affected half of the body insensitive to this stimulus. A shortened appreciation of the vibration of a tuning fork was associated with over-response to painful stimuli, independently of the unpleasant feeling-tone evoked by vibration.

[a] In some patients the consecutive contacts (especially with increasing strength) caused widespread tingling that made conclusive demonstration of the threshold impossible. Determination of tactile threshold was also prevented by the occurrence of involuntary (induced) movements, with accessory sensations misinterpreted as stimulation.

Table 4.3. Somatosensory findings in brain central pain (BCP) (sample series)

Greenspan *et al.* (2004)

Quantitative sensory testing (QST) in 13 consecutive patients (10 men, 3 women) with CPSP. MRI-confirmed CNS lesions

Clinical characteristics

Pain location	**Hemibody**	**Hemibody, sparing head**	**Upper extremity**	**Lower extremity**	**Patchy**
No. of patients	2	3	4	1	3
Visual analog scale	≤ 5	6–7	8–9	10	Mean
No. of patients	3	3	5	2	7.1 (2.0 SD)

No statistically significant difference for pain and detection thresholds among patients grouped by age, sex, side.

Psychophysical tests: thresholds assessed

- innocuous warm and cold (contact Peltier stimulator, 7 cm^2 or 9 cm^2)
- heat pain and cold pain (contact Peltier stimulator, 7 cm^2 or 9 cm^2, baseline temperature 35°C (heat) or 30°C (cold). Limits: 0–50°C)
- tactile (Semmes–Wienstein monofilaments, dorsum of the hand or of the feet)
- brushing allodynia (manual test, stiff brush)

Evaluation of thermal sensitivity: criterion of abnormal thresholds = mean ± 2 SD outside normative range. Thresholds as median values. Evaluation of laterality differences: normative data. In interpreting results of quantitative thermal sensory testing the side-to-side differences were considered more reliable, and a side-to-side difference > 95% CI in the direction of decreased sensitivity on the affected side was interpreted as hypoesthesia. If the side-to-side differences were not significant, then the results were evaluated in terms of the absolute threshold. Statistical assessment of the results both within populations and individual patients.

Sensory characteristics	**No. of patients**	**Reduced**	**Normal**	**Hypoalgesia, hypoesthesia**	**Allodynia**	**Indeterminate**[a]	**Present**	**Absent**
Cold threshold	13	11 (85%) [b]	2 (15%)					

Table 4.3. (cont.)

Sensory characteristics	No. of patients	Reduced	Normal	Hypoalgesia, hypoesthesia	Allodynia	Indeterminate[a]	Present	Absent
Cold pain threshold	13		2 (15%)	6 (46%)	3 (24%)[c]	2 (15%)		
Warm threshold	13	12 (92%)[d]	1 (8%)					
Hot pain threshold	13		10 (77%)	1 (8%)	(2 borderline)	2 (15%)		
Non-painful tactile threshold	10[e]		5 (50%)	5 (50%)		3 (not tested)		
Tactile allodynia (brushing)	13						7 (54%)	6 (46%)[f]

[a] Side-to-side differences not significant, and affected or unaffected threshold indeterminate at the greatest stimulus magnitude. Impossible to determine if the affected side was normal, hypo-, or hyperalgesic.
[b] Bilateral cold hypoesthesia with no laterality difference in 3 patients. Ipsilateral cold hypoesthesia (<< contralateral) in 3 other patients, with significant laterality difference.
[c] The most dramatic example of cold allodynia occurred in 1 of the 2 patients with normal cold detection threshold. The other 2 cases occurred in 2 patients with bilateral cold hypoesthesia with unilateral stokes contralateral to their allodynia and ongoing pain and the highest cold thresholds among patients with cold hyopesthesia.
[d] Bilateral warm hypoesthesia with no laterality difference in 2 patients (also with cold hypoesthesia). Ipsilateral warm hypoesthesia (<< contralateral) in 6 other patients, with significant laterality difference.
[e] Ongoing pain rating not different between patients with normal tactile threshold and hypoesthesia.
[f] Brushes non-painful, monofilaments irritating in 1 patient. No difference by side or age. Higher incidence in men (not significant) and in patients with normal tactile thresholds vs. tactile hypoesthesia (5/5 vs. 1/5, $p < 0.05$).

Tactile allodynia occurred more in cases with spared tactile pathways. Thermal, mechanical, and paresthetic descriptors of ongoing pain and pain rating did not differ between patients with normal and reduced tactile sensibility. The presence of tactile hypoesthesia did not correlate with the degree or quality of ongoing pain. All patients with insular lesions had tactile allodynia, but the incidence was not different from that occurring in other lesions.

Cold allodynia occurred in 2/11 patients (or 0/8 patients). Cold allodynia is significantly related to the *absence* of cold hypoesthesia; cold hypoesthesia is neither necessary nor sufficient for cold allodynia. Despite the large prevalence of cold hypoesthesia in CP patients, cold allodynia is relatively an infrequent event. After statistical analysis it is also concluded that patients with cold hypoesthesia may have burning or hot or cold ongoing pain, but not necessarily. Two patients with insular lesions (50%) had cold allodynia, but the incidence was not different from that occurring in other lesions. The insular lesions, however, did not extend fully to the suggested cortical termination of VMpo (dorsal margin of the insula or adjacent parietal operculum).

Warm and heat pain: QST revealed predominantly warm hypoesthesia and normal heat pain sensibility. Two patients showed borderline allodynia. Data do not fit the disinhibition hypothesis.

Tactile hypoesthesia: 50% of patients. Normal: 50% of patients. Tactile allodynia: to brushing: 54% of patients; to von Frey hairs: 8% of patients. Men showed a trend towards a higher incidence of brush allodynia. Tactile allodynia occurred significantly more often in cases with spared tactile pathways than those with normal tactile thresholds. Severity of pain was the same in both tactile normal and deficient groups.

The presence of tactile hypoesthesia did not correlate with the degree or quality of ongoing pain.

Cold hypoesthesia: in 85%of CPSP patients, some bilateral (either similar on both sides or with side prevalence).

Bowsher (2005a)

Review of 122 CPSP patients (seen between 1980 and 1990). MRI in 94 patients, CT scanning only in 2. QST in 112 patients (previously reported findings). Study on the proportion of CP patients showing allodynia. First report (according to the author) of "movement allodynia" (elicited by isotonic or isometric muscle contraction, occurring in a substantial number of CPSP patients). Report of a case of startle allodynia.

Table 4.3. (cont.)

Presence and type of allodynia (122 patients)[a]	
No allodynia	35/122 patients (29%)
Mechanical	50/122 patients (41%) pure: 34 patients (28%) + thermal (some form, usually cold): 9 patients + movement: 7 patients
Movement[b]	Alone: 10/122 patients (8%) Pure (pain *only* on movement): 6 instances Moderate background pain severely exacerbated by movement: 5 instances
Cold	Pure: 10/122 patients (8%)[c] + some other form of allodynia (usually mechanical): 11 patients [c]
Mechanical and acoustic startle	1 patient (pontine infarct)

[a] Percentages calculated by the author on 122 patients even though "the absence, or presence and type, of allodynia were tested and recorded in **108** patients."
[b] "Elicited by isotonic or isometric muscle contraction", "previously undescribed" but in 3 patients "pain *only* occurred when they moved the affected part (actively or **passively**)."
[c] "*Some sort* of thermal allodynia in 21 patients (17%)"; "intense burning sensation by a cold object in many patients."

Comparison of QST results (33 patients without allodynia, 31 with allodynia): greater affected/unaffected cold threshold difference in patients with cold + mechanical vs. pure cold allodynia (the difference "*almost reaches significance* ($p = 0.06$) [sic]"; **kind of statistical test not reported**), "*Very similar*" affected/unaffected differences for other modalities.

Lesion site and allodynia

	Infratentorial (brainstem) infarcts with crossed symptoms	Subtentorial lesions (crossed symptoms: 11 patients; contralateral symptoms: 7 patients)	Supratentorial (thalamic) lesions
Allodynia	9 patients	10/18 patients	Number of patients not reported
• pure mechanical	5 patients	3/11 + 2/7 patients (tactile) = 4/18	Number of patients not reported[a]
• mechanical + cold	2 patients (1 SAH)	1/11 (tactile and cold) = 1/18	Number of patients not reported
• pure cold	1 patients	2/11 patients = 2/18	Number of patients not reported[b]
• movement	1 patients	2/7 patients = 2/18	Number of patients not reported
• startle		1/7 patients = 1/18	Number of patients not reported
No allodynia	5 patients	5/11 + 2/7 = 7/18	5/5 patients (posterolateroventral tip of VPL) 9/24 patients VPL lesions

Table 4.3. (cont.)

Total	14 patients[c]	17 patients[c]

[a] Further rostral and dorsal lesions rather than lesion causing pure movement allodynia
[b] Tendency toward lesions in the dorsal part of the somatosensory relay nucleus (but very small number of good MRI scans)
[c] **Unexplained differences**. No radioanatomical differences between patients with or without allodynia.

Author's conclusion: these patients make up a not-inconsiderable proportion of CPSP patients (39.5% of CPSP patients with allodynia; 29% of all our CPSP patients).

Bowsher (2006a; includes **Bowsher *et al.* 2004)**

3 CPSP patients out of 5 with small restricted cerebral cortical infarcts, in all cases sparing SI (postcentral gyrus) (MRI). QST performed in all cases.

Findings (affected areas)	Patients with CPSP ($n = 3$)	Patients without CPSP ($n = 2$)
Spontaneous pain	Mild	Absent
Tactile thresholds	Unaltered	Unaltered
Sharpness (pinprick) perception	Absent	Unimpaired
Thermal perception (warmth, cold, and heat pain)	Impaired	Unimpaired or less impaired
Thresholds for mechanical pain (skinfold pinch)	Raised (2 patients)	Less raised
Sharpness, mechanical pain, innocuous temperature, noxious heat sensations	Greater deficit	Lesser deficit
Opercular-insular lesion (vs. subcortical lesion)		
Mechanosensory thresholds (von Frey, vibration, sharpness)	Notably lower	
Mechanical pain thresholds	Higher	
Thermal (all) thresholds	More elevated	
Warm/cold difference	Greater (in all subjects)	

Unexplained data disagreement (only for CPSP patients) in maximal affected/unaffected differences between 2006 and 2004 papers for touch (patients 1, 2), sharpness (patient 2), skinfold pinch (patient 2), warmth (patient 2), coolness (patient 2), warm/cold difference (patient 1), heat pain (patients 1, 2), cold pain (patient 2). Patients numbered as in the 2004 paper. No difference for pain free-patients.

No correlation between the presence or absence of CP with respect to damage to the spinothalamocortical pathway.

Author's conclusion: in the case of similar cortical lesions, either the presence or absence of spontaneous pain modifies the thresholds for some innocuous modalities, or the degree of deficit of some innocuous modalities determines whether or not central pain occurs.

Ofek and Defrin (2007)

Systematic study of 15 patients (2 women) with CP after CT/MRI-confirmed traumatic brain injury (Traumatic Brain Injury Patients, mean age 28 ± 10 years) compared with 16 traumatic brain injury patients without CP (Traumatic Brain Injury Patients, 24 ± 6 years) and 15 matched healthy controls. Other pain mechanisms (local injury, peripheral neuropathy, spinal injury) in TBIP patients excluded. Minimum duration of pain: 5 months after injury. Type and cause of injury in TBIP: blunt injury in 13, penetrating injury in 2; motor vehicle accident in 11, gunshot in 2, fall in 2. Mean duration of post-traumatic unconsciousness: 15 d. Hemiparesis in 11 patients, 8 independent walkers. No significant differences between groups in sex distribution, age, duration and severity of TBI, mechanism of injury, motor/mobility status.

Table 4.3. (cont.)

Evaluation tools: QST in the painful and pain-free body regions: warmth (WS) and cold (CS) sensation threshold, heat-pain threshold (HP), light touch threshold, graphesthesia, static allodynia, dynamic allodynia, mechanical wind-up pain, heat hyperpathia measured in hands and legs. Thermal stimulation: Peltier-based computerized thermal stimulator. Mechanical stimulation: Semmes–Weinstein monofilaments.

Pain intensity evaluation: Visual analog scale (VAS). Evaluation of the patient's pain experience: MPQ (+ derived measures: PRI, NWC, pain intensity)

Brain regions with MRI/CT visible traumatic lesion: **Parietal cortex** 8 (53%, statistically significant difference vs. TBINP, $p = 0.04$), frontal cortex 8 (53%), ventricle hemorrhage/enlargement 7 (46%), traumatic axonal injury 7 (46%), subarachnoid hemorrhage 6 (40%), temporal cortex 6 (40%), **corpus callosum** 3 (27%, statistically significant difference vs. TBINP, $p = 0.05$), brainstem 2 (13%), subdural hematoma 2 (13%), basal ganglia 2 (13%), cerebellum 1 (7%), occipital lobe 1 (7%).

Time between injury and pain onset: mean onset: 6.6 ± 9 months (range 0.5–30 months; pain onset within 1 month in 40% of patients, between 2 and 12 months in 50%, after 1 year in 10%).

Mean duration of pain: 16 months (range 6–66 months).

Location of pain: restricted to R body side in 10 patients, to L body side in 5 (additional central lower back pain in 1 case), present in the body side with a more severe motor and sensory deficit, dispersed across several body regions (mean of 5 body regions per patient). Most frequently reported painful areas: knee (93%), shoulder (80%), foot (73%), hand (53%), thigh (46%), lower back (46%), upper back (40%), head and face (40%), arm (33%). Pain on the entire body side in 2 patients. **Pain contralateral to the brain injury side in the 2 patients with penetrating injuries**.

Pain intensity: mean VAS score was 2.8 ± 2 (day test), worst pain: 5. NWC: 6.5 ± 3, PRI: 17.5 ± 8.

Pain descriptors: "it doesn't let the brain work"; exhausting, excruciating, irritating, "like real torture," "like non-stop exertion," pounding/throbbing, pressing, burning, cutting, "muscular effort-like," pricking, cool, cold, freezing, troublesome, numb, wretched, pressing, hot, burning (different qualities reported within different painful areas).

Aggravating factors: physical effort (active movement), cold weather, fatigue, touch, tension, immobilization, electrical nerve stimulation.

Alleviating factors: relaxation or rest, heating or warm weather, massage. Medications helpful in 4 patients.

QST results (statistically significant results)

	TBINP vs. control			**TBIP vs. control**		
Thermal thresholds [a]	**Higher thresholds**		**Notes**	**Higher thresholds**		**Notes**
	Hands	Legs	No side differences (similar thermal thresholds)	Hands	Legs	Abnormal thermal thresholds in the painful areas in 100% of cases
WS	$p < 0.001$	$p < 0.01$	Abnormal thermal thresholds in 44% of cases	$p < 0.001$	$p < 0.001$	Significantly higher in painful areas (hand: $p < 0.0001$, leg: $p < 0.0001$)
CS	$p < 0.01$	$p < 0.01$		$p < 0.001$	$p < 0.001$	Significantly higher in painful areas (hand: $p < 0.0001$, leg: $p < 0.001$)
HP	$p < 0.01$	$p < 0.01$		$p < 0.001$	$p < 0.001$	Significantly higher in painful areas

Table 4.3. (cont.)

	TBINP vs. control			TBIP vs. control		
Thermal thresholds [a]	**Higher thresholds**		**Notes**	**Higher thresholds**		**Notes**
						(hand: $p < 0.01$, leg: $p < 0.05$)
Touch thresholds [b]	Higher thresholds			Higher thresholds		
	$p < 0.05$	$p < 0.01$	Similar touch thresholds in both hands. Higher threshold in one leg vs. the other leg ($p < 0.05$)	$p < 0.05$ Similar touch thresholds in both hands	$p < 0.05$ Higher threshold in one leg vs. the other leg ($p < 0.05$)	No significant differences between the groups
Graphesthesia [b]	Slightly lower scores (difference not statistically significant)			Slightly lower scores (difference not statistically significant)		
	Similar scores in the two hands. No significant differences between the groups	More affected in one leg than the other ($p < 0.05$)		Similar scores in the two hands	More affected in one leg than the other ($p < 0.05$)	No significant differences between the groups

[a] Thresholds of WS, CS, and HP in the painful areas of TBIP also significantly higher than those measured in pain-free areas of TBINP; differences in WS, CS, and HP thresholds between the two body sides of TBIP also significantly larger than in TBINP.
[b] Touch and graphesthesia similarly affected in TBINP and TBIP

Incidence (%) of abnormal sensations

	TBIP		TBINP	
	Painful side	Pain-free side	One side	Other side
Hyperpathia	100*	27	44	25
Static allodynia	60*	0	6	0
Dynamic allodynia	47*	0	6	0
Wind-up pain	93*	33	25	25
Pathological sensations present	None: 0 Only one type: 0 Two types: 2 (13%) Three types: 6 (40%)		None: 8 (50%) Only one type: 5 (31%) Two types: 2 (13%) Three types: 1 (6%)	

Table 4.3. (cont.)

	TBIP	TBINP
	All: 7 (47%)	All: 0

* Statistically significant difference (comparisons between body sides and between groups)

Allodynia in all the TBIP and none of the TBINP ($p < 0.001$). Painful stimuli: cold temperature (water, air), crude touch, physical effort, movement. Dysesthesias in 27% of TBIP (streams of cold and electric-like sensations). Paresthesias in 53% of TBIP and 6% of TBINP ($p < 0.01$).

Authors' conclusions: damage to the pain and temperature system is essential for the development of pain in TBI patients (as demonstrated by the significant reduction of pain and temperature sensations but not necessarily of touch and graphesthesia in all painful regions). Unique clinical features: quality of pain (pricking and pounding/throbbing, rarely burning pain), movement allodynia in 100% of the patients, no differences between CP from blunt or penetrating injury in spite of the differences in the brain damage.

Maier *et al*. (2010)

DFNS (German Research Network on Neuropathic Pain) study aimed at exploring by means of QST the spectrum of sensory abnormalities in 1236 neuropathic pain (NP) patients. All diagnoses made and documented by a local center.

Central pain (= pain caused by a demonstrable lesion in the CNS in an area anatomically attributable to the lesion) **patients**: **51 (4.1%)**, 17 women, mean age 55 ± 13 years (19 patients < 50 years, 7 patients > 69 years), pain duration: ≤ 1 year in 11 patients (22%), > 1 year in 40 patients (78%); average pain intensity (NRS): 6.2 ± 2.6

QST standardized assessment within the affected and the contralateral control mirror body area: cold and warm detection threshold (CDT, WDT), paradoxical heat sensations (PHS) during thermal sensory limen (TSL) procedure, cold and heat pain thresholds (CPT, HPT), mechanical detection thresholds (touch [MDT] and vibration [VDT]), mechanical pain threshold (pinprick [MPT], blunt pressure [PPT]), mechanical pain sensitivity (MPS), dynamic mechanical allodynia (DMA), pain summation to repetitive pinprick stimuli (WUR: wind-up ratio) (i.e., 13 different thermal and mechanical tests). Assessment of negative (loss of function) and positive (gain of function) phenomena.

CP patients: high rate of PHS (26.0%); more frequent thermal sensory loss (CDT 49.1%, WDT 62.7%); frequent heat pain hypoalgesia alone (9.8%, not statistically significant) and pinprick hypoalgesia (MPT or MPS). QST parameters within the 95% CI and without relative abnormality: 10% of cases. At least one increased thermal or mechanical detection threshold (without thermal or mechanical hyperalgesia): about 40% of cases.

At least one decreased thermal or mechanical pain threshold, increased mechanical pain sensitivity, decreased pressure pain threshold or DMA (without thermal or tactile hypoesthesia): about 12% of cases. At least one positive sign combined with at least one negative sign: about 38% of cases (*from Fig. 2*). Leading combination of sensory signs: mixed loss without any hyperalgesia (27.5%). Second most frequent combination: mixed loss combined with only mechanical hyperalgesia (25.5%).

Frequency of different combinations of abnormal values (number of patients and %)

	No hyperalgesia	Only thermal hyperalgesia	Only mechanical hyperalgesia	Both thermal and mechanical hyperalgesia	Total
No loss of detection	5 (9.8%)	0	3 (5.9%)	2 (3.9%)	10 (19.6%)
Only thermal loss	3 (5.9%)	0	2 (3.9%)	1 (2%)	6 (11.8%)
Only mechanical loss	4 (7.8%)	0	0	1 (2%)	5 (9.8%)

Table 4.3. (cont.)

	No hyperalgesia	Only thermal hyperalgesia	Only mechanical hyperalgesia	Both thermal and mechanical hyperalgesia	Total
Mixed loss of detection	14 (27.5%)	2 (3.9%)	13 (25.5%)	1 (2%)	30 (58.8%)
Total	26 (51%)	2 (3.9%)	18 (35.3%)	5 (9.8%)	51

Frequency of abnormal values (number of patients and %)

	Gain: positive phenomena (gain of function)	Loss: negative phenomena (loss of function)
CDT	1 (2%)	25 (49%)
WDT	2 (3.9%)	**28 (54.8%)****
TSL	2 (3.9%)	**32 (62.7%)****
CPT	**3 (5.9%)***	5 (9.8%)
HPT	**5 (9.8%)***	9 (17.7%)
PPT	**8 (16%)***	7 (14%)
MPT	11 (21.6%)	12 (23.5%)
MPS	12 (23.5%)	**15 (29.4%)****
WUR	7 (16.3%)	–
MDT	–	25 (49%)
VDT	–	22 (43.1%)
PHS	13 (26%)	–
DMA	9 (17.7%)	–

* Significantly lower frequency within a QST parameter across etiologies.
** Sgnificantly higher frequency by two-sided configuration frequency analysis, without Bonferroni adjustment.

Spinothalamic function loss supported by the high incidence of negative signs for CDT, WDT, and MPT (but negative signs for MDT and VDT were frequent too).

Authors' conclusion: somatosensory profiles with different combinations of loss and gain are shared across the major neuropathic pain syndromes (*summary*). The analysis of QST parameters revealed a remarkable phenotypic heterogeneity across the major neuropathic pain syndromes, and thus confirmed two major predictions of the concept of mechanism-based classification of neuropathic pain (*text*).

Table 4.4. Somatosensory findings in cord central pain (CCP) (sample series)

Defrin *et al*. (1999)

Aim: to study the perception of acute pain over the hands and upper back (areas considered unaffected as cord injuries were restricted to T4–L3 segments) in 53 traumatic spinal cord injury (SCI) paraplegic patients suffering from chronic below-level pain (CP) vs. 18 healthy controls.

Type of SCI (patient groups)	Number of patients (mean age, years)	Average pain duration (years)	Results
Complete with pain (CSCIP)	21 (39.5 ± 9.7)	14.9 (range 2–35)	Warm or cold thresholds: no difference between any of the groups. Heat pain thresholds: significantly elevated only in CSCIP patients (stimulated area = 15.36 cm^2) or increased in all groups (stimulated area = 6.25 and 2.25 cm^2). Pain thresholds: higher in CSCIP patients than in all other groups. MPQ (CSCIP vs. ISCIP patients): higher PRI and larger NWC (only for the sensory dimension) in CSCIP patients. Area of chronic pain: 14.78% in CSCIP patients vs. 8.06% in ISCIP patients ($P<0.05$). Elevated heat pain thresholds, increased PRI(R) and NWC value in CSCIP patients with pain areas larger than the group average vs. CSCIP patients with smaller areas: (no such differences in ISCIP patients). Higher pain thresholds in CSCIP patients with pain rating above the group average than in normal controls. Heat-pain thresholds markedly reduced after DREZ lesion in 2 patients with diffuse constant burning below-level pain (+ paroxysmal electric-shock like pain in 1 patient) Average time between spinal injury and sensory measurements: 16.6 years (range 2–38 years).
Complete without pain (CSCINP)	10 (37.2 ± 10.8)		
Incomplete with pain (ISCIP)	15 (38.9 ± 9.2)	13.25 (range 2–36)	
Incomplete without pain (ISCINP)	7 (37.6 ± 9.1)		
Healthy controls	18 (35.6 ± 7.4)		

Authors' conclusion: only CSCIP patients show an elevation in pain threshold above the level of injury along with unchanged thresholds for warm and cold perception and a reduction in the perception of suprathreshold noxious stimuli (hypoalgesic state completely attributable to the change in pain threshold). Pain perception returns to normal values after pain relief. Pain intensity is significantly higher (elevation restricted to the sensory aspect of pain sensation) and the body area to which pain is projected is larger in CSCIP patients than in ISCIP patients

Ducreux *et al*. (2006): syringomyelia

46 patients with MRI-confirmed spinal syringomyelia

CP (= pain in an area of sensory deficit directly related to the SCI, not attributable to other condition, with specific characteristic descriptors): 31 patients (a subgroup with cold and/or tactile allodynia). No CP: 15 patients (+ 6 healthy volunteers, complementary fMRI study). Pain symptoms: spontaneous ongoing pain frequently associated with pain paroxysms (electric shocks, stabbing) and with allodynia in 20 patients.

Assessment tools: symptom intensity: NPSI; tactile allodynia (dynamic, paintbrush): VAS. Comparison of clinical and psychophysical criteria with NPSI/VAS.

CP patients ($n = 31$): demographic and clinical findings	
Sex distribution (F/M)	16/15
Mean age	50 ± 14 years
Mean dermatomal extension of deficits [a]	Warm: 13.1 ± 11.2; cold: 17.8 ± 13.2; pinprick: 16.4 ± 12.2
Mean dermatomal extension of pain [b]	5.8 ± 2.7
Spontaneous ongoing pain	11 patients (without evoked pain)
Allodynia (brush, pressure, cold,heat) and/or hyperalgesia [c]	20 patients (64%) (brush: 12 patients; cold: 11 patients; pressure: 7 patients; heat: 5 patients)
Pain location	Upper limb: 27 patients (+ neck: 7 patients); thorax: 5 patients; thorax and lower limb: 4 patients
Mean pain duration [a]	10.4 ± 8.3 years
Mean pain intensity (VAS, mm) [a]	56 ± 76
Pain quality (NPSI) [a,d]	Paresthesia/dysesthesia: 24 patients (77%); burning: 23 patients (74%); paroxysmal: 19 patients (63%); deep: 14 patients (45%)

[a] No relationship between pain intensity, duration, quality, and magnitude or extent of thermal deficits. No significant difference in thermal and mechanical deficits, graphesthesia, detection of movement direction impairment between maximal spontaneous pain area and adjacent lesioned but painless area.
[b] Painful area always located within the area of maximal thermal deficit, but more restricted.
[c] Allodynia to cold, pressure, or heat always associated with hyperalgesia to these stimuli.
[d] Deep pain: pressure/squeezing; paroxysmal pain: electric shocks, stabbing; paresthesia/dysesthesia: tingling, pins and needles.

Comparison of patients with or without pain: no statistically significant difference for age, sex distribution, duration of symptoms, etiology, extent of sensory deficits, thermal and mechanical detection thresholds (including vibration), impairment of graphesthesia and movement direction.

Comparison of patients with or without evoked pain and pain-free patients

	Patients without evoked pain (allodynia/hyperalgesia) ($n = 11$)	Patients with evoked pain ($n = 20$) [a]	Pain-free patients ($n = 15$)
Warm and cold detection thresholds (area of maximal deficit) [b]	Warm ≈ 48 °C Cold ≈ 12 °C (*Fig. 2*)	Warm ≈ 42.5 °C Cold ≈ 18 °C (*Fig. 2*) (less altered, $p < 0.01$)	Warm 46.5 ± 5 °C Cold 13.7 ± 6.5 °C
Extent of thermal deficit [b]	13.0 ± 5.4 dermatomes ($p < 0.05$)	6.2 ± 6 dermatomes (significantly lower)	14.7 ± 6.8 dermatomes ($p < 0.01$)
Unilateral or asymmetrical thermal deficit	82% of patients [c]	55% of patients ($p < 0.01$)	27% of patients

Table 4.4. (cont.)

	Patients without evoked pain (allodynia/hyperalgesia) ($n = 11$)	Patients with evoked pain ($n = 20$) [a]	Pain-free patients ($n = 15$)
Correlation between burning pain intensity (NPSI) and extent of thermal deficits	Warm: $\rho = 0.63$, $p < 0.01$ Cold: $\rho = 0.59$, $p < 0.01$	NS	NS
Thermal deficit (patients with cold allodynia vs. brush-evoked allodynia)		Less severe	
Warm and cold detection threshold (in the area of maximal deficit, patients with cold allodynia vs. patients with tactile allodynia)		Warm. 36.0 ± 3.7 vs. 43.4 ± 5 °C ($p < 0.01$) Cold: 25.0 ± 5.7 vs. 18.6 ± 8.2 °C ($p < 0.01$)	

[a] Less severe deficit in comparison with patients without allodynia or pain-free patients.
[b] Both magnitude and extent of thermal deficits less severe in patients with allodynia.
[c] Larger metameric extension of warm or cold deficits (and maximal thermal impairment) on the painful side.

Comparison of healthy people and patients			
Stimulus	**Healthy people ($n = 6$)**	**Patients with allodynia ($n = 6$)**	**Pain-free patients ($n = 6$)**
Cold		Cold allodynia	
22 °C	Moderate cold (never painful)	Painful in all patients (VAS 59 ± 24 mm) [a]	Not perceived
4 °C	Painful (VAS 56 ± 18 mm)	As above	Very weak/absent (never painful)
		Brush-induced allodynia ($n = 6$)	
Brush stimulation (hand)	Not applicable	Painful in all cases (mean VAS: 61 ± 21 mm) [b]	Not applicable

[a] Similar to that evoked by the 4 °C stimulus in healthy people. Pain described as deep and freezing, and sometimes burning/tingling.
[b] Pain described as burning (4 patients) and as electric shocks (2 patients).

Authors' conclusions: no significant difference in the magnitude or extent of sensory deficits between patients with and without NP (lesions of the spinothalamic pathways are not sufficient for developing CP). Patients with and without allodynia show different pattern of sensory deficits (mechanisms of CP are not univocal). Different sensory deficits in patients with cold and tactile allodynia suggest different pathophysiological mechanisms (in fMRI study: distinct patterns of brain activity associated with different subtypes of allodynia. Prefrontal cortex only area consistently activated by evoked pains. Alteration of high-level pain mechanisms might play a major role in allodynia due to central lesion.

Finnerup *et al*. (2007a)

21 SCI patients, 10 below-level pain (ongoing primary neuropathic pain (NP) at least two spinal segments below the lesion but allowed to extend rostrally, pain group), 11 without at-level or below-level NP/dysesthesia (pain-free group).
Pain duration ≥ 6 months, intensity ≥ 3 (on NRS: 0–10).
Assessment tools: MPQ, NPSI, pain localizationon (body chart), NRS, clinical examination, QST.

Clinical characteristics (no statistically significant differences between the two groups)

	Pain group ($n = 10$)	**Pain-free group ($n = 11$)**
Sex (F/M)	5/5	2/9
Age, years, mean (SD)	53.0 (14.2)	45.1 (14.5)
Mechanism of injury (non-traumatic: transverse myelitis, abscess, tumor, hemangioma, disk herniation)	Traumatic: 4 patients Non-traumatic : 6 patients	Traumatic: 5 patients Non-traumatic: 6 patients
Pain location	Below-level: 10 patients (extending to the at-level area: 2 patients) At-level (+ evoked pain/dysesthesia): 4 patients (at-level distinct from below-level pain)	
Allodynia (below-level, history)	8 patients (evoked pain/dysesthesia: 10 patients)	0
• Light touch allodynia • Cold allodynia • Warm allodynia	7 patients (dysesthesia: 3 patients) 6 patients 1 patient	Intermittent paresthesia (tingling or tight sensations): 6 patients
Median pain intensity (spontaneous below-level pain), NRS	6.5 (range 3–10)	
Quality of neuropathic pain (NPSI)	Burning: 9 patients Pressure/squeezing: 8 patients Paroxysmal: 5 patients Tingling/pins and needles: 9 patients	
Most common descriptors (MPQ)	Burning, pricking, squeezing, shooting, freezing + grueling, exhausting, annoying	

Table 4.4. (cont.)

Clinical examination/QST: pain evoked by a cold/warm thermo roll below-injury level: pain group, 4 patients (cold), 0 patients (warm); pain-free group: none. Paradoxical burning pain upon exposure to cold: 2 pain patients and 1 pain-free patient.

Results (QST/MRI): Similar reductions of mechanical and thermal detection thresholds below injury level in both groups. Intensity of pinprick hyperalgesia and brush-evoked dysesthesia below level correlate with the intensity of spontaneous below-level pain ($p = 0.012$, Spearman's correlation coefficient = 0.54, and $p = 0.005$, Spearman's correlation coefficient = 0.59, respectively). Higher but not statistically significant below-level evoked pain, decrease in thermal threshold and dorsal gray matter lesion in the pain group than the pain-free group. Loss of spinothalamic functions does not appear to be a predictor for SCI-CP.

Defrin *et al*. (2007a)

11 SCI paraplegic outpatients recruited from a rehabilitation center. 4 women, 7 men, mean age 54.6 ± 6.3 years. Injury restricted to T4–T12. 2 complete and 9 incomplete traumatic SCI. Treatment-resistant below-level pain (CCP).

Sensory status below the lesion

	Preserved	Mild alterations	Moderate alterations	Severe alterations	Not available
Mechanical sensibility	3 patients	3 patients	1 patient	1 patient	1 patient
Thermal sensibility	–	–	3 patients	6 patients	–

Complete SCI: 2 patients

Finnerup *et al*. (2007b)

30 patients: 10 SCI patients (7 complete, 6 traumatic) with diffuse below-level NP (below-level pain only: 2 patients; at- and below-level pain: 4 patients; at-level pain distinguished from below-level pain: 4 patients), 10 SCI patients without NP, 10 healthy controls. (NP: chronic pain in an area of sensory abnormality, onset < 6 months after the SCI [traumatic or disease-based, border zone at the thoracic level]). Baseline measurements: evoked pain to single (von Frey monofilament) and repetitive punctuate stimuli (2 Hz for 30 s), evoked pain, or dysesthesia to brush, cold sensation (acetone droplet), cold and warm detection, and cold and heat pain thresholds (Thermotest), skin temperature, skin perfusion, and resting sweat (autonomic assessment). Same measurements after topical capsaicin + measurement of: intensity of capsaicin-induced pain/dysesthesia, changes in ongoing NP (NRS), capsaicin-evoked flare, brush-evoked allodynia, and punctuate hyperalgesia (soft brush and von Frey filament).

Results (baseline tests and capsaicin-evoked responses below the injury level) in 9 SCI patients with **below-level pain**:

Evoked pain: not felt (complete lesion in most patients); thermal thresholds: cold and warm (52–10 °C) not detected. Autonomic measures: no differences among the groups ($p = 0.76$, Kruskal–Wallis test). Capsaicin-evoked flare: no differences among the three groups ($p = 0.26$, one-way ANOVA). Intensity of ongoing below-level NP during capsaicin application: unchanged in 7, increased in 1 (1 point on NRS), decreased in 1 (1 point on NRS)

Authors' conclusions: capsaicin applications (50 mg/mL, 150 µL) do not increase below-level NP (unlikely role of peripheral input from small afferent central SCI pain). Higher doses of capsaicin may show other results.

Felix and Widerström-Noga (2009)

Study aimed at assessing the test–retest reliability of quantitative sensory tests (QST) and examining the validity of QST measurements as indicators of NP in SCI patients with chronic NP: **at** (dermatome of the neurological LOI and 3 dermatomes below this level) and/or **below** (at least four dermatomes below the neurological LOI) level sharp, shooting, burning, stabbing, electric pain.

22 SCI-NP patients, 19 men. Only baseline values for 12; test–retest analysis from the 10 remaining patients + 10 healthy controls.

QST in all participants (assessment of functional integrity of somatosensory pathways). Mechanical detection threshold (MDT) and vibration detection threshold (VDT) to assess dorsal column function, and thermal detection thresholds (cool and warm) and thermal pain thresholds (cold pain and hot pain) to assess spinothalamic tract function. Test sites identified on anatomical landmarks (repeatability). Above level and below level sites (including NP areas) tested.

Results: *Test–retest reliability*: **SCI patients**: substantial reliability (ICCs 0.84 to 0.95) for MDT, VDT, CDT, and WDT. Fair reliability (ICCs = 0.50) for CPT and HPT. **Controls**: substantial reliability (ICCs 0.86) only for VDT. Moderate reliability (ICCs 0.63–0.70) for MDT, CDT, WDT, HPT. Fair reliability (ICCs 0.49) for CPT.

No statistically significant difference for MDT, VDT, ATDT, ATPT obtained in pain sites vs. non-pain sites.

Significant correlation between NPSI scores and ATPT values obtained within painful test sites ($r = 0.58$, $p < 0.02$).

Conclusions: the degree of reliability of QST in SCI-NP patients is similar to that seen in healthy controls. Thresholds for thermal and cold pain are more variable across sessions than other QST measures. Lower average thresholds (CPT and HPT) in painful areas significantly correlate to higher pain severity (NPSI), regardless of the location (at vs. below) or the severity (complete vs. incomplete) of injury. *Areas affected by severe NP may have more functionally intact nociceptive system than areas with less severe pain.*

ATDT, average thermal detection threshold; ATPT, average thermal pain threshold; CDT, cool detection threshold; CPT, cold pain threshold; HPT, hot pain threshold; ICC, intraclass correlation coefficient; LOI, level of injury; MDT, mechanical detection threshold; NPSI, Neuropathic Pain Symptom Inventory; VDT, vibration detection threshold; WDT, warm detection threshold.

Hari *et al*. (2009)

Study hypothesis: enhanced STT recovery is associated with neuropathic pain. 28 SCI patients. Comparison of both recovery of pinprick (STT function) and light touch (dorsal column function) scores (3-point scale) within the first year after SCI (first examination 13 ± 9 d post injury, second examination 324 ± 57 d post injury) among patients with and without CP (below-level pain, bNP) according to a structured interview. **Data analysis in 8 bNP patients** (5 men, mean age 46 ± 14 years, 5.1 ± 1.9 years between injury and interview, traumatic lesion in 6, ischemic in 2) and 8 patients without CP. Pain intensity rating: NRS. Current NRS = 0 in 2 patients (1 intermittent pain and 1 successful treatment). Statistical analyses of data of five segments below the last dermatome with normal sensory function.

Table 4.4. (cont.)

Recovery scores not analyzed: light touch in 3 patients, pinprick in 4 patients (2 with and 2 without bNP, scores decrease over time).

Results:

(1) STT function. CP patients vs. no-CP patients: statistically significant larger improvement of pinprick scores (Mann-Whitney U test, 0.045). *No statistically significant difference between early and late examination scores* (only tendency for larger STT dysfunction at the early examination in CP patients). CP patients: improvement of the pinprick scores within the first year after SCI correlated positively only with the current pain intensity (Spearman's $\rho = 0.783$, $p = 0.022$) but not with the maximal pain intensity.

(2) DC function. No difference between CP and no-CP patients. No correlation between pinprick and light touch scores.

Authors' conclusion: recovery of STT function and not the dysfunction per se is associated with the development of CP even if functional STT recovery does not seem mandatory for the development of CP (as CP was present in 50% of the patients with a decline in STT function). New therapies aimed at promoting sensorimotor recovery after SCI could simultaneously induce CP.

Hatem *et al*. (2010): Syringomyelia

Prospective study aimed at detecting a possible link between the presence and/or variety of painful neuropathic symptoms and functional and structural changes of the spinal cord in MRI-confirmed syringomyelia. 37 patients (25 women, mean age 46 ± 13 years). Mild to severe thermal (heat and/or cold) deficits of the cervicothoracic skin territories (mean dermatomal extension per hemibody: 7.2 ± 6.6). Shoulders and/or hands included in all cases. Stable syringomyelia for at least 2 years. 27 CP patients (patients with pain in an area of somatosensory deficit directly attributable to the cord injury, not related to any other condition, and with DN4 questionnaire score ≥ 4/10). Control group: 21 healthy volunteers.

Assessment tools: detailed clinical neurological examination, NRS (BPI), NPSI, SF-MPQ, QST, MRI + DTI–FT (C3–C4), LEPs, SSEPs. Stimulation sites: both hands and both shoulders.

Demographic and clinical data

	Patients with syringomyelia ($n = 37$)		
Thermal deficits			
Symmetric	17 (46%)	Asymmetric	20 (54%)

Area of maximal thermal deficit		Shoulder (L or R)		22 (59%)	Hand (L or R)	15 (41%)
Deficits of other modalities						
Vibration	23 (62%)	Tactile (von Frey hairs)	29 (78%)	Graphesthesia	11 (30%)	
Movement direction	6 (16%)	Joint position (fingers)	4 (11%)	Stereognosis (hand)	1 (3%)	
Patients with neuropathic pain ($n = 27$, 73%)						
Duration of pain		13±11 years				
Localization of pain		Unilateral		Hand and shoulder	8 (30%)	17 patients, pain on the side with the most extensive thermal deficit for warmth in 14 (82%), for cold in 15 (88%) cases
				Hand	5 (19%)	
				Shoulder	4 (15%)	
		Bilateral		Hands and shoulders	4 (15%)	10 patients
				Both hands	3 (11%)	
				Both shoulders	3 (11%)	
Maximal pain localization		Hand		12 patients	Shoulder	15 patients
Spontaneous pain		11 (41%) patients		Spontaneous and evoked pain	16 (59%) patients	

Table 4.4. (cont.)

			Brush-evoked pain	9 (33%)
			Cold-evoked pain	3 (11%)
			Cold- and brush-evoked pain	2 (7%)
			Cold- and heat-evoked pain	1 (4%)
			Cold-, heat- and brush-evoked pain	1 (4%)
Evoked pain in the hand or the shoulder in all but 2 patients. Area of maximal evoked pain coincident with that of maximal spontaneous pain in all but these 2 patients				
Mean pain intensity median (25th–75th percentiles, NRS)		6 (4–8)		
NPSI dimensions	Burning	23 (85%)	Deep	22 (82%)
	Paroxysmal	16 (59%)	Evoked	20 (74%)
	Paresthesia/dysesthesia	18 (67%)		
Significant correlation between the score of the "evoked pain" (NPSI) and intensity of both average pain ($p = 0.01$) and burning pain ($p = 0.003$) at the same site.				
Laser stimulation	Number of sites perceiving the stimulus	4 (18 patients, 49%) 3 (8 patients, 22%) 2 (4 patients, 11%) 1 (4 patients, 11%) 0 (3 patients, 8%)		
	Elicited sensations	burning, sharp, shooting or stinging		

Comparison of patients with and without NP

Comparisons of LEP, SSEP, and quantitative sensory testing (statistically significant differences only)

	Hand						Shoulder						
	Right			Left			Right			Left			*
	CP patients	NoP patients	Controls	CP patients	NoP patients	Controls	CP patients	NoP patients	Controls	CP patients	NoP patients	Controls	
LEP													
N240-P350 amp (mV)	14 ± 15	11 ± 13	29 ± 16	22 ± 18	6 ± 8	30 ± 18	20 ± 19	17 ± 22	35 ± 26	22 ± 18	6 ± 8	34 ± 23	CP vs. C, NoP vs. C
N180 latency (ms)	243 ± 46	270 ± 74	198 ± 21	214 ± 51	273 ± 48	196 ± 20	213 ± 42	236 ± 53	178 ± 30	213 ± 49	257 ± 54	177 ± 28	CP vs. C, NoP vs. C
Reaction time (ms)	691 ± 262	631 ± 246	414 ± 84	660 ± 357	866 ± 374	401 ± 87	530 ± 203	492 ± 224	318 ± 57	527 ± 234	1021 ± 855	327 ± 65	CP vs. C, NoP vs. C
QST													
WDT (°C)	40.1 ± 7.8	39.6 ± 7.6	32.4 ± 0.5	38.2 ± 7.1	40.6 ± 7.5	32.4 ± 0.7	41.6 ± 6.8	43.1 ± 6.9	32.9 ± 1.1	39.2 ± 6.7	43.2 ± 7.2	32.7 ± 0.9	CP vs. C, NoP vs. C
CDT (°C)	21.7 ± 9.2	23.8 ± 9.7	30.8 ± 0.5	24.4 ± 8.9	22.6 ± 9.5	31.0 ± 0.4	22.8 ± 8.7	21.3 ± 9.0	30.6 ± 0.5	23.1 ± 9.4	19.8 ± 9.4	30.8 ± 0.7	CP vs. C, NoP vs. C
HPT (°C)	46.9 ± 3.4	46.0 ± 3.1	43.5 ± 2.4	44.9 ± 4.3	45.7 ± 3.9	42.9 ± 2.7	46.7 ± 2.9	48.1 ± 3.2	44.1 ± 2.1	45.5 ± 4.1	47.9 ± 2.1	43.5 ± 2.1	CP vs. C, NoP vs. C
MDT (log N)	2.1 ± 1.0	2.3 ± 1.2	1.0 ± 0.3	2.0 ± 1.3	2.1 ± 1.3	1.0 ± 0.3	2.2 ± 1.1	2.3 ± 1.1	0.9 ± 0.1	2.5 ± 1.0	2.5 ± 0.9	1.0 ± 0. 3	CP vs. C, NoP vs. C

VDT (mm)	4.3 ± 6.0	3.1 ± 2.9	1.1 ± 0.8	5.0 ± 9.5	8.4 ± 10.9	1.2 ± 0.9	10.7 ± 11.7	12.2 ± 12.9	3.1 ± 1.3	9.0 ± 12.3	18.5 ± 14.3	3.4 ± 1.2	CP vs. C, NoP vs. C

CP: 27 patients; NoP (No pain patients): 10 patients; healthy controls: 21 patients. No differences between CP patients and NoP patients. (ANOVA). **No statistically significant differences between groups** for N240 latency, P350 latency (LEP), N120-P240 amp, N120 latency, P240 latency, reaction time (SSEP), CPT, MPT (QST).

*, statistically significant difference (ANOVA). WDT, warm detection threshold; CDT, cold detection threshold; HPT, heat pain threshold; CPT, cold pain threshold; MDT, mechanical (tactile punctate) detection threshold; MPT, mechanical (tactile punctate) pain threshold; VDT, vibration detection threshold.

CP patients and NoP patients indistinguishable on the basis of thermal/mechanical and vibration thresholds, LEPs, SSEPs, DTI–FT analysis. Only discriminating variable between CP patients and NoP patients: asymmetry of deficits [index of asymmetry = more asymmetric extension of thermal deficits in CP patients on clinical examination ($p = 0.02$) but not on LEPs and SSEPs]. Patients with spontaneous and evoked pain vs. patients with spontaneous pain only or NoP patients: STT function better preserved, lower levels of lemniscal dysfunction (= milder clinical somatosensory impairment), less structural spinal cord damage (DTI)

Chapter 5

Central pruritus

Central pruritus following CNS damage has not received adequate recognition as part of the spectrum of CP. This would justify the limited number of reports (Tables 5.1 and 5.2).

Pruritus can blend with pain or dysesthesias or present singly. Most likely, patients may complain of itching, but the treating physician may dismiss it until scratching makes the problem visible. In all patients, other causes of pruritus were excluded by thorough investigation and the only dermatological findings were due to scratching. Pruritus tends to be continuous, but may also present in paroxysms or bouts.

Both brain and cord lesions have been described. In the brain, stroke is the main trigger (6/35 CPSP patients in the series examined by Klit *et al.* 2011), while in the cord intramedullary masses are mainly responsible. Drug therapy is generally unsatisfactory, but surgery abolished the symptoms in two cases in the short term. Spontaneous resolution is also possible.

No sex preponderance is seen in brain cases, but females are over-represented in cord lesions.

Pruritus is also commonly observed in multiple sclerosis (e.g. Osterman 1976, Yamamoto *et al.* 1981), but has not received due attention in the literature. It does not differ from the itching seen after the conditions described above.

Table 5.1. Central neurogenic pruritus due to brain lesions (excluding multiple sclerosis, MS)

Authors	Sex/ age	Trigger	Onset	Sensory findings	Site	CT/MR	Drugs	Effect	Notes
King *et al.* (1982)	F 58	Subarachnoid hemorrhage (basilar tip aneurysm) wrapping. Also stenosis 90% right ICA	Postoperative, over several weeks	Pain temperature hypoesthesia	Left limbs, left trunk (both pruritus and hypoesthesia)	Hypodensity of posterior limb internal capsule/lateral aspect of frontal and temporal lobes (right)	Carbamazepine	Reduction in intensity, frequency and duration	Also occasional paroxysmal sensations of warmth in the same distribution as the pruritus. EEG: focus of intermittent slow activity + sharp waves + spikes in frontotemporal region. Episodes of pruritus *uncorrelated* with slow + sharp activity
Sullivan and Drake (1984)	M 43	*Nocardia* abscesses (2), frontal (right), no mass effect	Not specified	Pin sensibility decreased Occasional touch allodynia (perceived as pruritus)	Left limbs, left trunk (both pruritus and hypoesthesia)	No lesion on sensory axis	(1) Phenytoin + cyproheptadine (2) Carbamazepine	(1) Itch less paroxysmal but more persistent (2) Improved	EEG: mild diffuse slowing + irregular polymorphic right frontotemporal delta rhythm. Itching present during EEG recording, but *uncorrelated* to EEG changes. Further complaints: painful fits

Massey (1984)	M 36	Infarct	Not specified	Hemianesthesia	Left (hemisoma)	Hypodensity in MCA territory	5 of these patients treated with carbamazepine or amitriptyline. However, all 9 relieved at 3 months follow-up (in F 67, amitriptyline 50 mg + benadryl)		EEG: no focus associated with pruritus
	M 54	Hemorrhage	Not specified	?	Left (hemisoma ?)	Hypodensity in internal capsule			
	F 64	Infarct	Not specified	Hemianesthesia	Right (hemisoma)	Hypodensity in MCA territory (parietal)			
	M 72	Infarct	Not specified	Hemianesthesia	Left (hemisoma?)	Hypodensity in internal capsule			
	M 68	Infarct	Not specified	Hemianesthesia	Right (hemisoma?)	Hypodensity in internal capsule			
	M 61	Infarct	Not specified		Left (hemisoma?)	Hypodensity in MCA territory			
	F 62	Hemorrhage	Not specified	?	Right (hemisoma?)	Hypodensity in internal capsule			
	M 76	Infarct	Not specified	Pinprick sensibility decreased (left hemisoma)	Left forearm and leg (pruritus)	Hypodensity in internal capsule + MCA territory – focal			
	F 67	Infarct	Postoperative, over *c.* 1 month (carotid surgery)	Hemianesthesia (pruritus bilateral, worse on left)	Left hemisoma	Hypodensity in MCA territory + internal capsule			

Table 5.1. (cont.)

Authors	Sex/ age	Trigger	Onset	Sensory findings	Site	CT/MR	Drugs	Effect	Notes
Shapiro and Braun (1987)	F 74	Infarct	Days	Normal, except poor 2-point discrimination (on left)	Left ear, cheek, ala nasi, upper lip, neck, upper back, knee	Hypodensity (superficial) in parietal lobe	Amitriptyline (20 mg/day)	Significant but incomplete – spontaneous disappearance	
Summers and MacDonald (1988)	2 children	Brainstem glioma (+ neurofibromatosis)						Resolved in both cases after a course of radiotherapy	Chief complaint of severe, episodic, paroxysmal, unilateral facial itching
Procacci and Maresca (1991)	F 82	?	Not specified	Hyperpathia for 2 hours (needle scratch of skin)	Whole body (starting on left side)	Negative (also at MRI)	Antihistaminics + psychotropics	Ineffective	Intense pruritus, 2 years long, worse in the morning
Canavero *et al.* (1997)	M 37	Subarachnoid hemorrhage	2 weeks	Not available	Left nose and throat	Not available	54 drugs incl. amitriptyline at full dosage. Propofol test. IT baclofen	Ineffective. Diazepam 10–25 mg transitorily effective	
Kimyai-Asadi *et al.* (1999)	F 74	Right thalamic stroke	Several weeks	Normal (?)	Various localized areas of the left trunk and extremities	Right thalamic stroke	Topical therapies (moisturizers, emollients)	Alleviation of each episode of pruritus	Episodic pruritus. Right side spared. Oral medications refused
	M 69	Right MCA stroke	Several days	Left-sided hemiplegia	Left thigh	Infarction of the territory of MCA	Amitriptyline (50 mg/day)	Effective (or spontaneous resolution?)	Localized, unremitting pruritus, interfering with sleep. Pruritus resolved in a week
Seo *et al.* (2009)	F 56	Wallenberg's syndrome	3 weeks				Gabapentin + topical moisturizers	3 months later resolved (or spontaneous resolution?)	Pruritus over face and trunk.

An undetailed report by Andreev and Petkov describes pruritus of the nostrils (6 patients) as almost pathognomonic of a brain tumor infiltrating the base of the fourth ventricle (Canavero *et al.* 1997).

Table 5.2. Central neurogenic pruritus due to cord lesions (excluding multiple sclerosis, MS)

Authors	Sex/age	Trigger	Onset	Sensory findings	Site	Therapy	Effect	Notes
Kinsella *et al.* (1992)	F37	Syrinx C4–T5 plus solid mass T2–T3	7 years of left arm/shoulder constant pruritus (occasionally prickly and painful or like pins and needles). Somewhat relieved by scratching. Worsened by hot water 3 months later pain and weakness in left arm. 6 months later, gradual onset of interscapular pain and progressive tingling of the left hand	C5 LSC. Decreased pinprick sensation in the area of the rash only		Topical steroids	Improved	Declined surgery
Vuadens *et al.* (1994)	F 69	Cavernoma T1	Not specified	Dysesthetic area inner aspect right arm	6-year-long pruritus + also aching pain. Itch appeared late and preceded CP by at least 4 years	Not specified	Not specified	
Johnson *et al.* (2000)	F15 months	Pilocytic astrocytoma T4–8	Intense pruritus since age 4 months localized to T6/7 dermatomes			Surgery (90% resection)	Pruritus resolved immediately after surgery. Follow-up 3 months	

Table 5.2. (cont.)

Authors	Sex/ age	Trigger	Onset	Sensory findings	Site	Therapy	Effect	Notes
Kavak and Dosoglu (2002)	F36	Ependymoma C4–7	Burning pruritus for 1 year, C5–6 distribution bilaterally with hyperesthesia			Antihistamines, topical steroids, lubricants	No benefit	Refused surgery
Sandroni (2002)	F 55	Cavernoma T9–10	Sudden	Pain plus intense itch; then pain abated, and itch spread Itch appeared on the 9th year of symptoms (pain)	Mid-back (itch) Groin (pain); spread to whole lower abdomen below T9	5% lidocaine patch	Marked relief No response to H1 blockers and steroids Topiramate ineffective on both itch and CP Other AD/ AED ineffective	Previous episodes of typical CP in affected hypoesthesic areas, each spontaneously regressed
Dey *et al.* (2005)	M 54	Cavernoma C3–4	Gradual	Unilateral, focal itch (after pain)	Excision at first completely relieved both CP and itch. 3 months postop, neck and shoulder pain recurred, radiating down left arm to base of left thumb, spreading over 2 years to whole hand. Pain changed from intermittent and stabbing to constant and burning. Itch recurred 2 years postop	(1) 5% lidocaine patch, EMLA cream and gabapentin (2) Opioids (3) TCAs, SSRIs, AEDs (OXCBZ, CBZ, zonisamide, tiagabine, levetiracetam), IV lidocaine, stellate ganglion block with lidocaine (4) TENS + acupuncture	(1) Moderate relief of itch (2) Pain improved, but not itch (3) No effect (4) Itch worsened	Both itch and pain improved by distraction. Scratching temporarily relieved itch but worsened the pain. Some itch was felt deep within the biceps area of the upper arm; temporary relief without pain exacerbation by squeezing biceps Normal postoperative MRI

Magilner (2006)	F 6	Pilocytic astrocytoma C1–5	Neck itching worsened over several weeks to frank pruritus. Then right neck pain added, which grew in severity					Rapid worsening. Surgery. Result on pruritus unstated
Wiesner *et al.* (2007)	M 36	Ependymoma C1–7	(1) Constant burning itching of head, neck, shoulders, and arms worse on wearing clothes (2) Hypoesthesia and paresthesiae in both arms, worse on right			(1) Topical steroids/ antihistamines (2) Surgery	(1) No effect (2) Abolition (follow-up: 2 months)	
Crane *et al.* (2009)	F 18	SCI (C6 lesion, surgical treatment)	3 months after the injury	Episodic aching	Left C6 dermatomal distribution at the level of SCI	Gabapentin 300 mg nightly	Not tolerated	
			7 months after the injury	Burning pain Itching Touch allodynia	Bilateral legs Left arm Right arm	Gabapentin 4800 mg 4 qid + occasional bedtime oxycodone + TENS	Moderate relief	
			10 months after the injury	Constant pruritus	Left arm (more severe at night)	TENS	No relief	
			17 months after the injury	Pain + intractable itching	Dorsal left forearm and digits in C6 and C7 dermatomal Distributions	(1) Gabapentin 3600 mg tid + TENS + lidocaine patches (2) IV Bier block (200 mg lidocaine/ 100 μg clonidine/ 50 mg	(1) Good pain relief but itching still refractory (2) No relief (3) Relief for 2 days then	Negative response to Bier block rules out peripheral mechanisms for pruritus

Table 5.2. (cont.)

Authors	Sex/ age	Trigger	Onset	Sensory findings	Site	Therapy	Effect	Notes
						methylprednisolone/ saline (60 mL solution) (3) Left stellate ganglion block (10 mL ropivacaine) (4) Acupuncture (laser, needle)	prompt relapse (4) No effect	
			19 months after the injury	Itching (VAS 3; 10 at night)	Left arm			
			29 months after the injury	Unrelenting pruritus		Stellate ganglion catheter placement for 1 week	1 month relief, then milder pruritus relapse	Bedtime gabapentin dose increased to 1500 mg 34 months after SCI, pruritus unabated

Chapter 6

Natural history

Central pain may produce immense suffering ("a great burden"), even when intensity is low: its generally very unpleasant and irritating, largely constant character makes it incomprehensible to almost all sufferers. Patients can be completely disabled and CP may be so devastating as to override any other disability in the chronic stage. By dominating the sensorium, interfering with the thought processes, and undermining the morale, CP frequently alters mood, intellect, and behavior, with deterioration of personality, depression, and neurotic tendencies, interfering with rehabilitation and impairing daily activities and quality of life. Many patients with severe persistent pain undergo a progressive physical deterioration caused by disturbance of sleep and appetite, fatigue, a restriction in physical and daily activities, and they often become addicted to medications, which further contributes to general fatigue, increased irritability, and decreased libido and sexual activity. Pain significantly interferes with memory of positive events by disrupting their encoding and facilitates the memory of negative events through selective retrieval of those events. The social effects are devastating: divorce, social isolation, unemployment, drug abuse, and self-neglect are often seen. Chronic pain may impair the immune system and even alter insulin sensitivity. Some patients with severe persistent pain become so discouraged and desperate that they commit suicide, regardless of depression. CP is also a major financial burden.

There are no prospective, adequately powered, long-term studies on the natural history of CP. There are reports of both sudden disappearance after a further brain lesion (Chapter 20) and disappearance after removal of the inciting lesion (so-called **reversible central pain**: see Appendix).

Brain central pain

Generally speaking, BCP is a chronic pain, which usually stays with patients for the rest of their lives. On rare occasions, it may gradually subside even after prolonged periods (CPSP: Greenspan *et al.* 1997, Kim 1999). Garcin (1968) stated that regression of brainstem CP is exceptional, but a few cases have been seen. The CPSP case 1 of Michel *et al.* (1990) simply reported an abatement of his pain. Bassetti *et al.* (1993) described one patient who developed transient CP following cortical parietal stroke. Andersen *et al.* (1995) reported that in two patients CPSP disappeared spontaneously: one had evoked dysethesia and shoulder pain at 1 month and another, with a lower brainstem infarction, complained of ocular pain with a Horner syndrome (possibly the same patients reported in Klit *et al.* 2011). According to Schott (2001), CP can disappear spontaneously even after many years, temporarily or permanently, generally slowly, but he does not back up this assertion with personal or published evidence; however, he had a patient with unremitting CPSP for 15 years except for 8 hours of 100% relief during a flight. Slow disappearances would feature ever longer pain-free intervals, although, when present, pain would be as severe as ever. Garcia-Larrea *et al.* (2010) described one patient with an insular stroke who developed arm dysesthesias during the acute phase only: 2 months later, he was completely asymptomatic. Klit *et al.* (2011) reported that in 23% of their CPSP patients the pain had decreased over time since onset in either intensity or distribution, while 34% complained of increased pain.

Pain occurring acutely immediately after traumatic cortical injury (e.g., penetrating head injuries) – a lancinating pain felt by the patient at the very moment of injury – has been considered CP of cortical origin (Garcin 1937); it fades away rather quickly (hours to days).

Cord central pain

Although in some cases CCP lasts only a few months, if paraplegia pain persists for longer than 6–8 months

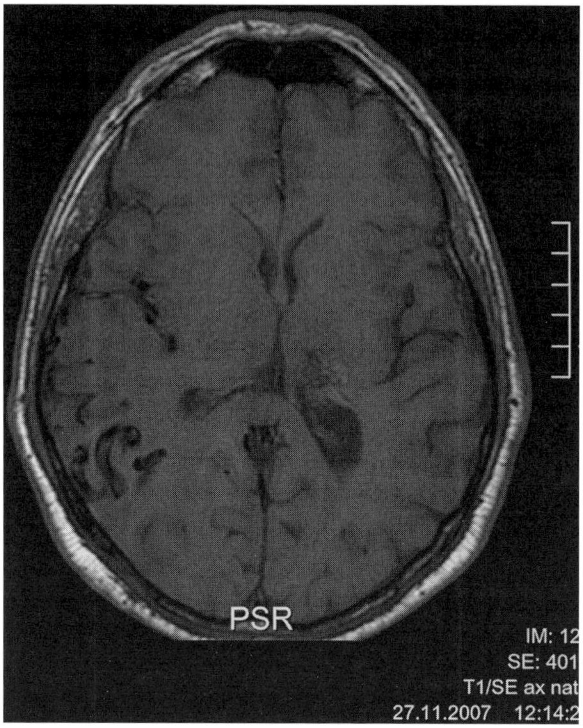

Figure 6.1. Thalamic cavernoma triggering central pain. Complete extirpation was achieved; not only was CP not improved, but it actually worsened on follow-up. Courtesy of Prof. Yasuhiro Yonekawa, Department of Neurosurgery, University of Zurich, Switzerland.

after the injury (the majority), it will become a long-term problem. Unlike BCP, which usually tends not to change significantly, except in degree, over time, CCP may change markedly, even dramatically, over the years: it may increase in severity for several years and even change in distribution and quality, sometimes dramatically. In one series, pain increased with the years in 73% of patients, ameliorated in 6%, and remained unchanged in 20% (Defrin *et al.* 2001). Some patients follow an aggressive course with intensity escalation, a few having an abatement of pain after a few years such that it becomes non-disabling (Beric 1999, Tasker 2001a). In another series, 40 of 217 patients still experienced pain in the long term (Davis and Martin 1947).

In Brown-Séquard's syndrome (hemisection of the cord), on the lesion side, intense pain spreading to the paralyzed, but not analgesic, limbs may be felt suddenly at the moment of injury, fading away in a few hours, days, or weeks: this is not CP (Garcin 1937, Riddoch 1938). CP associated with multiple sclerosis may often present during acute relapses and spontaneously vanish as the relapse clears (e.g., Portenoy *et al.* 1988). Some cases of CP recede after shunting for syringomyelia (e.g., Suzuki *et al.* 1985, Milhorat *et al.* 1996, Attal *et al.* 2004a) and it is reported that type I Chiari malformation-associated neurogenic pain (but not particularly sensory loss) responds well to surgery (Bejjani and Cockerham 2001, Meadows *et al.* 2001).

In patients with dysesthetic CP due to intramedullary tumors, symptoms tend to persist in many after removal (McCormick *et al.* 1990, Epstein *et al.* 1993). Surgical removal of intramedullary cavernomas may relieve CP initially, but many relapse at follow-up (Kim *et al.* 2006). Also, new CP can appear after excision of the mass (Canavero *et al.* 1994). Deutsch (2010) operated on five intramedullary cavernomas (four thoracic, one cervical): the intensity of the associated pain (likely CP) was reduced from visual analog scale (VAS) 8.6 to VAS 2 at 1-month follow-up, but relapsed to VAS 3.7 at 1 year. This is similar to what is seen in brain lesions, whose extirpation brings about some degree of tissue damage (Fig. 6.1).

Chapter 7

Central pain-allied conditions and special considerations

This chapter will review CP allied conditions (painful fits, Parkinson's disease) and focus on multiple sclerosis (MS) and syringomyelia. For a discussion of iatrogenic lesions, the interested reader should consult the first edition of this book (Canavero and Bonicalzi 2007a). Here, we simply recall how cordotomy for non-cancer pains led to CCP in 14% (6/42) in a large series (Ramadan *et al.* 1987).

CP allied condition 1: painful epileptic fits

Pain as a symptom of an epileptic seizure is rare (0.3–4.1%: Nair *et al.* 2001, Charlesworth *et al.* 2009), although the exact frequency remains to be determined (amounting to anywhere between *c.* 200 000 and *c.* 3 million patients worldwide, assuming an average pain prevalence of about 1%). Reports in children are exceptional.

Painful auras have been recognized as such for a long time, including atrocious tearing pains during jacksonian fits (De Ajuriaguerra 1937).

Pain generally accompanies simple partial attacks, with or without a jacksonian march, and with no side prevalence, in both adults and children. During the attack, the patient may complain of unpleasant sensations – numbness, pins and needles, intensely unpleasant but difficult to define, burning, cramping, aching, gnawing, throbbing, stinging, electric shock-like, stabbing, "like a thousand bee-stings," "like a sharp knife" – besides true pain. Pain may involve the whole hemisoma (or sometimes the *whole body or limbs bilaterally*), a limb or hemiface, combinations of these, or also spread contralaterally. Visceral pain and throbbing, pricking, or diffuse headache are part of the clinical spectrum. The usual cause is a tumor (meningiomas, gliomas, metastases, or abscesses), penetrating head trauma, stroke, or encephalitis. In many cases, it is idiopathic.

Penfield and Gage (1933) described the case of an epileptic woman in whom seizures were heralded by a sharp pain in the right lower quadrant of the abdomen, immediately followed by loss of consciousness. At operation, they found atrophy of a small convolution just posterior to SI and near the midline: galvanic stimulation of this area reproduced her pain and this was confirmed in another patient (case 5) with post-traumatic epilepsy and a normal cortex. They observed that "seizures beginning in the postcentral gyrus may be initiated by pain and discomfort in the opposite side of the body and without direct reference to the thalamus." Although the exact mechanism is unclear, the parietal region (contralateral SI and ipsi/contralateral SII) is the commonest site for lesions responsible for painful seizures. However, the site of the lesion may not always correlate with the site of the seizure during ictal pain, especially if the pain does not occur early in the ictal sequence. Bilateral EEG anomalies during painful fits are on record (Scholz *et al.* 1999). One epileptic patient had pain reproduced by neurosurgical stimulation of parietal BA5 (Scholz *et al.* 1999); another had a focal cortical dysplasia in the left middle cingulate cortex: she suffered from acute attacks of very painful, difficult-to-describe (but not burning), deep sensations in the right thigh, sometimes extending to the knee and lower leg (Roebling and Lerche 2009). In both these cases, however, propagation to SI cannot be ruled out. Importantly, there is no objective sensory deficit (e.g., Rétif 1963); instead, it seems clear that the decreased inhibition accompanying a seizure interferes with pain control mechanisms in certain cortical areas. This might account for the apparent intensification of paresthetic or dysesthetic sensations to the point of becoming painful, in some patients.

Tonic-clonic fits, sometimes accompanied by paroxysmal burning, lancinating, or even electric shock-like pain in the legs, glutei, or pelvis, both ipsilateral and contralateral to the fits, have been described for extramedullary tumors, multiple sclerosis, and transverse myelitis (McAlhany and Netsky 1955, Ekbom *et al.* 1968, Harrington and Bone 1981). Nathanson (1962) reported a patient with an extramedullary meningioma at T1 presenting with paroxysms of severe burning pain, lasting about 20 seconds in the left buttock and leg, with stiffening of the entire limb (the thigh slowly flexed on the hip as the leg partially extended). Pagni and Regolo (1987) reported the case of a woman who presented tonic-clonic spasms followed by clonic jerks in the left limb, along with pain in the glutei and in the anterior aspect of the leg: an anterior meningioma at T10 was found. In both cases, the attacks ceased within a few days of tumor removal. Miró *et al.* (1988) described paroxysmal pelvic pain, occurring 1–3 times a day, as a symptom of MS. Pagni and Canavero (1993) reported a case of a woman with paroxysms of pelvic pain resembling tic douloureux: the pain, which was at first itching and burning, became electric shock-like as the frequency of the attacks, which always lasted a few seconds, increased in time. MRI disclosed a dorsal extramedullary meningioma at T6–7. Carbamazepine – and, later, surgery – abolished the attacks. The dorsal columns are known to convey visceral nociception (Lenz *et al.* 2010). In spinal cases, focal demyelination induced by compression can induce hyperexcitable foci in the cord nociceptive fibers, and these foci may both discharge spontaneously and be triggered by mechanical distortion of the cord (Pagni and Canavero 1993).

CP allied condition 2: Parkinson's disease

Pain as part of Parkinson's disease (PD) was recognized by Parkinson himself (Garcin 1937). According to De Ajuriaguerra (1937), PD-associated pains "*siègent principalement aux membres, a la nuque et aux lombes, occupant surtout les articulations et les muscles sous forme de douleurs profondes parfois atroces ou survenant par crises d'élancements et de brûlures, surtout nocturnes. Elles sont souvent limitées au côté atteint dans les syndromes unilatéraux. Très souvent, ces douleurs précèdent les débuts apparents de la maladie . . . Il est plus rare de les voir persister tout le long de la maladie*" (principally affect the limbs, the nape and the loins, mostly at the level of joints and muscles as deep, sometimes atrocious, pains or shooting or burning painful paroxysms, mostly at night. They are often limited to the affected side in unilateral syndromes. Very often, these pains precede the onset of the disease . . . more rarely they persist indefinitely).

CP is said to be part of the pain spectrum reported by PD patients (Hanagasi *et al.* 2011: 12.7% !) According to some authors, the appearance of regional pain in some PD patients before the onset of motor disturbances supports this idea (e.g. Demchuk 2010). On the other hand, studies assessing sensory anomalies reject this conclusion (Table 7.1): in all instances, sensory thresholds were decreased, rather than increased, as is usual in CP. Förster (1927) believed that the striopallidal system exerts an inhibitory action on the thalamus. However, stereotactic lesions of the globus pallidus for the treatment of extrapyramidal motor disorders never originated CP. Honey *et al.* (1999) improved one of two PD patients with poorly localized, bilateral, often burning dysesthesias with pallidotomy at 6 weeks postoperatively, but none at 1 year; instead, cramping and deep aching pains responded to pallidotomy, with most patients relieved or improved at 1 year. Kim *et al.* (2008) found that 23/25 PD patients had their "central pain" relieved by bilateral subthalamic (STN) DBS; pain in the trunk and lower back was the least responsive. Paradoxically, at 6 months, one patient without previous "CP" developed it (!). This interpretation has been rejected (Gierthmuehlen *et al.* 2010): although some patients reported an improvement of pain with STN-DBS or L-DOPA, objectively pain sensitivity as assessed by QST was not altered by STN-DBS or L-DOPA, speaking against a direct modulation of CP processing by L-DOPA or STN-DBS in PD.

Special considerations 1: syringomyelia

Syringomyelia (in the spinal cord) and syringobulbia (in the lower brainstem) are cystic cavities filled with CSF-like fluid, varying from a small lesion in the dorsal part of the spinal cord over a couple of segments to huge cavities extending from the most caudal part of the cord into the medulla oblongata. The largest cavities leave only a thin layer of spinal cord tissue undamaged at the maximally cavitated regions; gray matter necrosis and wallerian degeneration are usually seen. Cavities are thought to arise in the center of the cord, which is where STT fibers cross the midline to reach their position in the ventrolaterally located STT. A lesion with this location will affect the sensibility to temperature and pain, i.e., a dissociated sensory loss will appear. Syrinxes may be associated with Chiari

Table 7.1. Parkinson's disease (selected series)

Djaldetti *et al.* (2004)				
36 patients with predominantly unilateral PD, 15 PD patients with response fluctuations, 28 age-matched healthy controls				
21 patients (8 women and 13 men) with hemi-PD and endogenous pain (initial symptom of the disease in 6 patients)				
Pain variability by time of day, duration, and location				
Pain quality: burning, itching, or tearing				
Pain site: usually localized to the more affected side (difficult to pinpoint in some patients)				
Mean VAS score: 48.9 ± 24.1 mm				
Subjective pain assessment: VAS, von Frey filaments (tactile thresholds), contact thermode for warm sensation (WS) and heat pain thresholds (HPTs)				
	Predominantly left-sided hemi-PD patients (15/21 patients)	**Predominantly right-sided hemi-PD patients (6/21 patients)**	**PD patients with fluctuations (15 patients)**	**Hemi-PD patients without pain (15 patients)**
	Pain side predominance			Symptoms side predominance
Left	6	1	11	3
Right	1	1	4	12
Bilateral	8	4	Painful sensations (mostly bilateral) in 12 patients	
Mean VAS score (mm)	51.5 ± 25.8	46.6 ± 27.3	55.7 ± 21.43 mm	
Quantitative assessment of pain perception				
Tactile threshold	No difference between patients in both patient groups and controls nor between sides			
WS threshold	No difference between patients in both patient groups and controls nor between sides		No side differences between "on" and "off" periods	
HPTs	42.6 ± 3.0 °C		No side differences between "on" and "off" periods	45.6 ± 2.8 °C ($p < 0.01$)
	PD patients with pain in the more affected side	PD patients without pain in the more affected side		
	41.4 ± 2.6 °C	43.7 ± 3.3 °C ($p < 0.0001$)		
The severity of subjective pain and HPTs on the affected side was correlated only with disease duration.				
Authors' conclusion: HPTs were lower in the PD patients than in controls and lower in the PD patients with pain than in those without pain. In the patients with unilateral PD, HPTs were significantly lower on the more affected side compared with the less affected side. As endogenous pain in PD patients is accompanied by increased sensitivity to some painful stimuli, basal ganglia abnormality may involve pain encoding.				

Table 7.1. (cont.)

Schestatsky *et al*. (2007)

Psychophysical and neurophysiologic study aimed at evaluating whether primary central pain (PCP) in PD may be due to a dysfunction of pain pathways or the processing of pain in the CNS. Study population: PD patients younger than 65 years, with predominantly unilateral signs (9 PD-PCP patients + 9 PD patients without pain [PD-NoP]) + 9 healthy controls. PCP diagnosed according to established criteria. Pain onset after the diagnosis of PD in all PD-PCP patients. Pain usually spontaneous, poorly localized, with exacerbations, usually more intense in the more affected side (whole hemibody involved in 6 patients, only the arm in 3). Mean VAS: 5.3. Most frequent descriptors: burning, itching, and tearing sensations.

Assessment: clinical characteristics of pain, thermal QST, LEPs, laser-induced sudomotor skin responses (l-SSRs) in *off* (after 14-hour discontinuation of all antiparkinsonian medications) and *on* conditions.

Results

***Off* condition** (PD-PCP patients vs. PD-NoP patients and controls): statistically significant differences in heat pain and laser pinprick thresholds due to lower thresholds (more affected side > less affected side) in PD-PCP patients (no significant differences between PD-NoP patients and controls). **LEPs**: N2 or P2 latencies: no differences between groups; N2/P2 amplitude: statistically significant difference (**higher** LEP amplitudes in PD-PCP patients vs. PD-NoP patients or controls). No differences between more affected and less affected side in any group of patients. **l-SSRs**: mean latency or amplitude of the first l-SSR: no differences between groups; statistically significant difference for l-SSR-HI and mean l-SSR amplitude (lower l-SSR-HI and a higher mean l-SSR amplitude in PD-PCP patients, more affected side > less affected side). No significant differences in any l-SSR variables between PD-NoP patients and controls. No correlation between mean l-SSR amplitude and pain scores.

***On* condition**: PD-PCP patients: lower pain-NOW scores and higher l-SSR-HI and lower l-SSR mean amplitude than in *off* condition (values still significantly different from those in PD-NoP patients and controls). Differences among groups no longer present for the other variables.

Authors' conclusion: Patients exhibited signs of hyperalgesia and lack of habituation of SSRs to repetitive pain stimuli (abnormal control of the effects of pain on autonomic centers?), attenuated by L-DOPA (possible dysfunction of dopamine-dependent centers regulating both autonomic function and inhibitory modulation of pain inputs), but **conduction along peripheral and central pain pathways *is normal* in PD patients with or without PCP**. Pain in these patients does not seem to be related to central sensitization or defective inhibitory control over afferent inputs.

Nègre-Pagès *et al*. (2008)

Cross-sectional survey aimed at assessing chronic pain in PD patients (prevalence, description, analgesic consumption). 450 PD patients, 425 with chronic pain (>3-month duration). Evaluation: clinical examination + self-reported questionnaires in a survey. Pains related or unrelated to PD identified according to predefined criteria. Comparison with 98 patients with other chronic disorders to assess if pain is more frequent in PD patients.

Chronic pain present in 278/450 PD patients. Pain unrelated to PD (osteoarthritis etc.): 111/425 patients (26%). PD-related pain: 167/425 patients (39.3%). PD as sole cause of pain (PD-pain direct group): 103 patients. PD aggravating other pains : 64 patients. PD-pain direct group: heterogeneous pain description (**resembling neuropathic pain** in 14 patients with normal sensory examination). PD-pain direct characteristics: more recent, more frequent after PD onset, less frequently worsened by physical effort, more frequently worsened during *off* episodes and better improved by antiparkinsonian drugs, more frequently located in the lower limbs and less frequently reported to doctors.

PD-related pain patient characteristics: younger at PD onset, with more motor complications and more severe depressive symptoms. PD pain more intense but less frequently reported to doctors and associated with less frequent analgesic consumption than non-PD pain. Pain twice as frequent in PD patients as in patients with other chronic disorders (after adjustment for osteoarticular comorbidities).

CP not specifically reported.

Table 7.1. (cont.)

Defazio *et al.* (2008)
402 consecutive PD outpatients with MMSE > 24 (mean age 67.4 ± 9.1 years) + 317 healthy matched controls (mean age 65.5 ± 10.4 years). Pain present at the time of study and lasting for at least 3 months in 281 PD patients and 199 controls ($p = 0.04$). **Central neuropathic pain** (CNP: burning, tingling, formication, or bizarre quality) reported by **18/402 PD patients** (4.5%) vs. 5/317 controls (1.6%, $p = 0.04$)
No reported relationship between L-DOPA-related changes in parkinsonian disability and NP.
402 patients: consecutive outpatients (148 women, Nov. 2006, to Mar. 2007) + healthy controls (outpatients' relatives, $n = 317$) frequency-matched to case patients. Pain assessors unaware of the study hypothesis. Pain classification: dystonic (i.e. associated with visible dystonia) and non-dystonic, including cramping (aching pain in muscles), arthralgic (stiffness after rest and pain with motion, confined to joints), peripheral neuropathic (pain in the territory of a root or nerve), **central neuropathic pain** (burning, tingling, formication, or bizarre quality). Headache and other facial pain not analyzed.
At study time, 281 PD patients (69.9%) vs. 199 controls (62.8%) reported experiencing pain for at least 3 months ($p = 0.04$). PD patients and controls differed for the presence of depression (67 vs. 19; $p = 0.001$) and medical conditions associated with painful symptoms (99 vs. 112; $p = 0.02$). Non-dystonic pain reported by 267 PD patients (66.4%) and 199 (62.8%) controls ($p = 0.28$). Cramping and CNP significantly associated with PD.
Frequency and distribution of CNP: PD patients 18/402 (4.5%); Controls 5/317 (1.6%) ($p = 0.04$). No obvious relationship between L-DOPA-related changes in parkinsonian disability and NP.
Authors' conclusion: the frequency of non-dystonic pain was similar in PD patients and controls, but cramping and central neuropathic pain subtypes were significantly associated with PD.
Brefel-Courbon *et al.* (2009)
9 patients. Comparison of results of cold pressor test during off and on conditions (random order) in 9 pain-free PD patients and 9 controls + analysis of rCBF (PET) during experimental alternate randomized noxious and innocuous stimuli. Results: pain threshold in *off* condition significantly lower in PD patients than in controls (8.0± 2.9 °C vs. 4.4 ± 3.8 °C; $p = 0.03$), significantly raised after L-DOPA administration (8.0 ± 2.9 °C vs. 4.6 ± 3.0 °C; $p = 0.007$, no variation in controls). No significant difference in pain thresholds in the *on* condition between PD patients and controls. rCBF: PD patients (*off* condition) vs. controls: significant increase (reduced after levodopa administration) in pain-induced activation in right insula and prefrontal and left anterior cingulate cortices.
Authors' conclusion: PD patients have a lower pain threshold (normalized after levodopa administration) and a higher pain-induced activation in nociceptive pathways (reduced by L-DOPA).
Barone *et al.* (2009)
1072 patients. Multicenter survey aimed at assessing the prevalence of non-motor symptoms (NMSs), their association with cognitive impairment, and the impact on patients' quality of life (QoL) in PD patients. 1072 consecutive patients: 647 men (60.4%, mean age 66.8 ± 9.6 years), 425 women (39.6%, mean age 68.2 ± 9.1 years), median PD duration 5.1 years. Evaluation tools: UPDRS-III, modified Hoehn and Yahr (HY) scale, MMSE, FAB, PDQ-39. Patient classification: (1) "naive" (10%, never taken dopaminergic agents); (2) "stable" (70.2%, dopaminergic treatment, no motor complications); (3) "complicated" (19.8%, motor fluctuations and/or dyskinesia under dopaminergic treatment). All patients evaluated during the *on* state.
Number of patients reporting pain: 653 (60.9%). Pain type: undefined in 223 patients (20.8%), leg pain in 406 patients (37.9%), abdominal pain in 61 patients (5.7%), related to drugs intake in 11 patients (1.0%), shoulder pain in 205 patients (19.1%). Pain significantly more prevalent in women (67.5% vs. 56.6%) and less frequent in the naive subgroup of patients. Prevalence of pain and disease stage (HY scale): overall: 653 patients (60.9%), HY 1: 85 patients (50.9%), HY 1.5–2: 302 patients (58.6%), HY 2.5–3: 218 patients (67.1%), HY 4–5: 39 patients (79.6%).
CP prevalence not specifically addressed.

Table 7.1. (cont.)

Beiske *et al*. (2009)
Home-ridden PD patients. 413 patients identified in an outpatient registry; 243 eligible patients (mentally and physically able to complete a structured interview); 176 included (41% women). Mean age 69 years (range 35–90). Response rate: 72% (176/243 but 87% [176/202] according to the authors). Pain assessment: Norwegian version of the BPI (variable of interest: pain severity index), SF-36, and semi-standardized questions.
Central neuropathic pain (CNP: boring, constant, ineffable and poorly localized, not limited to a dermatome or specific neural distribution) **reported by 15 patients (10%)**. Duration > 6 months in 80% of patients. 80% of patients reported CNP as related to PD and 40% as associated with motor fluctuations and alleviated by dopaminergic drugs. Only significant pain predictor: female gender.
Limitation of the study: diagnostic uncertainty (see examination protocol for CP).
Neurological examination + structured interview + standardized questionnaires. Pain reported by 146 (83%) patients Musculoskeletal pain reported by 70%, dystonic pain by 40%, radicular-neuropathic pain by 20%, and **central neuropathic pain** by 10% of patients. Mean score of BPI average pain (last 24 h): 3.39.
CNP duration (months)/% of patients: <1/0%; <3/7%; <6/7%; >6/80%; missing 7%. Percentage of patients reporting that the pain started after the diagnosis of PD: 80%
Authors' conclusion: nearly all CPSP and MS-CP patients have abnormal temperature and pain sensibility. Regrettably, we did not collect such data on sensibility among the patients with CNP. *Studies are therefore needed to demonstrate whether CNP in PD patients is associated with sensory changes or not.*

I malformation (30% of the cases), cervical disk disease/spondylosis, basilar impression, and communicating hydrocephalus; they may also be post-traumatic (only 5% of the cases with minor SCI develop a syrinx years later), generally following hematoma resolution, or due to infection, tumors, or iatrogenic lesions.

Roughly half or more of patients with syringomyelia suffer from a blend of at-level and below-level pains: dysesthesias, burning pain, pins and needles, stretching pressure of the skin, in most cases hyperesthesias, involving one arm (seldom both), neck, shoulder, and hemithorax, i.e., in the distribution of the suspended dissociated sensory loss. There is a female prevalence. Facial pain is frequently reported with syringobulbia. Spontaneous pain and subjective sensory disturbances may often precede by many years any other sign of this slowly progressing disease.

In 42/51 patients (Milhorat *et al.* 1996), the dermatomal pattern of pain overlapped with a segment of analgesia–anesthesia. Obvious trophic changes were seen in 15/51 patients (29%). Another series (Ducreux *et al.* 2006) showed that 27/31 patients suffered CP in the arm, 12 with additional pain in the neck or in the thorax, another 5 both in the thorax and the leg. CP extended over 2–10 dermatomes, unilaterally in 24. Spontaneous pain was single in 11 and associated to evoked pain in 20 (allodynia to brush 12, heat 5, and cold 11). Pain was described as burning in 23, deep (pressure, squeezing) in 14, paroxysmal (electric shocks, stabbing) in 19; paresthesias and/or dysesthesias (tingling, pins and needles) were reported in 24.

Quantitative sensory testing (QST) shows that all patients with syrinx have abnormal temperature and pain sensibility, mostly pronounced with total loss of temperature sensibility. Patients in advanced stages also have impairment of lemniscal sensibility. For instance, Attal *et al.* (2004a) performed QST before and after surgery (3 and 9 months) in patients with cervical and dorsolumbar syrinxes, most suffering pain. Thermoalgesic, but not lemniscal, deficits were found in all. Spontaneous pain was generally located within an area of thermal deficit, but its intensity was not correlated with the magnitude thereof. Surgery induced a significant decrease of the deficits (tactile more than thermal), but effects on pain were variable and not correlated with those on thermal sensibility.

Pain is especially common with post-traumatic syringomyelia. Nashold (1991), in his series of paraplegics with pain, found a spinal cyst in 60% of the patients, generally extending from the site of the spinal trauma rostrally, involving multiple segments of the normal spinal cord. In a few patients, at operation, two separate cysts that extended above and below the site of the trauma were found, but they were not interconnected.

Paraplegics who suffer from a traumatic syringomyelia often develop pain extending above injury level, but also referred to distant dermatomes, even many years after injury (15 in one of the patients of Durward *et al.* 1982), probably due to the slow enlargement of the spinal cyst and the subsequent pressure on the normal spinal cord above the level of the trauma; up to two-thirds of paraplegics with pain of delayed onset exhibit a syringomyelia. The pain is generally sharp or aching, electrical and burning in character; it is often located in the dermatomes adjacent to the injury level, but may expand to involve higher dermatomes. The paraplegic is often aware that his or her sensory level has risen, and, if a spinal cyst encroaches on the cervical spinal cord, motor deficits can occur in the arms. This pain may be activated along with diffuse visceral pain by infections of the urinary tract or by constipation. Continuous escalation in pain is the natural course. Shunting is generally ineffective in reversing the pain in a significant number of cases (Dworkin and Staats 1985, Milhorat *et al.* 1996, Kramer and Levine 1997).

Hydromyelia is a different condition from syringomyelia, having no electrophysiological alterations, yet two-thirds of the patients had pain, including burning neuropathic pain, in a large series (Roser *et al.* 2010). Apparently, these pains are very well managed without surgery.

Special considerations 2: multiple sclerosis

Multiple sclerosis (MS) is a chronic degenerative condition of the CNS of unknown etiology. CP as a symptom of MS has been recognized since the nineteenth century (De Ajuriaguerra 1937) (Table 7.2). Plaques of demyelination are most frequently found in the spinal cord, particularly in the dorsal columns, in the brainstem, and periventricularly in the forebrain. Yet, despite the difficulty in determining the exact location of the lesions that result in CP, due to widespread dissemination in the CNS, nonetheless, the topographical distribution of the symptoms and signs in MS (i.e., bilaterality of pain) appears to indicate that many of the MS lesions that cause CP are spinal (O'Connor *et al.* 2008, Svendsen *et al.* 2011).

CP is correlated with increasing age, EDSS, disease duration, but not sex. Some patients with MS have CP for a limited period during relapses (days to months); others have chronic CP.

MS-CP is generally dysesthetic, but also tingling, pins and needles, pricking, cold, or warm. As in all CPs, several other qualities, singly or in combination, may be present, particularly burning and aching; a pressing belt-like (girdle) pain at the level of the upper border of the lesion may also be seen. CP, when maximal, was generally described as tingling (59%), tiring (52%), taut (45%), burning, dull, and grueling (41% each) in one study (Svendsen *et al.* 2005). Intensity is often high. Pruritus is also part of the spectrum (Canavero *et al.* 1997). During relapses, it can affect any part of the body, in different combinations at different levels; in chronic stages, a great majority of those affected have pain in the lower extremities, about one-third in the arm, and one-fifth in the trunk, partially or totally, unilaterally (one-quarter) or bilaterally (three-quarters), hemipain being uncommon. Some patients experience CP before other symptoms, others complain of pain along with other symptoms and signs. It tends to be worst at night and to affect less disabled patients. The pain tends to be constant, but can be intermittent, deep more than superficial or both, and can radiate. CP can develop or worsen during a rise of temperature (exercise, sunbathing), so-called Uhthoff's sign. In one study (Svendsen *et al.* 2005), aggravating factors were cold in 12 patients, warmth in 5, same position for a long time in 11, body movement including walking in 6, physical strain in 6, touch (clothes, etc.) in 9, tiredness in 4, stress in 2, and loud noise in 1. Touch allodynia was most commonly reported in CP patients: these more often had cold and/or mechanical allodynia than patients with musculoskeletal pain (a statistically significant difference). The frequency of temporal summation tended to be higher in CP patients.

Nearly all patients have alterations in temperature and pain sensation in painful areas (O'Connor *et al.* 2008), with a greater incidence of thermal deficits in the feet than in the hands (Österberg and Boivie 2010); lemniscal pathways are also affected. Some patients experience paradoxical heat pain sensation evoked by noxious cold, a phenomenon also seen in pain-free patients. No association between CP and site of demyelinations has been found (Svendsen *et al.* 2011), although there was a trend toward a lower number of patients with lesions of the Vc-SI projection: thalamic lesions were seen in two (15%) CP patients.

In MS, facial pain is at first usually identical to idiopathic trigeminal neuralgia, with plaques involving the trigeminal root entry zone. Later, with

Table 7.2. Multiple sclerosis (selected series)

Hansen *et al*. (1996)

Study on the incidence of thermal sensory abnormalities and paradoxical heat sensation (PSpos) in patients with multiple sclerosis (MS, definite in 13, probable in 3, possible in 6). 13 women (6 definite MS). MRI in all but 2 patients (both with clinically definite MS); 34 healthy controls. Examination: bilateral dorsal hand and foot (thermal sensory analyzer, Marstock method).

Patients with definite MS (*n* = 13): *lesion location* (MRI) periventricular, 12 patients (+ brainstem/cerebellum in 1, + cord in 2); clinical signs of *somatosensory disturbances*: hypoesthesia or numbness (attributed to dorsal column function): 10 patients; thermhypoesthesia or hypoalgesia (attributed to STT function): 8 patients (both system dysfunction in 6 patients). *Paresthesia, hyperpathia, pain* in 1 patient (without somatosensory disturbances; normal SSEPs). Pathological SSEPs: 8 patients. PSpos: 9 patients. PSpos (TSL) (probable or definite) MS patients: 10/24, 3/34 controls (+ 1 excluded due to erratic responses).

Incidence of threshold abnormalities and PSpos

	Threshold abnormalities			PSpos	Induced warmth	Induced burning
	CDT	WDT	TSL			
Controls ($n = 34$)	2 (6%) (2F, 2H)	3 (9%) (1F, 2H)	3 (9%) (2F, 1H)	4 (12%) (4F)	TSL (4F)	
Patients ($n = 16$) (probable or definite MS)[a]	6 (37%) (4F, 2H)	9 (56%)[b] (6F, 8H)	6 (37%) (6F, 6H)	10 (62%)[b] (12F, 2H)	TSL (10F, 1H) CDT (2F)	TSL (1F, 1H)

[a] Incidence of PSpos significantly raised only in probable or definite MS patients
[b] Difference statistically significant, Yates corrected chi-square test. More than one affected site in several patients. On average, larger temperature changes needed for detection thresholds in PSpos patients
F, feet; H, hands.

Authors' conclusion: no current diagnostic significance of paradoxical heat sensation. As CNS lesions facilitate paradoxical heat sensation, temperature sensation is probably integrated at the thalamocortical level.

Österberg and Boivie (**2010**)

Single-center study. Questionnaire sent to 429 MS patients (283 women); 371 answers (86%), 7 patients excluded, 364 analyzed (85%). CP in 100 patients (27.5%), including 18 patients (4.9%) with trigeminal neuralgia (TN). Interview and neurological examination in 62 CP patients (MS-CP patients, 42 women, mean age at examination 52 years, mean EDSS 4.8, median 6.0, mean duration of pain 11 years, range 0.5–38) + 16 patients with MS with sensory symptoms but without pain (MS-NP patients, control group, 10 women, mean age at examination 47 years, mean EDSS 4.2, median 3.8, mean duration of sensibility disturbances 14 years, range 3–27).

Assessment tools: clinical testing (touch, cold, pinprick, dermolexia, kinesthesia) and QST (perception thresholds for vibration [Vibrameter], touch [von Frey filaments], warmth, cold, cold pain and heat pain [Thermotest)]; cut-off limits 50.0 °C and 0 °C). Tests performed on defined regions of the body, always including hands and feet. Comparisons between painful and non-painful regions. Index values used to grade the severity of the sensibility abnormalities and to compare the results on hands and feet.

MS-CP patients ($n = 62$)			
Pain location	Lower extremities 85% Upper extremities 34% **Trunk 27%**[a]	Pain side	Unilateral 27% Bilateral 73%
Pain qualities	Aching 45% Burning 42% Pricking 21% (2–4 pain qualities experienced by > 66% of patients) Both superficial and deep in 58% of cases	Sensory symptoms	Numbness 76% Hypoesthesia 61% Spontaneous paresthesia 55% Hyperesthesia 34% Evoked dysesthesia 24% Allodynia 10% After-sensation 7%

Pain as first sole symptom in 3 patients (5%). Pain onset in the same year as other MS symptoms in 34% of patients. VAS score range: minimal intensity: 28 (mean), maximal 68 (mean). Constant pain in most patients.
[a] Only statistically significant difference vs. controls, Fisher's exact test.

Perception thresholds in MS-CP patients and in controls

	MS-CP patients							Controls			
	Painful areas (PA)			Non-painful areas (NPA)			Statistical tests (PA vs. NPA)				Statistical tests (MS-CP vs. control)
	Mean	Median	SD	Mean	Median	SD		Mean	Median	SD	
Feet[a]											
Warmth (°C)	43.3	43.5	5.7	38.7	36.9	4.3	$p < 0.001$	40.9	40.0	4.6	$p < 0.05$
Cold (°C)	15.5	20.5	13.5	21.2	26.4	11.8	$p < 0.05$	23.5	26.3	8.3	$p < 0.01$
Difference limen (°C)	27.7	23.5	17.0	17.5	11.6	14.7	$p < 0.01$	17.5	13.5	11.3	$p < 0.01$
Heat pain (°C)	46.9	47.9	3.4	46.1	47.2	3.3	ns	47.3	48.1	2.3	ns
Cold pain (°C)	6.3	0.0	9.0	12.5	14.0	9.3	$p < 0.01$	7.6	7.7	8.0	ns
Touch (mg)	26 230	2200	78 091	1889	1100	1817	ns	5446	2200	6887	ns
Vibration (µg)	67.8	22.5	80.3	11.6	5.0	19.7	$p < 0.001$	61.2	30.0	64.5	ns
Hands											
Warmth (°C)	33.7	33.0	2.7	33.4	33.2	2.2	ns	31.9	31.6	2.2	$p < 0.05$
Cold (°C)	28.4	29.3	6.0	29.4	30.3	3.9	ns	28.7	28.4	1.4	ns

Table 7.2. (cont.)

Perception thresholds in MS-CP patients and in controls											
	MS-CP patients							Controls			
Difference limen (°C)	5.3	3.5	7.6	4.0	2.5	4.9	ns	3.2.	2.7	2.1	ns
Heat pain (°C)	41.5	41.2	4.1	41.7	41.5	4.1	ns	42.1	42.6	2.8	ns
Cold pain (°C)	13.0	13.9	6.4	14.9	14.0	7.3	ns	12.8	13.4	6.8	ns
Touch (mg)	1547	730	3940	904	200	2175	ns	10 741	2200	21 942	$p < 0.05$
Vibration (μg)	6.4	0.6	12.7	2.7	0.4	7.8	ns	23.3	2.3	51.5	nd
Extremities[a]											
Difference limen	2.5	3.0	1.2	1.7	2.0	1.1	$p < 0.001$	2	2.0	0.8	$p < 0.05$
Heat pain/ cold pain	1.1	1.0	1.0	0.4	0.0	0.8	$p < 0.001$	0.5	0.0	0.7	$p < 0.001$

	MS-CP patients	Controls	Statistical tests (MS-CP vs. control)
Abnormal sensibility to temperature and/or pain in the painful region	97%	81%	$p < 0.05$
Sudden burning sensation of heat (patients not perceiving non-noxious warmth but feeling heat pain)	19% (at the HP threshold)	13%	ns
Spasms (triggered occasionally by heat pain and cold pain)	10%		
Paradoxical heat pain evoked by noxious cold [a]	13%		
Paradoxical cold pain evoked by noxious heat [a]	1.6%		
Non-painful dysesthesiae from unpleasant stimulation	27%	44%	
Abnormal pinprick perception (painful region)	63%	81%	ns
Dysesthesiae or hyperalgesia to pinprick	11%	25%	ns

[a] Paradoxical sensations only found in the lower extremities

Authors' conclusions: the results support the general hypothesis that only patients who have lesions affecting the spinothalamocortical pathways run the risk of developing CP.

involvement of the descending root, pain becomes continuous and disagreeable and paresthesias appear. Some neurosurgeons report microvascular compressions in these patients, but others do not (Antic and Peric 2009). Microvascular compression is found in many normal subjects (Peker *et al.* 2009).

In MS (as well as cervical spondylotic chronic myelopathies and extramedullary tumors, both cervical and of the foramen magnum), an uncomfortable, not truly painful, sensation, closely resembling that produced by an electric current, can be elicited by the active or passive flexion of the head, and radiating from the cervical to the coccigeal region and to the four limbs, so-called **Lhermitte's sign** (Garcin 1968). It is seen in 9% (up to 40%) of MS patients (Solaro *et al.* 2004), and some classify it as intermittent CP (O'Connor *et al.* 2008): this is not so, as no patient needs treatment (in rare cases, low dose carbamazepine suffices).

Chapter 8

Diagnosing central pain

CP is pain due to a CNS lesion along the spinothalamoparietal path. Thus, an appropriate lesion must be demonstrated in such a location. At the same time, the presence of PNP, which may mimic CP (e.g., diabetic polyneuropathy in stroke patients), but also nociceptive musculoskeletal pains, occasionally occurring in the same body area, must be excluded. A common source of diagnostic uncertainty is that symptoms of CPSP regularly occur after a significant passage of time from the precipitating event, calling for careful interviewing.

Pain and dysesthesias have the same characteristics whatever the level or etiology. Similar symptoms can be caused not only by diseases affecting primarily the CNS, but also by lesions neighboring the neuraxis (e.g., extramedullary tumors, aneurysms, meningeal masses) and damaging the nervous tissue only secondarily. Sometimes pain is the presenting symptom and remains an isolated finding for a long time, as occurs in syringomyelia and, exceptionally, other diseases (e.g., spinal cord tumors).

CP is independent of non-sensory abnormalities, and these may be present at the moment of examination or may have subsided. In addition, the degree of pain and sensory abnormalities may not be necessarily correlated with the severity of other neurologic disabilities. The distribution of these abnormalities will overlap or contain the perceived location of the pain.

Particularly in spinal cord lesion cases, CP can be missed among other accompanying pains, or it may be misidentified as nociceptive pain *tout court*. CP appears in many disguises and therefore requires a meticulous diagnostic workup.

Mental status is usually normal, and CP patients are no more depressed or anxious than other chronic pain patients; psychiatric consultation is unnecessary. The psychological evaluation is usually done with the Minnesota Multiphasic Personality Inventory (MMPI), and other more detailed psychological tests (Hamilton, Beck, etc.) as indicated; elevation on the scales of depression, hysteria, and somatization may hint at a dysfunctional state.

The suggestion that neuropathic pains (including CP) be individualized as a specific group, based on common symptomatology across etiologies, must be rejected *tout court*: response to treatment – to name one – differs between CP and, e.g., postherpetic neuralgia or complex regional pain syndrome. There is a smorgasbord of **screening methods**, primarily aimed at non-specialists (Tables 8.1 and 8.2). However, these cannot replace clinical judgment, as they miss too many patients, and the tools that are available for evaluating chronic neuropathic pain are not specifically tailored to SCI patients (Calmels *et al.* 2009). We do not recommend their use outside research settings.

In our experience, diagnosis of CP will be secured in practically all patients by hewing to the following recommendations (Table 8.3).

STEP 1 The best way to get a history from a CP patient is to ask about all possible pain qualities, rather than leaving it up to the patient. No sensory descriptor is pathognomonic for CP. Shooting pain and tingling sensations are reported by about 50% of patients with musculoskeletal pain, and about 30% of patients with non-neuropathic pain complain of burning pain, and clinical examination therefore cannot be replaced by interview questions alone.

A comprehensive bedside examination should be performed, above all probing of somatosensory functions with cotton (touch sensation), an ice cube and a warm vial (temperature sensation), and a pin (pain sensation). Body distribution and any summations or gradients should be included in the description. Meticulous and repetitious questioning is required. Experience and subtlety are required for evaluation. A pain drawing filled out by the patient helps delineate the distribution of spontaneous pain (a pain diary assesses intensity fluctuations and, later, response to

Table 8.1. Screening and assessment tools for neuropathic pain

Tool	Description	Notes / drawbacks
Leeds Assessment of Neuropathic Symptoms and Signs (LANSS)	5 symptom items and 2 clinical examination items. Sensitivity 82–91% and specificity 80–94% (compared to clinical diagnosis). Validated as a self-report tool (S-LANSS, used in epidemiological studies)	Many items linked to clinical syndromes borderline to NP (e.g., CRPS); questions not specific to validated characteristic of NP, insufficient sensitivity and specificity to reliably distinguish NP from other chronic pain syndromes
Neuropathic Pain Questionnaire (NPQ)	Self-administered questionnaire, sensory examination not included. 12 items (10 sensory + 2 affective). Sensitivity 66% and specificity 74% (compared to clinical diagnosis). NPQ-short form: 3 items, similar discriminative properties	Pain etiologies not reported in the validation sample. Some items not NP-specific. Sensitivity and specificity justify its use when NP is already highly suspected. Said to be able to discriminate between NP and non-NP patients in a specialist pain clinic
Douleur Neuropathique en 4 questions (DN4).	7 symptom items and 3 clinical examination items. Easy to use. Sensitivity 83% and specificity 90% (compared to clinical diagnosis). Diagnostic tool strictly clinical. Used as a self-report questionnaire (only 7 sensory items) with similar results Highly discriminating in SCI patients	Developed and validated in French. A score ≥ 4/10 suggests NP. The DN4 questionnaire cannot establish the exclusive neuropathic nature of pain but can reliably confirm the presence of an NP component Not specifically tailored for CP
PainDETECT	9 items (self-report questionnaire). Sensitivity 85% and specificity 80% (83% of patients correctly classified to their diagnostic group)	Developed and validated in German
ID Pain	5 sensory descriptor items and 1 locator item (pain in the joints). Exact sensitivity and specificity not reported	Recommended cut-off score: 3 points (compared to clinical diagnosis, in the validation study 58% of the patients with NP scored > 3 vs. 22% of the patients with nociceptive pain and 39% of the patients with mixed pain)
Neuropathic Pain Specific Interest Group (NeuPSIG) grading system	Evaluation criteria: (1) pain with a distinct neuroanatomically plausible distribution; (2) history suggestive of a relevant lesion or disease affecting the peripheral or central somatosensory system; (3) demonstration of the distinct neuroanatomically plausible distribution by at least one confirmatory test; (4) demonstration of the relevant lesion or disease by at least one confirmatory test	Grading of certainty for the presence of NP: • definite NP: all (1–4) • probable NP: 1 and 2, + either 3 or 4 • possible NP: 1 and 2, without confirmatory evidence from 3 or 4 Relevant on a nosological and taxonomic level but hard to use in daily clinical practice
Standardized evaluation of pain (StEP)	10 physical tests and 6 questions	Validated to identify NP in patients with chronic lower back pain (axial = non-neuropathic, radicular = neuropathic). Clinical examination emphasized. Burning pain and other symptoms score negatively (in contrast with the other screening tools)
McGill Pain Questionnaire (MPQ) Short-form MPQ (SF-MPQ)	SF-MPQ: the most commonly used quality assessment tool	Not validated for NP assessment; no more sensitive to change than unidimensional intensity scales

Table 8.1. (cont.)

Tool	Description	Notes / drawbacks
SF-MPQ 2	SF-MPQ 2: recently developed, aimed at measuring neuropathic and non-neuropathic symptoms	SF-MPQ might be useful in the assessment of the sensory and affective dimensions of pain SF-MPQ 2 not fully validated
Neuropathic Pain Scale (NPS) Pain Quality Assessment Scale (PQAS)	NPS: used in several NP trials PQAS: derived from the NPS to overcome its limitations	NPS: first tool devoted to NP quality assessment. Several common NP qualities omitted; fully validated only in MS PQAS: not fully evaluated, no data about its use in blinded NP trials
Neuropathic Pain Symptom Inventory (NPSI)	Factorial structure, favoring the capture of different aspects (distinct mechanisms?) of NP	Originally validated in French. Particularly sensitive to treatment effect. Validity and reliability said to be established in patients with PNP and CP

Table 8.2. Minimal dataset of measures for clinical trials for pain after spinal cord injury (SCI)

Construct	Experts' recommended measures	Comments
Classification of pain after SCI	Proposed IASP Taxonomy or BR-SCI-PT	Low reproducibility between 3 investigators for the Tunks classification and IASP classification ($k = 0.33$–0.65); better agreement between investigators for the IASP classification (61–78%) than for the Tunks classification (45–48%) Cardenas classification: $k = 0.68$ (Cardenas *et al.* 2002) Bryce–Ragnarsson classification: mean $k = 0.70$ (0.55–0.91) (Bryce *et al.* 2007)
Pain intensity	0–10-point NRS (established validity)	There is no specific tool for evaluating pain (intensity or nature and various characteristics) in SCI patients. VAS or NRS admitted, SF-MPQ and NPSI recommended (Calmels *et al.* 2009).
Mechanical allodynia/ hyperalgesia	Brush or cotton wool and at least one high-threshold von Frey filament (unknown validity)	
Thermal allodynia/ hyperalgesia	Peltier-type thermotester (unknown validity)	
Neuropathic and nociceptive pain discrimination	LANSS (unknown validity)	
Change in neuropathic pain	NPS (unknown validity)	Multidimensional assessment tool not fully validated, lacks specificity, not very useful in daily clinical practice (Calmels *et al.* 2009)
Global improvement of pain	7-point PGIC (original Guy/Farrar) (adequate validity)	
Pain interference	SF-36 single question and MPI or BPI pain interference items (adequate validity)	No specific assessment tool available. Generic questionnaire (BPI) (Calmels *et al.* 2009)

Table 8.3. Examination protocol for central pain: Turin Advanced Neuromodulation Group (TANG) guidelines

PATIENT'S NAME AND ADDRESS
DATE
HISTORY
(1) Is pain the major or primary complaint? If not, indicate the alternative (e.g., weakness)
(2) Nature of primary neurologic disability (a) Primary diagnosis (e.g., stroke, tumor, etc.) (b) Location of disability (e.g., left hemiparesis)
(3) Date of onset of neurologic signs/symptoms • Date of onset of pain
(4) Description of pain (a) Location • Body area – preferably use pain drawing • Superficial (skin) and/or deep (muscle, viscera) • Radiation or referral (b) Intensity (0–10: VAS or NRS) • Most common intensity: at maximum; at minimum (c) Temporal features • Steady, unchanging • Fluctuates over (minutes, hours, days, weeks) • Paroxysmal features (shooting pain, tic-like) (d) Quality (e.g., MPQ) • Thermal (burning, freezing, etc.) • Mechanical (pressure, cramping, etc.) • Chemical (stinging, etc.) (e) Factors increasing the pain (cold, emotions, weather, sex, spasms, pressure sores, bladder infections, etc.) (f) Factors decreasing the pain (rest, drugs, etc.)
(5) Neurological symptoms besides pain (a) Motor (paresis, ataxia, involuntary movements) (b) Sensory (hypo/hyperesthesia, paresthesia, dysesthesia, numbness, pruritus, over-reaction) (c) Others (speech, visual, cognitive, mood, sleep, sex, etc.)
IMAGING AND OTHER STUDIES
(1) MRI/CT
(2) Angiography (traditional, CT, MR)
(3) fMRI/PET/SPECT
(4) SSEP/MEP/LEP
(5) Specialized exams (CSF assays, etc.)
TREATMENT HISTORY
(1) Oral drugs (specify doses)
(2) Neuromodulation
(3) Neuroablation
(4) Complementary and alternative medicine (CAM)

Table 8.3. (cont.)

SENSORY EXAMINATION
Preferably use sensory chart with the dermatomes. Indicate if modalities listed have normal, increased, or decreased threshold, and if paresthesias and dysesthesias are evoked.
(a) Vibratory sense (tuning fork, biothesiometer or vibrameter)
(b) Tactile (cotton wool, hair movement – include von Frey hairs if possible, nylon filaments – pressure algometry)
(c) Skin direction sense, graphesthesis
(d) Kinesthesia (joint movements)
(e) Temperature (specify how tested, e.g., Peltier's thermode, thermorolls) • Cold (noxious and innocuous); warm (noxious and innocuous)
(f) Pinprick (+ fast repetitive pricks)
(g) Deep pain (specify how tested)
(h) Allodynia • To mechanical stimuli (static: punctuate stimuli; dynamic: swab the skin with cotton several times) • To thermal stimuli (cold, heat)
(i) Hyperpathia (specify how tested)
(j) Other abnormalities like radiation, summation, prolonged after-sensation

therapy). Sensory testing should start in an unaffected area and should be compared to testing in the affected area, moving outward until skin that responds normally to stimuli is found (and vice versa when testing for evoked pains, in order to minimize the patient's exposure to painful stimuli).

Description of pain (quality, intensity, etc.) is usually assessed with several scales, the most common being the **Numerical Rating Scale** (NRS: 0, no pain; 10, worst imaginable pain) and the **Visual Analog Scale** (VAS). Outside of stroke populations, VAS is a reliable and accurate measure of pain and analgesia; however, verbal scales seem to be unsuitable in the presence of aphasia (more common in patients with left hemispheric stroke) and unilateral spatial neglect (mostly patients with right hemispheric stroke) (Benaim *et al.* 2007). Price *et al.* (1999) showed that people with stroke were less likely than an age-matched control group to correctly complete five subjective rating scales, including horizontal and vertical VAS. VAS was the most sensitive scale examined, but it had the greatest number of mistakes even in patients with posterior circulation stroke, the better-performing group. In conclusion, the use of VAS in any format as a self-report measurement tool after stroke should be approached with caution and by specialists only. The **Faces Pain Scale** (FPS) is a horizontal seven-point scale with schematic face depictions representing different level of discomfort (face 0, no pain; face 6, the worst possible pain). FPS was developed for children but is also used in cognitively impaired adults. FPS does not require speaking ability as patients simply select the face best describing their pain, but its horizontal disposition (VAS-like) could make it unsuitable in patients with unilateral spatial neglect, so theoretically a vertical version of the FPS could be used by all stroke patients (Benaim *et al.* 2007). As FPS, VAS, and NRS highly correlate, any of these three scales could be used for measuring pain severity in stroke patients, but it should be remembered that, as a gold standard for the assessment of pain in these patients is still lacking, it is possible that none of the three scales is valid. Benaim *et al.* (2007) recommend that clinicians select at least two different scales for use in daily practice (e.g. FPS and vertical colored VAS). Magnitude of CP may also be inferred indirectly by self-reports or interference with social, vocational, and daily life activities or directly from observable behavior, including facial grimace, and abnormal movement or posture.

Table 8.4. Tools for assessing central pain

Sensation (fibers)	Clinical testing	Quantitative sensory testing	Laboratory testing	Comments
Touch Vibration (Aβ)	Piece of cotton wool Tuning fork (128 Hz)	Von Frey hairs or Semmes–Weinstein monofilaments Electronic vibrameter	Nerve conduction studies (NCS) Somatosensory evoked potentials (SSEPs)	Nociceptive pathway function not assessed
Pinprick, sharp pain Cold (Aδ)	(Wooden) cocktail stick Thermoroller	Weighted needles Thermode (or probe operating on the Peltier principle)	(Late) laser-evoked potentials (Aδ-LEPs) Other EPs techniques (contact heat-evoked potentials, potentials elicited by a surface concentric electrode) No suitable laboratory tool for assessing cold	LEPs: easy and most reliable tool for assessement of the nociceptive pathway function, with high specificity but low sensitivity (increased by recently recommended normal limits) **Diagnostically useful in CP but currently not available in most centers** Other EPs techniques: diagnostic value not supported by evidence-based studies
Warmth Burning (C)	Thermoroller No clinically suitable method of assessing burning	Thermode (or probe operating on the Peltier principle)	Ultralate LEPs Contact heat-evoked potentials	Ultralate LEPs: related to C-fiber activation; recording technically too difficult for clinical applications. Insufficient available evidence for recommending any method of stimulation for assessing the C-fiber pathways. Clinical validation still lacking Usefulness in CP not assessed
			Microneurography, nerve biopsy, punch skin biopsy (IENF, intra-epidermal nerve fibers), pain-related reflexes	Useless in CP.
Evoked pain				
Dynamic mechanical allodynia		Standardized brush		Stroking skin
Thermal allodynia or hyperalgesia		Thermode		Threshold determination or pain to graded thermal stimuli
Punctate hyperalgesia		Von Frey monofilaments		Punctate stimulus
Static hyperalgesia		Pressure algometer		Mechanical pressure
Wind-up		Von Frey filaments		Temporal summation to punctate stimuli. Repetitive punctate stimuli (e.g., 2 Hz for 30 s)

Afferent function may on occasion be assessed by **differential blocks** implemented by either mechanical pressure (direct nerve compression or tourniquet ischemia) or injection of local anesthetics. Mechanical methods block fibers in order of size (Aβ, Aδ, and C) with recovery in the reverse order. These sequences are reversed for local anesthetic blocks. Such blocks help dissect the type of fibers subserving evoked pains, as each recognizes different mechanisms.

STEP 2 **High-field MRI** of the brain and cord is the neuroimaging technique of choice in all patients. It should reveal a CNS lesion that is consistent with the findings on neurologic examination. However, it cannot be relied upon exclusively in differentiating between complete and incomplete cord lesions.

STEP 3 When there is no clear-cut lesion visible on MRI, or when subtle sensory deficits cannot be confirmed by bedside sensory examination, a number of other tools may be used if available (Table 8.4), including **quantitative sensory testing (QST)**, **contact heat evoked potentials (CHEPs)**, and **laser evoked potentials (LEPs)**. LEPs, obtained by cutaneous stimulation of nociceptive fibers with pulses from an infrared or argon (or more tissue-damaging CO2) laser, will generally – but not always – reveal impaired conduction. LEPs may distinguish between CP and, e.g., fibromyalgia or psychogenic pain, and may also differ in patients with provoked pain and those with spontaneous pain only. However, neither QST nor LEPs are routinely used in the clinic, because they are time-consuming, the equipment is expensive, and results for QST may vary among examiners. Abnormalities may also be present in non-neuropathic pain states (e.g. fibromyalgia). Moreover, thresholds for thermal pain (cold in particular) vary more across sessions than other QST measures, with considerable variation from day to day. Some patients will show no sign of impairment at the time of examination: this does not exclude its presence initially. The use of QST protocols for diagnostic purposes or as outcome measures in persons with SCI and chronic pain has not been fully established, and little conclusive evidence exists regarding the use of QST in persons who have SCI and neuropathic pain (Felix and Widerström-Noga 2009).

Extreme caution should be employed when utilizing reflexive indices (e.g., nociceptive withdrawal reflex) as a measure of pain: verbal reports seem a more suitable tool to evaluate pain (Defrin *et al.* 2007a).

STEP 4 In doubtful cases, or in order to assess therapeutic response, **SPECT/PET** may be indicated as well as **pharmacological dissection** (Chapter 18). The propofol test is particularly useful in differentiating CP from (generally unresponsive) PNP and nociceptive pain in the cord trauma setting, but also the classic nociceptive shoulder pain of stroke patients.

It is unfeasible, on the basis of the topography and clinical characteristics of pain alone, to distinguish between cortical, subcortical, and thalamic lesions. Bilateral pain and dysesthesia referred to the limbs, although usually pointing to a spinal cord lesion, may be observed after unilateral brain lesions.

Section 3 Treatment

Ἰητρικὴ τεχνέων μὲν πασέων ἐστὶν ἐπιφανεςτάτη: διὰ δε ἀμαθίην τῶν τε χρεωμένων αὐτῇ, καὶ τῶν εἰκῇ τοὺς τοιούσδε κρινόντων, πολύ τι πασέων ἤδη τῶν τεχνέων ἀπολείπεται.

Medicine is the most distinguished of all the arts, but through the ignorance of those who practice it, and of those who casually judge such practitioners, it is now of all the arts by far the least esteemed.
Hippocrates, Nomos I, *1–4*

Chapter 9

Drug therapy

The reduction of pain is a prerequisite to rehabilitation, psychological treatment, and social/environmental modification. Unfortunately, CP remains one of the most ill-diagnosed and ill-treated entities among chronic pain syndromes, as proved by a simple review of the published literature. Why? Pain specialists hold wildly divergent opinions on available treatments: many rate as poor what others rate as excellent (Davies *et al.* 1991), with lack of consensus regarding management guidelines and lack of specialized expertise, and "a clear need for education in the use of particular treatments, *even* amongst those clinicians who regularly see this type of patient" (Ravenscroft *et al.* 1999). Worse still, many treatments that are considered first-line are associated with minimal relief (Cardenas and Jensen 2006). In the end, many patients change doctors because of inadequate relief.

Trial and error is the norm in the treatment of CP. As months or years go by, the typical CP patient finds no or unsatisfactory relief from the handful of drugs the average pain therapist knows and administers. Many patients end up intoxicated or develop important side effects, with addiction to opioids and benzodiazepines. Useless surgical procedures may also be attempted, usually without lasting relief. Even moderate enduring pain after any treatment can still be crippling. In a study of 70 patients suffering brain or cord CP, Sadosky and Dukes (2007) observed that, despite high adherence to drug therapy (91%), 63% still reported moderate pain and 22% severe pain. Ideally, the goal of treatment is the abolition of all pain, permanently.

We will attempt to comb out the most effective management strategies. An important caveat should be borne in mind: time is not an option. CP slowly "erodes" the will of patients, incapacitating the vast majority, sapping their resources, and must be treated aggressively, just like a "cancer of the soul." The best results for many patients will come from combination therapy in the very first place. Although many would object to prepackaged strategies for CP as a whole, we believe otherwise: pathophysiological evidence (see Section 4) strongly suggests a common substratum to all CPs. In addition, *pharmacologic dissection* helps guide therapy in the single patient.

General comments

Common to all controlled studies is the short follow-up (a few months at best), which is uninformative about long-term (years) efficacy.

The routine evaluation of clinical efficacy of a treatment is based on the use of so-called visual analog (VAS) or numerical rating (NRS) scales, supplemented by a (fantastically harlequinesque) cornucopia of others (Chapter 8). Although pain relief is more than just a change in pain intensity, such scales remain an important end-point for all assessments. Yet there is no universally accepted standard to define efficacy. Cut-offs change according to "expert" opinion: so it can be 1.8 (Hanley *et al.* 2006) or 2 or 3.3 points (Farrar *et al.* 2001, Turk *et al.* 2008) on an 11-point pain scale. Other indications have been suggested: for moderate pain, a 20% reduction on a 0–10 scale is minimal improvement, a 35% reduction is much improved, and a 45% reduction is very much improved; for severe pain, decreases on a numerical scale (NRS) have to be larger to obtain similar degrees of pain relief. In other words, the change in pain intensity that is meaningful to patients increases alongside the severity of their baseline pain (Cepeda *et al.* 2003; see also Mamie *et al.* 2000). Analgesic use as a measure of outcome is probably of poor value, as it may be complicated by dependency and coexistent nociceptive pains.

It has been said that loss of benefit is actually due to changes in the evaluative aspect of the patients' minds. Habituation involves central non-opioid frontal

Black Box. Gabapentin and pregabalin

"Killing the indigenous looks bad, but there's one thing that shareholders hate more than bad press and that's a bad quarterly statement. I didn't make up the rules." Mr Parker, in James Cameron's *Avatar* (2009)

In 2009, the *New England Journal of Medicine* divulged the details of how, over many years, Neurontin (gabapentin) had been brought to market through "misinformation and manipulation" (Landefeld and Steinman 2009). According to legal documents, a manufacturer's executive allegedly said: "We all know Neurontin's not growing for adjunctive therapy, besides that's not where the money is. Pain management, now that's money." Accordingly, a campaign was set up that involved the systematic use of deception and misinformation to create a biased evidence base and manipulate physicians' prescribing behaviors: (1) academic leaders received hundreds of thousands of dollars to promote Neurontin; (2) journals, living mostly off publicity, acquiesced to publish "pitch" articles; (3) negative trials were suppressed (Vedula *et al.* 2009). All participated in these campaigns: universities, hospitals, professional organizations, foundations, *in primis* in the USA. Neurontin's patent having expired, the manufacturer set its sights on a replacement, namely Lyrica (pregabalin), which is now receiving a similar treatment. In a *BMJ* editorial, the editors wrote:

> Like us, you have probably grown accustomed to the steady stream of revelations about incomplete or suppressed information from clinical trials of drugs and medical devices . . . Researchers for an official German drug assessment body charged with synthesising evidence on the antidepressant reboxetine encountered serious obstacles when they tried to get unpublished clinical trial information from the drug company that held the data . . . Once they were able to integrate the *astounding 74% of patient data that had previously been unpublished*, their conclusion was damning: reboxetine is "overall an ineffective and potentially harmful antidepressant" . . . This conclusion starkly contradicts the findings of other recent systematic reviews and meta-analyses published by reputable journals . . . The reboxetine story and similar episodes must call into question the entire evidence synthesis enterprise . . . our current evidence base . . . contains incomplete and questionable evidence (Godlee and Loder 2010).

Academic medicine is for sale ("drug promotion can corrupt the science, teaching, and practice of medicine"), and has been so denounced by two former editors of the *New England Journal of Medicine* (Angell 2004, Kassirer 2005) and others (Law 2006). Academic papers are often written by ghost-writers (Charlton 2008), with "academic leaders" acting as figureheads (case in point: ziconotide – see Chapter 16). Ghost-written manuscripts often downplay negative primary outcomes and emphasize other secondary outcomes and favorable subgroup analyses (e.g., a-posteriori analysis). Information is distorted to impress readers that something is noteworthy (so-called "spin"). In a representative sample of RCTs published over 1 year, more than 40% of the reports had spin in at least two of the study sections (abstracts, results, discussion, conclusions): reporting and interpretation were frequently inconsistent with the results (Boutron *et al.* 2010). Virtually all guidelines published by expert panels and involving drugs are under Big Pharma's direct control. One expert who is found often on these "pain drugs" panels is an American who works as a consultant for no fewer than 23 companies! Worst of all, false findings may be the majority or even the vast majority of published research claims (Ioannidis 2005): the greater the financial and other interests and prejudices in a scientific field, the less likely the research findings are to be true. Even "hot topics" are prone to this, as many competing teams want to be "the first."

Current medicine is one huge conflict of interest, and patients stand to lose the most. Many CP patients continue to take two or more medications despite poor analgesia: lack of treatment alternatives or lack of information cause them to maintain their insufficient drug protocol. Pain management and psychiatry are two of the most common "locales" for fraud. For instance, it has been proven that currently used antidepressants are in fact useless, being no more effective than an active placebo, and may actually be deleterious (Kirsch 2009, Whitaker 2010). Central pain too has become a "little house of horrors."

Who is to blame for this state of affairs? According to Kassirer (2005), doctors feel under-appreciated by society: inadequate respect and gratitude for their work, low pay, awful hours, high stress (whereas – for instance – soccer/football players are paid through the nose for kicking a ball). Secondly, patients expect fast (and possibly high-tech: Deyo and Patrick 2005) solutions to their problems, but medical science is not up to scratch. Why? Studies show that while the number of scientists has increased tremendously, the number of "geniuses" has not, i.e., the vast majority of scientists are mediocre and not very creative (and set upon stopping the few talented minds in order to uphold their power). It has been suggested that less endowed students, instead of taking up research, take up an administrative career and end up as heads, chiefs, or presidents (Sonnenberg 2007).

What can patients do? Become scientifically literate, for one, and stop believing that "if it's in print, it must be true."

and somatosensory cortex-dependent mechanisms (Rennefeld *et al.* 2010), and this fact must be considered. Perhaps modulating these areas might promote better effects.

CP commonly coexists with other types of pain (shoulder pain, musculoskeletal pain, etc.) and conditions (depression, anxiety, sleep disturbances, etc.) that impact quality of life. Patient education and support are critical, including careful explanation of the cause of CP and the treatment plan. Expectations must be addressed and realistic treatment goals established. The treating physician should focus on stress management, good sleep hygiene, physical therapy, and sex, among others.

Few head-to-head comparisons of different drugs are available, and different components (continuous versus evoked pains) may respond to different therapies.

Here we will list drugs that have been used for CP only; extrapolating from studies of peripheral neuropathic pains is unwarranted. When selecting a drug, one must consider the potential side-effect profile in that specific patient, potential drug interactions, comorbidities, cost, potential for abuse, and risk of overdose.

Individual variation in response is substantial and unpredictable. The approach is a stepwise process targeted to the most effective drug or combination with the fewest side effects. If only a partial effect is seen, one should add another drug with a different side effect. One may also combine a drug with quicker analgesia to a slower one. Underdosing must be avoided. A word of caution: summary NTT (number needed to treat) estimates provided in published meta-analyses are *not* a useful means of comparing the efficacy of different agents for the treatment of CP (Edelsberg and Oster 2009).

Although some believe that combination therapy may be more expensive, less tolerated, less adhered to, and also not additive (Norrbrink Budh and Lundeberg 2005), actually polypharmacy should be the norm in CP (especially for intrathecal combinations: Chapter 16). However, combinations for CP have not yet been addressed in a controlled manner.

As noted above, valuable time should not be wasted trying all possible effective drugs, and the clinician should focus on those with the best chances of success, over a defined timeline (Chapter 18). If these fail, neuromodulation should be rapidly undertaken.

Oral and parenteral drugs in clinical use

Tables 9.1–9.4 summarize the results of controlled and uncontrolled studies of oral and parenteral drugs used in the treatment of CP.

GABAergic drugs

The only parenteral drug assessed in a formal RCT is IV **propofol**, an IV anesthetic agent. Propofol effectively controlled CP at 0.2 mg/kg (one-tenth of the narcotic ED95 in humans), five times as effectively as pentothal at equipotent doses for CP. **Thiopental**, a barbiturate, is administered IV at 50 mg boluses up to 225 mg, and **thiamylal** at 50 mg IV every 5 minutes up to 250 mg: when effective, relief appears after 5–8 minutes and lasts several minutes. These drugs can be employed in drug dissection and for urgent pain control in a hospital setting.

Gabapentin in monotherapy satisfactorily relieved few patients (< 5% in our experience) and "gabapentin does not have proven utility as a monotherapy in the experience of ... [SCI] patients" (Ness *et al.* 2002). Another survey of SCI pain patients found that less than half of those who tried it were still using it, with *relatively low relief* (Cardenas and Jensen 2006) (see Black Box). In an RCT which also included nine CP patients, relief greater than 50% was seen in only 21% of patients (14% on placebo!) over 8 weeks (Serpell 2002). In SCI pain, clomipramine is more effective than gabapentin (55% vs. 48% of patients relieved: Reboiledo *et al.* 2002), and there is evidence that amitriptyline is superior to gabapentin and pregabalin, with similar rates of adverse events. Gabapentin should be used with caution in elderly and diabetic patients and abrupt withdrawal avoided. Gastrointestinal and CNS side effects are seen, along with weight gain, hypertension, impotence, urinary incontinence, myoarthralgias, and rarely Stevens–Johnson syndrome and suicidal ideation. If elected, start with 300 mg on day 1, 300 mg bid on day 2, 300 mg tid on day 3, then add 300 mg every 2–3 days in divided doses up to a maximum of 3600 mg. Maintain at effective dose for at least 2 weeks and then reevaluate.

Pregabalin is *not* recommended for the treatment of CP by the Scottish Medicines Consortium (July 2007: see *British National Formulary* March 2010, p. 277) and does not appear to be superior to gabapentin for pain management. Pregabalin should not be

Table 9.1. Controlled studies: oral drugs

Authors		Drug(s)	Final daily dose	No. of patients	Study design	Rating	Outcome	Notes	Conclusions
Davidoff *et al.* (1987b)	SCI	Trazodone HCl	150 mg	18	Randomized, double-blind, parallel, placebo-controlled (8 weeks)	Pain relief	Trazodone effects did not significantly differ from placebo	At- or below-level pain	NNT: 9 (95% CI 1.8–∞)
Leijon and Boivie (1989a)	CPSP	Carbamazepine Amitriptyline	CBZ: 800 mg AMI: 25 mg (morning) 50 mg (evening)	15	Randomized, double-blind, crossover (3 × 4 weeks, + 2 × 1 week washout), placebo-controlled	Daily pain intensity: verbal scale. Post-treatment global ratings. Comprehensive psychological rating scale	5/14 improved on CBZ 10/15 improved on AMI 1/15 improved on placebo	Double dummy (identical active or placebo). 80% men. Stepped increase to final dose of CBZ (starting at 100 mg 2 × day) and AMI (starting at 12.5 mg 2 × day). No follow-up. 1 dropout	AMI, but not CBZ, produced a statistically significant reduction of pain vs. placebo, CBZ only from 3rd week. NNT CBZ: 3.4 (95% CI 1.7–105). NNT AMI: 1.7 (95% CI 1.1–3.0). Higher plasma levels correlated with better analgesia NB: not confirmed in other studies
Drewes *et al.* (1994)	SCI	Valproate	VAL: up to 2400 mg	20	Double-blind, placebo-controlled, crossover (2 × 3 weeks, 2 weeks washout)	Pain relief: MPQ. Present pain (rating scale 1–5)	6/20 improved on VAL 4/20 improved on placebo	Low-quality study VAL: stepped increase starting at 600 mg 2 × day. Dose increased according to serum levels. 1 dropout. Blind status not clear (serum level measured)	No significant analgesic effect. NNT: 10 (95% CI 2.7–∞)
McQuay *et al.* (1994)	CPSP	Dextromethorphan	DEX: up to 81 mg	9	Randomized, double-blind, placebo-controlled, crossover. Integral *n*-of-1 design (2 × 10-day periods)	Pain relief, pain intensity, mood, sleep, global rating	0/9 improved on DEX 0/9 improved on placebo	19 patients with chronic pain. 1st treatment period: DEX 13.5 mg 3 × day; 2nd treatment period: DEX 27 mg 3 × day. No long-term clinical benefit	No significant analgesic effect for DEX

Vestergaard *et al.* (1996)	CPSP	Citalopram	CIT: 10–40 mg	9 CIT; 4 placebo	Randomized, double-blind, parallel, placebo-controlled		No dichotomous data	SSRI	No significant analgesic effect for CIT
Chiou-Tan *et al.* (1996)	SCI	Mexiletine	MEX: 450 mg	11	Randomized, double-blind, placebo-controlled, crossover (1 week washout, 2 × 4 weeks)	Pain relief: VAS, MPQ	No dichotomous data	SCI dysesthetic at- or below-level pain. 15 patients enrolled, 11 completed the study	No significant analgesia **Low-dose trial!**
Haines and Gaines (1999)	CP	Ketamine	KET: up to 100 mg/day PO	2 BCP, 3 CCP (1 MS)	*N*-of-1 randomized, controlled	Daily pain diary, VAS, Likert scale	No effect for KET during the unblended "run-in" period in any CP patient		Intolerable side effects in the whole group
Vestergaard *et al.* (2001)	CPSP	Lamotrigine	LAM: 200 mg	30	Randomized, double-blind, placebo-controlled, crossover (2 × 8 weeks, 2 weeks washout)	Pain relief: Likert scale. Global pain score. Stimulus evoked pain. Primary end-point: median pain score during the last week of treatment	12/30 improved on LAM 3/30 improved on placebo	Stepped increase to final dose of LAM (25 mg 1st–2nd week, 50 mg 3rd–4th week, 100 mg 5th–6th week, 200 mg 7th–8th week). Median pain score: LAM 200 mg: 5; placebo: 7. Significant reduction of cold allodynia. 1 patient withdrawn because LAM adverse events. ITT analysis (200 mg)	No significant effects at lower doses. LAM reduced pain score approximately 30%. LAM moderately effective for CPSP. NNT LAM: not available **Low-dose trial!**
Heiskanen *et al.* (2002)	CPSP	Dextromethorphan	DEX: 100 mg. Administration followed (4 h) by intravenous infusion of	2	Randomized, double-blind, crossover, placebo-controlled	Pain relief: VAS pain intensity, MPQ, QST	DEX had no effect on morphine analgesia. 8 patients responded to	Mixed population of 20 patients with chronic pain. DEX or placebo given 4 h prior to an IV	Results not broken down according to pain type

Table 9.1. (cont.)

Authors		Drug(s)	Final daily dose	No. of patients	Study design	Rating	Outcome	Notes	Conclusions
			morphine 15 mg				morphine after placebo	morphine administration (15 mg)	
Finnerup *et al.* (2002)	SCI	Lamotrigine	LAM: up to 400 mg	30	Randomized, double-blind, crossover, placebo-controlled (1 week baseline period, 2 × 9 weeks, 2 weeks washout)	Pain relief: change in median pain score from baseline	Categorical slight to complete pain relief (secondary outcome measure): 10/22 on LAM, 5/22 on placebo	At- or below-level pain. Slow LAM increase. 22 patients completed the study. LAM more effective in patients with brush-evoked allodynia and wind-up like pain (7/7 pain relief vs. 1/14 without). 3 patients withdrawn because of adverse events. ITT analysis (200 mg)	No statistically significant effect of LAM in the total sample. In 7/8 patients with incomplete cord lesions LAM was more effective than placebo on at- or below-level pain. NNT LAM (incomplete lesions, 50% pain relief): 12 (2–∞)
Cardenas *et al.* (2002)	SCI No CP in some patients	Amitriptyline Benztropine besilate (active placebo)	AMI: 10–125 mg 0.5 mg	(84) 26 SCI pain, 6 transition zone pain	Randomized, double-blind, placebo-controlled (6 weeks)	Pain relief: average pain intensity (NRS, 0–10). MPQ, BPI, FIM (functional independence measure), SWLS (satisfaction with life scale), CHART (Craig handicap assessment and reporting techniques)	No dichotomous data	84 patients. 44 patients AMI, 40 placebo. ITT analysis and study completers analysis	No significant differences between AMI and placebo in pain intensity (also with regression analysis for different types of pain) or pain-related disability. SWLS > in placebo group. Certain subgroups of patients may benefit. 18% of patients chose to continue AMI, but 5% chose to continue placebo. No significant difference in AMI/placebo side effects

Lampl *et al.* (2002)	CPSP	Amitriptyline extended release	AMI: 75 mg	19 AMI, 20 placebo	Randomized, double-blind, placebo-controlled (1 year)	Prophylactic treatment of patients with acute thalamic stroke to prevent CPSP	Primary end-point: occurrence of CPSP within 1 year	AMI was slowly titrated from 10 to 75 mg in extended release. CPSP in AMI group: 4/18 patients; CPSP in placebo group: 3/19 patients	The placebo group showed a pain rate of 21% within 1 year, vs. 17% in AMI group. AMI not beneficial in preventing the onset of CPSP
Tai *et al.* (2002)	SCI	Gabapentin	GBP: 1800 mg	7	Prospective, randomized, double-blind, placebo-controlled, crossover (2 × 4 weeks, 2 weeks washout)	Pain relief: NPS	**GBP = placebo** among pain descriptors (except "unpleasant feeling")	Results limited by the small sample size and **low maximum dosage of GBP**	**Non-significant** trend to benefit on unpleasant feeling, pain intensity, and burning sensation only
Harden *et al.* (2002)	SCI	Topiramate	TOP: 800 mg (titrated over 10 weeks)	9 (+ 5)	Parallel, randomized, placebo-controlled	Pain relief: VAS and descriptor scale	TOP = placebo (below 800 mg). TOP > placebo on descriptor scale but not VAS scale in final 2 weeks only at 800 mg	Many side effects at 800 mg	
Rowbotham *et al.* (2003)	CP	Levorphanol	LEV: 0.15 or 0.75 mg to a maximum of 21 capsules/day	23 (10 CPSP, 5 SCI, 8 MS)	Randomized, double-blind, dose-response (8 weeks)	Pain relief: VAS (0–10 cm). Primary outcome: mean pain rating	% reduction from baseline. Low strength: CPSP: 6; SCI: 13; MS: 9. High strength: CPSP: 16; SCI: 30; MS: 63	Patients who completed the study: 15. CPSP: 3/10 (mean pain reduction: 20%). SCI: 4/5 (mean pain reduction: 22%). MS: 8/8 (mean pain reduction: 27%). Low strength (mean pain reduction): CPSP: 14; SCI: 13; MS: 9. High-strength (mean pain reduction): CPSP: 23; SCI: 31; MS: 63	Capsules intake titrated by the patient. 7 of 10 patients with CPSP did not complete the study (reasons unknown). 27% of patients withdrew. SCI pain may have included CP. MS pain may have included dysesthetic pain

Table 9.1. (cont.)

Authors		Drug(s)	Final daily dose	No. of patients	Study design	Rating	Outcome	Notes	Conclusions
			Low strength: mean daily dosage: 2.7 mg High strength: mean daily dosage: 8.9 mg	5 CPSP, 2 SCI, 4 MS 5 CPSP, 3 SCI, 4 MS					
Morley *et al.* (2003)	NP	Methadone	MET: 10 or 20 mg/day	19 (2 CPSP, 1 transverse myelitis)	Randomized, double-blind, placebo-controlled	Pain relief (maximum pain intensity, average pain intensity, and pain relief): VAS	Average pain intensity MET vs. placebo (VAS). MET 10 mg: CPSP1: 59 vs. 65.8; CPSP2: 33.4 vs. 46.4; CCP: 47.8 vs. 42.8. MET 20 mg: CPSP1: 66.9 vs. 66.6; CPSP2: 26.6 vs. 47; CCP: not tested	All patients poor responders to traditional analgesic regimen	10 mg/day: not statistically significanct. 20 mg/day: statistically significant pain improvement. The analgesic effects extended over 48 hours
Wade *et al.* (2003, 2004)	MS SCI	Plant-derived cannabis medicinal extracts (CME)	Delta-9-tetrahydro-cannabinol/cannabidiol (THC, CBD), 1:1, or CBD:THC, sublingual spray doses of 2.5–120 mg/day	24 (18 MS, 4 SCI)	Consecutive series of double-blind, randomized, placebo-controlled single-patient crossover trials (2 weeks)	Patients recorded symptoms, well-being, and intoxication scores on a daily basis: VAS + NRS+Barthel index observer rating (at 2 weeks)	Pain relief associated with both THC and CBD was significantly superior to placebo	Self-administered sublingual spray. Dose titration against symptom relief or unwanted effects (hypo-tension, intoxication on rapid titration)	CME indicated for refractory patients. Unwanted effects predictable and generally well tolerated
Karst *et al.* (2003)	NP	CT-3 (analog of THC-11-oic acid)	CT-3: 80 mg	21 (8 women) Hyperalgesia in 21 cases, allodynia in 7 cases. Traumatic SCI (L1): 3 patients (pain in one or both legs). Post-surgical tethered cord (removal of IT	Randomized, placebo-controlled, double-blind crossover, two 7-day crossover treatments. CT-3 (20 mg bid for 4 days then 40 mg bid for 3 days). Identical	Pain relief: VAS, NRS. Vital signs, hematologic and blood chemistry, ECG. Trail-Making Test, Addiction Research Center Inventory–Marijuana scale. Adverse effects	VAS mean differences (3 h after intake of study drug): significant difference between CT-3 and placebo (mean [SD], −11.54 [14.16] vs. 9.86 [21.43]; $p = 0.02$). No	Concomitant analgesic use allowed. *Results in patients with CCP not reported separately*	CT-3 was effective in reducing chronic NP compared to placebo

				ependymoma at C4 to T1): 1 patient (whole-body pain below the shoulders)	capsule no. for placebo. Washout and baseline period (1 week). Analogous crossed over second 7-day treatment period		major adverse effects observed		
Svendsen *et al.* (2004)	MS-CP	Dronabinol	DRO: maximum 10 mg/day	24	Randomized, double blind, placebo controlled, crossover (2 × 3 weeks, 15–21 days; 2 weeks, 19–57 days; washout)	Median spontaneous pain intensity (numerical rating scale) in the last week of treatment. QST	Median spontaneous pain intensity significantly lower with DRO than placebo. Median pain relief score: VAS 3 vs. 0		DRO has a modest analgesia on MS-CP. NNT for 50% pain relief: 3.5 (95% CI 1.9–24.8)
Levendoglu *et al.* (2004)	SCI (complete, thoracic, and lumbar)	Gabapentin	GBP: maximum 3.6 g/day (gradually titrated dosage)	20	Prospective, randomized, double-blind, placebo-controlled, crossover (18 weeks; 4 weeks medication/ placebo titration, 4 weeks stable maximum tolerated dose, 4 weeks crossover medication/ placebo titration, 4 weeks stable maximum tolerated dose)	Pain relief: NPS, VAS (0–100), Lattinen's questionnaire (adapted)	GBP reduced intensity and frequency of pain, and improved quality of life. **Neuropathic pain descriptors not relieved: itchy, sensitive, dull, and cold**	All patients completed the study. Mean effective dose: 2235 mg. Dysesthetic pain included. *Below-level pain not specifically mentioned*	
Carlsson *et al.* (2004)	SCI	Dextromethorphan	DEX: 270 mg	2	Randomized, double-blind, placebo-controlled, crossover (2 separate administrations)	Pain relief: VAS (0–100)	No effect in 1 patient, 69% VAS reduction in 1 patient	Study population: 15 patients with neuropathic pain of traumatic origin. Most patients experienced adverse effects (none severe)	A single high dose of DEX has an analgesic effect (up to 30% pain reduction vs. placebo)

Table 9.1. (cont.)

Authors		Drug(s)	Final daily dose	No. of patients	Study design	Rating	Outcome	Notes	Conclusions
Notcutt *et al.* (2004)	MS pain	Cannabis extract	Wide range of dosing	16	Randomized, placebo controlled		Benefit at no fixed dose	Side effects comparable to psychoactive drugs	
Rog *et al.* (2005)	MS	Whole-plant cannabis-based medicine (CBM; delta-9-tetrahydrocannabinol: cannabidiol (THC:CBD))	THC 2.7 mg; CBD 2.5 mg (each spray). Gradual self-titration to a max. 48 spray/day	66	Randomized, double-blind, placebo-controlled, parallel group (5 weeks: 1 week run-in, 4 weeks treatment)	Daily pain and sleep disturbance (11-point numerical rating scale). NPS. Cognitive function, mood, MS-related disability, PGIC	Trial completed by 64 patients (97%): 32 CBM patients (2 withdrawn), 32 placebo patients. ITT analysis. Results at week 4 (mean change): pain intensity: CBM: −2.7 (95% CI −3.4 to −2.0); placebo: −1.4 (95% CI −2.0 to −0.8, $p = 0.005$). Sleep disturbance: CBM: −2.5 (95% CI −3.4 to −1.7); placebo: −0.8 (95% CI −1.5 to −0.1, $p = 0.003$)	Inclusion criteria: patients with spontaneous or evoked dysesthetic pain (burning, aching, pricking, stabbing, and squeezing) and patients with painful tonic spasms. CBM generally well tolerated (1 patient withdrawn because of adverse effects, but more patients on CBM than placebo reported dizziness, dry mouth, and somnolence)	CBM delivered via an oromucosal spray, as adjunctive analgesic treatment. Mean number of daily sprays: CBM 9.6 ± 6 (range 2–25), placebo: 19.1 ± 12.9 (range 1–47). THC: CBD ratio ≈ 1:1 (other cannabis-based compounds < 10%). CBM was superior to placebo in reducing the mean intensity of pain and sleep disturbance. PGIC: no difference between the proportion of patients rating themselves as "much improved" or "very much improved" in the CBM group (9/34) vs. placebo group (4/32). Cognitive side effects: limited to long-term memory storage

Siddall *et al.* (2006)	CCP (SCI)	Pregabalin		PGB: 460 mg (average, 3rd week; max. 600 mg)	70 PGB, 67 placebo (83% men). Pain at least 1 dermatome below LOI in 130 (94.9%). CP likely in 131/137 (95.6%) (indeterminate in 6) or in 125/128 (97.7%) with lesions above L2 (clinical conclusion)	Randomized, placebo-controlled, parallel groups, multicenter study. Baseline week + 12-week study (3-week titration period + 9-week fixed dose period). Flexible-dose PGB (150–600 mg/d) administered bid. ITT analysis; completion rate: PGB patients: 70%, placebo patients: 55%	Primary efficacy measure: end-point mean (last 7 days) pain score (NRS, patient's diary). Secondary end-points: pain responder rates, SF-MPQ, MOS sleep scale, HADS, PGIC. Tolerability and safety assessments. Additional analysis: % of patients with ≥ 30% and ≥ 50% pain score reduction (baseline vs. end-point = responder analyses), NNT	Mean end-point pain score: PGB patients: 4.62; placebo patients: 6.27 ($p < 0.001$). Mean treatment difference (pain at end-point), 1.53 (95% CI 0.9–2.1, $p < 0.001$, excluding patients with lesions at or below L2) in favor of PGB. Efficacy observed from the 1st week, lasting for the duration of the study. PGB significantly more effective than placebo (end-point assessments): SF-MPQ, ≥ 30% and ≥ 50% pain responder rates ($p < 0.05$), MOS and HADS improvements ($p < 0.001$ and $p < 0.05$), PGIC ($p < 0.001$). **NNT: 30% responder rate = 3.9; 50% responder rate = 7.1**. Severe end-point pain in 15.9% PGB patients vs. 43.3% placebo patients	In most patients below-level CP (IASP criteria). Baseline VAS > 4 cm required at admission. Mean pain duration about 10 years. Mean baseline pain score: PGB patients: 6.54, placebo patients: 6.73. % of patients taking medicationns at baseline: 95.6% PGB as add-on analgesic in 70% of patients (concurrent medications allowed at constant dose during the trial) Most common adverse events: transient somnolence and dizziness. Withdrawals due to side effects: 15 PGB vs. 9 placebo patients	**Biased paper**: **(1) Strong ties between authors and manufacturer** **(2) Industry-sponsored, possible, intentional (?) GBP withdrawal state in some patients** **(3) Unclear randomization/ allocation/ concealment** **(4) Possible understatement of side effects in PGB patients** **(5) At-level pain not clearly dissociable from below-level pain (1 dermatome below the LOI!)**

Table 9.1. (cont.)

Authors		Drug(s)	Final daily dose	No. of patients	Study design	Rating	Outcome	Notes	Conclusions
Harden *et al.* (2006)	MS-CP	Levetiracetam	LEV: 3000 mg	4 (MS)	Double-blind, randomized, crossover, placebo controlled 2-week baseline/ washout + LEV/ placebo + washout + crossover	Daily VAS, PPI, SF-MPQ	High daily pain variability in MS patients (analysis impossible)	Abstract. Pilot study. Never published as full paper	
Breuer *et al.* (2007)	MS-CP	Lamotrigine	LAM: 400 mg (max.)	12 (15 enrolled, 12 included in the efficacy analysis [at least 1st period of the study completed], 11 completed both periods)	Randomized, double-blind, placebo-controlled, 2-period, crossover pilot. 8 weeks double-blind titration period + 3 weeks maintenance period + 2 weeks tapering period + 2 weeks washout, 2 ×	BPI, NPS, MSQOL-54. Daily diary (SF-BPI, use of other analgesic drugs, changes in health, and occurrence of adverse events). Primary outcome measure: mean pain intensity score during the final maintenance week of each of the 2 study periods	LAM dose: 400 mg/d : 8 patients, 300 mg/d 1 patient, 100 mg/d 1 patient, 50 mg/d 1 patient. No statistically significant difference between LAM and placebo in pain-related outcomes (rate of responders: 5/11 LAM, 2/11 placebo) or QOL. Adverse events: 1 rash (herpes zoster). Withdrawals: 1 LAM and 1 placebo patient (mild adverse events, 1st period)	Preliminary study (feasibility and effect size for sample size determination) for a planned larger trial. 10 women. Mean age: 49.3 ± 11.7 years. Probable or definite MS + NP for at least 3 months Titration period: LAM dose increased until total relief, unmanageable adverse events or 400 mg/day	The results support neither the use of LAM in patients with MS-CP nor the need for a larger trial

Rintala *et al.* (2007)	SCI	Amitriptyline (AMI) Gabapentin (GBP) Diphenhydramine (antihistamine, active placebo)	AMI: 50 mg tid (max. dose) GBP: 1200 mg tid (max. dose) Placebo: 25 mg tid	38 (36 men), at- and below-level pain (42 patients needed to detect a VAS difference of 1.8 according to a sample size calculation made in the planning phase). 22 patients (58%) completed all 3 phases (26 GBP phase, 28 AMI phase, 25 placebo phase)	Randomized, controlled, double-blind, triple crossover. 6 groups, medication order: (1) GAP (2) GPA (3) AGP (4) APG (5) PGA (6) PAG. Each drug administered for 9 weeks 31 weeks duration: (1) baseline week; (2) daily drug dose gradually increased (first 4 weeks) then kept constant (if possible, 4 weeks); (3) medication gradually tapered off (9th week); (4) washout week (10th week)	Primary outcome variable: pain intensity (VAS + NRS); depression (CESD-SF), amount of medication taken for breakthrough pain, dropout rates, side effects, medication cost. Patients' evaluation: end of the baseline week, + weeks 2, 4, (6), 8, 10 (during each of the 3 medication phases)	Mean VAS ratings (week 8, 22 completers): AMI: 3.46 ± 2.09; GBP 4.85 ± 2.86; placebo 5.11 ± 2.54 (= AMI more effective than GPB, $p = 0.03$, or placebo, $p = 0.012$, t-test). High baseline CESD-SF patients: AMI 4.21, placebo 6.67 ($p = 0.035$), GBP 6.68 ($p = 0.061$). **GBP no more effective than placebo** ($p = 0.97$). Low CESD-SF patients: no significant difference among AMI, GBP, placebo	Patients with > 6 months NP pain, rated ≥ 5 on a VAS. Baseline VAS scores: low CESD-SF (< 10) patients: 4.61; high CESD-SF (> 10) patients: 7.41. Oxycodone + acetaminophen for breakthrough pain but no other pain medications allowed. Drug dosage reduced if needed (severe side effects). Non-significant trend suggesting AMI more effective than GBP in high baseline CESD-SF patients.. No significant differences in secondary outcome measures Monthly cost of medication: AMI \$1.76, GBP \$31.59. *Results on at-and below-level pain not differentiated*	**AMI was more efficacious than placebo and GBP** in relieving at- or below-level SCI pain. Results not attributable to dropout rates, order or dose of medications, amount of medication taken for breakthrough pain, or side effects

Table 9.1. (cont.)

Authors		Drug(s)	Final daily dose	No. of patients	Study design	Rating	Outcome	Notes	Conclusions
Silver *et al.* (2007)	Mixed NP incomplete SCI, MS	Lamotrigine	LAM: up to 400 mg/day	LAM: 111 Placebo: 109 SCI: 3 (2 LAM, 1 placebo) MS: 9 (7 LAM, 2 placebo)	Randomized, double-blind, placebo-controlled parallel group up to 14 weeks duration (including 8 weeks of dose escalation). Flexible LAM dose (200, 300, or 400 mg/day)	Primary end-point: mean change in pain-intensity (baseline to week 14). Secondary end-points: SF-MPQ, NPS, rescue medication use, CGIC, PGIC	No statistically significant difference in any of the pre-specified outcome efficacy measures between LAM and placebo	LAM as add-on drug (patients with NP inadequately controlled by gabapentin, TCA, or a non-opioid analgesic). Mean weekly pain score ≥ 4 on an 11-point NRS. *LAM effects on SCI and MS-CP unknown (results not broken down according to pain cause)*	
Vranken *et al.* (2008)	CPSP SCI	Pregabalin	PGB: 460 mg (starting dose 150 mg/day; average 600 mg/day in 9 and 300 mg/day in 8 patients)	76; 40 randomized. 19 CPSP (4 thalamic, 3 BS infarction, 12 strokes). 21 SCI (11 complete lesion). Patients arranged into 8 categories of different size based on sex, age, diagnosis (BCP, CCP). Study completed by 17 PGB patients and 16 placebo patients	Randomized, double-blind, placebo-controlled, parallel study, 4 weeks. Flexible-dose regimen, no base-line period, escalating doses of PGB (150, 300, and 600 mg/day) or matching placebo. If insufficient pain relief, 3-day interval titration until VAS reduced 1.8 points or max. 600 mg/day reached or intolerable side-effects	Primary efficacy measure: pain intensity (VAS). Tolerability, PDI, and EQ-5D (health status), SF-36 (quality of life). Mean end-point pain score: average of 3 VAS scores measured in the last 24 h of treatment) Predefined visits: baseline, start of the trial, end of weeks 1 and 4. Phone consultations at weeks 2 and 3	Mean pain intensity (VAS, ± SD) before and after 4 weeks of treatment: placebo: 7.4 (± 1.0) – 7.3 (± 2.0); PGB: 7.6 (± 0.8) – 5.1 (± 2.9). Statistically significant decrease in end-point mean pain score for PGB (VAS-score difference from placebo: 2.18, 95% CI 0.57–3.80; $p = 0.01$, t-test). No difference in pain relief between BCP and CCP. Statistically significant improvement for the EQ-5D, bodily	LANSS score > 12 and baseline VAS > 6 in all patients. Allodynia in 17+17 patients. *Gabapentin (if taken) discontinued at least 3 days before receiving PGB as add-on analgesic.* Concurrent medications allowed: opioids (53% of patients), ADs (20%), CBZ (10%), baclofen (10%.), NSAID. Withdrawal: 3 PGB and 3 placebo-treated patients (side effects)	**Flexible-dose PGB produced modest relief, as PGB patients still reported VAS 5 (mean) at end of trial *Possible (intentional?) GBP withdrawal state in some patients; randomization took place after all patients were recruited***

					Final dose maintained until end of study		pain domain of the SF36 (no statistically significant difference in the other domains) No significant difference in PDI		
Frank *et al.* (2008)	Myelopathy Spinal artery thrombosis SCI Transverse myelitis CP	Dihydrocodeine (DHC) Nabilone (NAB)	DHC 240 mg/day (max. dosage) NAB 2 mg/day (max. dosage)	96 randomized (73 included in the available case analysis, 64 included in the per-protocol analysis DHC/NAB group: 2 myelopathy, 2 spinal artery thrombosis, 1 SCI, 1 transverse myelitis, 10 CP NAB/DHC: 4 myelopathy, 4 transverse myelitis, 20 CP	Randomized, double-blind, controlled, crossover 14 weeks' duration (6 weeks of escalating treatment + 2-week washout period + 6 weeks treatment) Treatment allocation: random permuted blocks of 10. Sample size calculations (90% power to detect a difference of 60% in mean VAS, $p = 0.05$): 30 patients/ treatment	Primary outcome: pain difference (VAS) between nabilone and dihydrocodeine (last 2 weeks of treatment). Secondary outcomes: changes in mood, quality of life, sleep, and psychometric function (HAD score, SF-36 form, six psychometric tests). Side effects (questionnaire)	Mean baseline VAS score: 69.6 mm (range 29.4–95.2). on a 0–100 mm scale Available case analysis: mean score 6.0 mm longer for NAB than for DHC (95% CI 1.4 to 10.5). Per-protocol analysis: mean score 5.6 mm (10.3 to 0.8) longer for NAB. More frequent side effects with NAB but no major AEs for either drug.	Only patients with mean VAS > 40mm admitted to the study. Other analgesics allowed except for dihydrocodeine and cannabinoids. Pre-specified visits at weeks 0, 2, 4, 6, 8, 10, 12, 14. Trial not completed by 33 patients	DHC provided better pain relief than NAB and had slightly fewer side effects *Results not broken down according to pain type/origin*
Wilsey *et al.* (2008)	SCI-CP MS-CP PNP	Cannabis (delta-9 THC, smoked)	High-dose (7%), low-dose (3.5%), placebo cigarettes	38 (6 SCI-CP, 4 MS-CP)	Randomized, double-blind, placebo-controlled, crossover, mixed linear model analysis	Primary outcome measure: pain intensity (VAS). Secondary outcome measures: NPS, evoked pain variations (HPT, sensitivity to light touch), psychoactive side effects, neuropsychological performance	Analgesic response without effect on evoked pain. Minimal psychoactive effects + some acute cognitive effects (memory, at higher doses)	*Results not broken down according to pain type*	Cannabis may be effective at ameliorating NP. Use may be limited by its method of administration (smoking) and modest acute cognitive effects

Table 9.1. (cont.)

Authors		Drug(s)	Final daily dose	No. of patients	Study design	Rating	Outcome	Notes	Conclusions
Finnerup *et al.* (2009)	CCP (SCI)	Levetiracetam	LEV: from 500 mg bid to 1.5 g bid (week 3–5, max. dosage). Final dose reduced to 2 or 2.5 g/day if unacceptable adverse events LEV as add-on drug in 58% of patients	24/36 randomized SCI patients (17 at-level, 31 below-level; evoked pain in 15)	Randomized, double-blind, placebo-controlled, crossover, multicenter. 1-week baseline period + 2 × 5 weeks treatment periods (1-week washout period) Power calculation: 30 patients = power > 90% (α = 0.05)	Primary outcome: change in median daily pain score (NRS) from baseline to the last week of each treatment period. Secondary outcome: relief of overall, at-, and below-level pain, allodynia, spasm, and spasticity	LEV ineffective (primary outcome $p = 0.46$ [Kock's adapt. Wilcoxon test] and secondary outcome measures). Early discontinuation: 4 patients, only 4 weeks LEV: 3 patients. LEV generally without serious adverse events.	Computer-generated block randomization Usual (but no ADs) pain treatment continuation allowed (constant dose). Final dose at least 2 g/day for at least 2 weeks only in 24/36 randomized patients Also evaluated: no. of patients with 33% pain relief, sleep interference, use of escape medications, symptoms change (NPSI). LEV continued only by 2 patients after trial completion (1 at the 6-month follow-up)	LEV does not relieve NP or spasm severity following SCI Possible study limitation: heterogeneity of the group
Norrbrink and Lundeberg (2009)	CCP (SCI)	Tramadol	TRA: median max. dose 250 mg (range: 100–400 mg) TRA: 50 mg PO tid (starting dose); 50 mg increase	36; 35 included in the ITT analysis (at least 1 dose of medication assumed). 23 TRA, 12 placebo	Randomized (2:1 ratio), double-blind, placebo-controlled. 4 weeks. Mean treatment duration: TRA: 18.8 ± 10.8 days (range 1–30); placebo: 25.1 ±	Daily diary, CR-10 scale, MPI, HAD scale (mood), Li-Sat 9 (life satisfaction), quality of sleep, PGIC, side effects. Primary outcome measures: pain intensity, PGIC	Evaluation (4th week, TRA vs. placebo patients): significant improvement (but **small changes in median scores**) in pain intensity ratings (including	At- or below-level SCI pain, duration > 6 months, intensity > 3 on Borg's CR-10 scale. Baseline: pain + sensory modalities assessement	Slow individualized titration to minimize the risk of adverse events

			every 5 days (max. dose: 400 mg/day)		10.1 days (range 7–30)		pain severity on the MPI-S) and anxiety ratings. Favorable effect on the PGIC in 7/12 TRA patients vs. 1/11 placebo patients. Side effects in 91% of TRA patients vs. 58% of placebo patients. Substantial adverse events: 48% withdrawals in TRA patients vs. 17% in placebo patients	(including dynamic mechanical allodynia). Higher levels of pain in placebo patients Previous stable pain medication allowed (concomitant analgesic medication in 61% of TRA patients and 50% of placebo patients)	
Rossi *et al.* (2009)	MS-CP	Levetiracetam (500 mg tablets)	LEV: 3000 mg/day LEV dose reduced to 2 g due to adverse effects in 2 patients	20 (15 women): 12 LEV, 8 placebo	Single-center, prospective, randomized, single-blind, placebo-controlled 3 months 1 tablet bid (1st week), gradually increased to 3 tablets bid starting from the 4th week	VAS (pain intensity, evaluated for 3 consecutive months). EDSS (disability), HDS (depression), MSQoL-54 (quality of life) at study entry and at 3rd month. Changes in VAS > 2 cm considered clinically important.	Statistically significant mean VAS difference in LEV vs. placebo patients ($p < 0.05$, 2nd and 3rd month). Significant VAS reduction only in LEV patients over time ($p < 0.05$) Patients with VAS reduction > 2 cm (LEV vs. placebo): 1st month 18.2% vs. 12.5%; 2nd month 72.7% vs. 12.5%; 3rd month 81.8% vs. 14.3%; differences statistically significant ($p <$ 0.05) starting at 2nd month). Degree of pain reduction related to the severity of baseline pain	Patients non-responsive or intolerant to conventional medications (AEDs, TCAs, duloxetine, baclofen). Patients with trigeminal neuralgia, back pain, visceral pain, and painful tonic spasms not included. No adjunctive pain-relieving medications allowed. Pain type: LEV group: continous (C) 66%, intermittent (I) 17%, C/I 17%; placebo group: C 62.5%, I 37.5%, C/I 0%.	LEV well tolerated, beneficial against MS-CP, improves quality of life of MS patients

Table 9.1. (cont.)

Authors		Drug(s)	Final daily dose	No. of patients	Study design	Rating	Outcome	Notes	Conclusions
							only in LEV group ($p < 0.05$)	3 withdrawals (2 LEV, somnolence, MS relapse; 1 placebo, severe pain). ITT analysis not permitted. Overall rating of QoL significantly improved in LEV group	
Chitsaz *et al.* (2009)	MS-CP	Nortriptyline Self-applied TENS	NTP: 50 mg	59 patients. NTP: 30 patients TENS: 29 patients. Sample size calculation: 30 patients in each group = 80% power to detect (2-sided α = 0.05) a mean clinically relevant VAS difference (= 2 points)	Randomized, single-blinded, concealed treatment allocation 8 weeks NTP: 10 mg/day for 3 days, then 25 mg/day for 4 days, then 50 mg; TENS: tid, 20–30 mins + at occurrence of pain and/or sensory complaints. Electrodes 3 cm apart over the symptomatic area. 60 Hz, 40 μs, rectangular monophasic waves. Stimulus strength below the motor threshold, intensity level set to produce a tingling sensation	Structured interview, physical assessment, self-reported VAS, use of medication, adverse effects. Response to treatment assessed at 2, 4, and 8 weeks	**TENS = NTP**. Significant decrease in VAS (pain and/or sensory complaints) in both groups. VAS decrease (pain and/or sensory complaints, baseline vs. 8 weeks): NTP: from 4.9 ± 1.9 to 3.3 ± 2.1 ($p < 0.001$). TENS: from 5.3 ± 1.6 to 2.8 ± 1.5 ($p < 0.001$). Mean difference in VAS between the 2 groups (at 8 weeks follow-up): –0.5 (95% CI –1.5 to 0.5, ns). NTP generally well tolerated	EDSS ≤ 6, at least 2 years of MS Chronic and episodic pain and/or sensory complaints (including burning sensations, TN, numbness, or itching) of the upper extremities Only pain or sensory symptoms (e.g., paresthesia or dysesthesia) with unpleasant feelings included	Both NTP and TENS effective Given the side-effect profile of NTP, TENS may have some benefits over NTP Study limitations: lack of double blinding, relatively short follow-up, not placebo-controlled

Rintala *et al.* (2010)	SCI	Dronabinol Diphenhydramine (antihistamine, active placebo)	DRO: 20 mg/day Placebo: 75 mg Starting dose: DRO 5 mg/day, placebo 25 mg/day at bedtime. DRO + 5 mg every 3rd day up to 5 mg qid	7 below-level pain (2 women, 5 men); 4 paraplegic; 3 tetraplegic. Mean age 50.1 ± 8.3 years. Anticipated recruitment of 15 patients, with 11 completing both arms	Randomized, controlled, double-blind, crossover Upward titration: 12 days; stabilization phase: 7 days; maintenance phase: 28 days (steady dose of medication); downward titration: 9 days; washout phase: 7 days (breakthrough medication only); second study medication (same schedule)	Average pain intensity (BPI item = 0–10 NRS); side effects	5 patients analyzed. No significant VAS difference (DRO vs. placebo: baseline vs. end of the maintenance phase: 0.2 ± 0.84 vs. −1.8 ± 2.5, $p = 0.10$; maintenance phase: − 0.2 ± 0.67, vs. −1.40 ± 1.25, $p = 0.10$, Wilcoxon test). Most common side effects (both medications): dry mouth, constipation, fatigue, drowsiness	Pilot study. Patients with > 6 months NP, rated ≥ 5 on a VAS, at least 3 levels below the LOI. Average worst pain intensity: at screening 8.1 ± 1.6. 2 patients excluded due to too low baseline pain intensity (2 on a 0–10 scale) Oxycodone + acetaminophen for breakthrough pain but no other pain medications allowed. 2 withdrawals on DRO (in 1 case refusal to be switched to the 2nd medication)	**DRO no more effective than placebo for below-level NP**; side effects common Study limitations: very small sample size; measure of average pain intensity based on single reports; maybe inadequate washout period; reliance on self-reports by the patients; weaning off all current pain medications; occasional bits of missing data
Vranken *et al.* (2011)	CP (BCP, CCP; at-level pain also possible)	Duloxetine	DUL: 60 mg/day (8 patients) or 120 mg/day (15 patients); mean: 99.1 ± 29.2 mg/day	48 (24 DUL, 24 placebo)	Randomized, double-blind, placebo-controlled 3-step randomization (step 2: randomization by minimization) 8-week duration Flexible dose. Starting dose: 1 capsule/day (= DUL 60 mg/day or matching placebo). If insufficient pain relief (VAS reduction < 1.8): 2 capsules/day	Blinded visits at baseline, at the start and end of the trial (week 8). Telephone consultations at weeks 2, 4, and 6. Primary efficacy measure: pain intensity score (pain diary, self-recorded VAS, spontaneous and evoked pain). Mean pain score based on the average of 9 VAS scores Secondary end-points: health status and quality of life (EQ5D, PDI, SF-36, PGIC, QST	Mean pain intensity VAS (± SD) before and after 8 weeks: placebo 7.2 (± 0.8) vs. 6.1 (± 1.7) (15% pain reduction); DUL 7.1 (± 0.8) vs. 5.0 (± 2.0) (> 2 points on the VAS, 29.6% pain reduction). DUL vs. placebo: trend towards a statistically significant decrease in mean	Inclusion criteria: VAS ≥ 6, DN4 score > 3. Concomitant analgesic medication allowed if on a stable regimen apart from antidepressants (discontinued at least 30 days before entering study). No new analgesic therapies allowed during the trial DUL patients: mean age 50.4 ±	**No significant effect on pain intensity** Outcome cannot be attributed to high placebo response Study of sufficient power

Table 9.1. (cont.)

Authors		Drug(s)	Final daily dose	No. of patients	Study design	Rating	Outcome	Notes	Conclusions
					(= DUL 120 mg or placebo) Single downward dose titration after a 1-week interval allowed, then final dosage during the remainder of the study period. Sample size calculation: 24 + 24 patients = 90% power to detect a clinically relevant 25% decrease in mean VAS (from 7.3 [placebo] to 5.4 [DUL], assuming a common SD = 2 and using a two-group t-test with a 0.05 two-sided significance level)	[in the area with maximal pain: tactile pain threshold (static allodynia), brush-induced (dynamic) tactile allodynia, cold allodynia, mechanical static (punctuate) hyperalgesia, pinprick-evoked pain, pressure pain threshold]), safety of DUL. Data analyzed on an ITT basis. NNT (reduction of pain by at least 30% or 50%) reported	pain score ($p = 0.056$) No difference in response to DUL between SCI patients ($n = 18$) and CPSP patients ($n = 6$) ($p = 0.61$). NNT 30%, and 50% pain relief 3.4 and 24 Other statistically significant results (DUL vs. placebo): alleviation of dynamic ($p = 0.035$) and cold allodynia ($p < 0.001$), improvement for the bodily pain domain on the SF36 ($p = 0.035$). No difference in adverse effects between groups	9.4 years, mean VAS 7.1 (± 0.8), brain abscess 1 case, CPSP 5 cases, SCI 18 cases Placebo patients: mean age 50.4 ± 10.1 years, mean VAS 7.2 (± 0.8), CPSP 8 cases, SCI 16 cases. Dynamic tactile allodynia (brush) and cold allodynia significantly reduced by DUL ($p = 0.019$ and $p < 0.001$, respectively). No significant differences for static allodynia, pressure-pain threshold, mechanical static hyperalgesia (pinprick), other domains of the SF36, PDI, and EQ-5D. PGIC: DUL better than placebo ($p = 0.014$)	
Kim *et al.* (2011)	CPSP	Pregabalin (PGB)	150–600 mg/day PGB mean daily dose 356.8 mg (range 125.0–539.7) mg	219 (110 PGB [67 men], 109 placebo [70 men]) Study completed by 183 (83.5%) patients	13-week, randomized, double-blind, multicenter, placebo-controlled, parallel group	Primary end-point: mean pain score (last 7 available scores of the Daily Pain Rating Scale [pain score recorded on an 11-point NRS] while	Weekly mean pain score decrease: PGB patients from 6.5 (baseline) to 4.9; placebo patients	Eligibility criteria: stroke ≥4 months, CPSP ≥3 months, VAS ≥40 mm on the SF-MPQ	Pain reductions at end-point did not differ significantly between PGB and placebo Unexpectedly high placebo response

Computer-generated randomization, blinded 1:1 PGB-placebo ratio, randomized permuted block design 4 phases: 2-week screening and washout, 4-week dose adjustment (1 week PGB 75 mg bid, then 1 week PGB 150 mg bid, then 2 weeks PGB 150 mg bid or increase to max. allowed dose of 300 mg bid), 8-week maintenance, 1-week tapering (PGB 75 mg bid)	on study medication) Secondary end-point: DSIS, an 11-point NRS, weekly mean pain scores, proportion of patients with at least a 30% and 50% reduction in mean pain score, QANeP, NPSI, weekly mean sleep interference scores, MOS-sleep scale, HADS, SF-MPQ, VAS-Part B, EQ-5D, PGIC, CGIC + vital signs, adverse effects, treatment discontinuation, laboratory data, and concomitant medications	from 6.3 (baseline) to 5.0 Least-squares mean difference between groups = −0.2 (95% CI −0.7 to 0.4), favoring PGB; difference not statistically significant ($p = 0.578$). Results not modified by baseline insomnia status, neuropathic pain status, or pain severity 30% or 50% reduction in mean pain score at end-point not reached by the majority of PGB patients. Statistically significant ($p < 0.05$) improvements in secondary end-points (PGB better than placebo): MOS-sleep scale, HADS-A anxiety scores, CGIC (but $p = 0.049$) Adverse effects more frequent with PGB (discontinuation in 8.2% vs. 3.7% of placebo patients)	CPSP diagnostic criteria: medical history, physical examination, imaging findings, and conformance to Treede *et al.*'s criteria (*Neurology* 2008, **70**, 1630–5) Continuation of pharmacological therapies for pain or insomnia used in normal routine allowed	(mean pain score reduction ≥ 50% in 20.4% of patients) + pain reductions with placebo increasing gradually over time (loss of statistical separation between the 2 groups at 8 weeks: possible explanation of the positive results in the 4-week study reported by Vranken *et al.* 2008)

Table 9.2. Controlled studies: parenteral drugs

Authors		Drug(s)	Route/dosage	No. of patients	Study design	Rating	Outcome	Notes	Conclusions
Portenoy *et al.* (1988)	CP and others	Oral opioids		3 SCI, 1 syrinx, 1 spinal AVM, 2 CPSP				Results not broken down according to type	
Arner and Meyerson (1988)	CP and others	Morphine IV 15 mg		1 CCP	Randomized, single-blind, placebo controlled trial		Ineffective	Acute boluses. SCS and PVG DBS: ineffective	
Portenoy *et al.* (1990)	CP	Hydromorphone	6.39 mg IV	2 (1 brainstem CPSP)	Controlled trial		>50% relief at test (partial relief with oxycodone + acetaminophen)	NB: 80% of all pain relief when plasma levels were not at peak (**placebo effect likely**)	
Kupers *et al.* (1991)	CP and others	Morphine	0.3 mg/kg IV	4 CPSP, 2 SCI	Double-blind, placebo-controlled crossover study	Affective and sensory dimensions of pain sensation: 101-point rating scale	Statistically significant reduction of pain effect rating (from 62 to 43). Pain sensory rating not affected, with trend towards increasing		
Bainton *et al.* (1992)	CPSP	Naloxone	NAL: up to 8 mg in 20 mL vehicle	20	Randomized, double-blind, placebo-controlled crossover study	Pain relief: VAS, verbal pain scores	Transient pain relief: 3/20 with NAL, 4/20 with saline, 4/20 with both	Pain scores obtained immediately before and after NAL or saline injection. Subjective ratings followed for 2 weeks	No effect on CPSP

Hansebout *et al.* (1993)	SCI	4-aminopyridine (4-AP)	Escalating total dose from 18.0 to 33.5 mg (IV, 2 separated [2-week] infusions over 2 h)	8	Randomized, double-blind crossover study	Neurological motor and sensory evaluation	Significant temporary neurologic improvement, including reduction in chronic pain, in 5/6 patients with incomplete SCI. No effect was detected in 2 patients with complete and 1 severe incomplete SCI	Effects persisted up to 48 h after infusion	
Backonja *et al.* (1994)	CP	Ketamine	0.25 mg/kg (IV bolus over 5 min)	6 (2 CPSP)	Randomized, double-blind, placebo-controlled crossover study	Pain rating scale 0–10	Pain relief in CPSP patients. Ketamine: patient D: 50% (ongoing pain); patient F: 100% pain relief (ongoing allodynia, hyperalgesia). Placebo: patient D: 0%, patient F: modest		Pain relief lasting 2–3 h. Ketamine affected the evoked pain and associated after-sensation more than ongoing constant pain. Allodynia, hyperalgesia, and after-sensation improved. Side effects during single-dose injections mild and well tolerated
Canavero *et al.* (1995a)	CP	Propofol	0.2 mg/kg (single IV bolus); 0.3 mg/kg/h (continuous IV infusion)	8 CPSP, 8 SCI	Double-blind, placebo-controlled crossover study	Pain relief: VAS (0–10)	Effect lasting no more than 20 min (generally 10 min)	Continuous (6–24 h) IV infusion in propofol-responsive patients. Temporarily effective with hours-long post-effect	Pain and allodynia abolition in propofol-responsive patients. Propofol did not reduce non-CP, nor did placebo

Table 9.2. (cont.)

Authors		Drug(s)	Route/dosage	No. of patients	Study design	Rating	Outcome	Notes	Conclusions
Eide *et al.* (1995)	SCI	Ketamine (KET) Alfentanil (ALF)	60 μg/kg (IV bolus, + 6 μg/kg/min for 17–20 min) 7 μg/kg (IV bolus, + 0.6 μg/kg/min for 17–20 min) (3 infusions, 2 h apart)	9	Randomized, double-blind crossover study	Continuous and evoked pain relief	KET = ALF > placebo ALF = KET > placebo	Neither KET nor ALF significantly changed thresholds for the sensation of heat pain. No clear differential effects on at- and below-level pains	Both continuous and evoked pains were markedly reduced by KET and by ALF. Bothersome dizziness in one patient
Hamamci *et al.* (1996)	?	Calcitonin	1 × 100 IU/day (IM)	26	Placebo-controlled	Pain score	Pain score of the calcitonin group was significantly lower than that of the control group	Post-stroke patients with hemiplegia and "reflex sympathetic dystrophy." 4-week study. 26 patients received calcitonin, 16 saline	Uncertain diagnosis. CPSP in some patients?
Dellemijn and Vanneste (1997)	CP	Fentanyl Diazepam	FEN: 5 μg/kg/h (mean dose: 873 μg) DIA: 0.2 μg/kg/h (mean dose: 52.1 mg)	3	Randomized, double-blind, active placebo-controlled-crossover study (drugs infused at a constant rate for a maximum of 5 h)	Pain relief: rating scales (including unpleasantness)	Maximum relief of pain intensity was better with FEN than with DIA (66% [95% CI 53–80] vs. 23% [12–35]) or with saline (50% [36–63] vs. 12% [4–20]). FEN CP patients responders: 1/3. Placebo CP patients responders: 0/3	Mixed population of 53 patients with neuropathic pain. DIA as active placebo. Saline as inert placebo. 2 consecutive double-blind infusions: FEN + DIA and FEN + saline	DIA had no clinically significant effect on pain intensity and pain unpleasantness. The beneficial effect of FEN was independent of the type of neuropathic pain and the degree of sedation. FEN therapy produced

									equal relief of pain intensity and pain unpleasantness. DIA and saline did not reduce either pain index. Side effects more common with FEN than with DIA or saline. No severe side effects. The clinical characteristics of neuropathic pain do not predict response to opioids.
Mailis *et al.* (1997)	SCI	Sodium amylal	4–7 mg/kg (IV infusion, 7–10 min, max. dose 500 mg or 50 mg/kg)	1	Placebo-controlled study	Pain relief: VAS. Sensory testing	VAS reduction from about 6 to about 4. Dramatic reduction of allodynia. Substantial reduction of hyperalgesia	17 NP patients. 1 patient with C4 myelopathy (AVM)	No benefit on deep pain. Sympathetic block responder
Potter *et al.* (1998)	SCI	Fampridine-SR (sustained release 4-amino-pyridine)	12.5 and 17.5 mg bid (PO, 2-week treatment period +1 week washout)	26	Randomized double-blind dose-titration crossover study	Patient satisfaction, sensory scores, motor scores	No statistically significant benefits on measures of pain	Incomplete SCI in all patients	
Attal *et al.* (2000)	CP	Lidocaine	5 mg/kg (IV infusion over 30 min)	6 CPSP, 10 SCI (5 syrinx, 3 SCI, 2 spondylotic myelopathy)	Randomized, double-blind, placebo (saline)-controlled	Pain relief: VAS (0–10), global assessment, QST	Pain relief > 50%: 11/16 with lidocaine; 6/16 with placebo. 3 had no benefit or worse pain vs. 8 with placebo. 2	Post-study follow-up: 12 patients took oral mexiletine (400–800 mg/day) for 4–12 weeks. 30–50%	Significantly greater pain relief starting 15 mins post-injection and lasting up to 30 mins after the

Table 9.2. (cont.)

Authors		Drug(s)	Route/ dosage	No. of patients	Study design	Rating	Outcome	Notes	Conclusions
					crossover study		patients had more relief with placebo. Burning totally/partially relieved in 6 vs. 2 (placebo), paresthesias abolished in 8/11 vs. 2/11. In 5 patients (62%), allodynia reduced ≥ 50% by lidocaine (vs. 1 by placebo), in 4 by 100% for up to 1 h post-injection (never with placebo)	relief in 3 patients (2 lidocaine responders, 1 placebo responder). No improvement in 8 patients (6 lidocaine responders). Intolerable side effects from long-term mexiletine. Difference between lidocaine and placebo: moderate. In 7 patients refractory to all previous treatments, spontaneous pain responded less to lidocaine	end. With lidocaine, significant brush-induced allodynia and static mechanical hyperalgesia reduction. No effect on thermal evoked pains. In 2 patients, 30–50% relief for 2–10 days. NNT: 5 (SCI patients). Side effects in two-thirds of patients
Attal *et al.* (2002)	CP	Morphine	16 mg IV (mean dosage, range 9–30)	15 (9 SCI, 6 CPSP)	Randomized, double blind, placebo (saline) controlled, crossover	Pain relief: VAS (1–100), QST	No significant difference in pain reduction between morphine and placebo. 3 patients 100% relieved at the end of injection (vs. 1 with placebo), 2 for > 2 h, 1 patient	Morphine effect correlated with decreased responses to suprathreshold thermal stimuli (general antinociceptive activity). Following the completion of the study all	Morphine significantly reduced brush-induced allodynia but had *no effect on static mechanical and thermal evoked pains*. **Ongoing pain was not significantly**

							worsened by morphine. 1 syrinx patient with prominent mechanical allodynia 100% relieved	patients began to take sustained oral morphine (mean dosage: 93 mg; range 60–140 mg) in a long-term study on efficacy and side effects	**reduced**, but 7 patients (46%) responded to morphine. The effects of IV morphine correlated with those of oral morphine at 1 month. Oral morphine was effective only in 3 (2 SCI, 1 CPSP)/ 14 patients (1 lost to follow-up) at 12–18 months with 50–75% relief, starting from week 1 and peaking at week 4. Morphine PO less tolerated than IV
Kalman *et al.* (2002)	MS	Morphine	Up to 1 mg/kg over 20 min, continuous IV infusion	14	Single-blind, placebo (saline)-controlled study. Followed by naloxone	Pain relief: VAS	4 patients were opioid responders (no pain relief from placebo, > 50% pain reduction with morphine, and > 25% pain increase with naloxone). Effective dose: 43, 47, 50, and 25 mg		Morphine is effective only in a minority of patients (29%) and only at high doses. Same results reported by these authors in discussion for CPSP
Canavero and Bonicalzi (2004a)	CP	Propofol	0.2 mg/kg (single IV bolus)	44 (23 CPSP, 21 SCI)	Randomized, double-blind, placebo-controlled crossover study	Pain relief: VAS (0–10); NVS (0–4)	Pain relief (spontaneous pain intensity reduction > 30% or allodynia reduction > 50%): 24/44	Study aimed at validating IV subhypnotic propofol as a diagnostic test for CP	Propofol was significantly superior to placebo in reducing the intensity of spontaneous

Table 9.2. (cont.)

Authors		Drug(s)	Route/ dosage	No. of patients	Study design	Rating	Outcome	Notes	Conclusions
							patients with propofol, 6/44 patients with placebo		ongoing pain (for up to 1 h after the injection) and of both mechanical and cold allodynia. In a few cases, only the evoked components were abolished
Kvarnstrom *et al.* (2004)	SCI	Ketamine Lidocaine	0.4 mg/kg (IV infusion over 40 min) 2.5 mg/kg (IV infusion over 40 min)	10	Randomized, double-blind, three-period, three-treatment, placebo-controlled crossover study	Pain relief: VAS. QST, traditional sensory tests	Positive response (50% reduction in VAS score during infusion): 5/10 patients with ketamine, 1/10 patients with lidocaine, 0/10 patients with placebo. Temperature thresholds: no changes. Sensibility: no changes	Primary objective of the study: to examine the analgesic effect of ketamine and lidocaine on SCI below-level pain. Secondary objective: to assess sensory abnormalities to identify responders. Sensory assessments do not predict response to treatment	Ketamine but not lidocaine showed a significant analgesic effect in SCI-CP. Pain relief not associated with altered temperature thresholds or other changes of sensory function. Lidocaine and particularly ketamine were associated with frequent side effects
Finnerup *et al.* (2005)	SCI	Lidocaine	5 mg/kg (IV infusion over 30 min)	24	Randomized, double-blind, placebo-controlled crossover study	Pain relief: VAS. QST	Neuropathic at- and below-level spontaneous pain: (1) significantly reduced in all patients ($p < 0.01$) (2) significantly reduced in 12	26 patients with NP at or below level enrolled, 2 dropped out before any treatment. Evoked pain in 12 patients. No evoked pain in 12 patients.	SCI at- and below-level pain reduced by IV lidocaine irrespective of the presence or absence of evoked pain Lidocaine usually not suited for

							patients with evoked pain ($p < 0.01$) (3) significantly reduced in 12 patients without evoked pain ($p < 0.048$) No difference in number of patients with pain reduction ≥ 33% between patients with ($n = 6$) and without ($n = 5$) evoked pain. At-level brush-evoked dysesthesia significantly reduced. Median pain reduction: about 35%. NNT for 50% pain relief: 3	Adverse effects: IV lidocaine, 19 patients; placebo, 1. No correlation between maximal plasma concentration and maximal pain relief or pain intensity. Non-significant decrease in cold allodynia, pinprick hyperalgesia, or pain evoked by repetitive pinprick	long-term treatment
Vranken *et al.* (2005)	CP	S(+)-ketamine	50 or 75 mg daily (transdermal iontophoretic administration)	33 (8 CPSP, 1 MS, 1 PD, 3 thalamic lesion, 4 brainstem lesion, 16 SC lesion)	Randomized, double-blind placebo-controlled study	Pain intensity: VAS Health status (PDI, EQ-5D) Quality of life (SF-36). Safety assessment	No statistically significant differences in VAS between ketamine (both dosages) and placebo Pre- vs. post-treatment VAS scores: placebo group: 7.1 vs. 6.4 ketamine 50 mg: 7.3 vs. 6.2 ketamine 75 mg: 7.3 vs. 5.7 No improvement in health status or QoL from ketamine 50 mg	1-week trial Appropriate dose from an open-label preliminary study Sample size and power calculated pre-study (with 33 patients, power 0.8 for estimated VAS differences) Only mild and spontaneously resolving adverse events without differences between	Iontophoretic S(+)-ketamine no more effective than placebo; 75 mg/day of S(+)-ketamine improved health status and QoL

Table 9.2. (cont.)

Authors		Drug(s)	Route/ dosage	No. of patients	Study design	Rating	Outcome	Notes	Conclusions
							Significant improvement in PDI, EQ-5D and SF-36 (except for the role-physical functioning and general health perception) from ketamine 75 mg	ketamine and placebo groups	
Sang *et al.* (2006)	CCP	Fosphenytoin Lidocaine Saline (placebo)	F: 12 mg phenytoin equivalents/kg vs. 4 mg/kg vs. 2mg/kg lidocaine vs. saline, all infused IV over 15 min	17 (7 complete [CL], 10 incomplete [IL])	Randomized, double-blind, placebo-controlled crossover study	21-point log-linear Gracely scale. Primary end-point: % change from baseline pain intensity (analyzed with linear model containing sequence, subject within sequence, period and treatment)	Mean pain intensity: 12 (4–16)/20. In the F 12 mg arm, peak reduction in mean pain intensity was 50% at 45 min following the start of infusion with a significant reduction of pain vs. placebo in ongoing pain over the entire testing period (mean % change from baseline over 4 h, 31%, $p = 0.007$). Trends only for fosphenytoin 4 mg/kg and lidocaine. CL patients had mean 18% improvement ($p = 0.007$) and IL patients 40% ($p = 0.017$).	Abstract Study completed by 17/17 enrolled patients (all analyzed). Side effects well tolerated	Sodium blockers for CP supported
Mailis-Gagnon *et al.* (2009)	SCI	Sodium amobarbital IV	AMO: mean dose 253 mg (range 190–350)	SCI 5 patients (according to the authors: at- and below-	Retrospective, single-blind, placebo-controlled	Evaluation of spontaneous pain and sensory abnormalities	Case 3: pain decrease: AMO: from 6 to 0; LID: from 5 to 0.	Case 3: No transitional zone, no sensation below T10,	Overall results: **AMO superior to LID**

		Lidocaine IV	LID: mean dose 297 mg (range 200–450)	level pain in cases 1 and 2; **pure below-level pain in case 3 (M, 28 years [T10 fracture, motor/ sensory deficit at T10–11]);** at-level pain in cases 4 and 5	(IV normal saline)	(anesthesia to light touch, pinprick, and cold), variations before and after each infusion	No change in sensory abnormalities	pain in both legs
Amr (2010)	SCI	Ketamine IV (KET) [+ Gabapentin PO (GBP)]	Group I: KET 80 mg/day (5 h infusion) for 1 week [+ GBP 300 mg tid] Group II: placebo infusion [+ GBP 300 mg tid]	40 with post-traumatic SCI NP Complete lesion in 8+6 patients	Randomized (1:1), controlled, double-blind	Pain intensity changes (VAS at: baseline, daily during treatment, weekly for 1 month post-treatment) Side effects	Baseline mean VAS scores: GI: 84.2, GII: 83.7 mm. Pre- vs. post-treatment VAS scores: statistically significant reduction in both groups ($p < 0.05$) during all the study periods, more pronounced in GI than in G II ($p < 0.0001$) during the infusion week + 1st and 2nd post-infusion weeks. No statistical difference between the groups at 3rd ($p = 0.54$) and 4th weeks ($p = 0.25$). No major adverse effects	Patients already taking GBP. Midazolam (2–5 mg) prior to infusion. Small sample size **Useless study: no. of patients complaining of CP and/or at- or below-level pain unknown; diagnostic criteria for NP not reported; results not broken down according to pain type**

Table 9.3. Uncontrolled studies: oral drugs

Authors	Pain type: no. of patients	Drug(s)	Dosage	Study design	Pain rating	Outcome and notes	Conclusions
Fine (1967)	Epileptic pain (post-stroke): 5	Phenytoin, phenobarbital				All relieved	Paroxysmal pain responsive
Albert (1969)	MS-CP: 6	Carbamazepine	600 mg			4 definite reliefs	Paroxysmal and burning pain responsive
Espir and Millac (1970)	MS-CP: 7	Carbamazepine				No data for true CP	Paroxysmal pains responsive (placebo ineffective)
Gibson and White (1971)	SCI pain: 2	Carbamazepine	Case reports			Partial to very good relief at 4–8 months (never 100%)	Effect on lancinating, pulsatile pain; burning at low level remains
Cantor (1972)	CPSP: 2	Phenytoin	Case reports			Partial benefit at 150 mg in both, in 1 patient at 1 year	
Mladinich (1974)	CP, brainstem	Phenytoin				Benefit	
Agnew and Goldberg (1976)	CPSP: 8, plus 2 other non-CP pain patients	Phenytoin	Full dosage	Case series	Charts for pain estimation	Incomplete data. Marked improvement: 3; minimal improvement: 2; unchanged: 2; pain worsened: 3	Return of pain on stopping phenytoin in improved patients
Heilporn (1978)	SCI-CP (diffuse pain): 11	Melitracen (150 mg PO), flupenthixol (3 mg PO/day) plus TENS				8 patients benefited	
Gimenez-Roldan and Martin (1981)	Tabetic pain: 6	Carbamazepine		Case series		IV penicillin vs. carbamazepine. 1/6 pain relief with penicillin, 5/5 pain relief with CBZ	
Clifford and Trotter (1984)	MS-CP: 12	Tricyclics		Case series		100% relief in 8, partial in 3; non-burning dysesthesia relieved	1 patient 100% relieved by PO baclofen; 1 relieved only by phenol spinal block
Schott and Loh (1984)	CPSP: 5	Physostigmine, piridostigmine				2 long-term reliefs	

Koppel (1986)	CPSP (thalamic): 2	Amitriptyline	50 mg/day	Case reports	Not available	Improved at this dose (higher dose worsened!) Follow-up: 13 months.	
Bowsher and Lahuerta (1987)	Tabetic pain	Valproate				Effect on lightning pain	
Tourian (1987)	CPSP: 10	Doxepin (75–200 mg/day) plus propanolol 82 mg/day)				About 50% long-lasting relief	Propanolol potentiates doxepin
Scharein *et al.* (1987; IASP congress 1987, S469 A109) Zangemeister *et al.* (1987; IASP congress 1987, A592)	CP: 50	Carbamazepine	Not available	Case series	Not available	12/50 CP patients (24%) sufficiently relieved	
Moulin *et al.* (1988)	MS pains	Amitriptyline, imipramine, carbamazepine	Up to 100 mg	Case series		Poor results for true CP	One-third of patients had no thermoalgesic impairment
Portenoy *et al.* (1988)	MS-CP: 3	Opioids; tricyclics (amitriptyline, imipramine)		Case series		Partial relief from PO opioids; high dose imipramine in 1 but not another; amitriptyline highly effective in 1	Drugs ineffective in 2 cases: doxepin, CBX, PHT, clonazepam, valproate, tryptophan, fluphenazine
Hampf and Bowsher (1989)	CPSP	Distigmine plus AD	Not available				
Awerbuch and Sandyk (1990)	CPSP: 9	Mexiletine	Up to 10 mg/kg/day, 4-week period	Case series	5-point scale	Days 1–3: 150 mg; days 4–6: 300 mg. At least moderate relief in 8/9 patients	Mexiletine may be a safe and effective agent in the management of thalamic pain and possibly other paroxysmal pain syndromes of central origin
Michel *et al.* (1990)	CPSP: 3 CPSP: 5	Fluvoxamine Clonazepam	Not available Not available	Case series (12 patients)		1 partial pain relief, 1 scarce effect, 1 no effect Partial pain relief in 2 patients, scarce effect in 2, no effect in 1	

Table 9.3. (cont.)

Authors	Pain type: no. of patients	Drug(s)	Dosage	Study design	Pain rating	Outcome and notes	Conclusions
Maurer *et al.* (1990)	CP: 1	Delta-9 THC (5 mg) plus codeine (50 mg)				More effective than placebo on painful dysesthesias	
Takenobu and Hori (1990; IASP congress 1990, S493]	CPSP: 13	Carbamazepine	Not available	Case series	Not available	Effective in several cases	1 CCP patient: SCS abolished it
Tourian (1991)	CP: number not available	Baclofen PO (80 mg) with/ without clonidine (0.4–1 mg/day)				Relief in some patients	
Sanford *et al.* (1992)	SCI-CP: 1	Amitriptyline (AMI), carbamazepine (CBZ)	150 mg/day, 400 mg/day			Some relief with AMI, substantial relief of burning and paroxysmal pains by adding CBZ at 3 years	Effect only by combining both drugs, not singly
Lema *et al.* (1992)	Caudal ependymoma: 1	Opioids NSAIDs Amitriptyline	Not available Not available 50 mg/day	Case report	VAS	No relief No relief No relief	TENS: no relief
Fenollosa *et al.* (1993)	SCI: postal survey of 380 patients, 38% of whom responded	Amitriptyline + clonazepam + NSAIDs, or amitriptyline + clonazepam + 5-OH-tryptophan + TENS, or amitriptyline + clonazepam + SCS, or morphine (continuous IT administration)	Not available	Case series review	Pain relief	"Satisfactory relief" in 35% of the patients who responded 80% global success	IT morphine very safe and useful in selected patients Rest phase between tiers: 15–90 days
Edmondson *et al.* (1993)	CP: 4	Mexiletine PO		Case series		Previous effective lidocaine infusion. 2 continued taking the drug and reported excellent relief at 12 months; 2 had intolerable side effects	
De Salles and Bittar (1994)	CPSP: 1	Carbamazepine				Partial relief	

Bowsher (1994)	CP: number not specified	Mexiletine PO				Effective in several patients	
Zachariah *et al.* (1994)	SCI: 3	Divalproex sodium				Relief in 2	1 dropped out
Canavero and Bonicalzi (1996)	CPSP: 3; CCP: 1	Lamotrigine	From 50 mg/day PO to 200 mg tid	Placebo-controlled in 2 patients	Patient self-reports and pain scores	Pain relapse after switching to placebo or drug discontinuation in 3 patients. Amitriptyline added in 1 patient with more effective analgesia	
Sist *et al.* (1997)		Gabapentin				Mixed pain population, including CP patients; gabapentin effective	
Samkoff *et al.* (1997)	MS-CP: 1	Gabapentin	300 mg tid		Not available	Dramatic improvement sustained for 6 months of follow-up	Baclofen, AMI and CBZ: either incomplete relief or adverse effects
Houtchens *et al.* (1997)	MS: 25	Gabapentin	300–2400 mg/day	Case series		Best response on throbbing pain/needles, least effect on dull aching pain	
Zylicz (1997)	CPSP: 1	Methadone	From 5 mg bid to 30 mg/day (gradual increase)	Case report	Patient's report	Previous trial with IV morphine, from 2.5 to 6 mg/h, continuous infusion	Effective. AMI, dexamethasone, CBZ, paracetamol (acetaminophen) ineffective
Wood and Sloan (1997)	CP	Ketamine		Case report		Effective	
McGowan *et al.* (1997)	CP (brainstem): 16	Amitriptyline		Case series		2 patients: 100% relief; 14 patients: partial relief	Prompt relapse upon weaning
Carrieri *et al.* (1998)	CPSP: 1	Lamotrigine	100 mg bid	Case report		Pain relapse on stopping lamotrigine	
McCleane (1998a)	MS	Lamotrigine	25 mg/day up to 200 mg/day	Placebo-controlled, double-blind (2 × 8 weeks, 2 weeks washout)	Pain relief	31 patients. 22 patients completed the study. 3 adverse events. Effective	
McCleane (1998b)	MS: 1	Lamotrigine	50 mg/day up to 200 mg/day	Case report		100% relief; relapse upon cessation; again 100% control but discontinuation for rash	Tramadol not effective. Carbamazepine partially effective

Table 9.3. (cont.)

Authors	Pain type: no. of patients	Drug(s)	Dosage	Study design	Pain rating	Outcome and notes	Conclusions
Attal *et al.* (1998a)	CP: 7; CPSP: 2	Gabapentin	Up to 2400 mg		Spontaneous ongoing pain: VAS (1–100). Paroxysmal pain: number of daily attacks	Mixed pain population, including CP patients. Gabapentin starting dosage: 600 mg. Study duration: 6 weeks. Spontaneous ongoing pain and daily attack number: significant decrease at 6 weeks. Significant reduction of brush-induced and cold allodynia	Results not broken down according to pain type
Merren (1998)		Gabapentin	Up to 2700 mg/day	Case series		Mixed pain population, including CP	**Best responses occurred in patients with peripherally mediated pain**
Ness *et al.* (1998)	Cord CP (SCI/MS): 6	Gabapentin	900 mg/day or more (according to pain relief)	Case report	VAS	No benefit in 3 patients. Long-term benefit (reduction of pain score of at least 3) after 6 months in 3. **True CP not very responsive**	
Mercadante (1998)	SCI: 3 (A: cauda, B: iatrogenic after dorsal SCS, C: CCP)	Gabapentin	Up to 2400 mg		VAS	B: severe somnolence, then slow titration to 1600 mg: VAS from 10 to 6 C: titrated to 2400 mg + tramadol 400 mg/day: VAS from 8–10 to 3–6	B: tramadol, baclofen, morphine, NSAIDs, benzodiazepine ineffective C: codeine, acetaminophen, tramadol, NSAIDs, antidepressants, benzodiazepine ineffective
Dahm *et al.* (1998)	MS-CP (1 CP)	Opioids	Not available	Case report	VAS	No enduring benefit	
Takano *et al.* (1999)	CPSP: 2	Amantadine	50–150 mg/day			Not available	Previous response to IV ketamine
Cianchetti *et al.* (1999)	MS: 21 (15 with burning paresthesias)	Lamotrigine	25 mg/day increased slowly to a maximum of 400 mg/day	Case series	Patients' report, verbal scale	Marked improvement in 3, moderate improvement in 5 (of 15 MS-CP patients). Globally, 13/21 100% improved, 11 with sustained benefit at > 1 year	Lamotrigine is effective in controlling painful paroxysmal phenomena in MS patients

Enarson *et al.* (1999)	Mixed pain population, including CP: 21	Ketamine	Starting dose 100 mg/day, titrated upward. Median final dose 220 mg/day	Case series review		Titration upward by 40 mg/day until efficacy was reached, or until side effects became limiting. Intolerable side effects: 9 patients. No effect: 4 patients. Equivocal responses: 4 patients. Long-term treatment in 4 patients (100–500 mg/day)	Demographic data not shown. More effective if pain < 5 years
Fisher and Hagen (1999)	SCI: 1	Ketamine	10 mg tid, titrated upward up to 25 mg tid	Case report	VAS	IV followed by SC ketamine as starting treatment. Haloperidol added. Pain relief from 5/10 (8/10 at night) to 3/10	
Sakurai and Kanazawa (1999)	MS-CP: 14	Lidocaine, mexiletine	Lidocaine infusion: 6–8.8 mg/kg/h over 30 min, then 2–2.8; mexiletine: 300–400 mg/day	Case series		Effective in most. Placebo not or scarcely effective	Almost complete abolition of painful tonic seizures. Lidocaine > mexiletine, although both effective. In 1 patient, no benefit from CBZ (400 mg), valproate (800 mg), and clonazepam (2.5 mg). Truncal more resistant than limb dysesthesias
Van Bastelaere and De Laat (1999)	SCI-CP: 1	Lamotrigine	600 mg	Case report		Pain abolition	3600 mg morphine ineffective
Kapadia and Harden (2000)	SCI-CP: 1	Gabapentin	1800 mg/day	Case report	VAS, MPQ	Good control	Opioids, CBZ, tricyclic antidepressants, and TENS ineffective
		Doxepin	100 mg				
Vick and Lamer (2001)	CPSP: 1	Ketamine IV	0.2 mg/kg bolus	Case report	VAS	Marked relief	CBZ, PHT, GBP, amantadine, IV lidocaine, opioids, TCA ineffective
		Ketamine PO	50 mg			Relief (VAS 3) at 9 months	
D'Aleo *et al.* (2001)	MS-CP	Topiramate	200–550 mg	Case series		Three reliefs (none 100%); 1 dropped out	

Table 9.3. (cont.)

Authors	Pain type: no. of patients	Drug(s)	Dosage	Study design	Pain rating	Outcome and notes	Conclusions
Shimodozono *et al.* (2002)	CPSP: 31	Fluvoxamine	25–125 mg/day	Open label	VAS	After 2–4 weeks significant VAS decrease, from 7.7 to 6	Significant effect only if stroke < 1 year
Canavero *et al.* (2002a)	CPSP: 3; syringomyelia: 1; cord lesions: 3 BCP: 1; CCP: 1 CPSP: 1; CCP: 1; plus 2 other CP	Topiramate Amantadine Dextrometorphan	Up to 600 mg/day Up to 100 mg 100–1000 mg		VAS	No effect. Pain worsened in 3 patients Pain worsened 2 moderate reliefs, 20% benefit	
Canavero *et al.* (2002b)	CPSP: 3; syringomyelia: 1; SCI: 2	Reboxetine	Up to 10 mg/day	Single-blind, prospective	VAS	Pain reduction. >50% (cut-off limit for analgesia): 1 patient (treatment disclosure); <50%: 2 patients; none: 3 patients	Reboxetine (selective noradrenaline reuptake inhibitor) does not appear to exert major analgesic effects in CP
Bowsher (2002)	CPSP: 64	Amitriptyline				Modestly significant correlation between onset of therapy and efficacy (>50%): 89% of those beginning treatment within 6 months of onset achieved target benefit vs. 42% starting it >1 year from onset	
Bitanga *et al.* (2002)	CPSP (8.8% of population); CP (8.3%); myelopathic pain (3.6%); brainstem pain (0.2%)	Gabapentin	300–1200 mg/day in 92%	Open-label prospective non-comparative post-marketing study of 1214 Filipinos	VAS	CPSP: from VAS 68 to 19 CP: from VAS 69 to 18 Myelopathic pain (CCP?): from VAS 77 to 16	**2 week-long (!) very low-dose study (!)** **Criteria for diagnosis undefined!**
Chen *et al.* (2002)	CPSP: 1	Gabapentin				Significant pain relief and function improvement within 2 weeks	
Putzke *et al.* (2002)	SCI: 27	Gabapentin	1800–3600 mg/day (in 2	Case series follow-up	Pain rating scale	6 discontinued. 21 had ≥ 2 VAS reduction at 6 months. 3 years later, 10/14 responders still benefited.	Below-lesion CP: 8 benefits, 4 failures. Rectal-

			cases < 900 mg)			Below-lesion pain: 8 responders, 4 non-responders	perineal CP: 4 benefits, 2 failures. Complete SCI: 3 benefits, 2 failures. Incomplete SCI: 11 benefits, 5 failures. Burning pain: 9 benefits, 4 failures. Non-burning pain: 5 benefits, 3 failures
To *et al.* (2002)	44 NP SCI patients identified, 38 with data (28 men). 19 paraplegic and 16 tetraplegic (= 35). 24 chronic pain (> 6 months) in 24, acute in 9 (= 33).	Gabapentin	2400 mg/day (median mainte-nance dose, range 900–4800 mg/ day)	Case series (retrospective review, data retrieved from medical records)	Pain relief (VAS or verbal description prior to and during treatment [1, 3, 6 months])	Significant VAS decrease in 76% of patients % of cases with available VAS data: baseline: 74%, 1 month: 68%; 3 months: 50%; 6 months: 57% VAS values in **11 patients** with data at all four measurement points: pretreatment 8.86, at 1 month 5.23, at 3 months 4.59, at 6 months 4.13 ($p < 0.001$); significant curvilinear trend ($p < 0.001$). Verbal description: from "unbearable" to "liveable"	**Study limitation according to the authors (!):** **VAS and pain observations made in an uncontrolled and non-standardized manner; incomplete VAS set (four) for many patients (the study was not a formal clinical trial); GBP results not broken down according to pain type (chronic or acute), location, level of SCI, completeness of injury, comedications taken (this being a particularly confounding finding)**

Table 9.3. (cont.)

Authors	Pain type: no. of patients	Drug(s)	Dosage	Study design	Pain rating	Outcome and notes	Conclusions
Cohen and Abdi (2002)	BCP: 1	(1) Dextro-metorphan (2) Gabapentin (3) Mexiletine (4) Clonidine	(1) 60 mg PO tid, then to 90 mg PO tid	Case report	VAS	(1) VAS from 9 to 6 (+ oxycodone: VAS from 6 to 4; 6 months later: VAS 3) (2) Mild relief (3) No relief (4) No relief	
Falci *et al.* (2002)	SCI-CP: 41	Tricyclics Antiepileptics Baclofen Klonopin Opioids	Not available	Case series	VAS	No benefit (opioids at most taking the edge off the pain)	Some patients refractory to IT opioids, baclofen, clonidine, local anesthetic or SCS
Jenkins *et al.* (2002)	SCI: 12	Oxcarbazepine	Up to 900 mg/day (phase I) and up to 1500 mg (phase II)	Case series	Not available	Moderate relief overall in 7/12, and 7/7 in those with allodynia	
Ahn *et al.* (2003)	SCI: 31	Gabapentin	1800 mg/day or maximum tolerated dose	Case series	VAS	Comparison among patients with different duration of symptoms (< 6 months and > 6 months)	Gabapentin may be effective in SCI patients whose duration of symptoms is < 6 months. Patients with duration of symptoms > 6 months showed a significant but lesser decrease
Kamano (2003)	CPSP (brainstem): 1	Amitriptyline	Not available	Case report	Not available	Neither helpful nor tolerated	
		Mexiletine	Not available			"Some effect"	
Widerström-Noga and Turk (2003)	SCI	Opioids PO Antiepileptics	Not available	Case series	Not available	33.3 reported their pain was considerably better, and 23.8% reported it eliminated	Both classes most effective drugs among all classes tried. Differential effect on CP unreported
Willoch *et al.* (2004)	CPSP: 2	Morphine PO	Not available	Case series	Not available	Poor effect	

Takahashi *et al.* (2004)	CPSP: 2 (both of immediate onset)	Zonisamide	200 mg/day	Case report		Patient 1: "pain well controlled" (follow-up 5 months). Patient 2: VAS reduction from 7 to 2 (follow-up 1 year)	No side effects
Attal *et al.* (2004b)	CPSP: 1; SCI: 4	Dronabinol	2.5 mg bid up to 25 mg/day (maximum dosage)	Case series	VAS, MPQ, number of painful attacks	Consecutive patients. Side effects in all. No significant effect on ongoing pain and evoked pains	
Sakai *et al.* (2004)	MS: 1	Ketamine	20 mg increased to 40 mg/day PO	Placebo-controlled	VAS	Effective on severe pain and allodynia. Pain reduction from IV lidocaine (3 mg/kg) and oral mexiletine (300 mg/day)	
Norrbrink Budh and Lundeberg (2004)	SCI: 90	31 patients: opioids 14: NSAIDs 11: antiepileptics 10: antidepressants	Not available	Survey	Various scales	Opiates more effective in younger patients **Patients with neuropathic pain (at- or below-level pain not defined) had less relief** with opiates than patients with nociceptive or mixed pains	
Rasmussen *et al.* (2004)	BCP: 6; CCP: 10	Imipramine (IMI) or gabapentin (GBP)	IMI: ≥ 50 mg/day. GBP: up to 2.4 g/day	Case series	Numeric Pain Rating Scale. 4-point scale (0–25%, 26–50%, 51–75%, or 76–100% global pain relief)	Primary end-point: global pain relief. Pain relief in CP patients: (IMI / GBP) 0–25%: 0 BCP, 2 CCP / 0 BCP, 2 CCP 26–50%: 1BCP, 4 CCP / 0 BCP, 2 CCP 51–75%: 3 BCP, 0 CCP / 2 BCP, 0 CCP 76–100%: 0 BCP, 0 CCP / 0 BCP, 0 CCP	Good outcome of therapy with IMI or GBP is not predicted by definite evidence of nervous system lesion or by the presence of abnormal sensory phenomena. Study's results do not support a mechanism-based approach in classifying and treating pain
Henkel and Bengel (2005)	Wallenberg: 1	Gabapentin and amitriptyline	Not available	Case report	VAS	Marked reduction of pain	Opioids ineffective. Iatrogenic streptococcal meningo-encephalitis following cervical myelography

Table 9.3. (cont.)

Authors	Pain type: no. of patients	Drug(s)	Dosage	Study design	Pain rating	Outcome and notes	Conclusions
Seghier *et al.* (2005)	CPSP: 1	Amitriptyline, gabapentin	75 mg, 2400 mg	Case report	VAS	40% reduction	
Raza *et al.* (2005)	CCP (post-thoracic meningioma surgeries)	Gabapentin	Not available	Case report	Not available	No effect	
Montes *et al.* (2005)	CPSP: 1	Carbamazepine Gabapentin, lamotrigine, oxcarbazepine, amitriptyline, bromazepam, paracetamol (acetaminophen)-codeine, IV morphine IV ketamine	Not available	Case report	VAS	Initial response, but rapid relapse No effect Increased burning	
Canavero and Bonicalzi (2005a)	BCP: 9; CCP: 7	Mexiletine (MEX), gabapentin (GBP)	MEX: up to 1000 mg; GBP: up to 3600 mg	Case series	VAS	68.75% of patients had ≥ 50% reduction, 1 less than that, 1 made worse, 2 intolerant	3 stopped due to side effects after initial benefit. 50% of patients had at least 50% relief up to 12 years
Bowsher (2006a)	CPSP (post-SAH): 1	Cannabis (smoked)	Not available	Case report	Not available	Some relief	
Cardenas and Jensen (2006)	CCP: 117	(1) NSAIDs (2) Baclofen (3) Opioids (4) Benzodiazepine (5) Gabapentin (6) TCA (7) Carbamazepine (8) Phenytoin (9) Mexiletine	Not available	Survey	VAS	(1) >50% of patients still use (VAS −3.73 points) (2) *c.* 60% still use (VAS −3.42 points) (3) *c.* 60% still use (−6.27 VAS points) (4) *c.* 50% still use (−4.51 VAS points) (5) *c.* 40% still use (−3.32 VAS points) (6) *c.* 20% still use (−2.9 VAS points) (7) *c.* 20% still use (−2.17 VAS points: **least of all**) (8) >20% still use (−2.58 VAS points) (9) 100% still use **(−6 VAS points)**	If we compare the length of relief, broken down into weeks, months, years, best effects were respectively obtained with: TCA, mexiletine, TCA Relief for years: marijuana smoking
Solaro *et al.* (2007)	12 MS patients (8 women) with painful paroxysmal symptoms (PPS);	Oxcarbamazepine (OXCBZ)	600–1200 mg/day (mean dosage 1033 mg/day)	Open-label pilot study, 3 months minimum follow-up	"Three-point scale" (0–3) Clinical evaluation at T0 (study entry), T1 (pain	Complete and sustained pain statistically significant relief in 9/12 patients (75%) 2 drop-outs (adverse effects)	Previous ineffective treatment with gabapentin, CBZ, baclofen, TCAs

	paroxysmal dysesthetic disturbances in 5 patients				relief), T2 (3 months after beginning of study)	**A 0–3 scale is a FOUR-point scale. Results analyzed by means of an unreported statistical test**	
Djaldetti *et al.* (2007)	PD-related pain (costant stabbing, aching, tension, and burning): 23 Pain in limbs (15 patients), shoulder (7), neck (4), chest (1), teeth (1), waist (2), whole body (1)	Duloxetine	60 mg once-daily	Open-label study	VAS, BPI, SF-MPQ, PDQoLQ, UPDRS motor part, QST (pre- and post-treatment completion)	Non-PD-related causes of pain ruled out. PD treatment optimized Subjective effect on pain: abolished in 2 patients, markedly alleviated in 6, mildly to moderately alleviated in 5 (= beneficial effect in 13/20 patients, 65%). Only mean VAS, BPI, and SF-MPQ scores significantly decreased (*unknown statistical test*). Duloxetine ineffective in 7 patients. Study discontinued (intolerable side effects) in 3 patients	No placebo control
Murphy *et al.* (2007a, 2007b)	CCP (SCI: 104 compliant patients [51 pregabalin, 53 placebo] without serious treatment-associated adverse events in a previous RCT)	Pregabalin	150 mg bid [*sic!*] within 1 week of concluding RCT Dosage adjustments: 150–600 mg/day Mean final weighted dosage: 388 mg/day	Open-label study. 9-month extension study [see Siddall *et al.* (2006)] Quarterly drug holidays (3–28 days) Treatment restart in case of pain relapse Treatment withdrawal if no pain relapse	SF-MPQ (efficacy); adverse events, clinical and laboratory assessments (safety)	Abstract, never published as full paper. 1 patient not treated, 60 patients completed the study, 43 discontinued End-point mean improvements: SF-MPQ: (sensory −0.7 ± 5.8, affective −0.3 ± 2.8, total −1.0 ± 8.1); VAS (−7.9 ± 25.2); PPI (−0.3 ± 1.2). Pain "very much" or "much" worsened (during drug holidays) in 88 patients. No pain relapse in 3 patients	Pregabalin demonstrated sustained analgesic effect ≥ 1 year in patients with CCP 14.6% of patients withdrew because of adverse events: higher than primary study!
Que *et al.* (2007)	SCI CCP: 1	Baclofen	25 mg/day	Case report	VAS	No significant analgesia	
		Diazepam	2 mg/day			No significant analgesia	
		Tramadol SR	100 mg/day			No significant analgesia	
		Gabapentin	300 mg bid			VAS −30%	
Rog *et al.* (2007)	MS-CP: 63/66 patients enrolled in the RCT (95%), 14 men (22%);	Delta-9 tetrahydro-cannabinol/ cannabidiol (THC/CBD)	THC/CBD oromucosal spray (27 mg/mL: 25 mg/mL).	Uncontrolled, open-label non-comparative, effectiveness	Primary end-point: number, frequency, type of adverse events.	Study aimed at establishing long-term tolerability and effectiveness profiles for THC/CBD Mean final NRS-11 (RCT): THC/CBD 3.8, placebo 5.0	THC/CBD effective, with no evidence of tolerance in 28 selected MS-CP patients who

Table 9.3. (cont.)

Authors	Pain type: no. of patients	Drug(s)	Dosage	Study design	Pain rating	Outcome and notes	Conclusions
	mean age, 49 ± 8.4 years (range 27–71)		Dosage titrated to maintain the existing analgesia 6.5 sprays/day (mean), mostly after 4 p.m.	and tolerability indefinite-duration extension study (follow-up of the patients who completed an RCT: Rog *et al.* 2005) Mean duration of the study: 463 ± 378 days (median 638, range 3–917). Treatment duration >1 year: 34 patients (54%); until the end of the study: 28 patients (44%) (mean duration of treatment 839 ± 42, median 845, range 701–917)	Secondary end-points: NRS-11 NP score changes, laboratory results, vital signs, trial drug usage, intoxication VAS scores	Mean final NRS-11 in the 28 (44%) patients who completed the follow-up study: 2.9 ± 2.0 (range 0–8.0, change from the RCT baseline – 3.4 ± 1.8, range – 7.0 to – 0.1). Adverse events in 58 patients (92%, moderate in 49 [78%], and severe in 32 [51%], among them ventricular bigeminy and circulatory collapse in 1 patient) Most commonly reported adverse events: dizziness (27%), nausea (18%), feeling intoxicated (11%). Withdrawals (due to adverse events): 17 patients (25%)	completed 2 years of treatment Adverse events were common but of mild to moderate severity
Wine *et al.* (2007)	MS-CP	Nabilone	0.5 mg at night + upward titration	Case series	Neuropathy Pain Scale (0–100)	From 51.5 to 35 (mean)	
Canavero and Bonicalzi (2007a)	CP	Levetiracetam	500 mg	Unpublished observations	VAS	No effect	
Maarrawi *et al.* (2007a)	CPSP (2 capsulo-thalamic, 2 capsulo-lenticular, 1 juxta-thalamic, 1 thalamic, 2 brainstem)	PO morphine and dextro-propoxyphene	Titration to effect	Case series	Not available	No response and/or severe side effects in 5 patients and mild effect in 3 patients	

Ramachandran *et al.* (2007a)	CPSP: 1	Methadone oxycodone Phenytoin Gabapentin Amitriptyiline NSAIDs Benzodiazepine	Not available	Case report	VAS	No benefit (all)	
Carroll *et al.* (2008)	CP: 3	Mexiletine (MEX)	150–900 mg	Case series	Not available	Benefit (?)	Test infusions with lidocaine identify patients most likely to continue MEX therapy. MEX may have a clinical niche
Wasner *et al.* (2008a)	CCP: 12 (11 traumatic, 1 cord infarction)	Amitriptyline Oxycodone Pregabalin	Not available	Case series	Not available	Inadequate analgesia (all)	
Hans *et al.* (2008)	At-level NP due to extirpated epidural cord metastasis	Lidocaine 5% patches	Not available	Case report	Pain relief	Within 4 h after the first patch application, neuropathic symptoms started to disappear. After 12 h, patient had become completely pain-free. This topical treatment was continued for several weeks with lasting analgesic efficacy	
Shankar *et al.* (2008)	Thalamic AVM, with SAH. Radio-surgery + shunt: 1	Lamotrigine Dilantin Gabapentin Opioids TCA SSRI	Not available	Case report	VAS	No significant relief No significant relief No significant relief Unsatisfactory Unsatisfactory Unsatisfactory	
Lee *et al.* (2009)	CCP: 1	Gabapentin Amitriptyline Oxycodone	2700 mg/day 25 mg/day Not available	Case report	VAS	No benefit	
Pickering *et al.* (2009)	CPSP: 1	Nortryptiline Gabapentin Nabilone Opiates Pregabalin	60 mg/day 1800 mg/day Not available Not available Not available	Case report	VAS	No effect No effect No effect Little benefit Little benefit	

Table 9.3. (cont.)

Authors	Pain type: no. of patients	Drug(s)	Dosage	Study design	Pain rating	Outcome and notes	Conclusions
Hanihara *et al.* (2009)	CPSP (thalamic hemorrhage): 1	Sulpiride, amitriptyline	100 mg/day, not available	Case report	Not available	Sulpiride 100 mg/day plus amitriptyline improved her delusions within 3 months	CP and delusion linked?
McGeoch *et al.* (2009)	CPSP (thalamic): 1	Hydrocodone	Not available	Case report	VAS	No effect	
Solaro *et al.* (2009)	16 MS patients (10 women) with painful paroxysmal symptoms (PPS); TN: 2 patients, paroxysmal dysesthesias: 7 patients + others	Pregabalin (PGB)	75 mg gradually increased to 300 mg (max. dosage). Mean dosage: 154 mg/day	Open study	"Three-point scale" (0–3). Clinical evaluation at T0 (study entry), T1 (pain relief), T2 (3 months after the beginning of the study)	Complete and sustained statistically significant pain relief (–2 VAS points in 9 patients, incomplete relief in 4, drop-outs: 3 patients) Follow-up: 3 months **A 0–3 scale is a FOUR-point scale. Results analyzed by means of an unreported statistical test**	Gabapentin up to 2400 mg/day and CBZ up to 1200 mg/day, baclofen and TCA: side effects (7 patients) or no effect (9 patients)
Kishi *et al.* (2009)	CPSP, thalamic: 1	Clonazepam	0.5 mg /day	Case report	Not available	No effect	
Jiang *et al.* (2009)	SCI: 28	COX-2 inhibitors	Not available	Case series	VAS	–23.3%	Pains not specified
		Amitriptyline + Carbamazepine + COX-2 inhibitors				–54.5%	
		Amitriptyline + gabapentin + neurotropin/ COX-2 inhibitors				–65.8%	
Karakulova and Novikova (2010)	Syrinx pain: 34	Gabapentin	300 mg tid	Case series	Not available	Reduction of pain	
Lampl *et al.* (2010)	CPSP (5% of mixed group)	Pregabalin	Titrated to effect	Case series	VAS	Not available	Follow-up: 4 weeks (too short!) **Positive effect on global group likely biased by 19% with herniated sciaticas whose natural history is towards resolution!**

Kim *et al.* (2010)	CCP: 1	Opioids Gabapentin Amitriptyline	Not available 1800 mg/day 10 mg/day	Case report	VAS	Ineffective Unsatisfactory Unsatisfactory	
Tanei *et al.* (2010)	MS-CP: 1	CBZ Morphine Amitriptyline Gabapentin Diazepam	800 mg/day 30 mg/day 60 mg/day 1800 mg/day 4 mg	Case report	VAS	Transient reliefs (all)	
Mori *et al.* (2010)	MS: 19	Pregabalin and/or gabapentin Levetiracetam	Not available Not available	Case series	VAS and others	Ineffective in 18 Ineffective in 4	
Calabrò *et al.* (2010)	SCI: 1	Topiramate	150 mg/day	Case report	Not available	Dramatic improvement of painful ejaculation	Pain refractory to AD/AEDs
Hamauchi *et al.* (2010)	CCP (iatrogenic)	Ketamine PO	Not available	Case report	Not available	Ketamine test challenge: analgesia. Daily ketamine for 6 months: effective analgesia	NSAIDs, clonazepam, gabapentin: no effect

Barrera-Chacon *et al.* (2011)	SCI	Oxycodone (OXY)	Not reported (!)	54, paraplegic or tetraplegic (≥ 2 months) assessable patients (57 recruited)	Observational, prospective, multicenter study 3-month follow-up	Pain intensity and characteristics (VAS; DN4 scale), pain impact on activity and sleep (Lattinen scale); quality of life (EQ-5D); concomitant treatments, treatment-related adverse events	Study completed by 48 patients. OXY added to AEDs in 83% of cases. Statistically significant ($p <$ 0.001) pain relief (VAS reduction from 7.1 ± 1.3 to 4.3 ± 1.7), decrease in Lattinen total score (from 13.2 ± 3 to 7.7 ± 3.4), and increase in index of preference values (from 0.26 to 0.62) Non-significant EQ-5D VAS increase (p = 0.06). At least one treatment-related adverse event in 53.7% of patients (most frequently constipation)	Pain classified according to Siddall *et al.* (2000: below-level = located diffusely below the level of injury). Note (Table 2): above-level pain in 3 patients, at-level in 7 patients, below-level in 44 patients = 54 patients: apparently no patient had pain at more than one level	OXY, mostly in combination with AEDs, decreases pain intensity in SCI patients, improves health-related QoL, and diminishes the impact of pain on physical activity and sleep

Table 9.4. Uncontrolled studies: parenteral drugs

Authors	Drug(s)	Route/dosage	Pain type; no. of patients	Study design	Other details	Outcome
Di Biagio (1959)	Atophanyl	IV	CP: 2	Placebo-controlled		Great relief in 1, 0% in another
Plotkin (1982)	Morphine	IV, 1.5 mg/min up to 30 mg	Thalamic pain: 1; SCI: 3	Case series	Some control attempted, partially single-blind. Pain relief evaluated by a 10-point scale. Several days between morphine and pentobarbital test. Morphine followed by naloxone 0.8 mg. "Morphine saturation test method" as per Hosobuchi	Results not broken down according to pain. No response to morphine
	Pentobarbital	IV, 25 mg/min			Pentobarbital administered until the patient is on the point of unconsciousness, at which time pain should totally disappear if central	
Boas *et al.* (1982)	Lidocaine	IV, 3 mg/kg (infusion 240 mg)	CP, thalamic: 1		90% relief (transient)	1.5–2 mg/kg enough for CP
Edwards *et al.* (1985)	Lidocaine	IV	CP		Benefit	
Budd (1985)	Naloxone (NAL)	IV, 4–8 mg	CPSP: 13		Abatement of pain and hyperpathia in 7 patients (relief ranging from 4 days to 2.5 years) [IASP congress 1987, S252, A481: 25 CP patients, NAL 12 mg IV bolus; 20 patients improved]	Endo-opioids reduce CBF after stroke (inhibit locus ceruleus with release of norepinephrine): NAL reverses and increases cerebral perfusion.
Fatela *et al.* (1987; IASP congress 1987, A394]	Clomipramine	IV, 25–100 mg, then 125 mg qid	CPSP: 1	Case series	No effect	
Ray and Tai (1988)	Naloxone	IV, 0.4 mg titrating weekly to 12 mg (in 500 mL of Na/lactate); 12 mg	CPSP: 2	Case reports	Patient 1: 1st course: partial relief for 6 months; 2nd course: greater relief for 6 months; 3rd course: 100% relief for 6	Patient 1: amitriptyline + valproate effectve for 3 years, then relapse. Haloperidol + clomipramine: failure.

		for another 2 weeks			months; 4th course: 100% relief Patient 2: 1st course: considerable but incomplete relief for 4 months	
Bowsher (1989)	Naloxone	IV, 0.8 mg	Cordotomized patients with mirror pain		Increased pain in one-third and induced it in one not suffering pain	
Tasker *et al.* (1991)	Penthotal	IV, 50–225 mg (average: 136 mg)	BCP/CCP	Case series	73% responders	CP is not dependent on opiate mechanism; 55% of CCP cases responded to morphine, but only the evoked pains and less frequently lancinating pains, *rarely steady pain*
	Morphine (some also fentanyl)	IV, 15–18 mg			0% responders	
Arner and Meyerson (1991)	Morphine	IV, 70 mg over 45 min	BCP: 1	Single case in letter	No effect	CP unresponsive to opioids
Backonja and Gombar (1992)	Lidocaine	IV, single infusion	BCP: 6; CCP: 2	Case series	3 BCP benefited over 8–20 weeks; partial relief in 2 SCI cases	
Edmondson *et al.* (1993)	Lidocaine	IV, initial bolus: 50–100 mg + continuous infusion for 48 h	CPSP: 4	Case series	All patients reported some relief within the first 12 h of infusion. Subsequent oral mexiletine trial: 2 patients had excellent relief at 1 year, 2 stopped because of intolerable side effects	
Galer *et al.* (1993)	Lidocaine	IV, 5 mg/kg/h for 60–90 min	CP: 13	Retrospective series	1 excellent relief, 3 partial reliefs, 9 0% reliefs	
Nagaro *et al.* (1995)	Lidocaine	IV, 1.5 mg/kg in 1 min	CP and PNP	Case series	VAS assessed 5, 15, and 35 min after the infusion: pain decreased to less than 50% of pre-infusion value in more than 75% of cases of thalamic pain	SCI pain relatively refractory

Table 9.4. (cont.)

Authors	Drug(s)	Route/dosage	Pain type; no. of patients	Study design	Other details	Outcome
Migita *et al.* (1995)	Thyamilal, morphine	See Yamamoto *et al.* (1997), below	CP: 2	Case report	Patient 1: barbiturate and morphine ineffective Patient 2: barbiturate effective, morphine ineffective	
Yamamoto *et al.* (1997)	Morphine, then naloxone	IV, 3 mg every 5 min up to 18 mg	CPSP: 39 (thalamic 25, extra-thalamic 14, brainstem 0)	Case series	Study evaluating the effect of IV morphine (day 1), IV thiamylal (day 2), and IV ketamine (day 3). A few patients fell asleep with barbiturate. Threshold of significance: ≥ 40%. No differences between thalamic and suprathalamic cases. All ketamine-responsive cases except 1 also sensitive to thiamylal, but 4 cases resistant to ketamine responded to thiamylal	1 thalamic and 1 suprathalamic patients (of 3 sensitive to IV morphine) relieved at long term by oral morphine 30–120 mg/day All patients refractory to imipramine (75 mg), maprotiline (60 mg), bromazepam (12 mg), ibuprofen (600 mg) Pain worsened by ketamine in 2 patients
	Thiamylal	IV, 50 mg every 5 min up to 250 mg				
	Ketamine	IV, 5 mg every 5 min up to 25 mg	CPSP: 23			
Kumar *et al.* (1997)	Morphine	IV, 25 mg	CPSP: 5; CCP: 3	Case series of DBS	0% relief in all	
Koyama *et al.* (1998)	Amobarbital (AMO)	IV, 50 mg	CPSP: 1	Case report	CP after loss of his left upper extremity. AMO IV was followed by 300–400 mg/day AMO PO	IV (but not PO) AMO was effective in reducing CP, although similar plasma concentration levels were reached PO and IV
Canavero and Bonicalzi (1998a)	Propofol	IV, 0.2 mg/kg	SCI: 1	Review with case report	Reported the efficacy of IT midazolam in 1 SCI-CP patient	All drugs proposed as diagnostic test
	Lidocaine	IV, 3–5 mg/kg in 30 min				
	Ketamine	IV, 60 µg/kg + 6 µg/kg/min				

	Midazolam Baclofen Fentanyl Alfentanil Clonidine	IT, 1–2.5 mg IT, 50 μg IV, 50 μg IV, 0.6 μg/kg + 6 μg/kg/min IT				
Waijima *et al.* (2000)	Thiopental	IV, approximately 1 mg/kg	SCI: 1	Case report	IM butorphanol, saline and atropine sulfate as a placebo, IT morphine HCL, mexiletine, IV lidocaine ineffective IV thiopental, fentanyl, butorphanol, ketamine, midazolam, droperidol, sevoflurane-oxygen anesthesia quite effective	Original CP decreased after 16 subarachnoid blocks with local anesthetic. IV thiopental was the most effective treatment in CP. CP worsened by spinal anesthesia
Trentin and Visentin (2000)	Lidocaine	IV, 4 mg/kg over 30 min	CP: 16	Case series	44% responded; after 45 min, lidocane = placebo	**Later good response to mexiletine PO**, but not amitriptyline
Chatterjee *et al.* (2002)	Herbal cannabis	1 "joint" daily	CPSP: 1	Case report	Complete pain relief and marked improvement in dystonia from smoked cannabis (3-month follow-up)	Right hemiplegic painful dystonia (left-sided idiopathic caudate atrophy). 3 temporarily successful thalamotomies performed. Partial response to morphine plus buproprion and amitriptyline (VAS reduction from 9/10 to 4/10)
Cahana *et al.* (2004)	Lidocaine	IV, 5 mg/kg (in 150 mL saline) over 30 min without a bolus. 2 daily cycles for 5 days at a 6 month interval	CP (post-infective pontine lesion): 1	Case report	Persistent spontaneous pain and frequency of pain attacks reduction was observed immediately, 1, 3, and 7 days and 1, 2, and 3 months after treatment in all body areas but the chin	Persistent pain relief after repeated IV lidocaine infusions. CP unresponsive to amitriptyline, nortriptyline, carbamazepine, oxcarbazepine, gabapentin, valproate, lamotrigine, baclofen, and clonazepam
Cohen and DeJesus (2004)	Ketamine	PCA device (2.7 mg/h basal; same dose on demand)	CCP (syrinx): 1	Case report	1 year later, pain dramatically decreased, opioids significantly reduced	Previous high-dose opioids ineffective

Table 9.4. (cont.)

Authors	Drug(s)	Route/dosage	Pain type; no. of patients	Study design	Other details	Outcome
Nuti *et al.* (2005)	Morphine	IV test	CP: 7	Case series	No significant effect	
Iranami *et al.* (2006)	Tramadol	IV, 50 mg over 15 min	CPSP: 1	Case report	100% relief for 5 h (!?). Then 6-day trial of codeine 20 mg PO plus milnacipran (25 mg) bid: 100% relief (!?) and full relapse upon cessation of 1 day (!?). Restarted, again with full analgesia *within hours* (!?). Full analgesia for 10 months. Study: 6 days ON + 1 day OFF + continuous therapy ON	AMI/CBZ: no effect. NB: this patient appears to be a full placebo responder
	Thiopental	IV, 50 mg			No relief	
Bharadwaj and Danilychev (2006)	Hydromorphone	IV, 24 mg/h	CPSP: 1		No analgesia	
	Add-on: lidocaine	2 mg/kg over 20 min followed by 1mg/kg/h infusion			100% analgesia. Hydromorphone down 50%. Death 2 weeks later, pain-free	
Hans *et al.* (2007)	Adenosine	IV, 3 mg IV, 5 mg, then continuous infusion over 90 min	MS-CP: 1		Significant reduction of spontaneous dysesthesias+ mechano-thermal allodynia Prolonged relief for up to 6 weeks Treated for 14 months without tolerance	Gabapentin 900 mg/day: some pain reduction, but intolerable side effects IV lidocaine (4 mg/kg): stopped for bronchospasm
Lee *et al.* (2009)	Lidocaine Ketamine	IV tests	CCP: 1	Case report	No benefit	
Tanei *et al.* (2010)	Ketamine	IV infusion (60 mg) bimonthly	MS-CP: 1	Case report	Transient benefit	

Sakas *et al.* (2011)	Morphine Barbiturate Ketamine	Not available	CPSP: 1	Case report	Transient benefits	Gabapentin: transient benefit
Kern *et al.* (2010)	Lidocaine patch	Not available	SCI (1 patient) + mixed group	Case series	Not available	The probability of benefiting from therapy in the presence of allodynia was about 10-fold higher compared to patients without. Females responded better.
Guetti *et al.* (2011)	Buprenorphine	Transdermal TDS 35 μg/h every 84 h	CPSP: 1	Case reports	VAS 2 after 1 month. Stopped after 10 applications due to side effects	Gabapentin 2 g and oxcarbazepine 900 mg plus tramadol 400 mg/day: ineffective

used in severe congestive heart failure. Abrupt withdrawal must be avoided. Side effects derive from CNS, visual, renal, cardiac, and gastrointestinal toxicity. As with gabapentin, Stevens–Johnson syndrome and suicidal ideation are rarely seen. If elected, start with 25 mg and increase by 25 mg every 2–3 days in divided doses up to 600 mg. In a 9-month-long open-label extension of an RCT targeting CP, 14.6% of the patients withdrew because of adverse effects (serious in 3.9%, all after the 3-month duration of the RCT!) (Murphy *et al.* 2007a, 2007b). This drug has been approved as an anxyolytic, which might justify its continued use in some patients. It has a faster onset of effect than gabapentin.

Valproate and **oral baclofen** at orally tolerated doses (< 60 mg/day) are ineffective in the vast majority of patients. **Benzodiazepines** generally have no effect or increase pain compared to controls (Menefee *et al.* 2000); we note that in France oral clonazepam is often given for painful paroxysms. Use of sedative drugs is associated with a 36% increase in overall mortality risk, with the highest risk in patients aged 55–74 years (Belleville 2010).

Antiglutamatergic drugs

The only antiglutamatergic drug available for clinical use so far is **ketamine**. However, ketamine is a drug of addiction with neurotoxic effects (particularly with intrathecal/epidural administration) and unpleasant psychiatric side effects. Renal damage and cystitis are part of the spectrum. Rapid-acting routes of administration (e.g., intranasal) should be avoided and doses kept as low as possible. Psychotomimetic effects appear to be most common in anxious and apprehensive individuals. Oral ketamine can (rarely) induce hepatic failure; it has a low bioavailability (*c.* 15%) and is rapidly metabolized to the much weaker norketamine. At low dose (30 mg), it has morphine-sparing qualities (Bell 2009). Plasma concentrations can be increased (3.6 times) by administering 500 mg of clarithromycin 1 hour before ketamine (Hagelberg *et al.* 2010); it also affects the metabolism of midazolam. Long-term subcutaneous ketamine may lead to painful indurations. S-ketamine may – or may not – have fewer side effects than racemic ketamine. Ketamine is best reserved for parenteral in-hospital administration for urgent pain control and pharmacologic dissection.

Oral NMDA blockers (**dextrometorphan, riluzole, memantine**) have no or only modest analgesic effects and many side effects: they are not advised in the routine treatment of CP. Selective AMPA/kainate blockers (e.g., **tezampanel**) have yet to be tested on CP; these too are associated with side effects (e.g., hazy vision, sedation).

Sodium channel blockers

Intravenous **lidocaine** has been administered at doses of 1 mg/kg (over 10 minutes) to 5 mg/kg (over 30 minutes to 5 hours) diluted in saline, sometimes via a pump. Pressure and ECG monitoring are mandatory. Dysarthria and somnolence call for immediate suspension, and lidocaine is contraindicated with Adams–Stokes syndrome or severe atrioventricular heart block. The most frequent minor side effect is dizziness during infusion. Lidocaine can suddenly worsen/trigger the symptoms of multiple sclerosis (Sakurai and Kanazawa (1999), possibly due to a different distribution of ion channels in demyelinated axons.

Lamotrigine must be increased slowly (!), starting with 25 mg once daily for 14 days, then increased to 50 mg once daily for a further 14 days, and then increased by a maximum of 50–100 mg every 7–14 days up to 500 mg (on occasion even 800 mg daily), if tolerated. Side effects include rash, hypersensitivity syndrome, CNS and visual symptoms and signs, arthralgia, and suicidal ideation. Serious skin reactions (i.e., Stevens–Johnson syndrome and toxic epidermal necrolysis), rarely with fatalities, have developed, especially in children, mostly in the first 8 weeks. Consider withdrawal if rash or signs of hypersensitivity syndrome (which includes multiorgan dysfunction) develop. Concurrent valproate increases plasma concentration.

Mexiletine is only available through "special-order" manufacturers or specialist importing companies: consult the manufacturer's leaflet for special precautions of use. Dosage is given in Table 18.1.

Carbamazepine has so many contraindications and cautionary notes attached that, in view of its overall scarce efficacy on CP, it should be avoided *tout court* (except for the treatment of trigeminal neuralgia and other paroxysmal symptoms of multiple sclerosis). *Oxcarbazepine* is said to have less hepatic enzyme-inducing potential. Carbamazepine (but not lamotrigine) is known to result in adverse effects that mimic an MS exacerbation (Ramsaransing *et al.* 2000, Solaro *et al.* 2005).

Experience with **zonisamide** (also a T-type Ca^{2+} channel blocker) and **lacosamide** (which is arrhythmogenic) is scarce. **Levetiracetam**, whose mechanism of action is unknown, and **topiramate** (also a $GABA_A$ agonist/AMPA antagonist), which has a high withdrawal rate, are not particularly effective.

Aminergic drugs

Amitriptyline and all tricyclics are contraindicated in patients with myocardial infarction, arrhythmias (particularly heart block), mania, acute porphyria, and severe liver disease. Use with caution in hyperthyroidism, pheocromocytoma, epilepsy, diabetes, prostatic hypertrophy and urinary retention, chronic constipation, glaucoma, and suicidal patients. Elderly patients are particularly susceptible to many of these side effects, with an increase of falls: low initial doses should be used, with close monitoring, particularly for psychiatric and cardiac side effects. Overdosage can be fatal. Side effects are myriad and include cardiac, CNS (including sedation), antimuscarinic, endocrine (including sexual dysfunction), and many others. However, once elected, the patient should be encouraged to persist with treatment, as some tolerance to these side effects seems to develop. They are reduced if low doses are given initially and then gradually increased, but this must be balanced against the need to obtain analgesia as fast as possible. Tricyclics should not be stopped abruptly. A systematic review did not find an increased risk of adverse cardiovascular outcomes in high-risk patients (Swenson *et al.* 2006), and doses < 100 mg do not appear to be associated with sudden death (Ray *et al.* 2004). If elected, start with 10–25 mg daily at bedtime (they are sleep-inducing) and increase slowly every few days up to 150 mg if necessary, under cardiologic surveillance. Analgesia can appear days to 5 weeks after initiation, regardless of dose, and can increase slowly, even if plasma levels are stable: a trial of efficacy should never last less than 2 months, barring intolerable side effects (with at least 2 weeks at maximum tolerated dosage). After suspension of therapy, analgesia is lost gradually, but slower than expected from plasma levels. Artificial saliva is indicated to counter mouth dryness. Although some congeners may be better tolerated (e.g., **nortriptyline** and **clomipramine**), amitriptyline (and perhaps **imipramine**) appears to be the most effective of all aminergics (e.g., **desipramine**, **duloxetine**). Selective serotonin reuptake inhibitors (SSRIs) (e.g., **fluoxetine**), serotonin–norepinephrine reuptake inhibitors (SNRIs) (e.g., **venlafaxine**, **milnacipran**), and selective norepinephrine blockers (e.g., **reboxetine**) are currently not indicated for CP for lack of or trivial benefit.

Opioids and cannabinoids

Intravenous **morphine** (and congeners) relieved none or only few patients with CP, and only at very high doses:

> Prolonged high-dose opioid therapy may be neither safe nor effective . . . Long-term use of opioids may also be associated with the development of abnormal sensitivity to pain [which] has much in common with the cellular mechanisms of neuropathic pain . . . Prolonged opioid use may result in reduced fertility, libido and drive and in immunosuppression especially in susceptible patients . . . Opioid therapy may increase the burden of care (Ballantyne and Mao 2003).

A meta-analysis (Noble *et al.* 2008) found that many chronic pain patients discontinue long-term opioid therapy due to adverse effects or insufficient analgesia. At 1 year, withdrawal rates were 52–88% for oral opioids and 43–67% for transdermal; withdrawal rates for both oral and transdermal opioids in the studies with longest follow-up were 88% at 18 months (95% at 4 years for transdermal opioids). The evidence that oral opioids reduce pain long-term in the relatively small proportion of patients who continue treatment is weak (Noble *et al.* 2008). Whereas cognitive function is preserved in patients taking stable moderate doses of opioids, this can be impaired for up to 7 days after a dose increase. A ceiling dose (*c.* 195 mg of morphine daily) may vary in the single patient, and those receiving high doses rarely report satisfactory analgesia or improved function (Ballantyne and Mao 2003). If the patient is on oral morphine, 2–3 months may be necessary for complete washout. **Methadone** may be less immunosuppressive than morphine, but it has a higher risk of respiratory depression due to accumulation. The risk of opioid misuse, abuse, or addiction ranges between < 5% and 50%. Constipation does not habituate, which calls for a concurrent bowel regimen. Physical dependence is seen in all patients.

Tramadol is less efficacious than morphine, and can lower the seizure threshold and precipitate the serotonin syndrome in combination with SSRIs and SNRIs.

The place of opioids (including tramadol) in CP management is restricted to very few patients, who can tolerate their long-term side-effect profile in the face of satisfactory analgesia (Canavero and Bonicalzi 2003a).

Naloxone has not proved analgesic in an RCT. One notes the impossibility for an agonist and its antagonist to have therapeutic effects on the same disease, barring unknown mechanisms of action.

Studies on **cannabis** and **cannabinoids** (both natural and synthetic) have been assessed in a meta-analysis:

> In terms of efficacy, [they] display a positive and moderate short-term trend toward a reduction in the intensity of pain in chronic patients, but the same cannot be said for the harms. In this case, the results call into question the possibility of this therapy being efficacious over long periods of time ... in longer-term trials (4–5 weeks) ... cases of acute psychosis were observed ... harmful effects on brain tissues ... such studies might well be *overestimating the intervention's efficacy and underestimating its adverse events* ... cannabis and its derivates tend to accumulate in adipose tissues. This, in turn, acts as a reservoir that continuously releases them, possibly resulting in more potent effects in regular users (Martin-Sanchez *et al.* 2009).

Cannabis users are more likely to meet the criteria for a lifetime psychiatric diagnosis, and perform less well on several neuropsychological tests. Inhaled cannabis can exacerbate extant psychiatric conditions (e.g., schizophrenia) and can impair MS patients: neuroprotection and immunosuppression are seen at levels beyond what is achievable in clinical practice (Semple *et al.* 2005, Arnett 2008, Wang *et al.* 2008).

Efficacy on CP is very limited (Attal *et al.* 2004b, Rintala *et al.* 2010). Unlike opioids, cannabinoids appear to improve sleep.

Chapter 10 Neuromodulation

Perhaps we can now envision a day in which, with the use of stimulation techniques, we can take advantage of the brain's natural modes of organization and reinforce them in time of need, whether to control pain, . . . epileptic . . . discharge, or . . . tremor.
Ervin et al. *(1966)*

Neuromodulation is the next step when drug therapy fails. In view of the continuing efforts aimed at neural reconstruction in the human central nervous system and thus the "physiological" reversion of pain, and progress in neuromodulation, there is little room left for ablative procedures, which have low long-term efficacy and a high incidence of permanent, disabling complications, including new or worsening of pre-existent CP, as ablation only adds further damage.

Neuromodulation can be achieved through electrical stimulation of the damaged nervous system or intrathecal drug infusion through implanted pumps.

A brief history of the electrical modulation of pain

The interested reader is referred to Mottelay (1922). The analgesic effect of electrical stimulation has been known since ancient times. For instance, Scribonius Largus, a Roman physician (AD 50), reported that a freedman of the emperor Tiberius called Anthero was cured of the gout by shocks received from the electric fish *Torpedo* (the numbing fish of Aristotle); Dioscorides advised the same treatment for inveterate pains of the head, and similar applications are alluded to by Galen. The eighteenth century witnessed a resurgence of this technique, despite strong opposition. With Italy's Luigi Galvani and Alessandro Volta in the nineteenth century, electrotherapy was poised to make progress. Giovanni Aldini, Galvani's nephew, first treated a depressive patient with a primitive cranial stimulating apparatus (the forerunner of transcranial direct current stimulation) with benefit (Fig. 10.1). He was also the first to prove that a human brain in a fresh cadaver could be stimulated to obtain motor responses. His demonstrations in London and elsewhere circa 1800 sparked the fantasy of the time and led to Mary Shelley's novel *Frankenstein*.

In the nineteenth century, several physicians treated pain with custom-made electrotherapy machines, e.g. Duchenne de Boulogne, who published a classic book in 1855, and Hermel, who treated neuralgias with "electro-puncture."

In 1892, Sir William Osler wrote in the neuralgia section of his highly acclaimed textbook (pp. 962–3):

> The continuous current may be used. The sponges should be warm, and the positive pole be placed near the seat of the pain. The strength of the current should be such as to cause a slight tingling or burning, but not pain.

Riddoch (1938) noted that CP could sometimes be diminished by concomitant stimulation through faradization in the abnormal or adjacent normal body parts.

Electroconvulsive therapy, first introduced in 1938 by Italy's Ugo Cerletti, was also applied for pain control.

Mazars *et al.* (1960) first reported attempts to stimulate the somatosensory pathways, particularly the neospinothalamic tract at its termination in the thalamic sensory relay nuclei, for the treatment of chronic neurogenic pain. Their theoretical framework was the theory of Head and Holmes, which held that CP might be the consequence of an imbalance between protopathic and epicritic sensory functioning: stimulation of the thalamic sensory relay nuclei would presumably increase the epicritic component and hence inhibit the protopathic inflow (an anticipation of the later gate control theory). Acute thalamic stimulation was later found to suppress the aversive behavior in patients with facial postherpetic neuralgia (White and Sweet 1969).

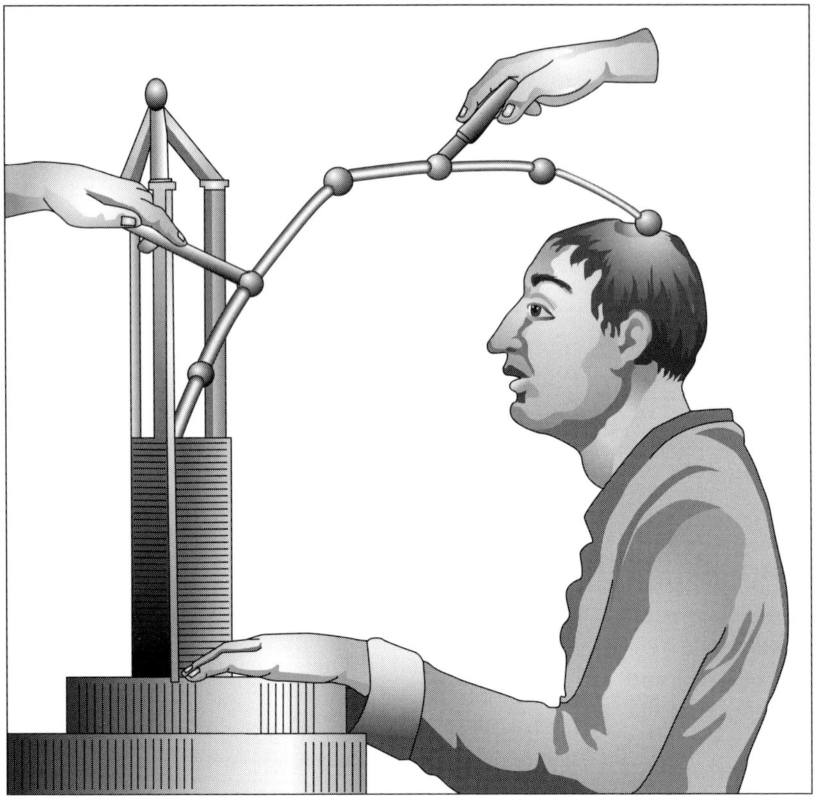

Figure 10.1. First application of non-invasive cortical stimulation in a depressed patient. Adapted from Aldini 1803.

However, the real interest in deep brain stimulation (DBS) for the treatment of chronic pain in humans arose in the 1970s. The discovery that electrical stimulation of the rat midbrain could produce profound analgesia without the concurrent administration of drugs, and Melzack and Wall's gate control theory, according to which stimulation of large-diameter fibers is capable of inhibiting nociceptive information, paved the way for most electrical neurostimulation procedures (although this construct has been rejected as a viable mechanism of analgesia).

Initial attempts at spinal stimulation hark back to the 1940s (Martini *et al.* 1943, Ajmone-Marsan *et al.* 1951). Unfortunately, these did not lead to direct clinical application. The gate control theory of pain inspired Shealy to implant the first dorsal column stimulator in a cancer patient. Almost simultaneously, Shimoji *et al.* (1971) in Japan also developed an epidural stimulator for chronic pain relief. Transcutaneous electrical nerve stimulation (TENS) was first introduced in the 1960s as a screening procedure for spinal cord stimulation.

Surgical motor cortex stimulation was first tried in 1988 by Tsubokawa and his group in Japan, and in 1995 another Japanese group first reported on the effects of non-invasive cortical stimulation on CP (see Chapter 11).

A note on mechanism of action

How electrical neuromodulation actually works remains unknown, despite a plethora of neuroimaging and electrophysiological data (see following chapters). The latest and, in our view, most fecund approach has been delineated by Montgomery (2010) for deep brain stimulation (DBS), but it applies similarly to all other stimulatory interventions:

> Although the prevailing view is that neurological disease is caused by a deficiency or a surplus of neurotransmitters, DBS reminds us that . . . neurological and psychiatric disorders can be seen as "misinformation" related to the pattern of electrical activities in and among neurons. The old saws of clinical neurology that there are "positive"

> symptoms . . ., "negative symptoms" . . . and "disconnection" symptoms need to be updated based on symptoms related to misinformation. The information and misinformation in the brain most likely is primary and proximately represented in the electrical activities of neural systems. Neurotransmitters are the messengers not the message and it is the message that is of paramount importance.

In his view, the brain is an ensemble of nested and interconnected, poly-synaptic re-entrant neuronal oscillators which can be understood inside an informational (Shannon-like) framework. The theory posits that a re-entrant oscillation that amplifies the signal through resonance must be stimulated long enough to have a resonance effect, which comes with a latency for the effect. The stimulation frequencies must match the fundamental frequencies in the targeted oscillators to be clinically effective.

One type of misinformation is a low signal-to-noise ratio, whereby actual information is buried in noise. This ratio can be improved by stimulation-driven resonance amplification. Resonance then depends on the stimulating frequency relative to the fundamental carrier frequency of the neural oscillators involved.

A second type of resonance amplification is stochastic resonance, i.e., adding noise to a signal to improve the signal-to-noise ratio. Although the noise added to the signal has to be of a certain bandwidth, the advantage of stochastic resonance is that the fundamental frequencies of the underlying neural oscillators do not have to be known precisely. Since trying to replicate the normal patterns of spike trains remains beyond our current capabilities, another approach is to overwrite the misinformation with no information, e.g., by stimulating the neurons to fire in a highly regular manner (so-called information ablation).

In sum, continuous and regular stimulation imparts no information, but may convert misinformation into no information or at specific frequencies resonate with and amplify the signal above the background noise, thereby increasing the information content.

Chapter 11

Cortical stimulation

Non-invasive cortical stimulation

The reader is referred to Canavero (2009, 2011) for full discussion and technical details. Repetitive transcranial magnetic stimulation (rTMS) and transcranial direct current stimulation (tDCS) are non-invasive techniques with a benign side-effect profile and are easy to administer. Patients are awake, alert, and sit or lie comfortably during treatment sessions, which are roughly 20–30 minutes long. In most studies, the primary motor area (MI) has been the main target of stimulation, but the primary somatosensory cortex (SI) can also be effective. Certainly, the large electrode used for tDCS (5 × 7 cm) involves both MI and SI. The target has been located either with conventional techniques or neuronavigation, and confirmed by neurophysiological means (i.e., the ability to elicit motor evoked potentials – assessed by electromyography and/or observation of twitches – in a muscle group corresponding to the affected body region).

Efficacy

A meta-analysis concluded that 64% (54.6% at follow-up) of chronic pain patients responded to extradural cortical stimulation (ECS) versus 40% of patients responding to non-invasive stimulation (weighted responder rate of 72.6% for ECS vs. 45.3% for rTMS/tDCS) (Lima and Fregni 2008). A review of all studies (Tables 11.1 and 11.2) shows that several patients did not deviate from baseline visual analog scale (VAS) ratings. In some TMS studies, reductions in pain ratings were also noted among patients in the sham conditions, and, in some trials, these did not differ significantly from pain-rating reductions noted with active treatment (O'Connell *et al.* 2010). This may have been due to inadequate tilting of the coil in sham conditions, producing unintended cortical stimulation sufficient to produce analgesic effects. In the case of tDCS, sham stimulation is easier to administer. On the other hand, studies in which post-treatment VAS ratings and patients are inadequately assessed over time may fail to detect treatment effects, particularly if analgesia is delayed a few days. This may detract from the overall impression of efficacy.

There is no uniformly effective frequency of stimulation, and both high (10–20 Hz) and low (0.2–0.5 Hz) frequencies can be effective. Each person shows variable cortical excitability, and this must be assessed at the individual level. The effect of TMS may start within minutes, but the duration of analgesia after a single session is usually brief (5 minutes to 8 days). Some authors emphasize how repeated sessions on consecutive days may lead to cumulative effects lasting beyond the time of stimulation, which could be exploited clinically in patients awaiting surgical implantation (Lefaucheur 2008). Unfortunately, differences in mean VAS ratings reported in all studies before and after treatment can be misleading, influenced by a large change in only a small subset of patients. Furthermore, significant differences were obtained even with small reductions in the VAS after rTMS treatment (O'Connell *et al.* 2010). Thus, non-invasive cortical stimulation cannot be recommended for chronic treatment at the present time, except in an unpredictable fashion in some highly responsive patients. tDCS does not appear to offer superior efficacy over rTMS.

Mechanisms of action

CP is subtended by an anomalous oscillatory loop between SI and the sensory thalamus (see Chapter 26). ECS and rTMS may rebalance such oscillatory activity, by restoring defective intracortical inhibition (GABAergic), in parallel with pain relief. Propofol, a pure GABA agonist, renormalizes cortical and thalamic activity (Canavero and Bonicalzi 1998a, 2007a) and its effects correlate with TMS analgesia (Canavero *et al.* 2002c, 2003). Cortical stimulation

Table 11.1. Non-invasive cortical stimulation: Transcranial magnetic stimulation (TMS)

Authors/date	Stimulation site/ type of coil	Parameters of stimulation	Study design	Type of CP (number of patients)	Outcome measures	Outcome: comparison with placebo, effect duration
Migita *et al.* (1995)	MI corresponding to pain distribution	0.2 Hz (circular coil) 1 train of 16.7 min (200 pulses) 80% stimulator output	No sham	Cerebral palsy + talamotomy (1), putamen hemorrrhage (1)	VAS	Pt 1: 30% reduction of pain; Pt 2: 0%; 1 responder (50%). Effect duration: 1 hour *Same effect seen after extradural cortical stimulation*
Canavero *et al.* (1998)	MI and SI corresponding to pain distribution	0.2 Hz (circular coil) 200 pulses 65–100% stimulator output	No sham Propofol	3 CP (2 CPSP, 1 postsurgery BCP)	VAS	CP: 1 responder (33%) Propofol matched TMS results in whole series (CP+PNP) *Extradural cortical stimulation (MI or SI) matched propofol and TMS results (one patient not implanted surgically)*
Canavero *et al.* (2002c, 2003) (new patients) (Two identical publications)	MI corresponding to pain distribution F8 and double cone	0.2 Hz 1 train of 16.7 min (200 pulses) 100% stimulator output (SO)	Sham Propofol	CPSP (5), SCI (4)	VAS	3 patients: 26–75% reduction of pain (both spontaneous and allodynia) for 1/4/16 hours 1 patient: 100% abatement of allodynia for 30 min (not spontaneous pain) 2 patients: worsening of pain 3 patients: no effect Pain relief strongly correlated to propofol-induced pain relief ($p = 0.002$)
Rollnik *et al.* (2002)	MI corresponding to pain distribution Circular and double-cone coils	20 Hz 20 trains of 2 s (800 pulses) 80% RMT		SCI (2)	VAS	4% reduction of pain (sham: 2%) in whole series (CP+PNP) $p > 0.05$ vs. angled coil 6 responders (50%) Duration of effect: 6 days
Khedr *et al.* 2005	MI corresponding to pain distribution F8	20 Hz 10 trains of 10 s (2000 pulses), 5 consecutive sessions (1 week)	Parallel	CPSP (24)	VAS and other scales	45% pain reduction (sham: 5%) in whole group (CP+PNP) $p < 0.001$ vs. angled coil rTMS: 21 responders out of 28 Sham: 5 responders of 20

Table 11.1. (cont.)

Authors/date	Stimulation site/ type of coil	Parameters of stimulation	Study design	Type of CP (number of patients)	Outcome measures	Outcome: comparison with placebo, effect duration
		80% RMT				Duration of effect: ≥ 2 weeks after the last session
Hirayama *et al.* (2006) Saitoh *et al.* (2007)	MI corresponding to pain distribution, plus somatosensory, premotor and supplementary area F8 Neuro-navigated	5 Hz 10 trains of 10 s (500 pulses), one session 90% RMT 1/5/10 Hz 500 pulses	Crossover	CP 14 (4 putaminal, 7 thalamic, 1 brainstem stroke, 2 SCI)	VAS and other scales	BCP (12 patients): 4 patients no response, 1 patient made worse, 7 patients: 37.5% reduction of pain (range 12.5– 66.7%) CCP (2 patients): 52.6% and 20% reductions of pain Cauda lesion: 80% reduction of pain Duration of effect: 2–3 days in 1 patient only; in all others relief for max. 3 hours *CPSP has low response to rTMS* BCP: 5/10 (but not 1) Hz afforded > 30% pain relief 10 Hz rTMS > 5 Hz rTMS BCP more refractory to rTMS than SCI pain/PNP *rTMS may predict response to extradural cortical stimulation*
Irlbacher *et al.* (2006)	MI corresponding to pain area F8	5 Hz/1 Hz 500 pulses, 5 consecutive days in 1 week 95% RMT	Crossover	Thalamic (3) or brainstem (7) stroke, SCI (3)	VAS	5 Hz / 1 Hz / sham rTMS: 5% / 6% / 10% reductions of pain (= negative study) in whole group (CP+PNP) $p = 0.06$ (5 Hz rTMS) / 0.08 (1 Hz rTMS) vs. sham coil 2 responders (7%) whatever the type of rTMS
André-Obadia *et al.* (2006)	MI corresponding to pain area F8 Neuro-navigated	20 Hz / 1 Hz 20 trains 0f 4 s/1 train of 26 min (1600 pulses), one session each 90% RMT	Crossover	Thalamic/ thalamocapsular (8) or brainstem (2 : 1 dropout) stroke, cervical SCI (1)	VAS and other scales	Immediate pain abatement in all patients, whatever the frequency 20 Hz / 1 Hz / sham rTMS: 11% reduction of pain / 2 % increase of pain in several patients up to + 27% / 8% reduction of pain. No

						significant difference between 20 Hz and sham stimulation Relief after 20 Hz = relief after sham Superiority of 20 Hz vs. sham stimulation *only* for prediction of response to ECS Level of significance set at 10% reduction of pain: this would make this study a negative one according to criteria adopted in other studies! Duration of effect: *c.* 1 week ***Patients treated with extradural cortical stimulation. CP+PNP: 6 of 11 patients (55%) benefited. 5/11 responders to 20 Hz TMS benefited, vs. 1/5 non-responders. 1/6 responders to 1 Hz TMS benefited from MCS***
Defrin *et al.* (2007b)	MI corresponding to pain distribution F8	5 Hz 10 trains of 10 s (500 pulses), 10 sessions of 15–30 min (2 weeks) 115% RMT		SCI-CP (11) (T4/12 levels, 2 complete, 9 incomplete)	VAS / NRS / MPQ	27% pain reduction (sham: 37%) at the end of the treatment $p > 0.05$ vs. sham coil 30% of responders (sham: 10%) in the follow-up period only (2–6 weeks after the last session), *not* acutely
Lefaucher *et al.* (2001a, 2001b, 2004a, 2006a, 2006b, 2008) Lefaucher (2008) **NB: strong suspicion of data duplication in multiple papers**	MI corresponding to pain distribution F8	(A) 10 Hz 20 trains of 5 s (1000 pulses) 80% RMT (B) 10 Hz / 0.5 Hz 10 Hz / 0.5 Hz rTMS: 20 trains 0f 5 s / 1 train of 20 min (1000 / 600 pulses) 80% RMT (C) 10 Hz	Crossover	(A) Thalamic stroke (7) (B) Thalamic stroke (6), brainstem lesion (6) (C) Thalamic stroke (12), brainstem lesion (12), SCI lesion (12) (D) Thalamic (5) or brainstem (4) stroke, SCI (5)	VAS	(A) 10 Hz rTMS: whole group (CP+PNP) 31% (sham: 11% pain increase) $p = 0.01$ vs. sham coil 8 responders (57%), *c.* 1 week Significant but transient reduction in pain (B) 10 Hz / 0.5 Hz / sham rTMS: (whole group: CP+PNP) 20% / 4% / 7% $p = 0.001$ vs. sham coil (10 Hz-rTMS) 7 responders (39%) Duration of effect: transient (C) Whole group (CP+PNP): 23% reduction of pain (sham: 8%)

Table 11.1. (cont.)

Authors/date	Stimulation site/ type of coil	Parameters of stimulation	Study design	Type of CP (number of patients)	Outcome measures	Outcome: comparison with placebo, effect duration
		1 session , 20 trains of 5 s (1000 pulses) 80% RMT (D) 10 Hz 20 trains of 10 s (2000 pulses) 90% RMT (E) 10 Hz / 1 Hz 10 Hz / 1 Hz rTMS: 20 trains of 6 s / 1 train of 20 min (1200 pulses), one session 90% RMT (F) 10 Hz / 1 Hz 20 trains of 6 s / 1 train of 20 min (1200 pulses) 90% RMT (G) 10 Hz 20 trains of 10 s (2000 pulses) 90% RMT		(E) Thalamic (8) or brainstem (2) stroke, SCI (4) (F) Thalamic stroke (13), SCI (10) (G) Thalamic or cortical stroke (10), SCI (6)		$p = 0.0002$ vs. sham coil 22 responders (37%) Duration of effect: transient (D) 10 Hz rTMS (painful zone area / adjacent zone, no sham): 15% / 32% 7 responders (19%) / 20 responders (56%) Duration of effect: *c.* 1 week (E) 10 Hz / 1 Hz / sham rTMS: 32% / 11% / 10% reductions of pain $p = 0.002$ vs. sham coil (10 Hz rTMS) 12 (55%) / 3 (14%) / 3 (14%) responders Significant reduction in pain only after 10 Hz rTMS (F) 10 Hz / 1 Hz / sham rTMS: 24% / 5% / 10% reductions of pain $p = 0.002$ vs. sham coil (10 Hz rTMS) 20 (43%) / 4 (9%) / 9 responders (20%) (G) Whole group (CP+PNP) 26% reduction of pain (sham: 10%) $p = 0.009$ vs. sham coil 11 responders (34%)
De Ridder *et al.* (2007)	SI (primary somatosensory area) F8	1–20 Hz 90% RMT		Neurogenic pain (8)	VAS	5 patients relieved (62%) 1 Hz >> 20 Hz > sham
Goto *et al.* (2008)	MI (contralat.)	5 Hz 10 trains of 10s		CPSP (17) (9 putamen, 7 thalamus, 1	VAS	1 patient worsened, 4 patients no effect whatsoever, 6 patients ≤ 30% pain reduction, 3

		50 s inter-train intervals 90% RMT		corona radiata), hemisoma pain (8) 5 patients had no paresis, 7 mild to moderate, 2 severe (plegia in none)		patients 31–50% reduction, only 3 patients had 51–70% relief Efficacy independent of motor deficit DTI study Responders had higher delineation ratio of the corticospinal tract and thalamocortical tract. This latter delineation ratio was more significantly different between responders and non-responders than the former delineation ratio. The thalamocortical tract plays an important role in analgesia (previous studies suggested an intact pyramidal tract)
Kang *et al.* (2009)	MI (hand area), right F8	10 Hz 20 trains of 5 s 80% RMT 5 days in a row	Sham-controlled (sham after 3 months)	SCI, below-level (11)	NRS	At 1 week no difference between treatments Worst pain only: −14.1% (treatment) at 1 week and +6.85% (sham) (no change during 5 day stimulation) 3 weeks later: −20.7% (treatment) vs. −7.89% sham): non-significant (trend only)

Table 11.2. Non-invasive cortical stimulation: Transcranial direct current stimulation (tDCS)

Authors/ date	Stimulation site/type of coil	Parameters of stimulation	Study design	Type of CP (number of patients)	Outcome measures	Outcome: comparison with placebo, effect duration
Fregni *et al.* (2006)	Left MI (10–20 C3 contact)	2 mA anodal 5 sessions of 20 min on 5 consecutive days	Parallel groups	SCI (11 + 7 sham)	VAS and other scales plus medication use	58% relief in 63% of patients, but only 37% at long-term follow-up (statistically insignificant) Marginal significance of active vs. sham stimulation Duration of effect: ≥ 2 weeks Unilateral stimulation afforded bilateral benefit
Boggio *et al.* 2009	MI (10–20 C3/4) 7 × 5 cm (+ supraorbital sponge)	Anodal 2mA for 30 min	Double-blind, crossover, RCT Sham: tDCS OFF after 30 sec (itching induced) Dual-channel TENS unit on most painful part using 2 5 × 5 cm rubber electrodes, 6 cm apart, square pulse of 150 μs at 4 Hz for 30 min Active treatment: tDCS + TENS ON simultaneously	CPSP (thalamic) (3)	VAS + cognitive / mental scales	Patient 1: active tDCS + TENS: VAS from 10 to 5, active tDCS: VAS from 7 to 5; sham: VAS from 9 to 9 Patient 2: active tDCS + TENS: VAS from 5 to 0; active tDCS: VAS from 4 to 3; sham: VAS from 2 to 2 Patient 3: active tDCS + TENS VAS from 7 to 4, active tDCS VAS 10 to 8, sham: 6 to 7 (!)
Soler MD *et al.* (2010b)	MI	2 mA anodal 10 sessions of 20 min on 5 + 5 consecutive days (weekend off)	Double-blind, sham-controlled, parallel groups: (1) tDCS with walking visual illusion (2) tDCS with control illusion (3) Sham tDCS with visual illusion (4) Sham tDCS with control illusion	SCI (below level) (39 patients split in 4 groups) 2 patients in the tDCS+visual illusion also had at-level pain Assessment: before, after last day of treatment, after 2 ,4, and 12 weeks 1 dropout (tetraplegic with pain increased by visual illusion)	NRS (0–10) and other scales (mood, anxiety, sleep, daily life routines)	Only 30% of patients in tDCS+VI and 30% in tDCS groups reached 30% relief. Another 4 patients in the first group (but none in the latter) improved 20–30% Global impression on last day of treatment: very much/much improved: 5 patients tDCS +VI, 3 patients tDCS, 1 patient VI. Best: tDCS+VI (−29.7%, at last day of treatment). Best at 2 weeks: tDCS+VI Best at 4 weeks: no differences. Best at 12 weeks: tDCS+VI (greater maintenance of improvement) VI group: improvement after last day of treatment lost at follow-up

Table 11.2. (cont.)

Authors/ date	Stimulation site/type of coil	Parameters of stimulation	Study design	Type of CP (number of patients)	Outcome measures	Outcome: comparison with placebo, effect duration
						tDCS and placebo groups: NO effect. 3 patients in tDCS+VI group: better response than best placebo responder, just like tDCS alone, but here 2 patients showed later worsening **Continuous pain**: no effect in any group at any time. tDCS +VI improvement at end of treatment not maintained **Paroxysmal pain**: tDCS+VI and tDCS improved, but lost by 4 weeks (tDCS already at 2 weeks). VI: no effect. **Mechanical allodynia**: improved only by tDCS+VI at 4 weeks. **Dysesthesias**: improved by tDCS+VI up to 4 weeks, and VI Other scales improved best by tDCS+VI (>> VI alone)
Soler D *et al.* (2010)	MI	2 mA anodal 10 sessions of 20 min + virtual reality	Phase II, double-blind, RCT	CCP (40)	–	Greater benefit than each technique alone. Benefit especially on evoked/ paroxysmal pain. Long-lasting effect
Mori *et al.* (2010)	MI 10–20 EEG IS C3/4	2 mA anodal 20 min/day for 5 consecutive days	Blinded study, sham-controlled	MS (10 + 9 sham)	VAS	At day 5: –45.5% At 3 weeks: –63.17% (mean improvement) with 6 (60%) responders (50%+ VAS reduction) Placebo: –23.7% (low due to inadequate blinding, i.e., itching) Electrode 5 × 7 cm; lower threshold of efficacy: 0.6 mA for the 35 cm^2 sponge. Blinding with 2 mA more difficult (3 mA is already painful): this may justify high degree of benefit
Antal *et al.* (2010)	MI (hand area). 4 × 4 cm sponge	Anodal (1 mA) 20 min/day for 5 days	Randomized, double-blinded,	CPSP (1 patient	VAS	Not available for this patient Carbamazepine might decrease the effects of anodal

Table 11.2. (cont.)

Authors/ date	Stimulation site/type of coil	Parameters of stimulation	Study design	Type of CP (number of patients)	Outcome measures	Outcome: comparison with placebo, effect duration
	5 × 10 cm sponge over contralateral orbit		crossover, placebo-controlled single-center trial	in a mixed group)		stimulation after a single session of tDCS **Unilateral tDCS may be sufficient for patients with pain on both sides** Severity and therapeutic refractoriness of symptoms can correlate negatively with placebo response

can engage GABA mechanisms, as shown by tracer studies (Canavero *et al.* 2006a). Renormalization of the corticothalamic generator is paralleled by restoration of function in previously altered resting state networks and transmitter systems, including structures involved in the motivational-affective aspects of pain (the cingulate, prefrontal, and orbitofrontal cortices). It has been demonstrated that rTMS disrupts cortico-cortical signal propagation by silencing the output of any neocortical area whose afferents are electrically stimulated (Logothetis *et al.* 2010), and thus SII/insula and ACC, among others. rTMS does not alter the RIII reflex, thus excluding descending inhibitory systems (Nahmias *et al.* 2009). Opioids are not involved in rTMS-associated analgesia, as naloxone does not reverse it (Canavero 2009). Pain activated by C fibers, but not Aδ, may respond to slow rTMS (Leo and Latif 2007), and this may explain differential results.

tDCS appears to exert a neuromodulatory effect (anodal increasing neuronal excitability, cathodal dampening it), but its exact mechanism remains to be elucidated (Canavero 2009).

Can TMS help select patients for ECS?

The first to suggest that a trial of TMS could predict analgesia following ECS were Migita *et al.* (1995). We soon found this to be the case (Canavero *et al.* 1998, 2002c, 2003, Canavero and Bonicalzi 2002). Others confirmed these findings in single case reports or small series (Lefaucheur *et al.* 2004a, André-Obadia *et al.* 2006, Saitoh *et al.* 2007). While there is a consensus on the relation between a positive effect after TMS and subsequent analgesia with ECS, a negative TMS trial should not rule out ECS, as trunk and leg pain may be less targetable with TMS (Lefaucheur 2008). We found a relation between TMS and propofol, and suggested that the propofol test may predict analgesia with ECS (Canavero *et al.* 1998, 2002c, 2003, Canavero and Bonicalzi 2002, 2005b, 2007a).

Other techniques

A mention should be made of *cranial electrotherapy stimulation* (CES). Capel *et al.* (2003) applied CES 2 hours twice a day for 4 days in 14 SCI patients (versus 13 patients submitted to sham stimulation) in a double-blind fashion. There was a mix of neuropathic and musculoskeletal pains. Improvement was minimal (active +49% vs. placebo +41%). Tan *et al.* (2006) applied CES (ear-clip electrodes, 100 μA) in a double-blind RCT in 18 SCI patients. There were no significant differences in four BPI pain intensity subscale items or in composite pain intensity scores, and no significant changes in 10 BPI pain interference subscale items. There was a non-significant change in daily pre- and post-session pain intensity ratings, which was larger for neuropathic (especially average pain and least pain) than musculoskeletal pain. Globally, there was an 11% change, much less than in the former study. In sum, CES does not seem to be significantly effective for SCI-CP (see also O'Connell *et al.* 2010).

Invasive cortical stimulation

The reader is referred to Canavero (2009, 2011) for full discussion and technical details. The procedure is performed under local or general anesthesia. One or

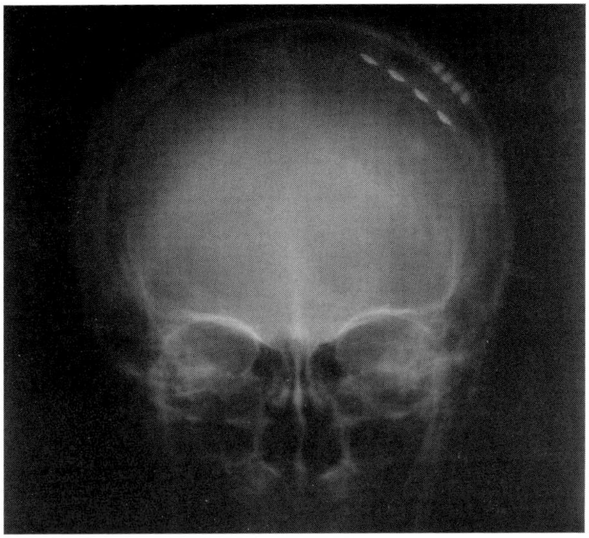

Figure 11.1. AP skull view showing a stimulating paddle positioned over MI.

two stimulating paddles are positioned on the dura overlying the motor or sensory cortex, either through burr holes or by means of a small craniotomy or craniectomy under fMRI and/or neuronavigational conditions, and, if effective parameters are found after a test period, they are hooked up to a subclavear pacemaker (Fig. 11.1). A subdural implantation may be elected in cases of pain involving the foot and distal leg, but should be avoided in general as it carries a risk of brain hemorrhage-related mortality and permanent morbidity. Most reported cases have received MI stimulation, generally extradurally, although bipolar stimulation, with the paddle placed perpendicularly to the central sulcus, is the same as distinct monopolar stimulation of MI and SI. Two parallel eight-contact paddles on SI and MI have been employed.

The belief that only a cathode can activate cortical neural tissue, and that the anode placed over the cortex is indifferent, is wrong: when MCS is applied bipolarly, neuronal activity may be evoked under both the cathode and the anode (bifocal stimulation), which implies that *SI is engaged* (Wongsarnpigoon and Grill 2009). Besides, modeling suggests that, when MI ECS is applied bipolarly, the neural activity evoked near the cathode may affect the activity near the anode – and vice versa – via their intracortical connections (likely an inhibitory interaction). Canavero and Bonicalzi (1995) reported the first case of effective SI ECS, and other cases followed. Best results are seen when the stimulating poles overlie parts of cortex corresponding to painful body parts (generally face, arm, chest, leg, singly or in combination), although data suggest that precise, "millimetric," somatotopic localization of the electrode may not be required. In addition, the leg area often extends, at least partially, on the convexity.

Efficacy

Globally, more than half of all reported patients with CP of brain origin were relieved more than 40% on a VAS scale at long term. Patients with CCP were also relieved, but the number of treated cases (about 20) is too small for any definite conclusions (Table 11.3). Concurrent drugs can be reduced or even stopped in many cases. A suggestion of greater response of evoked versus spontaneous pain is not confirmed in most series, and MI ECS does not relieve non-painful paresthesias.

What is rather puzzling is the observation that some groups report both good short- and long-term results, some have excellent initial results with a loss of benefit within weeks or months, some have scarce or no results at all. Failure rates in the literature fall between 12% and 84%. However, the majority list as treatment failures cases improving by < 30–40%, when in fact there are several patients who are actually satisfied with 20–40% relief, at least for a time, due to improved functional ability and quality of life; conversely, others may sometimes report high levels of pain reduction, yet fail to demonstrate any functional improvement. Certainly, changes in VAS scores alone often do not reflect the true effectiveness of a particular therapy, and they are clearly inadequate for determining benefits with regard to functional capacity, quality of life, and so on (discussed in Chapter 9). Nonetheless, explaining such variable results is not easy. Localization of stimulation target can be ruled out. Groups that meticulously explored the whole target cortex with intraoperative stimulation and used sophisticated localization technology (neuronavigation, evoked potentials, etc.) achieved either excellent or poor results in the same proportion. Inadequate neurostimulator programming (too short or too few contact combinations tried) is certainly a reason in some cases, and so is a team's lack of experience with neuromodulatory techniques and, above all, chronic pain management. A few groups ascribe

Table 11.3. Invasive cortical stimulation

Author(s)	Type of pain (number of patients)	Results (follow-up)	Notes/parameters
Tsubokawa's group			
Tsubokawa's group *Pain* 1990; Suppl 5, S491 (abs. 952)	CP (thalamic) (7)	Excellent (5: no drugs needed) or good (2: some drugs needed) pain relief *(abstract: effective in 75% of cases (> 7 months))*	**First report of MCS for CP (1988)** MCS vs. thalamic stimulation. MCS is more effective than thalamic stimulation. Improvement of motor function in some patients MCS improved movements of the painful limbs. Pain subsided within a few minutes 5–10 min ON, 4–5 h relief 5–6 times daily, then 2–3 times daily
Tsubokawa *et al.* (1991b) See also *Acta Neurochir Suppl (Wien)* 1991; **52**, 137–9	CPSP (12) (6 thalamic lesion, 3 putaminal lesion, 1 pontine hemorrhage, 2 other lesions)	Complete pain relief in 5/12 patients (1 year), considerable pain reduction in 3/12 patients (1 year). Long-term benefit in 8/12 patients (> 1 year)	Intermittent stimulation effective in 5/12 patients. No seizures; pain relief at stimulus intensities below movements threshold. Paresis improvement. Pain improvement in barbiturate-sensitive, morphine-resistant patients. Disappearance of the analgesic effect in 3 patients, with reappearance after revision of electrode placement
Tsubokawa *et al.* (1993) See also Tsubokawa *et al.* Pain 1993; **58** (Suppl), 150	CPSP (11) (8 thalamic stroke, 3 putaminal hemorrhage (+ small lesion in the posterior limb of the internal capsule))	Pain relief: **Immediate**: Excellent (> 80%): 6/11 (54%) Good (60–79%): 2/11 (18%) Fair (40–59%): 1/11 (9%) Poor (< 40%): 2/11 (18%) **Long-lasting**: Excellent (> 80%): 5/11 (45%) Good (60–79%): 0/8 Fair (40–59%): 0/8 Poor (< 40%): 3/8 (37%) (2 years)	Barbiturate-sensitive patients: 5 (+3?)/11; morphine-resistant patients: 10 (+1?)/11. Stimulation of area 4 ipsilateral to the inciting lesion. 1-week test period. Fair and poor responders not implanted. Satisfactory immediate pain relief in 8/11 patients (73%). Gradual effect reduction over several months in 3/8 patients. Long-term response in barbiturate-sensitive and morphine-resistant patients (also for Vc DBS). No pain-relieving effect by high-frequency postcentral stimulation (11/11 patients): in 2, worsening of pain, similar to their spontaneous ones. In 3 patients, areas rostral to MI stimulated without relief. Non-painful paresthesias unrelieved. 5–10 mins ON at a time – no stimulation at night 50–120 Hz 100–500 μs
Katayama *et al.* (1994)	CPSP (6; lateral medullary infarct)	MCS in 3 patients. Pain relief: 2/3 > 60%; 1/3 > 40% (4 months)	Pain relief > 40% in 1 patient previously unsuccessfully treated by Vc DBS. No satisfactory pain control by thalamic stimulation in any patients

Table 11.3. (cont.)

Author(s)	Type of pain (number of patients)	Results (follow-up)	Notes/parameters
Yamamoto *et al.* (1997)	CPSP (39) (25 thalamic stroke, 14 suprathalamic stroke)	28 MCS Excellent/good (50–100%) pain relief: Thalamic patients: 10/19 (53%) Suprathalamic patients: 3/9 (33%) (difference not significant) T+ or K+ & M+: 2/4 (50%) T+ or K+ & M–: 10/14 (71%) T– & K– & M+: 0/2 (0%) T– & K– & M-: 1/8 (13%) Overall: 13/28 (46%) (12 months)	Suprathalamic stroke = infarct or hemorrhage of the posterior limb of internal capsule, or parietal lobe, sparing the thalamus. No patients with midbrain or medullary lesions. MCS test period: 1 week 8/39: morphine responsive 22/39: thiamylal responsive 11/23: ketamine responsive Thiamylal+ketamine sensitivity + morphine resistance may predict a positive effect of MCS
Katayama *et al.* (1998) Includes: Katayama *et al.* *Stereotact Funct Neurosurg* 1997, **69**, 73–9 Tsubokawa *et al.* Abst. 3rd Int Congress INS. Orlando, 1996, p. 123 Includes all patients from previous publications	CPSP (31) (20 thalamic stroke, 8 putaminal hemorrhage, 3 lateral medullary infarction)	Early satisfactory (> 60%) pain relief: 23/31 patients (74%). Long-term efficacy (≥ 2 years): 15/31 patients (48%)	Damage of the posterior limb of the internal capsule in patients with putaminal hemorrhage. Previous ineffective SCS. Pain relief > 60%: 13/18 patients (73%) with no or mild motor weakness (70% of patients with inducible muscle contraction); 2/13 patients (15%) with moderate or severe motor weakness (difference statistically significant). Satisfactory pain control in 14/20 patients (70%) with inducible muscle contraction but in only 1/11 patients (9%) without inducible motor contractions ($p < 0.01$). No relationship between pain control and presence of hypoesthesia, dysesthesia, hyperpathia, allodynia, or disappearance of SSEP N20 wave plus stimulation-induced paresthesias, or motor performance improvement. 3 patients with MCS or DBS became pain-free without stimulation for years (all 3 getting initial excellent relief at progressively longer stimulation intervals during intermittent stimulation). 1 subcutaneous infection, 3 seizures during testing at intensities higher than muscle threshold. 10–20 mins ON at a time 20–50 Hz 100–500 , most at 200 µs 2–8 V

Table 11.3. (cont.)

Author(s)	Type of pain (number of patients)	Results (follow-up)	Notes/parameters
Yamamoto *et al.* (2000)	Small thalamic stroke, then action tremor, then Vim DBS, then cardioversion, then CPSP	50% relief over 2 years	Thiamylal/ketamine responsive, morphine resistant
Katayama *et al.* (2001)	CPSP (45)	Satisfactory pain control: SCS: 7% of patients; DBS: 25% of patients; MCS: 48% of patients	DBS and MCS in 4 patients. Better result: MCS 1/4, DBS 2/4
Fukaya *et al.* (2003) Includes: Katayama *et al. Acta Neurochir Suppl* 2003, **87**, 121–3	CPSP (31)	Unsuccessful MCS in 2 CPSP patients reporting abnormal pain sensation after stimulation of the motor cortex (see Chapter 22)	Experimental study on conscious somatosensory response during surgery for electrode placement
Paris group			
Nguyen *et al.* (2009) Includes: Nguyen *et al. Acta Neurochir Suppl* 1997, **68**, 54–60 Nguyen *et al.* (1999) Nguyen *et al. Arch Med Res* 2000, **31**, 263–5 Nguyen *et al. Neurochirurgie* 2000, **46**, 483–91 Drouot *et al.* (2002)	CPSP (32) BCP (thalamic abscess) (1) BCP (head injury) (2) SCI (9) **1993–2004**	> 60% relief: 13 40–60% relief: 15 < 40% relief: 7 Mean improvement on VAS 53%, on MPQ 56.7%, on WBPQ 62.7%, on MQS 32.9% Not available (in a previous series of 4: < 40% in a paraplegic patient (18 months); 100% (visceral pain + substantial reduction of diffuse pain) in a tetraplegic patient (22 months), another improved > 40%, one failure) Follow-up (global): 29–170 months	Progressive loss of effect in some patients reversed in most by correct repositioning of paddle 3 h ON and 3 h OFF (12 h/day) 40 (25–55) Hz 82.5 (60–180) μs
Nguyen *et al.* (2008) (with Velasco's group in Mexico)	CPSP (3)	Patient 1: –16% Patient 2: –38% (both hemisoma CP) Patient 3 (face CP): – 80% Follow-up: 1 year (stable benefit)	Benefit *not* due to placebo effect. MCS decreased MPQ affective subscore Drugs down 55% (patient 3) Improved QoL
Lyon group			
Nuti *et al.* (2005)	CP (27)	Follow-up: 2–104 months (mean 49 months)	Parameters:

Table 11.3. (cont.)

Author(s)	Type of pain (number of patients)	Results (follow-up)	Notes/parameters
Includes all previous publications: Peyron *et al.* (1995) Garcia-Larrea *et al.* (1997) Garcia-Larrea *et al.* (1999) Mertens *et al.* *Stereotact Funct Neurosurg* 1999, **73**, 122 Sindou *et al.*, *9th World Congress on Pain*, Book of abstracts, 1999 Montes *et al.* (2002)	Ischemic lesions (11) (3 thalamic (Vc), 4 medulla, 2 cortical parietal, 1 parietal/ insula/ACC, 1 parietal/ insula) Hemorrhagic lesions (11) (1 thalamic (Vc), 1 thalamus/midbrain, 5 capsulothalamic, 1 capsulolenticular/ insula, 3 cortical parietal) Frontoparietal trauma (1) SCI (discal hernia-associated myelopathy) (3) Spinal conus AVM (1) **1992–2003**	Pain relief: BCP: Excellent (> 70%): 3 Good (40–69%): 8 Poor (10–39%): 8 Negligible (0–9%): 4 CCP: Excellent: 0 Good: 3 Poor: 1 Negligible: 0 Decreased analgesic intake: 52% of patients (complete withdrawal 36%); unchanged: 45% of patients, unavailable data: 3%. Decrease/withdrawal of analgesic in 10/11 poor responders (Contradictory results, as noted by authors) Favour re-intervention: 70% of patients	0.5–5V (mean 1.5 V), 30–80 Hz (mean 45.5 Hz), 60–330 µs (mean 140 µs), ON 30–120 min, OFF 15min – 24 h 5–6 h of stimulation each day Prospective evaluation of MCS. Long-term outcome evaluated by means of: (1) % pain relief, (2) VAS, (3) postoperative VAS decrease, (4) reduction in drugs intake, (5) yes/no response for being operated again **MCS efficacy not predictable by motor status**, pain characteristics, lesion type, QST, SSEP/LEPs, pain duration, BCP vs. CCP, presence of evoked pain No subjective sensations during active stimulation Partial epileptic seizures in 3 patients in the early postoperative stage or during trials for increasing intensity. 1 speech disorder and 1 motor deficit resolved spontaneously Long-term relief predictable from early pain relief 1–2 paddles, 3 subdural MCS may have adverse cognitive effects. The risk may increase with age (> 50 years)
Turin Advanced Neuromodulation Group (TANG)			
Canavero and Bonicalzi (1995)	CP (2) (1 CPSP, 1 syringomyelia)	Pain relief: 30–50% in syringomyelia patient (2 years); no relief in CPSP	Syringomyelia patient: parietal somatosensory stimulation. Spreading of pain to contralateral side and vanishing of analgesia at 2 months. Modest propofol response CPSP patient: propofol unresponsive
Canavero *et al.* (1999)	CPSP (1; thalamocapsular stroke)	Effective short-term pain relief (allodynia disappearance and 50% reduction of burning pain) (5 weeks)	Propofol-responsive patient. Painful supernumerary phantom arm during MCS and lasting 6 months after stimulator switch-off. Pain relapse after 5 weeks
Canavero and Bonicalzi (2002, 2007c) Includes: Canavero *et al.* (1998) Canavero *et al.* *Neurol Res* 2003, **25**, 118–22	CP (5 CPSP, 2 SC pain) + 1 algodystonia **1993–2003**	Effective (30–100%) pain relief with MCS/PCS in 2/7 patients. Long-term efficacy (4 years) in 2 patients (BCP and MS-CP). Ineffective MCS in 4/7	Effective SI stimulation in 1, then resubmitted to MCS with same benefit plus 50% opioid reduction (however, patient unsatisfied and explanted). Overall efficacy: 3/7 CP patients, all propofol-responsive. Ineffective MCS in 4/7 CP patients, all propofol-

Table 11.3. (cont.)

Author(s)	Type of pain (number of patients)	Results (follow-up)	Notes/parameters
			unresponsive, but 1 who could not be assessed due to intermittent nature of pain. Algodystonia: temporary benefit
Saitoh's group			
Hosomi *et al.* (2008) Includes all previous publications, including: Tani *et al.* (2004) Saitoh *et al. Neurosurg Focus* 11 (3), article 1, 2001 Saitoh *et al. J Neurosurg* 2000, **92**, 150–5	CPSP (thalamic) (10) [+1 patient relieved without stimulation]	4: no initial relief; 6: 21–90% initial relief (mean: 55.6%) [late relief at 14–75 months: 10–80% (mean: 31.6%)]. 1 explant due to enduring benefit from CS manipulation.	Pharmacological test with phentolamine, lidocaine, ketamine, thiopental, morphine, placebo. Ketamine-sensitive patients seem to be good candidates for MCS **Some pain reduction by SI stimulation** Ineffective prefrontal stimulation First report of bilateral cortical stimulation for SCI pain. 4 months interval between implants 2 serious ICH, with 1 vegetative. 2 infections subdural approach, 1–2 plate electrodes within central sulcus, in 9 patients 1 plate in interhemispheric fissure, extradural ECS in only 2 patients **Globally: initial VAS score reduction in BCP: 42%; late relief: 26% at 1+ year** 3–4 periods ON (30 mins each) a day, followed by 5–6 h benefit in OFF 25–50 Hz, 200 μs, 0.9–5 V
	CPSP (putaminal) (3)	All 3 relieved initially 60–75% (mean: 65.3%) [late relief at 13–88 months: 15–60% (mean: 41.6%)]; 1 explant (15% relief patient)	
	CP (brainstem: 3 stroke, 1 injury)	1: no relief 3: 25–63% initial relief (mean : 42.6%) [late relief at 33–73 months: 15–50% (mean: 35%)	
	CPSP (temporoparietal) (1)	30% initial relief, then 10% at 72 months	
	CCP (SCI) (2) **1996–2005**	50–89% initial pain relief (60–65% late relief at 27–75 months); 1 explant	
Other groups			
Tasker *et al.* (1994)	CPSP (1, large suprathalamic infarct)	Substantial pain relief with *ipsilateral to pain MCS*; gradual abatement over 6 years; relief with *subdural* stimulation over a few months.	Contralateral MCS due to a lack of sufficient MI on the affected side. Stimulation-induced ipsilateral paresthesias
	CPSP (2) (1 with AVM)	1 relief, 1 failure	
Hosobuchi (1993) Includes:	CPSP (5) (1 post-removal of parietal cortical AVM, 1 brainstem infarction, 3 thalamic lesion)	Pain relief: Initial: 5/5 excellent	Efficacy dramatically reduced in 2 thalamic pain patients, to 0% in 1 patient and 30% in 1 patient 2–6 months after implantation

Table 11.3. (cont.)

Author(s)	Type of pain (number of patients)	Results (follow-up)	Notes/parameters
Stereotact Funct Neurosurg 1992, **59**, 76–83 Abstr. IASP congress 1993		At 2–3 months: 4/5 excellent (> 50%), 1 fair. At 9–30 months: 3/5 excellent (thalamic, parietal, brainstem)	1 h ON/6 h OFF 20–30 Hz, 180–260 μs, 3–5 V
Meyerson *et al.* (1993)	CPSP (3) (2 thalamic hemorrhage, 1 brainstem infarction)	Pain relief: None: 3/3	In spite of multipolar electrode grid in 1 and relocation of paddle in another Most patients had one or two seizures during test stimulation Painful sensations at the electrode site in 2 patients 1 epidural clot leading to aphasia 20–30 mins ON 5 times a day; 50 Hz, 300 μs, amplitude 20–30% below motor threshold
Dario *et al.* Long-term results of chronic MCS for CP. Abstr. 9th World Congress on Pain, IASP Press, 1999, A185. Includes: Dario *et al.* *Riv Neurobiol* 1997, **43**, 625–9	CPSP (2 thalamic stroke, 1 brainstem stroke)	70% pain relief in 1 thalamic patient (3 years) Gradual abatement of pain relief over 2 years 60–90% relief. Then 50–70%, then 20–30% at 3–41 months (average: 27 months)	**All patients propofol-responsive** 2–2.5 V, 120–210 ms, 50–75 Hz, continuous mode
Franzini *et al.* (2003) Includes: Franzini *et al.* Abstr. XLVIII Congresso SINCH, Copanello, 1999 Franzini *et al.* *J Neurosurg* 2000, **93**, 873–5	CPSP (3: A, B, C)	Satisfactory (30–50%) pain relief: patients A (> 4 years) and B (> 2 years) Short-term pain relief (6 months): patient C	**2 responders propofol-sensitive.** Pain abolition after a second stroke in patient B. Unsatisfactory pain relief (30%) by further stimulation in patient C. Complete abolition of thalamic hand
Herregodts *et al.* (1995)	CP (thalamic) (2)	Immediate pain relief: > 50% in both patients Long-lasting pain relief: 1/2 (full relapse in 1 at 4 months)	1 h ON every 6 h
Migita *et al.* (1995)	CPSP (2) (A: putaminal hemorrhage; B: post-20 months stereotactic thalamotomy)	Pain relief: 70–80% in patient A (1 year) No relief in patient B	Patient A: morphine and barbiturate unresponsive. 30% pain relief with TMS Patient B: previous 6 months effective Vc DBS. Barbiturate responsive, morphine and TMS unresponsive
Fuji *et al.* (1997)	CPSP (2 thalamic infarction, 5 hemorrhage)	Satisfactory pain relief: 6/7 patients (1 month)	Lesions included internal caspule, Vc, and pulvinar (MRI confirmed, 5 patients).

Table 11.3. (cont.)

Author(s)	Type of pain (number of patients)	Results (follow-up)	Notes/parameters
		Unsatisfactory pain relief: 5/7 patients (3 months).	Early electrode removal in 1 patient after unsatisfactory test stimulation 30 mins ON, 10–100 Hz, 200 μs, 3–8 V
Barraquer-Bordas *et al.* (1999)	CPSP (1; capsuloinsular hemorrhage)	MCS trial ineffective (motor response elicited)	Hemisoma burning pain, + evoked pains. DBS reduced CP for 5 months and evoked pains, until glioma displaced electrode with relapse and death
Kuroda *et al.* (2000)	CPSP (1; evacuated putaminal hematoma)	MCS ineffective. Later **SI/SII** CS **effective** for 4 years	
Roux *et al.* (2001)	CPSP (2) SCI (1) Myelopathic pain (1)	Both > 80% relief 60% relief 90% relief Follow-up: 6–14 months	
Mogilner and Rezai (2001)	SCI (1)	Relief (not broken down) (mean follow-up 6 months)	30 mins – 2 h ON 5–10 times/day, 110 Hz, 210 μs, 2–8 V
Rodriguez and Contreras (2002)	SCI (post-cervical ependymoma removal) CP (1)	Evoked pain dramatically improved Steady burning pain moderately relieved (2 months)	Third-party analysis of results. Tremor improvement. No reduction of analgesic intake after MCS. 5 Hz, 450 ms, 7.1 V, ON 2 h, OFF 3 h, 0–/2+
Nandi *et al.* (2002) Includes all patients reported in: Carroll *et al.* (2000) Smith *et al. Neurosurg Focus* 2001; **11**(3), article 2	CPSP (7) (1 cortical stroke, 3 thalamic stroke, 2 brainstem stroke) Gunshot brainstem injury (1)	Appreciable pain relief: 1 patient, cortical (4 years); 2 patients (weeks to months)* No relief: 4 patients (thalamic, brainstem) *Brainstem injury: 50–60% (31 months): 1 patient	**The only patient where it was tried: propofol-sensitive** Pain disappearance for 5 months after stimulator switched off in the responder Enduring benefit in 1 patient only
Frighetto *et al.* (2004)	CPSP (1)	Relief (no details given)	Previous ineffective thalamotomy
Henderson *et al.* (2004)	CPSP (1)	Relief, then loss, then new relief (?) after intensive reprogramming	
Brown and Pilitsis (2005)	CPSP, Wallenberg (1) CPSP, thalamic (1)	0% pain relief VAS 10 to 8; MPQ from 65 to 32 (both sensory and affective scores)	Follow-up max. in whole series (PNP and CP): 10 months **Contrary to Nguyen, they conclude that precise, somatotopic localization of the electrode may not be required, because the optimal inter-electrode distance determined during cortical mapping and afterwards with subjective patient evaluation of pain control was fully 3 cm**

Table 11.3. (cont.)

Author(s)	Type of pain (number of patients)	Results (follow-up)	Notes/parameters
			Intraoperative neuronavigation and cortical mapping for stimulation site targeting. Strength and discriminative sensation improvement from MCS in 3 patients with facial weakness and sensory loss. Dysarthria improvement in 1 patient More than 50% reduction in pain medication dose *Continuous* stimulation 40 Hz, 90–240 μs, 2–8 V
Slawek *et al.* (2005)	CPSP, brainstem (1)	20% VAS reduction; withdrawal of narcotic and decrease of non-narcotic medications, ability to introduce rehabilitation and improvement of sleep	Follow-up: 4 months No side effects
Savas and Kanpolat (2005)	CP (1)	0% relief during test stimulation	
Gharabaghi *et al.* (2005) Includes: Tirakotai *et al.* (2004)	CPSP (hemorrhage) (3) CP, insular (1)	70–100% relief (follow-up: 6–18 months) 90% relief (follow-up: 24 months)	Frameless neuronavigation. ***Single burr hole and vacuum headrest***. Awake patient. No complications Third-party evaluation Volumetric 3D MRI with superimposed fMRI data plus intraoperative electrical stimulation
Pirotte *et al.* (2005) Includes: Pirotte *et al.* *Neurosurg Focus* 2001, **11** (3)	CPSP: 3 subcortical 2 capsular 1 brainstem 1 MS pain 1 cervical syrinx 1 SC ependymoma **1998–2003**	Pain relief (%): 100%/50%/worsening 83%/failure (both plegic) 87.5% 100% 70% Failure	50–75% drug dosage reduction among responders 3rd party evaluation **Plegia *not* an unfavorable prognostic factor** 1 h ON every 4 h 40 Hz, 100 μs 1–5 V
Rasche *et al.* (2006a) Includes: Tronnier VM. *Schmerz* 2001, **15**, 278–9	CPSP(thalamic) (7) **1994–2005**	3 responders (–31%, –41%, –62%) 2/7 patients placebo responder Duration of positive effect: 2, 4, 1.5 years Relief of dysesthesia, allodynia, and hyperpathy in 2 CPSP patients (patients were able to touch the	50–85 Hz, 210–250 μs, 4.5–6.0 V, **continuous stimulation, then intermittent**. Double-blind test trial . VAS evaluation **Single burr hole**, neuronavigation Paddle parallel to central sulcus No sensation evoked by stimulation. Minor changes of parameters during follow-up Immediate or almost immediate (30–60 mins) pain reduction after turning the MCS on. After-effect: 30 mins to hours

Table 11.3. (cont.)

Author(s)	Type of pain (number of patients)	Results (follow-up)	Notes/parameters
		painful area without having painful sensations)	
Tronnier and Rasche (2009)	CPSP (11)	4 patients: > 50% relief Follow-up: up to 15 years	
Son *et al.* (2006)	BCP (traumatic) (1)	90–95% relief of spontaneous burning pain in arm and lower trunk, 70–80% relief of burning pain, heaviness, and deep pressure-like pain in leg, 50% relief of heaviness and deep pressure allodynia in foot Follow-up: 1 year	**Severe motor deficit in distal arm and leg.** Subdural electrode for arm pain; extradural paddle for leg pain parallel to the course of the superior sagittal sulcus 21 Hz, 210 µs, 0.8–2.5 V 0–/3+ , *continuous stimulation* (arm electrode) 30 Hz, 210 µs, 2–2.5V 0–/2+ *continuous stimulation* (leg electrode) After-effect: 5 mins
Ito *et al.* (2006)	CPSP (3)	Almost total relief in 2, improved in 1	Paddle parallel to MI Relief dependent on motor function
Sokal *et al.* (2006)	CP (thalamic) (1)	Decrease of pain	
Cioni and Meglio (2007)	CPSP (thalamic) (4) SCI (2)	Pain relief (50–60%): 1/4 patients, but unsatisfactory relief at 1 years 1 > 40% relief, 1 failure	Extradural multipolar (16–20) grid in all plus electrophysiologic mapping; several combinations assessed over 12 h
Molet *et al.* (2007)	CPSP (thalamic) (3) CCP (paraplegia) (1)	Benefit in some	CP and PNP series: results not broken down
Arle and Shils (2008)	2 post-stroke pain (PSP) patients (P5 58 years, P7 64 years) 3 mixed pain and movement disorders (PSM) patients (but according to their Table 2: P1 64 years, P2 61 years, P4 64 years, P6 49 years = 4 patients)	1 CPSP < 20% at 17 months 1 CPSP > 60% at 30 months PSM: good result: P2, 36-month follow-up; fair results: P1, 39-month follow-up, P4, 34-month follow-up; poor result: P6, 23-month follow-up P5: good pain control in her upper extremities and face, but less pain control in her leg region, minimal control of a **third-limb sensation**.	2 intraoperative seizures 1 postoperative programming seizure. No further seizure with voltage < 4.0 V *Continuous stimulation* 60–130 Hz, 60–400 µs, 2–7 V

Table 11.3. (cont.)

Author(s)	Type of pain (number of patients)	Results (follow-up)	Notes/parameters
Velasco *et al.* (2008)	CPSP (thalamic) (1)	60% relief (allodynia disappeared, hyperalgesia decreased) at 1-year follow-up	Double-blind randomized trial Hypoesthesia unchanged. 40–130 Hz, 90 µs, 2–3.5V
Shabalov *et al.* (2008)	SCI (cervical) (1)	VAS reduced > 50%	V 1–5.5; 20–50 Hz, 60–210 µs (whole group)
Mondani *et al.* (2008)	CPSP (2) MS (2)	50–80% benefit at 3 months	Subdural strips
Delavallée *et al.* (2008)	CPSP (3) (1 thalamic ischemia, 1 MCA hemorrhage, 1 MCA ischemia)	Poor result (pain relief < 40%): P2 (VAS 9 vs. 6) Excellent result (pain relief 100–80%): P4: (VAS 8 vs. 1), P6: (VAS 9 vs. 1) Follow-up: mean 54 months (range, 19–69 months) for whole group (CP + PNP)	Subdural strips. Octopolar electrode. **One severe motor deficit was satisfactorily relieved** P2: Initial satisfactory pain relief, rapidly diminished to poor relief. System dysfunction/lead mobilization ruled out Parameters of stimulation: P2: 80 Hz, 210 µs, 3.0 V, 30 min, several times/day; P4: 50 Hz, 210 µs, 2.1 V, 60 min, once/day; P6: 60 Hz, 210 µs, 2.0 V, 30 min, once/day
Finet and Raftopoulos (2009)	CPSP (1)	Initial satisfactory analgesia, rapid loss of effect (poor result)	**Subdural** octrode in interhemispheric fissure in front of CS
Vesper (2010)	CPSP (1)	> 50% relief	rTMS predictive
	CP (post AVM irradiation) (1)	100% relief Follow-up: 1–4 years	
Tanei *et al.* (2010)	MS-CP (1)	Test: > 50% VAS relief 60% relief Follow-up: 6 months	ON 1 h OFF 2 h 0/1+ 2/3, 6.5 V, **> 100 Hz** Reduction of preoperative drugs (+ ketamine stopped)
Fagundes-Pereyra *et al.* (2010)	(1) CPSP (5) (2) Traumatic BCP (2) (3) MS (1) (4) Tumoral BCP (1) (5) SCI (1) **1994–2002**	(1) Relief: 30%, 35%, 50%, 50%, 70% (2) Relief: 50%, 80% (3) Relief: 32% (4) Relief: 50% (5) Not available Follow-up: 12 months	First 7 patients: single burr hole; 3 later patients: craniotomy Paddle perpendicular to central sulcus. Negative pole on MI, positive pole on SI **Presence of motor deficit** or duration of pain: **insignificant factors** Patients with < 40% relief intolerant of MCS interruption! Decrease of effects in some patients CP group: VAS preop. 7.8, postop.: 3.82 ($p < 0.00001$) (courtesy of Fagundes-Pereyra 2011) 45–130 Hz, 45–210 µs, 2–5.3V, monopolar or bipolar stimulation

Table 11.3. (cont.)

Author(s)	Type of pain (number of patients)	Results (follow-up)	Notes/parameters
Sakas *et al.* (2011)	CPSP (thalamic) (1)	MI CS: 40% VAS reduction SI CS: 0% MI+SI: 90% VAS relief (face) 70% (arm) < 10% (leg) Follow-up: 2 years	2 eight-polar paddles in direct contact with MI and SI Interdural positioning, subdural interface
Tanei *et al.* (2011)	CPSP (8) CCP (tumor) (1) brainstem CP (MS, Chiari I) (2) **1999–2009**	CPSP: 80–100% relief (2 patients) 60–79% relief (4 patients) < 40% relief (2 patients) other CP: 60–79% relief (3 patients)	Single burr hole. 1 week trial. VAS assessment. ON 1 h, OFF 2 h Statistically significant difference in mean frequency between thalamic (55 Hz) and brainstem-cord CP (106 Hz) (3.04 vs. 6.68 V; 180 vs. 308 μs) DBS + MCS in 2 cord CP patients: additive effect
Lefaucheur *et al.* (2011)	CPSP (6)	VAS scores were 0, 0, 0, 2, 4.5, and 8 (initial: all > 7) at 1 year	Surgery (average length 320 mins!). 1 week of parameters search. Postoperative stimulation off for 1 month followed by a single-blind randomized phase (1 month) with stim OFF (3 patients) or ON (3 patients), then 10 months of open label. No crossover. Safety, not efficacy study Octopolar round paddle Assessment: VAS, BPI, MPQ, SIP, MQS, PGIC 2 patients had IPG explanted for infection and then reimplanted 6 months later. Final parameters: 40–50Hz, 60 μs, 2–6V. Continuous in 4 patients, cyclic in 2. In the randomized, blinded arm, only 1/3 patients with stim ON reported > 50% VAS relief Open label: improvement increased over time but significant only after 6 months

their success to elimination of non-responders to subacute therapeutic stimulation from those receiving long-term stimulation, which amounts to a sizeable population. Accordingly, some neurosurgeons are enthusiastic about the technique, whereas others are rather cold or downright negative. It may be that ECS is performed at many more centers than those which publish, and most of the failures go unreported, with only series with good results being published. This spurred the search for prognostic markers, and some have been proposed:

(1) An intact or nearly intact corticospinal motor function has been touted as a favorable prognostic sign, with about 75% of patients without major motor deficits receiving benefit, but several exceptions are on record (Table 11.3).

(2) Severe sensory changes not modified by MI ECS represent a predictor of unfavorable outcome, whereas improvement in sensory deficits that appears during the subacute therapeutic trial is followed by a favorable outcome (Drouot *et al.* 2002, Velasco *et al.* 2008). Exceptions to the rule

exist, and at least three cases of CP improved by ECS in spite of almost total lack of sensory cortex are on record (Peyron *et al.* 1995, Nguyen *et al.* 1999). Normal or near-normal sensory thresholds do not always portend a favorable outcome.

(3) Response to non-invasive stimulation (e.g., rTMS) may identify patients who will get successful stimulation, but this is not an absolute criterion (see above).

(4) Drug dissection protocols may help identify responders. The first one was proposed by Tsubokawa's group (Table 11.1): doses of 3 mg of morphine are injected every 5 minutes up to 18 mg, followed by naloxone 0.2 mg bid, followed by thiopental 50 mg IV bolus every 5 minutes up to 250 mg and ketamine 5 mg IV bolus up to 25 mg. Canavero and Bonicalzi (2002, 2007a, 2007c) developed the subhypnotic propofol test, in which the patient is injected in a single-blind fashion with 1.5 mg of Intralipid or similar white fat solution and after 20 minutes with 0.2 mg/kg IV bolus of propofol.

(5) We introduced parietal cortex stimulation on the basis of neuroimaging data (Canavero and Bonicalzi 1995), the first report of neuroimaging-directed brain stimulation. However, functional neuroimaging has not yet been evaluated in a clinically meaningful fashion.

(6) Successful ECS may be impossible in patients with a large surface of the cortex destroyed (e.g., stroke) and in those with a cortex distant from the dural surface (subdural hygroma, post-stroke atrophy, etc.). However, Canavero (2009) has made a strong case for ipsilateral (to pain) ECS.

There is no significant statistical difference between results obtained in thalamic or cortico-subcortical brain CP patients. Coverage of restricted painful territories (e.g., chest) should not be taken as contraindicating ECS, even though no sensorimotor phenomena are elicited during test stimulation. Paddles have been placed parallel to the rolandic fissure or perpendicular, with similar results. What is clear is that, despite some claims to the contrary, subdural implantation does not seem to improve results and may actually be less effective than extradural implantation: for CP, benefit at 1 year was only 26% in the largest series (Hosomi *et al.* 2008). Pain relief is not associated with age, sex, presence or absence of cerebral lesion, treated painful region, or pain laterality. Some authors offer ECS if the mean VAS score is 6 or more, but this is moot.

Therapeutic ECS does not generally induce any motor activation, even at a high voltage, or any sensory phenomena in a majority of patients. Thus blinded controlled studies are feasible. All studies performed to date exclude a placebo effect as the primary basis of analgesia (Canavero and Bonicalzi 2002, Rasche *et al.* 2006a, Velasco *et al.* 2008).

Absolute exclusion criteria for ECS include: major depression accompanied by suicidal thoughts or gestures, major psychosocial stressors (job dissatisfaction, marital problems, etc.), major personality disorders, alcoholism, and drug addiction. Hemisoma pains do not represent a contraindication, as these can be managed with two strip electrodes combined.

Programming includes a wide range of stimulation parameters (each patient is different and no indications are possible), with voltage varying from 0.5 V to 6 V up to 10.5 V (mean 3.8 V), pulse width varying from 60 μs up to 500 μs (mean 251.2 μs), and frequency varying from 5 Hz to 60 Hz (often 25–50 Hz, mean 51.1 Hz) up to 80 Hz and 130 Hz. Chronic stimulation can be cyclical (battery-sparing) or continuous. When cyclical, the duration of each stimulating session varies, anywhere from 5 minutes to 9 hours, 1 to 10 times a day. The choice of stimulation parameters also depends on the presence of the so-called post-effect. Many, but not all, patients have their pain relieved or improved immediately or within 5–60 minutes during intraoperative stimulation for periods ranging from several minutes to hours or several days without further stimulation. This effect has a tendency to abate over time and by the second month may stabilize at several minutes to a few hours.

Analgesia also can fade over time. Repositioning of the electrode or intensive reprogramming may restore benefit in some cases, although at a lower level than before. Tolerance and fatigue are proposed mechanisms of such effects. Granulations and fibrosis around the contacts have been found in some failures (e.g., Canavero and Bonicalzi 2002, Hosomi *et al.* 2008): surgical curettage may restore benefit.

Adverse and unusual effects

Permanent disabling morbidity (including epilepsy and intracerebral hemorrhage) and mortality have not been reported for the extradural approach, while there is a small such risk for the subdural approach. The most common adverse effect reported in the literature consisted of short generalized seizures, all of which were observed during the initial testing phases. The literature does not reveal cases of epileptic seizures during chronic treatment for CP (Canavero and Bonicalzi 2002). Antiepileptic medications are – or are not – administered for 1–6 months. Caution, however, is to be exercised when adjusting parameters, even long after stimulation has been instituted. Infections are possible (but not meningitis/encephalitis) and so are hardware failures. Two early reports (from Stockholm and Paris) reported two extradural hematomas, one of which had to be surgically removed, but this complication has not been reported since. Worsening of the original pain via ipsilateral or contralateral stimulation of MI/SI has been observed sporadically, and one of our CP patients developed a painful supernumerary phantom arm after MCS (Canavero *et al.* 1999).

Analgesia via ipsilateral stimulation is on record. No major modification of cortical somatotopy is seen in these patients, but bilateral benefit from unilateral stimulation is possible and focal stimulation of the hand area also relieved hemisoma pain in one case (Canavero 2009).

A handful of patients with excellent initial analgesia and increasing periods of post-effect have not relapsed for years after switching off the stimulating apparatus, a sign of neuroplastic phenomena induced by MCS in SI.

Mechanism of action

Neuroimaging studies of invasive cortical stimulation suffer from limited statistical power due to small number of patients, shortcomings of region of interest (ROI) measurements, inhomogeneity in patients' pains (CP versus PNP), group analyses versus single patients, type of cortical stimulation (extradural vs. subdural), target (MI vs. SI), and neuroimaging protocols (SPECT vs. PET vs. fMRI).

The data available are contradictory (Box 11.1, Fig. 11.2a,b).

While the Lyon group found no cortical activation whatsoever below the electrode, i.e., in MI or SI, in all their studies, Saitoh's group observed MI activation, Canavero and Bonicalzi (1995) rCBF changes in SI,

Box 11.1. Neuroimaging studies of invasive cortical stimulation

(1) **Tsubokawa *et al.* (1991a)** studied seven CP patients with ^{131}I-amphetamine SPECT, 4–10 days after implantation of a motor cortex stimulator. The rCBF showed a marked increase (+ 150–200%) in the stimulated cortex (MI/SI) and the ipsilateral thalamic and brainstem area, along with pain abatement. The skin temperature as assessed with thermography in the painful area increased to almost the same level as that in the contralateral non-painful area.

(2) **Canavero and Bonicalzi (1995)** found that parietal cortex stimulation renormalized a locus of SPECT hypoperfusion in the parietal cortex in one patient suffering CCP. Renormalization went along with analgesia. In another CP patient, MI ECS renormalized SPECT thalamic hypoperfusion, while providing analgesia **(Canavero *et al.* 1999)**.

(3) MI ECS has inhibiting effects on SI/MI cortex as well as contralaterally, as reported in an fMRI study of phantom pain **(Sol *et al.* 2001)**.

(4) **Saitoh *et al.* (2004)** submitted a right-sided CPSP patient to subdural MI CS, with excellent analgesia (VAS 8 to 1) after 30 minutes of stimulation. $H_2(15)O$ PET pre – and post-stimulation revealed significant rCBF increases in left frontal areas (BA9 and 11, BA32) and the left thalamus and decreases in temporo-occipital areas (right BA22 and left BA19). The efficacy of MI CS was mainly related to increased synaptic activity in the thalamus, whereas all other changes were related to emotional processes. The same authors performed $H_2(15)O$ PET (resolution: $4 \times 4 \times 5$ mm at full width at half-maximum [FWHM]) on six patients during right-sided 25–40 Hz CS (three with CP and three with brachial plexus avulsion (BPA) pain, all left-sided) **(Kishima *et al.* 2007)**. The PET study was performed 1–3 years after implantation. Stimulation was stopped more than 12 hours before PET. Six PET scans were performed before subdural MI CS. MI CS was run for 30 minutes and six PET scans were performed after onset of analgesia and then analyzed, considering all patients together, with the SPM software. Comparison of rCBF before and after MI CS showed significant rCBF increases after MI CS in the left posterior thalamus (pulvinar) and left posterior insula. No areas of significant rCBF decrease were identified. By comparing early post-MI CS scans with pre-MI CS scans, the authors found significant rCBF increases in the left posterior insula and the right orbitofrontal cortex (BA11) and significant *decreases* in the right BA9 and the *right BA4*. By comparing late post-MI CS scans with pre-MI CS scans, the left caudal ACC (BA24) showed significant increases, while comparison of early post-MI CS with late post-MI ECS scans brought out significant rCBF increases in the left SMA (BA6). Unlike the Lyon group's findings (see below), the ipsilateral (to MI ECS: right) thalamus was not affected. Results were not differentiated between central and peripheral neuropathic pain.

(5) The Lyon group (**Peyron *et al.* 1995**) reported on two patients with CP (both spontaneous and evoked), one with a right mesencephalic infarct with left leg pain (spontaneous and evoked) and one with a left parietal infarct sparing the thalamus, with right hemisoma pain, barring the face. In case 1, PET at rest showed no cortical abnormality, but right thalamic hypoperfusion (–9%). During MCS, CBF was increased in brainstem, orbitofrontal cortex (OFC), right thalamus, and cingulate cortex (CC): 30 minutes after discontinuation, persisting CBF changes were seen in OFC and CC. In case 2, PET at rest showed widespread CBF decrease in left parietal cortex (–35%) and hypoactivity in left thalamus (–10%), this latter being normal on MRI. During MCS, CBF was increased in brainstem, OFC, left thalamus and CC, while the parietal cortex asymmetry was unmodified. Analgesic effects in both patients lasted at least 30 minutes after stopping MCS and this was accompanied by sustained CBF changes, particularly in the thalamus. CBF increases were of the order of 7–9%. An important sustained CBF increase was seen in patient 2's brainstem, while in patient 1 it was delayed, of lesser intensity and shorter duration (patient 2, but not patient 1, also showed modulation of nociceptive flexion reflexes RIII). No change was seen in SI. Thalamic CBF changes were almost superimposable in both patients, but pain relief was satisfactory only in one patient, in whom there was also brainstem activation. CBF changes in OFC and anterior CC (ACC) were stronger and more sustained in the patient with less pain relieving-effect of MCS than the other. **Garcia-Larrea *et al.* (1997**) studied seven CPSP and three PNP (BPA pain) patients who underwent contralateral MI ECS (in three medially, i.e., subdurally). $H_2(15)O$ PET was performed before, during (5 and 20 minutes) and 30 minutes after a 20-minute session of stimulation. Results were not differentiated between CP and BPA. There was no significant difference in rCBF between the two controls or the two stimulation conditions. The only locus of significant CBF increase during MI ECS was observed in the motor thalamus. Sizeable but insignificant CBF increases during MI ECS were seen in the left insula, BA24–32, and upper mesencephalon (plus a rCBF decrease in BA18–19 bilaterally). No significant change was seen in MI (SI could not be resolved with their machine). All changes were reversible upon stopping MI ECS, although BA24 and mesencephalic changes persisted or even increased slightly after stoppage of MI ECS. They compared three patients with 80–100% relief and four with less than 40% relief. Mean thalamic CBF was enhanced in both groups, with a similar time course, albeit rCBF increase was greater in those with > 80% relief. In contrast, mean CBF in BA24–32 appeared to increase during MI ECS only in patients with good relief and to decrease in poor responders, even in individual analyses.

The same group (**Laurent *et al.* 1999**, **Garcia-Larrea *et al.* 1999**) evaluated 10 patients with CP and BPA (likely including the above-mentioned patients, although time from implantation to PET does not correspond). MI ECS was stopped 24 hours before PET. Four consecutive scans were first recorded (A). Then PET was recorded at 5, 15, 25, and 35 minutes after switching on MI ECS (B). MI ECS was subsequently stopped and PET recorded at 15, 30, 45, 60, and 75 minutes after MCS had been turned off (C). MI ECS (B vs. A) was associated with increased rCBF in rostral ACC contralateral to the electrode. During MI ECS stoppage (C vs. A) there was strong activation up to 75 minutes after MI ECS discontinuation of rostral ACC, orbitofrontal cortex, basal ganglia, and brainstem. MI ECS (B+C vs. A) was associated with decreased blood flow immediately below the electrode. Images of CBF changes in the brainstem did not cover the localization of the PAG. They did not find MI ECS activation of SI, a possible consequence of the spatiotemporal resolution limits (12 mm) of their PET machine. The low-threshold analysis (Z-score ≥ 3.5) of the two-step procedure yielded some regions of significant CBF increase: the whole thalamus (ipsilateral to MI ECS), the ACC (mostly contralaterally to MI ECS, plus midline), orbitofrontal areas, a region comprising the insula and descending towards the inferomedial temporal lobe – including amygdala (exclusively contralateral to MI ECS) and the subthalamic-upper brainstem region (ipsilateral to MI ECS). The second (high-threshold) step of the analysis (Z-score ≥ 4) restricted the above results spatially and limited the anatomical region of significant CBF increase to thalamic VL ipsilateral to MCS, with extensions to VA and subthalamic region. Vc was outside the region of increased CBF in both high- and low-threshold analyses. The sequence included condition A (CBF assessed basally, 15 minutes before MI ECS with stimulator turned off for 18 hours), conditions B and C (two consecutive scans performed respectively after 5 and 20 minutes of continuous MI ECS), and condition D (scan 30 minutes after MI ECS discontinuation). Pain ratings during PET were 4.8 ± 2.6 during condition A, 4.3 ± 2.9 and 3.69 ± 2.8 in conditions B and C, and 3.69 ± 2.8 in condition D. In spite of a trend to pain decrease from A to D, differences were not significant. As far as rCBF changes are concerned, in all cases there was an abrupt CBF increase during the first scan under MI ECS (5 minutes after onset) which remained stable during PET 20 minutes after MI ECS onset. These effects were reversible 30 minutes after MI ECS interruption in all sites, except in ACC, where rCBF had not yet reverted to pre-stimulation values 30 minutes after MCS discontinuation: here two spots of increased rCBF appeared in right and left ACC/orbitofrontal boundaries (despite unilateral analgesia!) and stayed almost so after switching off the stimulator. No significant change related to MI ECS was observed in SI or MI. CBF decreased in BA18–19, and this was totally reversible upon discontinuation of MI ECS. In CP and BPA patients with > 80% versus < 20% relief, while lateral thalamic CBF appeared to increase in all patients (albeit to a greater extent in those relieved: 15% vs. 5%), BA32 CBF increased in responders (+ 5% at 20 minutes), but decreased in non-responders (–10% at 20 minutes); upon close scrutiny, this does not seem a strong finding, as in their two reported CP cases this was not the case.

Garcia-Larrea *et al.* (2006) submitted to MI ECS a patient with left facial CP due to a left medullary infarct. Although the territory with sensory loss was much wider in the right non-painful than in the left painful side, PET showed significant rCBF reduction in the right thalamus, contralateral to the small painful area. 40 Hz MCS afforded 60% relief and PET showed renormalization of the thalamic anomaly.

Peyron *et al.* (2007) explored the post-stimulation period using an enlarged temporal window (as long as PET studies allow). Nineteen morphine-naive patients suffering BCP (13 patients), cord central pain (4 patients), or brachial plexus avulsion (2 patients) received 35 Hz (180 μs/2.5 V/cyclical) MI ECS (paddle parallel to rolandic fissure) and subsequent PET scans. Analgesic drugs were not discontinued, other than fast-acting opioids for at least 12 hours before exam. PET resolution was 7 mm. Patients were blinded to MI ECS status (*on/off*). After acquisition of baseline scans, the next four scans were acquired at 5, 15, 25, and 35 minutes after MCS onset. MI ECS was then turned off again and five further scans were recorded at 15, 30, 45, 60, and 75 minutes. Data were analyzed using SPM2 software and also considered for a functional connectivity analysis (FCA), which examines the temporal correlation of neural events between distributed brain areas. Mean pain relief was 10–40% in eight patients, 60% in six and > 80% in two. Results of *on* versus baseline and *off* versus baseline were as follows. Only a limited activation of the pregenual (pg) ACC (anatomically connected to MI) contralateral to MI ECS was found in the *on* versus baseline comparison. The large majority of activations were found in the *off* versus baseline subtraction in the ipsilateral premotor cortex, the contralateral pgACC (descending pain control) and midcingulate (noxious processing) and supplementary motor area (SMA), pallidum, putamen, and periaqueductal gray (PAG). Most of the rCBF changes that correlated with long-term analgesia occurred during the 75 minutes subsequent to MI ECS stoppage (after 35 minutes of effective stimulation). There was a correlation between rCBF changes and analgesia in the *on* condition in mid cingulate cortex (MCC) and pgACC (BA32/24) contralaterally to MCS and in prefrontal cortices (BA10) bilaterally. There was a trend for the mid cingulate to be activated in the *on* condition with a persisting activation in the *off* condition, while the pgACC still showed increased activity in the *off* condition. Regions whose rCBF increased relative to baseline during MI ECS and correlated positively with analgesia in the *off* condition (after stoppage of MCS) included a large ACC activation, extended from the posterior MCC and anterior MCC to the pgACC bilaterally, contralateral OFC and SMA, ipsilateral cerebellum and posterior cingulate cortex, prefrontal cortices and basal ganglia bilaterally, hypothalamus, upper mesencephalon (PAG) and lower pons. These activations were maximal in the *off* condition and correlated with average analgesia. In contrast to the findings of Saitoh's group (see above), MI rCBF below the electrode was not found to change or correlate with pain scores at any time, nor was SI. In the FCA, responses that correlated with analgesia with MI ECS *on* were found to correlate also with CBF changes in other subdivisions of lateral prefrontal cortices, in contralateral OFC, pgACC, anterior insula, putamen, and lower pons. In the *off* condition FCA, significant covariations were found between pgACC and basal ganglia, pgACC and brainstem, pgACC and posterior cingulated cortex. Basal ganglia covaried together bilaterally, but also with posterior cingulate and insular cortices. CBF changes in mesencephalon and lower pons covaried with basal ganglia and with pgACC. The authors concluded that a network comprising the ACC/OFC/medial thalamus and PAG – the same as seen during ECS induced analgesia by other procedures – appears to be the final common pathway of analgesia elicited by ECS (ACC and PAG being opioid-rich areas) and becomes activated *only* after MI ECS is discontinued. MCC and pgACC activities did not correlate with current pain relief, but with the amount of analgesia obtained after several cycles of MI ECS. The perigenual and subgenual ACC are associated with mood alterations and the production of affective states: they are part of a "ventral affective system" involved in the identification of the emotional significance of a stimulus, production of affective states, and automatic regulation of emotional responses, and also comprise the amygdala, anterior insula and ventral striatum. The mid-posterior cingulate cortex instead is concerned with pain unpleasantness. This study failed to replicate the authors' previous finding of a significant thalamic rCBF increase, except in the FCA. They concluded that MI ECS-related thalamic activation is phasic and short-lasting, likely a trigger for other activations, and may be averaged out when 35 minutes of MI ECS are lumped together and analyzed as a whole.

The same group (**Maarrawi *et al.* 2007a**) submitted a subgroup of the above patients (seven central pain, one trigeminal peripheral neuropathic pain) to PET with ^{11}C-diprenorphine PET, basally and after 2 months of chronic MI ECS. The two preoperative scans performed at a 2-week interval did not show significant differences. Medications were kept unchanged. Data were analyzed with SPM99. Voxel-wise comparison of preoperative and postoperative PET scans showed a significant decrease of opioid receptor binding postoperatively. Buprenorphine binding decrease (group level analysis) concerned the posterior part of the midbrain (PAG) (–25.6%), anterior middle cingulate cortex (–21.2%), lateral prefrontal cortex (–23.3%), and cerebellum (–18.3%). VAS decreases and binding decreases correlated significantly in PAG and anterior MCC (in PFC, there was only a trend). One CP patient got minimal relief from MI ECS (VAS 8 to 7) and decreases were 16.3% in PAG, 10.3% in aMCC, 10.11% in cerebellum, and 17.2% in PFC. The CP patient with the best relief (VAS 8 to 2 on MCS) showed decreases respectively of 37%, 30.3%, 22.2%, and 25.5%, which would seem to confirm that the magnitude of decreases significantly correlated with degree of analgesia. Yet the largest decreases were seen at PAG and PFC levels in a patient who had a VAS 7-to-2 relief, at aMCC level in the patient with the best analgesia, at cerebellar level in one with a VAS 8-to-5 change. The authors suggest that binding decreases were not due to loss of opioid receptors (as seen in some studies of CP), but to increased endogenous opioid secretion and resulting decreased receptor availability to exogenous diprenorphine and a possible reactive down-regulation and internalization of receptors. The authors' conclusion was that MCS triggers endogenous opioid secretion in part of the remaining medial pain system unaffected by opioid receptor loss in CPSP. The involved circuit would include MI that projects to PAG which in turn projects to ACC. However, their conclusion is nixed by poor opioid responsiveness of CP (Chapters 9 and 16).

They **(Garcia-Larrea *et al.* 1999)** also recorded CO_2 laser evoked potentials (LEPs) and flexion nociceptive reflex (RIII) in a subgroup of these same patients. LEPs (amplitude and latency of each component) and RIII (surface) were studied with MI ECS turned off, on and at least 30 minutes after MI ECS interruption. LEPs were obtained after stimulation of both the painful and the intact side, while RIII was obtained after stimulation of the painful side only. In one patient, after stimulation of the non-affected side, LEP amplitudes of the vertex component decreased significantly during active stimulation. In the group as a whole, after stimulation of the non-affected side, LEP amplitudes tended to decrease under MI ECS, although not statistically significantly. RIII was not modified in the three conditions. Electrophysiological responses did not correlate with VAS. There was a lack of any significant acute change in somatosensory evoked potentials (SSEPs) during MI ECS in any of the recorded patients with central lesions. None of the four patients whose nociceptive reflexes remained unmodified by MI ECS was satisfied with the attained analgesia. Although the seven patients with CP had sizeable epidural SSEPs during intraoperative monitoring, only four retained scalp-recorded SSEPs of sufficient amplitude to permit assessment of MI ECS effects. Parietal somatosensory responses up to 50 ms post-stimulus did not exhibit any significant change in amplitude, latency, or topography in relation to MI ECS. Thus, significant modulation of spinal nociceptive reflexes was seen during MI ECS in three of the seven patients, while it was unchanged in four. Modification thereof corresponded in every case to attenuation of the responses during MI ECS. Two of three patients with MI ECS-related reflex attenuation experienced good to very good relief, while the third reported > 60% abatement of allodynia during MI ECS, but only 30% of spontaneous pain.

Tsubokawa *et al.* (1991a) in MI, and Sol *et al.* (2001) in SI and MI bilaterally. Importantly, analogous studies conducted during MI ECS for Parkinson's disease clearly revealed cortical changes below the electrode (fully reviewed in Canavero 2009). Parenthetically, orthodromic activity increases brain metabolism, whereas antidromic activity does not (Montgomery 2010), possibly explaining some negative studies. As concerns the thalamus, Peyron *et al.* (2007) found no thalamic rCBF changes, whereas in their previous studies they did (Garcia-Larrea *et al.* 1997, 1999, 2006). Thalamic metabolic changes have been reported by Tsubokawa *et al.* (1991a), Canavero *et al.* (1999), Saitoh *et al.* (2004), and Kishima *et al.* (2007); CP relief is accompanied by thalamic renormalization (Pagni and Canavero 1995, Canavero *et al.* 1999).

As will be shown in Section 4, an impressive quantity of data points to an unbalanced reverberatory loop active between the sensory cortex and the sensory thalamus as the basis of CP. It can be hypothesized that invasive cortical stimulation acts locally by engaging inhibitory interneurons in the MI/SI dipole and the long corticothalamic reverberating loop, with subsequent fall-out effects on other brain regions, both through indirect transsynaptic effects and through direct anterograde or retrograde activation of white matter projections (rostral [perigenual] ACC and PAG, insula, etc.). The so-called ventral affect system cannot be considered central to analgesia, since cingulotomy in CP is either ineffective or has an effect on pain affect only (i.e., the pain is still there, but no longer bothersome; see Appendix). Similarly, an

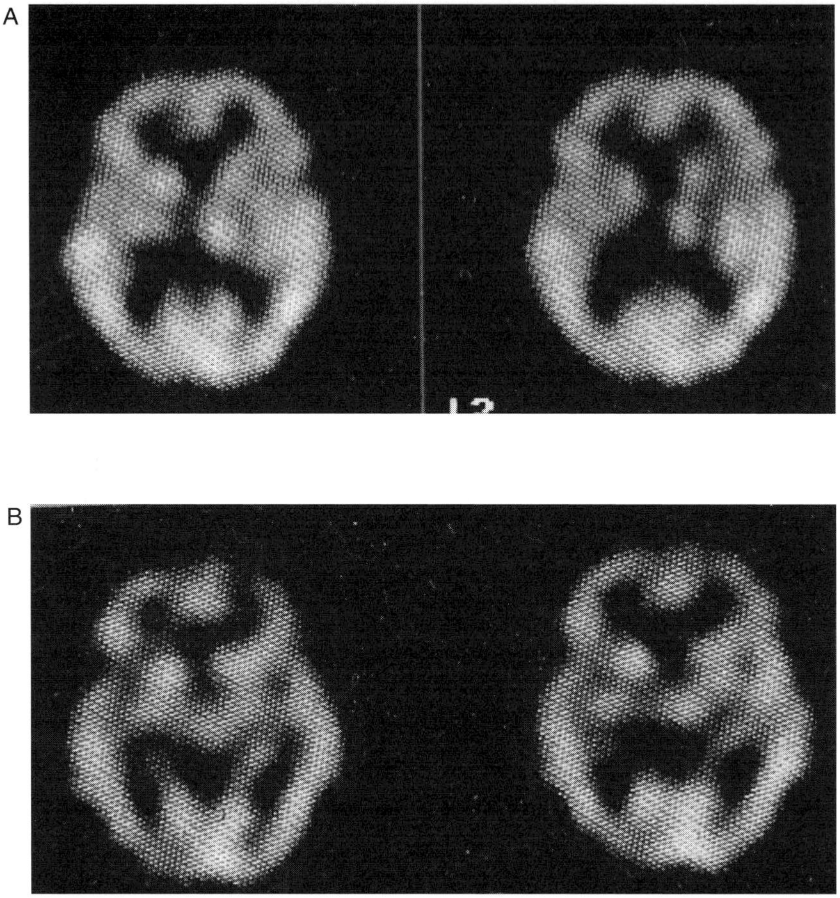

Figure 11.2. High-resolution SPECT scans showing (A) thalamic hypoperfusion in a patient with CPSP. (B) Motor cortex stimulation renormalized it, alongside analgesia. *See color plate section.*

increase of opioids as the basis of ECS analgesia is nixed by the almost complete lack of effect of opioids for CP (Chapters 9 and 16).

MCS increases the overall magnitude of post-movement β-synchronization and SSEPs; these increases are significantly correlated with analgesia. It also improves somatosensory input processing at cortical level, influencing the pain-inhibitory function of the system that mediates activation of non-noxious somatosensory neurons (Reyns *et al.* 2008). Importantly, propofol may both relieve CP and restore normal sensation in human patients (Canavero 2009). In any case, an intracortical mechanism of action is central.

Sensation and motricity are tightly coupled. Movements are known to increase the threshold for detection and decrease the perceived intensity of somatosensory stimuli, including those at a painful level (active movements having greater and more consistent effect than passive movements) without need of attentional or cognitive contributions (Brodie *et al.* 2009). Humans perceive forces they exert as weaker than identical forces acted upon them: in fact, a corollary discharge of the effort attenuates the subject's sensory feedback and pain interferes with mental representations of movement (see references in Canavero and Bonicalzi 2007a). Tonic painful input leads to inhibition of MI and SMA during motor performance on the painful side (and the contralateral one – though less so) (Binder *et al.* 2002). TMS studies show that under normal conditions sensory afferents limit the activity of inhibitory neurons in MI, and that after pure thalamic sensory stroke, MI intracortical inhibition is increased (Liepert *et al.* 2005). In one scenario, the CP generator tonically inhibits MI, but, if this is too intense, CS may not be able to engage inhibition itself. Finally, a relatively high stimulation frequency can induce a tonic depolarization and cortical inactivation effect, which is known to inhibit thalamic relays.

Fields and Adams (1974) first reported analgesia in humans by means of stimulation of subcortical motor fibers in the internal capsule. However, given that in humans there are few descending fibers from MI or SI to the superficial dorsal horn (Schoenen and Grant 2004), ECS cannot act by descending direct inhibition to the spinal cord.

Chapter 12

Deep brain stimulation

Despite initial optimistic reports, it has become clear that deep brain stimulation (DBS) is not as successful as was initially hoped. The clinical data do not fit with promising animal findings, and large discrepancies are noted between the results of different neurosurgical groups.

The targets for DBS include thalamic Vc nuclei and/or the posterior limb of the internal capsule, the caudal medial thalamic areas around the third ventricle, including CM-Pf and the junction of the third ventricle and the sylvian aqueduct (rostral ventral PAG, caudal ventral PVG). CP is generally treated by contralateral Vc stimulation, which is effective only unilaterally. The internal capsule (posterior limb) may be used if thalamic tissue is unavailable (e.g., after an infarct or encephalomalacia). Some groups simultaneously stimulate the PVG area and Vc (Fig. 12.1).

Mechanism of action

The mechanism or mechanisms of action of DBS are largely unknown, but it is increasingly clear that it depends on the electrical excitation of neural elements and not on their suppression, with antidromic activation playing a starring role (Montgomery 2010). Unfortunately, the variability of the axons' orientation limits the value of computational models of DBS.

PAG/PVG

Young and Chambi (1987) used a double-blind, placebo-controlled study design and found no evidence that PAG/PVG-induced analgesia in humans is mediated by an opioid mechanism. In a study, low- (1–20 Hz) and high-frequency (50 Hz) stimulation of the PAG neither produced relief nor reproduced pain in eight patients with thalamic CPSP, one with tumor thalamic CP, one with SCI pain, and one with tabes dorsalis, despite a modest-to-significant increase in CSF endorphin levels (Amano *et al.* 1982): this increase was interpreted as a psychological response. Actually, the contrast medium (metrimazide) used for the ventriculography, not PVG DBS, appears to be responsible for the elevated estimation of beta-endorphins (Fessler *et al.* 1984).

Aziz's group found that pain suppression is frequency-dependent (Nandi *et al.* 2003, Nandi and Aziz 2004). During 5–35 Hz PVG stimulation, the amplitude of thalamic field potentials (FPs) was significantly reduced, and this was associated with pain relief; at higher frequencies (50–100 Hz) there was no reduction in the FPs and pain was made worse. A post-effect of 5–15 minutes (depending on duration of stimulation) was seen in FP reversal upon switching off the stimulator. The FPs were of very low frequency (0.2–0.4 Hz) in Vc: their amplitude was much stronger OFF or with ineffective (50 Hz) stimulation than with analgesic 5–35 Hz stimulation. This suggested a fairly direct neuronal circuit between PVG and Vc mediated by reticulospinal neurons. All patients were also stimulated in Vc, alone or simultaneously with PVG. The PVG FPs were independent of both the pain scores and the state of stimulation of Vc. In non-responders, there was no flattening in the slow-wave thalamic FPs across different frequencies of PVG stimulation. This group (Pereira *et al.* 2007) submitted three CP patients to DBS and studied them with ^{99}mTc-HMPAO SPECT fitted to standard Talairach space at a 10% threshold. All patients were scanned ON- and OFF-DBS with an interval of 2 days, 4–7 months after surgery, and results compared. A wide array of cortical and subcortical regions were either activated or deactivated without a common thread among patients. Considering just the 30% threshold suggestive of very large rCBF differences and only effects during stimulation versus no stimulation, their patient 1 (PVG DBS) showed right SI/MI (3.3%) and left PFC (0.2%) plus brainstem (0.5%) hypoperfusion, patient 2 no anomaly, and patient

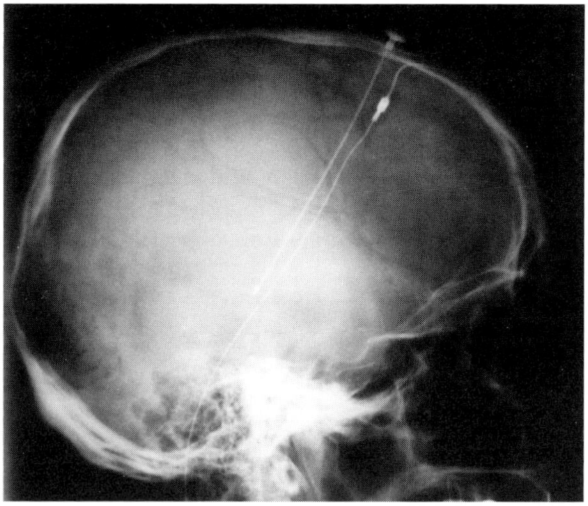

Figure 12.1. Skull radiograph showing a deep brain stimulation apparatus in place.

3 right hemispheric subcortical hypoperfusion. These authors tried to link these rCBF changes to areas thought to be involved in analgesia, but the findings do not lend themselves to any kind of reasonable analysis.

Vc

Vc DBS does not activate the endogenous opioid system (or other descending fiber tracts) (see full discussion in the first edition of this book: Canavero and Bonicalzi 2007a). Since the thalamocortical loop works more like a non-linear dynamic system that is not solely based on a firing-rate code, DBS may actually work by rebalancing a skewed oscillatory pattern (Chapter 26).

Neurometabolic studies have been published. These studies reported stimulator-induced signal increases to be higher than task activations (maximum 2%). Heiss *et al.* (1986) studied one CPSP case with PET. At rest (pain condition), the lowest metabolic rate was in the infarcted thalamus; some areas showed decreased glucose consumption in the otherwise normal ipsilateral cortex. A second PET during DBS (off-pain condition) revealed markedly decreased glucose metabolism in most brain regions. Rezai *et al.* (1999) scanned (fMRI) two patients who had steady-burning CP due to traumatic SCI (a third had PNP). PVG DBS – in contrast to Vc DBS – did not activate SI, but the cingulate cortex (compare with Vim DBS for tremor). Low-frequency stimulation of PVG led to activation of the medial thalamus (compare with Nandi *et al.* 2003). Activations near the electrode were written up to a possible local, non-specific CBF increase rather than neural pathway activation. At paresthesia-evoking intensities Vc DBS resulted in the activation of SI in all three pain patients. In most cases, areas of cortical activation corresponded to the homuncular somatotopy of paresthesias (3 V, 75–100 Hz, 150–200 μs). With no paresthesias, SI was not activated. In addition to SI, there was activation of thalamus, SII and insula. In a similar study, Duncan *et al.* (1998) submitted five patients with neuropathic pain (perhaps inclusive of CP) to Vc DBS. All had obtained relief for more than 3 years to reduce a placebo confounding role. Three patients were relieved, while two had no immediate relief. They reported that < 100 Hz Vc DBS increased rCBF in and near the thalamus and some cortical areas, the effect being more prominent with continued stimulation. Their data did not support activation of tactile thalamocortical pathways being the sole mechanism underlying successful Vc DBS. Their most prominent cortical rCBF increase was in ipsilateral anterior insula, both with *and without* relief, although somewhat stronger with relief. Patients perceived both paresthesiae and cold and warmth during stimulation. The close proximity of microstimulation sites evoking tactile and thermal sensations indicates that bipolar stimulating electrodes could easily stimulate neurons within both the insular and SI pathways. They also observed a **non-significant** trend toward activation in ACC with Vc stimulation. Davis *et al.* (2000) studied two patients with CCP (plus three other neuropathic pain cases) submitted to Vc/ML stimulation. The first was a paraplegic suffering from unilateral leg pain: he obtained 100% relief after 30 minutes of stimulation. This analgesia disappeared immediately upon cessation of DBS. Follow-up was 9 months. On PET day, he was on amitriptyline, baclofen, diazepam, and oxycodone. The second suffered from spinal arteriovenous malformation (AVM)-related CP to the left leg. Follow-up was 16 months. Analgesics were retained for 12 hours before PET. There was 0% relief at follow-up, but some relief immediately postoperatively (thalamotomic effect?). Paresthesias were strongest at the beginning of stimulation and subsided as stimulation continued. There was **no** clear relationship between the degree of stimulation-evoked pain relief and the magnitude of rCBF change in either region of the ACC (BA32–24). Activation of posterior ACC was detected after 30 minutes of DBS, but not at the onset of stimulation, in contrast to the ACC, which was activated throughout the period of DBS. Thus, posterior ACC was not related to direct activation from thalamus, but to other structures. Duncan *et al.* (1998) also noted that some of their DBS-induced activations were stronger after 30 minutes of DBS than at DBS onset. In contrast to this study, patients in Davis's study did not experience thermal sensations during DBS and **no insula activation** was seen. Lack of activation of SI-SII could be explained by low statistical power (only two responders), paresthesias in different body regions, thus activating different portions of SI-II, or diminishing paresthesias in the course of DBS. Other CBF changes may have involved other cortical and subcortical areas.

Other areas

Mayanagi and Sano (1998) state that "patients with chronic pain of thalamic or spinal origin failed to experience pain relief with hypothalamic DBS-like stimulation." Stimulation of the Koelliker–Fuse nucleus, a pontine satellite of the locus coeruleus and the major source of catecholamine-containing fibers to the spinal cord, has been attempted in CP cases. No reports exist for septum, caudate, or other brain targets.

Efficacy

Results of DBS for CP remain unsatisfactory. Two large studies have been conducted with the aim of FDA approval: the Medtronic 3380 study ended in December 1993 (20 BCP and 9 SCI patients), and the 3387 trial ended in May 1998 (Coffey 2001). Among CP patients, 11 CPSP were implanted and eight internalized, one post-tumor removal CCP patient and one MS-CP patient were implanted and internalized, four other unspecified CP patients were implanted and three internalized. Neither study achieved the prospectively defined success criterion of at least 50% of the patients reporting at least 50% relief at 1 year. Withdrawals and dropouts amounted to 70–73% of the patients at some follow-up intervals.

These two studies emphasized the limits of DBS studies. All relied on patients' self-reporting and, given the absence of blinding, this may have upped the response rates: the potential for at least short-term placebo responses is substantial, considering the elaborate nature of the surgical procedure, the mysterious electronic technology involved, and the close interpersonal relationship that develops between the pain patient and the attending clinician. Importantly, patients reported the presence of paresthesias even in placebo conditions (the ability to induce paresthesia in the painful area is considered important for target localization!). No control groups were ever included and no report described a systematic trial of different or deliberately ineffective stimulation parameters. Different components may respond differently. Follow-up in many studies has not exceeded 2 years. Cases reported as successful after a few weeks or months carried the same analytical weight in some reviews and meta-analyses as those followed for years. The proportion of patients who underwent system internalization using the same stimulation target for the same diagnosis varied from 0% to near 100% at different centers. The interval before the recurrence of pain after initial pain relief varied from days to years; reports with the shortest follow-up did not encounter the phenomenon, skewing the final impression. Some successes may have simply been due to "regression to the mean," i.e., spontaneous downward fluctuations of the pain. Although animal experiments predicted facilitation or cross-tolerance between DBS and opiate or neurotransmitter drugs, no such effects were observed when various drugs or stimulation holidays were used to prevent or treat tolerance in humans. In case of failure some patients were restudied and retrospectively diagnosed as hysterical or having non-organic pain (!). From the surgical standpoint, the PAG/PVG region responsible for analgesia is small, and thalamic size also varies considerably from patient to patient. Extreme precision is needed for deep stimulations, otherwise results will be jeopardized. Marchand *et al.* (2003) suggest that for some patients DBS can be helpful in reducing clinical pain, but the effect is *moderate*, as with SCS. Besides, a *strong placebo effect may be involved in the efficacy of any form of DBS, and placebo effects can last even for up to 5 years.* Interestingly, Wolksee *et al.* (1982) found no statistically meaningful difference between Vc and sham stimulation.

DBS is not totally safe. Surgical complications include infection (0–15%), intracranial hemorrhage (0–10%), stroke (0–2%), and death (0–4.4%) (Bronstein *et al.* 2011).

Table 12.1 summarizes the results of published studies of DBS.

Table 12.1. Deep brain stimulation (DBS)

Author(s)	Type of pain/number of patients	Target	Results/notes
Mazars *et al.* (1976)	Thalamic lesion (3 patients)	Vc (bilateral in SCI) or IC	Failure
Mazars *et al.* (1979) Includes all previous papers by this pioneer group on the topic **First group to stimulate the thalamus, starting 1960**	Brainstem lesion (6 patients) SCI (4 patients) BCP/CCP	 PAG/PVG	Relief in 5 Relief in 4 Poor results
Richardson and Akil (1977a, 1977b) Richardson *et al.* (1980)	SCI (paraplegia) (5 patients, then 19)	PAG/PVG	Significant pain relief in 2 (18 months). 1 patient previously submitted to failed rhizotomy/cordotomy Further series: good relief at 1 year in 6 patients AANS Congress, A836: Stimulation of nuclei cuneatus/gracilis via surface electrodes. 5 CCP patients: relief in 3, reduction in 1, failure in 1 (follow-up: not available) Ventrolateral PAG DBS for opioid-responsive intractable pains
Lazorthes (1979)	CP (thalamic) (28 patients) SCI (8 patients)	Vc	Successful pain relief in 5 Successful pain relief in 2
Schvarcz (1980)	CP (thalamic: 2 patients; partial SCI: 3 patients; postcordotomy: 1 patient)	Medial posteroinferior thalamic areas	Pain relief (deep background pain and hyperpathia): > 75% (but never 100%) relief: 2 50–75% relief: 2 Failure: 2 Hyperpathia abolished, deep background pain only reduced. No reversal by naloxone. Follow-up: 6–42 months
Mundinger and Salomão (1980)	BCP (incl. CPSP) (5 patients)	IC/ML (4) Pulvinar (1)	> 70%: 1; 50–70%: 1; 50%: 3 (1 pulvinar) (max. follow-up: less than 2 years). No relief at longer term.
Mundinger and Neumuller (1982)	SCI (5 patients)	IC/ML (3) Pulvinar (1) PAG/PVG (1)	0%, 50%, and 50–70% > 70% 50% (except one, follow-up shorter than 2 years)
Ray and Burton (1980)	CPSP (thalamic) (1 patient) CCP (iatrogenic) (2 patients)	CM-Pf	> 50% relief in all, drugs not stopped, effect abates in time
Plotkin (1982)	CP (thalamic) (1 patient) SCI pain (1 patient) SCI pain (2 patients)	Vc Vc PVG	0% success (?) 0% (?) 0% (?) (follow-up: 6–42 months)

Table 12.1. (cont.)

Author(s)	Type of pain/number of patients	Target	Results/notes
Dieckmann and Witzmann (1982)	CP (thalamic) (5 patients)	PVG/Vc	5 *slight* late reliefs (6 months – 4.5 years)
Andy (1983)	CPSP (2 patients)	Right CM-Pf and left CM stimulation	Good or excellent results (follow-up: up to 18 months)
Broggi *et al.* (1984)	CPSP (thalamic) (2 patients)	Vc	40–60% pain relief (12–18 months)
Turnbull (1984) Includes: Shulman *et al.* (1982) and other previous papers by this author	CP (including SCI)	Vc	Of limited efficacy, particularly ineffective in SCI pain. 1 patient with brainstem stroke relieved over a few years. **1 BCP patient relieved but soon DBS no longer necessary due to pain disappearance**
Namba *et al.* (1984)	CP (thalamic and putaminal stroke: 9 patients; extrathalamic subcortical: 1 patient; MS-CP: 1 patient)	IC (8) IC + Vc (1) IC + Vc + ML (1)	At discharge: 100% (3), 50–95% (3), fair (drugs needed, 2), 0% (3; 1 with thalamotomy, pulvinotomy, mesencephalotomy). Best stimulating point for analgesia not in the center of posterior limb but in most posteromedial part (area triangularis)
Frank *et al.* (1984)	SCI pain (1 patient)	Vc	Poor result
Tsubokawa *et al.* (1985 Katayama *et al.* (2001) Includes all CP patients submitted to DBS by Tsubokawa's group	CP above brainstem (8 patients) Myelopathic CP	Vc PAG PAG Vc	Short-term relief: 80% in 2/8 patients, 60–80% in 3/8 patients, < 60% in 3/8 patients Long-term relief: 33% No relief No relief 60–80% relief in 2
Hosobuchi (1986) Includes all previous published patients	BCP (cortex, thalamus, brainstem) (13 patients) Paraplegia CP (8 patients) Postcordotomy CP (9 patients) **1970–1984**	Vc, lemniscal, PAG	8 early successes, 5 failures; 6 late successes, 2 failures 3 early successes, 5 failures; 2 late successes, 1 failure 8 early and late successes (75–100% relief); 1 early bleeding PAG DBS: ineffective; lemniscal: 36% success Follow-up: 2–14 years
Heiss *et al.* (1986)	CPSP (thalamic) (1 patient)	Vc (likely, not specified)	Pain relief (follow-up: unavailable)
Levy *et al.* (1987) Includes Fields and Adams (1974), Adams (1977–1978)	(1) CP (25 patients)	(1) Vc or IC	(1) Test stimulations: 14 VPL, 11 VPM, 6 IC. Pain relief sufficient for internalization in VPL: 9/14 patients (64%); in VPM: 9/11 patients (82%); in IC: 1/6 patients. Initial success rate: 56%; long-term pain relief: 24%
	(2) SCI-CP	(2) Vc or PAG/PVG	(2) 14 electrodes implanted (7 Vc, 7 PAG/PVG) in 11 SCI patients. Pain relief sufficient for internalization in 2/11 patients (18%)

Table 12.1. (cont.)

Author(s)	Type of pain/number of patients	Target	Results/notes
	(3) CP, thalamic (3 patients) (4) Paraplegia pain (7 patients) (5) Postcordotomy CP (5 patients)	(3) PAG/PVG (both in 3) (4) PAG/PVG (5) PAG/PVG	(3) No persistent (> 6 weeks) pain relief (4) Unsatisfactory pain relief, no internalization (5) 7 electrodes implanted; 2 internalizations; no persistent pain relief (0%) 6 Vc and 2 PAG/PVG electrodes implanted; 2 Vc and 1 PAG/PVG electrodes internalized. 3/5 patients (60%) with initial successful stimulation, 2/5 (40%) long-term pain relief. Follow-up: 24–168 months; paresthesias independent of analgesia, not vice versa **CP relief approaches 30% (rate close to that expected from placebo)**
Siegfried (1991) Includes all previously published personal cases	CP, thalamic (19 patients) Partial SCI pain (17 patients) **1973–1989**	Vc PVG Vc	Long-term: 5 very good, 7 good, 3 fair, 4 poor. Better results in parathalamic lesions than true thalamic lesions Pain relief in 3 5 very good, 8 good, 3 fair, 1 poor DBS for MS-CP: effect lost in time
Crisologo *et al.* (1991)	Case 1: thalamic stroke with left pain; 6 months later, left stroke with right pain	Vc	Insignificant relief
Tasker *et al.* (1991, 1992) Includes all published cases from Toronto Western	CP (12 patients) CCP (13 patients) (complete lesion or incomplete lesion unresponsive to SCS)	Vc/IC PVG Vc (mostly bilateral)	Relief in 5 (3 with evoked pain: 2 relieved), failure in 7 (6 with evoked pain: stimulation painful in 3) PVG either ineffective or inferior to thalamic stimulation with the exception of 1 CCP patient whose severe allodynia and hyperpathia disappeared acutely after 5–10 min of PVG stimulation. Steady pain relief > 50%: 20% of patients; 25–50%: 16% of patients Intermittent pain relief: 0% Evoked pain relief 25–50%: 16% of patients Global: relief in 3 PAG DBS nearly always unpleasant. PVG DBS useful only for allodynia/hyperpathia in BCP. Paresthesia-producing DBS often painful in BCP Congress abstract: BCP (17 patients): 47% internalized, 35% of all cases with pain relief. Follow-up: 8–46 months CCP (16 patients): 38% internalized, 25% of all cases with pain relief. Follow-up: 23–48 months
Gybels *et al.* (1993)	CP (thalamic) (5 patients)	Vc	3/5 patients initial pain relief; 1/5 long-term benefit

Table 12.1. (cont.)

Author(s)	Type of pain/number of patients	Target	Results/notes
	SCI pain (5 patients)		Short-term pain relief in 3/5; long-term pain relief in 2/5 patients
	Postcordotomy CP (1 patient)		Failure
Hariz and Bergenheim (1995)	CP (thalamic) (6 patients)	Centrum medianum	4/6 relief; follow-up: 16 months
Young *et al.* (1995) Includes all patients appearing in previous publications	BCP (14 patients) CCP (12 patients) **1978–1993**	Unilateral PAG + Koelliker–Fuse nucleus (1 patient)	CP, thalamic. Failure
		PVG + Koelliker–Fuse nucleus (2 patients)	Excellent pain relief in 2 patients suffering from SCI-CP (follow-up 2 years and 8 months, respectively). In 1 patient cessation of stimulation after 2 years was not followed by a full-fledged return of pain. Additive effect from PVG-Koelliker–Fuse nucleus simultaneous stimulation (but KF > PVG)
		PAG/PVG	Excellent or good pain relief from PAG/PVG DBS only in 35% of patients (median follow-up > 7 years)
		Vc ± PAG/PVG	(From previous series) Excellent pain relief (Vc): 1; partial relief (Vc + PAG-PGV): 9; ineffective: 6 (Of SCI patients, 4 had ≥ 50% relief at 2–60 months) Apparently unsatisfactory long-term results from PVG stimulation in CCP Analgesia onset: within minutes; long after-effect in some patients
Kumar *et al.* (1997) Includes all patients from 1990 paper	CPSP (thalamic) (5 patients)	Vc (1) IC (4)	Short- and long-term (3.4 years) successful (50–75%) pain relief in 1; early failures (0–50% pain relief) in 4
	SCI pain (3 patients)	Vc	Early successful pain relief (51–100%): 1; early failures (0–50% pain relief): 2; late failures (2 years): 3 Analgesia within 10 min (bipolar stimulation); duration of pain pre-DBS not prognostic
Barraquer-Bordas *et al.* (1999)	CPSP (1 patient)	Vc DBS	Partial relief (analgesic reduction) of spontaneous and evoked pain. MCS ineffective. Pain full relapse after tumoral electrode displacement
Blond *et al.* (2000)	CP (brainstem or suprathalamic origin) (6 patients)	Vc DBS	Unsatisfactory results. Paroxysmal pain refractory
	SCI (3 patients) (Eur. Coop. Study) **1985–1997**		Pain relief > 50%: 1/3 patients

Table 12.1. (cont.)

Author(s)	Type of pain/number of patients	Target	Results/notes
Phillips and Bhakta (2000)	CPSP (1 patient)	PVG	Improvement
Krauss *et al.* (2001)	CPSP (thalamic stroke) (1 patient)	CM-Pf + Vc	Failure
Katayama *et al.* (2001)	CPSP (12 patients)	Vc (± ML)	3 patients (25%) relieved ≥ 60% on VAS scale at long term. All 3 patients thalamic-infrathalamic!
Romanelli and Heit (2004)	CPSP (1 patient)	Vc DBS	100% relief over > 55 months with several changes of parameters
Nandi and Aziz (2004) Owen *et al.* (2006)	CPSP (14 patients) (+ 1 patient) (5 cortical, 8 thalamic, 1 pontine, 1 IC) Other CPs (5 patients) **1995–2005**	Vc + PVG (16 patients) PVG (1 patient) Vc (1 patient)	In 1 patient, trial PVG DBS provided 0% relief 12 patients seen for an average of 16 months (3–36 months). 1 patient had less than 3-month follow-up. 11/14 were satisfactorily relieved and opted for IPG. 13/19 consecutive CP patients had satisfactory control with PVG and/or Vc DBS. Trial relief maintained over an average 16 months in all but 2 patients. Vc stimulation alone reasonably suppressed the pain in 4 patients (MS, tractotomy, post-SAH stroke, Chiari); however, in the first 2, paresthesias were intolerable. In the other 2 PVG DBS alone was superior. Combined Vc-PVG DBS was never synergistic and worsened the pain in 2 patients Their Fig. 2 with results on 14 patients (2 patients not shown, having less than 3-month follow-up): 3 patients not implanted (2 having less than 10% relief but 1 40%: why not implanted?). In 7 relief at follow-up was slightly better than test relief but in 4 it was less, in 1 case half of it; never 100% relief or somewhat less Final series of CPSP patients only (2006): 15 patients, evaluated with VAS, MPQ, PRI(R). Patients with Vc strokes only implanted in PVG-PAG; average follow-up: 27 months but results plotted *at 2 years; mean relief (VAS) for cortical strokes 42%; for all others 54%*; opposite results with PRI(R) (!) Wide range of improvements, from slight worsening to 91.3% improvement. 7 patients stopped all analgesics Post-effect: for over 24 hours **Severe burning hyperesthesia most responsive. Most patients preferred PVG DBS to Vc DBS (results thus refer mostly to PVG DBS)** Once burning abates, patients note the background crushing, aching sensation more strongly (past authors may have exchanged this phenomenon for tolerance and relapse)

Table 12.1. (cont.)

Author(s)	Type of pain/number of patients	Target	Results/notes
Owen *et al.* (2007)	CPSP (18 patients)	PVG (+ in a few Vc, 1 Vc without PVG)	6 failed trial, 12 implanted Mean improvement: 49 ± 28%, 3 patients lost to follow-up; of 9 remaining patients: 2 had 80–100% relief, 1 had 60–79% relief, 2 had 40–59% relief and 4 had < 40% relief (poor); i.e., 4/9: > 50% relief 2 failed trial, 1 implanted but poor relief
	SCI (3 patients)		?
	MS (1 patient)		Mean follow-up : 44.5 months (range: 1–76 months) for whole group of CP plus others VAS scale inadequate: this shows loss of effect in time, but if DBS turned off pain rebounds. Authors believe that remaining pain becomes more intrusive with time and patients score the pain higher, rather than loss due to tolerance
Pereira *et al.* (2007)	CPSP (thalamus, cortex) (2 patients) CCP (post-syrinx decompression) (1 patient)	Best trial and final target: right PVG, right VPL, left PVG and VPL (no difference)	At 1 year, 43%, 34%, 34% VAS reductions; 65%, 32%, 5% MPQ reductions *N*-of-1 (at 1 year) number of correct answers (of 10): patient 1 not available, patient 2 = 6, patient 3 = 10. Mean VAS ON/OFF: patient 1 not available, patient 2 = 54ON/88OFF, patient 3 = 80ON/90OFF In MPQ, reduction mainly due to sensory changes All patients on opiates, 1 on Neurontin. 1 patient stopped all analgesics and 1 reduced opiates
Pereira *et al.* (2008)	CPSP (21 patients) **2000–2006**	Vc + PVG	15 patients reported benefit (71%), mean VAS scores initially improved 43%, reducing to *19% at 1 year* and then with time (up to 5 years), suggesting tolerance MPQ indices more improved than VAS, in particular in the sensory domain. Allodynia most improved, burning, lancinating Parameters changed over time to maintain efficacy and overcome tolerance, average frequency and voltage both decreasing significantly with time with average PW unchanged Good positive correlation between frequency and voltage found
Rasche *et al.* (2006b)	CCP (11 patients): (A) Myelopathy (2 patients) (B) Brown-Séquard (1 patient) (C) Tetraplegia (1 patient) (D) Post-DREZ (1 patient) (E) Paraplegia (4 patients) (F) Conus SCI (1 patient) (G) Syringomyelia (1 patient)	In each patient, implantation of 2 leads (PVG+Vc)	(A) 0–25% and 25–50% VAS reduction over 3–5 years (B) Immediate / = trial stimulation / failure (C) 0–25% relief over 5 years (D) 75–100% relief after 6 months (E) 3 immediate failures, 1 0–25% relief over 2.5 years (F) Immediate failure (G) Immediate failure

Table 12.1. (cont.)

Author(s)	Type of pain/number of patients	Target	Results/notes
	CPSP (11 patients)		9 immediate failures, 1 25–50% relief over 2.5 years, 1 50–75% relief over 1 year. Some benefit on allodynia after PVG DBS, no effect on spontaneous burning pain and intermittent lancinating attacks. No effect on rectal, genital, or perineal pains (best parameters: 40–70Hz in PVG, 60–90Hz in Vc). Supra- and subthreshold Vc DBS usually *increased* the original pain (sometimes also PVG DBS). Combined DBS superior to single-lead stimulation, yet a clear dose–response relationship could be found in a few patients only. Only 54 out of > 2500 pain patients considered possible candidates for DBS. Stimulation can produce no effects and so placebo stimulation is possible. ALL double-blind stimulations. Internalization only if test DBS produced at least 50% relief with decrease of drugs. No narcotics allowed during test trial. Ventral PAG DBS: opioid-mediated, after-effect, gaze paralysis oscillopsia; dorsal PVG DBS: not opioid mediated, not well tolerated (fear, anxiety, etc.), no after- effect. In paraplegia cells in the representation of the anesthetic body part had no RFs, in others there was a mismatch between RFs and PFs
Hamani *et al.* (2006)	CPSP (8 patients)	Vc (+ PAG/PVG in 3)	4 patients with insertional effect (lasting 0.5–7 months); 4 patients with > 50% benefit on test trial: only Vc, not PAG/PVG stimulation. 0% long-term benefit (benefit lost within 6 weeks to 11 months). 5 Vc, 3 Vc + PAG/PVG.
	BCP (gunshot brain injury) (1 patient)	Vc	Insertional effect lasting 18 months (so DBS not tried yet)
	CCP (Chiari/syrinx) (1 patient)	Vc + PAG/PVG	Insertional effect: 4 months >50% relief on trial. 50% VAS relief 1 year later Stimulation in PAG/PVG elicited a pleasant warmth
	MS-CP (2 patients) Vc	Vc	1 insertional effect (2 months) 1 failure, 1 successful test (>50%), 63% VAS relief at 4 years
	SCI (4 patients)	Vc (bilateral) (+ PAG/PVG in 1 patient)	No insertional effects. 3 patients drew benefit on test stimulation *only* from Vc stimulation. All 3 still relieved at 2 months, 1 and 5 years. However from two other tables and text it seems only 1 patient was still relieved at long term (5 years; benefit 50% and 63% in legs from Vc DBS)
	1992–2004	NB: in hemisoma pains, one electrode extended into ML	Best relief in effective cases: 2 nearby contacts, 2.1–5 V, 90–300 μs, 100–130 Hz

Table 12.1. (cont.)

Author(s)	Type of pain/number of patients	Target	Results/notes
		Patients with tactile allodynia also implanted in PAG/PVG	Test period of 5 days: 25–120 Hz, 60–250 μs, up to 10 V, monopolar and bipolar stim. for each electrode Common feature in successful cases at long term: prompt, clear-cut response during the postoperative stimulation trial, Vc elicited a pleasant tingling in affected body part plus improvement of pain
Spooner *et al.* (2007)	CCP (C4 complete) (1 patient)	Right PVG + 2 DBS electrodes in the bilateral cingula (midsection)	1-week test trial. PVG reduced the pain from VAS 8 to 4, cingular DBS from VAS 8 to 3, lidocaine infusion dose reduced more with PVG than cingular DBS, mood improved more by cingular than PVG DBS. No sensation evoked at any time. Implanted for cingular stimulation only. Follow-up, 4 months: significant pain reduction, lidocaine reduced 55% without side effects. 1 year later death from pneumonia. Initial therapy: subcutaneous lidocaine plus intrathecal baclofen, **clonazepam**, and hydromorphone, with partial relief, but respiratory weakness and somnolence
Chodakiewitz and Rinaldi (2007)	(1) BCP (post-benign brain tumor removal) (3 patients) (2) CPSP (1 patient) (3) SCI (2 patients)	Vc	(1) All excellent pain relief at 6 months – 5 years (2) Excellent pain relief at 6 months (3) Tetraplegia: excellent relief Paraplegia: minimal relief Follow-up: 7–10 years
Franzini *et al.* (2008)	CPSP (1 patient)	Internal capsule (post. limb) adjacent to Vc	40% pain reduction (2 years) Pain recurrence (IPG exhausted). After IPG replacement, lesser pain relief. 3 years later traumatic BPA + SCI
Pickering *et al.* (2009)	CPSP (1 patient) right temporo-posterior parietal and insula; IC; VL	PVG/PAG	6 weeks later: global pain score: from 10 to 4; cold remained 10, deep pain gone, superficial pain from 10 to 7, all others improved 30–50%. Patients' assessment: 70% improved (allodynia improved to VAS 4–5 on left side and VAS 0 on right side). Sensory deficits improved: almost complete resolution of previous left hypalgesia and hypoesthesia. 2 V, 240 μs, 5 Hz. Fast reversal of analgesia upon cessation (minutes). Full relapse 4 months after implantation. Parameters adjusted with relief recaptured, then new relapse 1 year later (DBS not switched off by patient, so some relief possible) Globally: benefit for 9 months **Opioids cannot account for renormalization of sensory function**.

Chapter 13

Spinal cord stimulation

Spinal cord stimulation (SCS) can be achieved via surgical or percutaneous implantation of stimulating electrodes (Fig. 13.1). A definitive pacemaker is applied after a suitable test period, generally in the presence of paresthesias projected on the painful territory.

Mechanism of action

Activation of a dorsal horn spinal gate is excluded, since SCS has no or only insignificant effects on acute pain. SCS may modulate local spinal networks, but also thalamocortical areas: the amplitude of evoked potentials in the human somatosensory cortex (Larson *et al.* 1974) and thalamic centromedian nucleus (CM) (Nyquist and Greenhoot 1973) is reduced by SCS; SCS also reduced the firing rate (including bursting) of thalamic CM neurons, with a post-stimulation effect of a few hours, at parameters achieving partial relief, in a patient with mixed nociceptive–neuropathic–central pain (Modesti and Waszak 1975). Blair *et al.* (1975) found an attenuation of later SSEP components, with little effect on early components, during SCS-induced analgesia. Gildenberg and Murthy (1980) reported on two chronic pain (non-CP) patients who developed post-cordotomy dysesthesias. Both were submitted to SCS with minimal or only partial pain relief (20–40 Hz). Evoked potentials (EPs) were recorded from CM-Pf and Vc prior to stereotactic thalamotomy. On acute stimulation of the dorsal columns, EPs were recorded from CM-Pf and VPL, with little distinction between the two, but delayed responses were seen only in CM-Pf. EPs recorded from Vc were coincidental with therapeutic SCS becoming painful. This short latency EP was unaffected by SCS. Instead, in CM-Pf, two late responses at 80–150 ms on stimulation of either contralateral or ipsilateral median nerve occurred, and these were modified by SCS, with an after-effect of several minutes. Another late sudden EP (500 ms) was obliterated by SCS. Curiously, the late EP on stimulation of the median nerve could be modified by SCS even at a lower thoracic level (nixing the gate control theory and suggesting another gating mechanism, presumably in the brainstem). The more diffuse longer-latency EPs from CM-Pf were consistent with a more diffuse multisynaptic pathway due to C-fiber

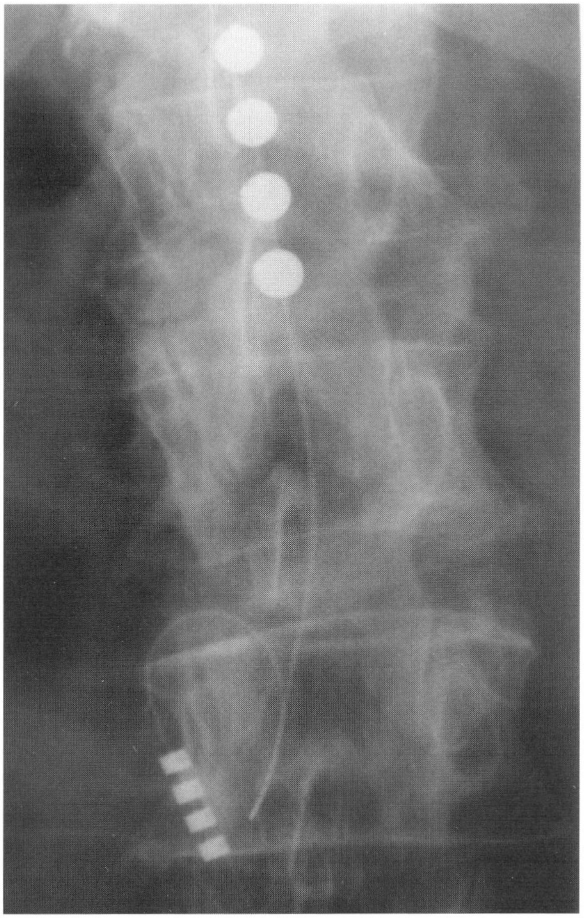

Figure 13.1. X-rays showing positioning of a spinal stimulating paddle (laminotomy).

activation and were recorded from both sides (!). They calculated a conduction velocity 200 m/s, which does not correspond to any known pathway, and may be unique to humans.

Tasker's group (Kiriakopoulos *et al.* 1997) reported on a SCI pain patient who described paresthesias and relief of her left leg pain at 2 V, but not 1 V: fMRI showed increased activity in the right sensory cortex at 2 V compared to 1 V stimulation. In an fMRI study of non-CP patients, Rasche *et al.* (2005) found that SCS elicited BOLD activations in the cingulate gyrus, thalamus, prefrontal cortex, SI, and SII. Pain reduction by SCS resulted in a reduction of functional activity in these areas. Similarly, in another fMRI study of non-CP patients, Stancak *et al.* (2008) found increased activation of the mesial MI (foot and/or perineal region) and BA5, contralateral posterior insula (BA13), and ipsilateral SII, plus deactivations in bilateral MI and ipsilateral SI corresponding to the upper limb and a small deactivation in the ipsilateral temporal pole. Kishima *et al.* (2010) conducted a PET study (resolution $4 \times 4 \times 5$ mm; SPM2) during SCS (max. 10V, 10–85Hz, 210–450 μs, for 30 minutes; after-effect >2 hours) and OFF stimulation for at least 12 hours before PET. There were two CPSP (putaminal) patients, one CCP (spinal infarction), and one SCI, plus five non-CP patients. Results were not broken down according to pain type. Pre/post comparisons revealed activations significantly correlated with analgesia in ipsilateral BA9/BA6 and bilateral BA8 (no rCBF decreases were detected, nor changes in SI/MI); changes were also seen in the thalamus. A TMS study found that SCS influences NMDA-mediated intracortical facilitation and concluded that clinical effects of SCS are at least in part of cortical origin (Schlaier *et al.* 2007).

SCS may modulate several transmitters and peptides (5-HT, acetylcholine, glycine, adenosine, GABA). In consideration of the efficacy of different GABA agonists, a role for both $GABA_A$ and $GABA_B$ receptors can be envisioned. Paradoxically, thyamilal, which is also a GABA agonist, antagonizes the inhibitory effects of SCS on dorsal horn activity in humans (Tanaka *et al.* 2009).

Efficacy

A prerequisite for successful pain relief by SCS is blanketing of the painful area by paresthesias, but evoked paresthesias do not guarantee pain relief, and evoked sensations can also be outside the painful area.

Marchand *et al.* (1991) provided the first placebo-controlled study of SCS for chronic pain (other than CP). The conclusion was clear-cut: reduction in clinical pain is small (less than 30%), and patients submitted to SCS all reported that they felt some sensations, when in fact the stimulator was not activated. Even today, there is a lack of high-quality evidence, no double-blind randomized trial (admittedly rather difficult to set up in this context) and serious flaws in blinding, recruitment, and assessment in nearly all studies.

When pain is below the lesion, SCS can be effective only if the corresponding dorsal column(s) retain sufficient functional value. If the territory below the lesion is totally anesthetic, SCS will not work. As a matter of fact, if the dorsal columns are totally interrupted, electrodes – even if implanted above the lesion – cannot stimulate the degenerated lemniscal fibers. Imaging and measurement of SSEPs may be useful to check integrity of the dorsal columns. Poor results are seen with complete lesions and intermittent and burning pain. Instead, SCS appears to be effective in some patients with incomplete lesions, painful spasms, at-level pain, or post-cordotomy pain. Most studies report a decline in efficacy of SCS over time. Generally, the best results have been obtained with multipolar electrodes, with laminotomy epidural placement (Carter 2004), when electrodes are localized above the pain segments, if stimulation paresthesias and pain segments are superimposed, and when the pain is localized rather than diffuse.

SCS can also induce new constant, painful dysesthesias or burning skin sensations, unrelated to actual stimulation, and which may either abate or linger years after removal of the stimulating apparatus (Enggaard *et al.* 2007).

SCS is generally a safe technique, but exceptionally an epidural hematoma can be induced necessitating urgent removal.

In conclusion, only a few BCP patients and a minority of well-selected CCP patients who show at least partially preserved SSEPs may obtain relief in the long term (years). Where appropriate, SCS may be enhanced by sacral nerve stimulation (Table 13.1).

Table 13.1. Spinal cord stimulation

Author(s)	Type of pain/number of patients	Results/notes
Nashold and Friedman (1972)	SCI pain (leg pain) (6 patients)	Excellent: 1/6 patients (follow-up: 11 years) Partial: 4/6 patients (mild analgesic still required) Unsatisfactory: 1/6 patients
Nashold (1975)	**CPSP (3 patients)**	Initial pain reduction with stimulation of the trigeminal tract in the upper cervical cord
Urban and Nashold (1978)	**CCP (3 patients)**	Pain relief: 1; unsuccessful test stimulation (no paresthesias): 1; lost to follow-up, but initial pain relief: 1
Sweet and Wepsic (1974, 1975)	Postcordotomy dysesthesia (7 patients)	Good relief: 2
	MS (3 patients)	Good relief: 1
	SCI pain (4 patients)	Failure
	Myelopathic pain (7 patients)	Failure *Hyperpathia never relieved*
Hunt *et al.* (1975)	Radiation myelitis CP (1 patient)	0%
Long and Erickson (1975)	SCI-CP (1 patients)	Failure
	Postcordotomy CP (2 patients)	Failure
Lindblom and Meyerson (1975)	SCI pain (2 patients)	1 early success
Sedan and Lazorthes (1978)	CCP (postcordotomy pain: 14 patients; SCI: 16 patients)	Postcordotomy pain: review of Sweet, Shelden, Nashold and Long reports (14 patients) SCS results: excellent: 3/14 patients; bad: 1/14 patients; failure: 10/14 patients SCI pain: review of Sweet and Long reports (16 patients) SCS results: excellent: 1/16 patients; fair: 2/16 patients; failure: 13/16 patients (**at least 1 patient with above-lesion SCS**) *No screening test in any patient.* BCP in anybody's experience: SCS totally ineffective
Rosen and Barsoum (1979)	MS	Good relief in 20%, 0% in 60% of patients
Richardson *et al.* (1980)	Paraplegia pain (10 patients)	**SCS rostrad to lesion**. Pain relief > 50% from test stimulation: 5 (3 with incomplete cord lesion) At 1-year follow-up: 4/5 lost to follow-up (2 patients died, 1 lost after 3 months); 1/5 pain relief (presumably from recovered lesion) Failure of test stimulation in 5 patients (3 with complete cord lesion)
Moraci *et al.* (1982)	SCI (1 patient)	Good relief. Follow-up: 10 months
Demirel *et al.* (1984)	CP (10 patients)	Positive trial test in 6/10 patients. No late results
Vogel *et al.* (1986)	CP (3 patients)	No response to trial stimulation in all

Table 13.1. (cont.)

Author(s)	Type of pain/number of patients	Results/notes
Wester (1987)	MS-CP (3 patients) SCI-CCP (3 patient) Tumor CCP (1 patient)	Benefit at 15 months (median; range: 4–60 months): 0% MS-CP, 33% SCI-CCP, 0% tumor CCP Comment: global effect restricted, dwindling effect in time, "**DCS not of any great help**"
Mittal *et al.* (1987)	CP (8 patients)	Positive trial test in 3 patients. Persistent pain relief (3 months, 8 years): 2 patients
Ikei and Uno (1987)	CPSP (thalamic) (1 patient)	Benefit. Follow-up: not available
Beric *et al.* (1988)	CP	SCS may worsen CP with absent STT function and preserved DCs
Buchhaas *et al.* (1989)	SCI pain (7 patients)	6/7 good or very good relief at 3–72 months
Krainick and Thoeden (1989)	CCP (4 patients; transverse spinal lesions: 2 patients, other spinal injuries: 2 patients; incomplete conuscauda lesion: 4 patients; tetraspasticity after cervical disc operation: 2 patients)	Initial pain relief in all patients; no long-term follow-up Overall (CP plus other pains) long-term (2–3 years) results: 50–75% pain reduction in 39% of patients. ≥ 60% had complications requiring removal of the stimulator
Michel *et al.* (1990)	CPSP (parietal) (5 patients)	50% pain relief in 2
Cole *et al.* (1987, 1991)	CCP (4 patients)	0% (1 worsened)
Devulder *et al.* (1991)	(1) SCI (2 patients) (2) MS-CP (1 patient)	(1) Failures (neurosurgical implantation, unipolar electrodes, monopolar SCS) (2) 100% relief (no drugs; percutaneous implantation Multipolar electrode, bipolar stimulation, 2.2 V, 210 μs, 70 Hz)
Simpson (1991)	Thalamic CP (9 patients)	3 significant, 3 modest, 2 no benefit, 1 worsened (one after initial modest benefit)
	Post-thalamotomy CP (1 patient)	Worsened
	Painful paraparesis, paraplegia, and hemiparesis (10 patients)	6 complete/partial, 1 non-substantial, 2 failures (1 worsened) (Relief: significant (complete or partial pain relief, with significant effect on medication and lifestyle, praise of the apparatus by the patient), modest (no substantial benefit, no significant change in medication, activity, sleep pattern), failure) Long-term follow-up data not available for single disease. Median overall follow-up: 29 months (2 weeks – 9 years)
Simpson (1999)	CP (thalamic) (1 new patient)	Worsened Conclusion: SCS relief very unlikely in complete SCI and reasonably likely in partial SCI; unlikely in BCP
Spiegelmann and Friedman (1991)	CCP (SCI, MS) (6 patients)	Positive stimulation test: 4 patients. Long-lasting 50–100% pain relief: 3 patients. Mean follow-up: 13 months (3–30 months). No further pain relief after a change in the distribution of paresthesias in 1 SCI pain patient

Table 13.1. (cont.)

Author(s)	Type of pain/number of patients	Results/notes
		(initial 1 year benefit). TENS was not predictive (TENS failures could respond to SCS, as found by many other groups)
Ohta *et al.* (1992)	SCI pain (4 patients)	At 1 week, 100% relief in all. However, at 3–5 months, no relief in 3, while in the fourth 70–80% relief at 19 months only when SCS turned on
Tasker *et al.* (1992) Tasker's group	SCI complete (11 patients) SCI incomplete (24 patients)	Steady (burning or not) pain unrelieved in 80% of patients. 25–50% relief in 20% of patients. Intermittent or evoked pain unrelieved in 100% of patients. All cases drawing benefit had T10–L2 lesions (22/24 implants): steady pain relief ≥ 50% in 27% of patients and 25–50% in 14% of patients. Intermittent pain unrelieved. 25–50% evoked pain relief in 25% of patients. Of cases relieved, two thirds had T10–L2 lesions Authors' conclusions: SCS is more effective for relief of steady pain (36%) than of intermittent (0%) or evoked pain (16%) (statistically significant difference). SCS is ineffective even for steady pain in cases with complete lesions (20% relief) Follow-up: > 1 year Failures usually associated with an inability to induce paresthesias in the area of pain, due to severe cord lesions inducing dorsal column atrophy (dieback), difficulty in accessing the epidural space (trauma or previous surgery), difficulty in producing paresthesias over the large area of patients' pain. **Failures not due to intrinsic resistance of CCP to SCS**.
Kim *et al.* (2001)	BCP 12 patients CCP 20 patients	Pain relief > 50% for 1 year only in 1 Positive stimulation trial: 7 patients; test worsened pain in 2 patients with evoked pain (just like Vc DBS in BCP patients with allodynia). Early failures (pain relief < 50% within 1 year of implantation): 2/7 patients (early success probably a placebo effect); late failures (past 1 year): 3/7 patients Long-lasting (mean follow-up: 3.9 years, range 0.3–9 years) > 50% pain relief: 2/7 patients Drug reduction not specified, nor enhanced ability to work
North *et al.* (1991, 1993)	SCI pain (11 patients) **1972–1990**	Permanent implants in 90% of cases. Benefit only in those with well-circumscribed, segmental pain at or just below injury level; diffuse pains were *all* failures SCI patients showed slightly longer latency to effect (15 vs. 12.9 min) and much shorter persistence of pain relief than FBSS (26.5 vs. 155 min)
Shimoji *et al.* (1993)	(1) BCP (9 patients) (2) SCI (12 patients)	(1) 3 had > 50% relief on test. Follow-up (> 1 year): only 2 patients: VAS relief 30% and 20%

Table 13.1. (cont.)

Author(s)	Type of pain/number of patients	Results/notes
	(3) Tabes dorsalis (3 patients)	(2) 5 patients had > 50% relief on test. Follow-up (> 1 year): only 3 patients VAS relief 60%, 50%, 30% (3) 3 had > 50% relief on test **SCS: 1.6–8 Hz (!)**, 30 min at the time
Italian cooperative study (Broggi *et al.* 1994)	Paraplegia pain (23 patients)	Failure in all implanted patients within 1 year of surgery, despite initial benefit in several in this highly select group
Van de Kelft and De La Porte (1994)	SCI (8 patients)	Not stated
Cioni *et al.* (1995) Includes all previously published cases of Meglio's group in Rome (*PACE* 1989, **12**, 709–12; *J Neurosurg* 1989, **70**, 519–24)	SCI pain (25 patients)	Pain due to trauma or surgery at all spine levels. 75% relief at the end of the test period: 40.1% of patients. Patients with more than 50% pain relief at a mean follow-up of 37.2 months: 18.2%. Better results in patients with painful spasms and constrictive pain in the transitional zone and with incomplete thoracic lesions. Below-level burning pain unrelieved **Authors' conclusions**: the relative integrity of the dorsal column is an important prerequisite for analgesia. 0% benefit without paresthesias evoked in the painful area **SCS not effective in treating true SCI-CP**
Lazorthes *et al.* (1995) Includes all patients operated on and previously published by both Lazorthes and Siegfried	SCI pain (101 patients)	SCI pain included traumatic paraplegia pain, iatrogenic lesions, or following cord tumor surgery, herpetic myelitis, and spondylotic damage Successful pain relief: • short-term: 50–58% of patients • long-term: 30–34% of patients **Authors' conclusions**: CCP and even more BCP respond poorly to SCS, with increasing degrees of denervation. Analgesia is much less significant for SCI-CP or iatrogenic CP following surgery on the cord (e.g., for tumor). Failures due to degeneration of lemniscal fibers
Barolat *et al.* (1995, 1998)	SCI pain (11 patients)	Short-term successful pain relief: 45% of patients. 55% of patients never experienced any pain relief (half never felt paresthesias in the painful area) Long-term successful results only in 27% of patients, with good (> 50%) pain relief in 2/11 patients and moderate (25–50%) pain relief in 1/11 patients **Authors' conclusions**: results of SCS on SCI pain have been disappointing in the vast majority of patients
Peyron *et al.* (1998)	CPSP (Wallenberg) (3 patients, with evoked pain)	Failure
Anderson and Burchiel (1999)	CPSP	CPSP not particularly responsive to SCS

Table 13.1. (cont.)

Author(s)	Type of pain/number of patients	Results/notes
Ravenscroft *et al.* (1999)	SCI (1 patient)	Relief
Tseng (2000)	SCI pain (1 patient)	Relief at 19 months
Katayama *et al.* (2001)	CPSP (45 patients)	All submitted to test stimulation. Satisfactory relief if VAS reduced ≥ 60%. Only 3 (*c.* 7%) attained this level of analgesia at long term (all thalamic or infrathalamic; none suprathalamic)
Eisenberg and Brecker (2002)	CCP (post-spinal cord tumor removal) (1 patient)	Relief for 9 months **Above-lesion SCS**
Warms *et al.* (2002)	SCI (9 patients)	Only 2 still using it at long term
Sindou *et al.* (2003)	CCP (30 patients) (9 MS, 7 trauma, 5 spinal tumor, 5 syrinx, 4 spondylotic myelopathy)	Long-term results (mean follow-up: 18.8 months, range 11.2–19.2 months): pain relief > 50% (and minimal drug use): 12/30 patients (40%) All patients had incomplete spinal cord damage (CP patients with complete spinal cord damage or midline pain excluded). SCS: paddle. Previous TENS course, but results not given. No differentiation between end-zone pain and diffuse CP. At least some retained sensibility in the painful areas and normal or near-normal SSEPs in most responders
Quigley *et al.* (2003)	Spinal cord/root compression (4 patients) MS (4 patients) Paraplegia pain (3 patients) **1989–2000**	Relief ≥ 50% in 4 SC-root compression, 3 MS, and 0 paraplegia pain (doctor's assessment), 2/3, 2/3, and 0/2 (patients' assessment) **General anesthesia, laminotomy in most patients**, > 80% receiving a quadripolar plate. Almost 60% inserted at T9–12. Then C1–4, C5–7, T5–8. 62% radiofrequency, 38% IPG. Test: 5-day, retrospective study via questionnaire. No routine antibiotics Majority of *all* patients used the SCS every day for about 12 h, 21% only during exacerbations, 10% did not use it any more. Average time from implantation to data collection: 4.2 years 64 revision operations out of 102 patients, due to electrode complications, generator complications, connecting lead fracture. Global infection rate was 4.9% (2/5 patients needed explantation). Globally (CP plus all other pains), patients who had used SCS for 5 years or more had lower levels of substantial pain relief compared to those using it for less (65% vs. 81%). It is unclear if this is due to tolerance, an initial placebo response, hardware failure, or some other phenomenon
Rogano *et al.* (2003)	CCP (12 partial lesion patients)	VAS from 9.9 to 3.6 (no details given) Minimum follow-up: 6 months (mean 19.1 ± 13.5 months)
Kumar *et al.* (2006)	(1) MS-CP (19 patients) (2) SCI pain (15 patients)	(1) Initial pain relief: 17/19 patients. Long-term success (50–100% relief): 15/17 patients

Table 13.1. (cont.)

Author(s)	Type of pain/number of patients	Results/notes
Includes all patients operated on and previously published by this group		(2) Initial pain relief: 7/15 patients. Long-term success (50–100% relief): 5/7 SCI patients Mean follow-up, whole series (including CP): 97.6 months Limb pain considered to be due to cord injury. Favorable response in SCI patients with incomplete paraplegia and with below-level CP. No benefit with SCS in patients with complete paraplegia and both at- and below-level pains
Kim *et al.* (2006)	CCP (cavernoma) (1 patient)	Failure
Kim SH *et al.* (2007)	Conus infarction (1 patient)	SCS: T11–2. VAS down (from 10 to 5) on trial (1–2+, 320 μs, 54 Hz, 4.2 V). VAS down to 3 in limbs but not in external genitalia and urethra (VAS 9) 4 years later, **sacral nerve stimulation**: VAS 3 (1–2+, 240 μs, 31 Hz, 6.4 V) 1 year later, global VAS 2–3
Sitzmann *et al.* (2007)	SCI (below-level only) (6 patients)	4 improved and implanted. At 1–6 years, > 50% relief. ML preservation (SSEP-confirmed) essential
Lee *et al.* (2009)	CCP (post-T5 meningioma removal) (1 patient)	Dual (T1/T2) SCS: trial (400–450 μs, 30–50 Hz, 4.3–4.7 V): VAS from 9 to 1. Allodynia disappeared. Follow-up: 8 months. VAS 1 in right distal leg, 4 in upper back and right flank. Gabapentin 900 mg/day. Lifestyle much improved Short follow-up; appears to be relapsing (VAS from 9 to 1 to 4)
Moens *et al.* (2009)	CCP (tethered cord) (1 patient) (intense burning, dysesthesia and hyperalgesia in buttock and right posterior thigh)	T12 SCS. Excellent pain relief, drug reduction. < 0.2 V, 60 Hz, 240 μs Follow-up: not available Several untethering surgeries
Pickering *et al.* (2009)	CPSP	Failure (T11/12)
Burkey and Abla-Yao (2010)	MS-CP (1 patient)	Octrode left of midline centered at C4–5. Test: no relief One octrode placed over lateral recess epidurally at C6–7 (C7 DREZ/Lissauer's tract stimulation effective for C6 dermatome pain!) + a second octrode placed medially adjacent and slightly rostral. 1 month after trial and lead removal, definitive SCS (80 Hz, PW 200 μs, contacts 3+/4–5–, 2.1mA, guarded stimulation for 12 h). Worst pain (evenings) from 7 to 6, least pain from 1 to 1, average pain from 5 to 2, right now pain from 4 to 1. Major improvement in general activity, mood, walking, work, relations with people, enjoyment of life, less in sleep. Heat hypoalgesia improved. Follow up: not available
Kim *et al.* (2010)	CCP, below-level (post- T3–4 schistosoma granuloma resection) (1 patient)	C1–3 SCS: > 50% benefit on test. Then analgesia from day 4 onwards. IPG. 9 months later, pain down 63%. Previously used drugs maintained

Table 13.1. (cont.)

Author(s)	Type of pain/number of patients	Results/notes
Aly *et al.* (2010)	CPSP (30 patients) Putaminal hemorrhage: 12 patients Thalamic hemorrhage: 9 patients Brainstem stroke: 3 patients Others: 6 patients Allodynia: 60% Hyperpathia: 37% **2002–2009**	Retrospective study. C4–7 SCS or T9–12 SCS. Trial: 2–7 days. VAS, PGIC (patient's impression) scales. 1.5–6 V, 210–350 μs, 10–50Hz Test stimulation: 15 poor (< 30% relief), 6 fair (30–49%), 9 good (> 50%) results. Median VAS from 8 (5–10) to 6 (1.5–10) after trial Only 10 patients (33%) opted for permanent implantation (7 with good test analgesia, 2 fair, and 1 poor (this one was satisfied with 25% reduction). All thalamic or putaminal strokes! Latest follow-up: 1 with < 6 months implantation, one 6 months implantation (subjectively minimally improved) 8 patients: no patient very much improved on PGIC, 3 failures, 6 much improved (VAS reduced 50–57% at 12–62 months) Age, sex, arm vs. leg, CP duration, cause of CP, evoked pains, motor weakness: none related to outcome In sum: 20% of CPSP patients relieved < 60% on VAS scale at long term (cf. Katayama *et al.* 2001, above)
Tomycz *et al.* (2011)	CPSP (brainstem) (1 patient)	Cervicomedullary junction paddle. Trial : 100% relief; implanted Long-term relief: not available Telephone assessment

Chapter 14

Transcutaneous electrical nerve stimulation

Transcutaneous electrical nerve stimulation (TENS) is applied at high frequency (80–150 Hz: *conventional* TENS), aimed at activation of myelinated cutaneous sensory fibers, or low frequency (short trains of impulses at 1–4 Hz over the motor nerves: *acupuncture-like* TENS). Stimulation must be directed over the most painful region; dual-channel stimulators should be employed to cover a large body area with pain.

Mechanism of action

TENS can apparently reduce CP only if the dorsal column–medial lemniscal (Aβ) pathways are uninjured or only mildly so (i.e., paresthesias are evoked). The exact mechanism of analgesia is unclear. Murakami *et al.* (2010) applied high-frequency TENS (100 Hz) for 15–30 minutes in healthy individuals and found in their magnetoencephalographic (MEG) study that it modulates excitability of a limited area of MI, but wider areas of SI (3b/a), i.e., beyond the representational map corresponding to the stimulated cortex, with further evidence of lateral inhibition in SI.

Efficacy

While certainly much less expensive than brain and spinal stimulation, and with almost no adverse effects, TENS cannot cover wide body areas and requires prolonged use several times a day, basically hampering a patient's daily activities. While a trial may be warranted before other more invasive procedures are contemplated, usually during drug therapy, few patients gain long-lasting pain relief, either with BCP or with below-level CCP. However, TENS may relieve some SCI patients with muscular or at-level pain. TENS is ineffective for MS-CP (Table 14.1).

Table 14.1. Transcutaneous electrical nerve stimulation (TENS)

Author(s)	Type of pain/number of patients	Results/notes
Banerjee (1974)	Below-level CCP (5 patients)	100% relief at short term (30 min tid) Effect lasted 8–10 h
Long and Hagfors (1975)	Pain secondary to CNS injury	TENS relatively ineffective
Davis and Lentini (1975)	SCI-CP (11 patients) plus other SCI neuropathic pains	2 successes, 2 partial successes, 18 failures; 4/4 failures for cervical lesions, 5/11 successes for thoracic lesions and 50% success for conus-cauda lesions
Hachen (1978)	SCI pain (39 patients)	Complete/almost complete relief: 49%; moderate improvement: 41% At 3 months, 28% and 49% respectively
Heilporn (1978)	SCI pain (3 patients)	Failures
Guilmart (thesis, detailed in Sedan and Lazorthes 1978)	BCP (2 patients) SCI-CP (9 patients)	1 relief Failures Conventional TENS
Long *et al.* (1979)	CP of any origin	Unresponsive to TENS in the majority of patients; response when seen not maintained over long-term. TENS usually worsened hyperesthesia
Eriksson *et al.* (1979, 1984)	(1) BCP (7 patients), CCP (11 patients) (2) CP (brainstem/face) (5 patients)	(1) Acupuncture-like TENS (6 patients), conventional TENS (12 patients) BCP: pain relief (continued for 3 months) in 5; CCP: pain relief at 3 months in 7 (in 6, at-level only, not below-level). Relief probably in incomplete lesions (2) Not broken down from group: probably some reliefs
Sindou and Keravel (1980)	BCP (thalamic) (5 patients) CCP (17 patients)	Failures Relief in 2 (late follow-up not specified)
Bates and Nathan (1980)	BCP (thalamic) (12 patients) CCP (16 patients) (2 post-cordotomy, 8 intrinsic spinal cord lesions, 6 syringomyelia and syringobulbia)	8 stimulated beyond 1 week. Stimulation up to 8 h/day; up to 70 Hz. 0/8 helped by TENS. Strong intensities increased pain 10 stimulated beyond 1 week. Detailed results not given Globally, of 235 patients with chronic pain and 160 passing test, 20–25% used TENS at 2 years or more of follow-up, sometimes only to help them over crises of pain
Ray and Tai (1988)	CPSP (1 patient)	Temporary relief
Portenoy *et al.* (1988)	MS-CP (2 patients)	Failures
Leijon and Boivie (1989b)	CPSP (15 patients)	Pain relief from conventional or acupuncture-like TENS in 4 (3 after 2 years): 20%/57% VAS reduction; 3 patients (2 brainstem infarction, 1 unknown lesion site) still relieved after 2 years. All 3 with retained lemniscal conduction

Table 14.1. (cont.)

Author(s)	Type of pain/number of patients	Results/notes
		Wallenberg's syndrome: 1 patient. High-frequency TENS for facial pain used without effect on arm and leg pains; the reverse 30 months later High- and low-frequency TENS had approximately equal effect in the other 2 patients (1–7 hours) The study applied rigid schedules not taking into account the varying distribution of pain and the subsequent need to apply the electrodes over the region with the most intense pain
Tulgar *et al.* (1991)	CPSP (1 patient)	0% relief after conventional (70 Hz) constant and burst stimulation (80 μs-long trains of pulses, each train consisting of eight 90 Hz pulses [repeated 1.3 times per second]) (A) VAS from 48 to 43 for 1 h after high rate frequency TENS (from 90 Hz to 55 Hz over 90 ms, 1.3 times/second) (B) VAS from 50 to 40 for 1.5 h after low rate frequency TENS (from 60 to 20 Hz over 90 ms 1.3 times /second). In sum: ineffective
Tasker (2001a)	CP	TENS seldom useful in patients with pain over a wide area of the body Possibly useful for facial pains
Kabirov and Staroselseva (2002)	CCP (syrinx) (14 patients)	30–100% relief in 12 (TENS 10 sessions, 60 min each)
Norrbrink Budh and Lundeberg (2004)	SCI (29 patients, 24 with neuropathic pain alone or with other pains)	Relief: 28% (very good results: 3%) **Efficacy of TENS in the range of gabapentin and amitriptyline!**
Nuti *et al.* (2005)	CP (>10 patients, including 3 Wallenberg CPs)	No significant analgesia
Cardenas and Jensen (2006)	CCP (41 patients)	Type of pain that was experienced and relieved not studied! 41 patients used it at some time, only 4 still using it. Average VAS relief: 3.08 points
Schyns and Coutts (2007)	Neuropathic pain (CP?) (5 patients × 3 groups)	RCT, placebo-controlled (A: 40 Hz/100 μs; B: 110 Hz/100 μs; C: placebo) Home treatment, 4 h/day for 14 consecutive days No statistically significant effects (trend for improvement on most measures (BPI, NPSI, NRS), with differences between frequencies)
Norrbrink (2009)	SCI (24 patients) (7 at-level pain, 6 below-level, 11 both)	12 patients: 80 Hz TENS; 12 patients: 2 Hz (bursts) TENS, tid for 2 weeks. 2-week washout, then crossover for 2 weeks. TENS on areas of preserved sensibility or just above. Results calculated as ITT. **No control group!** No differences whatsoever between high- and low-frequency TENS, no effect whatsoever on MPI,

Table 14.1. (cont.)

Author(s)	Type of pain/number of patients	Results/notes
		HDS, sleep scale, LiSat-9. 9 patients (38%) did not complete whole study. **Some patients had pain worsening!** 5 patients (21%) had ≥ 2 units reduction on NRS, 7 (29%) in worst pain intensity and 8 (33%) in pain unpleasantness. Of 15 patients who completed whole study, 5 rated one mode and 5 both modes good to very good; 5 patients had no benefit. Of the 4 patients who completed only one 2-week session, 3 no benefits and 1 good result. 6 patients (25%) continued treatment: 5 had good to very good effect after at least one test session and 1 a rather good effect from both modes, with a ≥ 2-unit VAS abatement in 3 patients
Pickering *et al.* (2009)	CPSP (1 patient)	Failure
Chitsaz *et al.* (2009)	MS	See Table 9.1

Chapter 15

Other stimulation techniques

Gasserian ganglion stimulation

This was introduced in 1978 by Steude. Presumably, the efficacy depends on an intact afferent pathway in the periphery along which nerve impulses generated by stimulation can reach the trigeminal nuclei in the brainstem and continue transsynaptically up to the cortex. Its place in the treatment of CP is virtually non-existent (Table 15.1).

Vagal nerve stimulation

There are no reports as far as CP is concerned, but it is anticipated that it will not impact the management of CP.

Electroconvulsive therapy (ECT)

Unilateral and bilateral ECT has been employed for pain control (Canavero and Bonicalzi 2001a).

Mechanism of action

Salmon *et al.* (1988) found no significant correlations between endorphin levels and ECT in CP; they also noted no placebo effect. The α4 subunit of $GABA_A$ receptors may be implicated in the clinical effects of ECT (see the first edition of this book: Canavero and Bonicalzi 2007a).

ECT likely has direct, acute effects on the cerebral cortex. In the words of Von Hagen (1957), "electroshock therapy may produce its effect . . . from a reduction in the influence of the cortex on . . . reverberating . . . [circuits]", and we proposed that ECT interferes with a corticothalamic reverberation mechanism (Canavero 1994, Canavero and Bonicalzi 2001a). Seizures may be a natural example of spontaneous ECT: case 3 of Bornstein (1949) reported that a phantom sensation slowly shrunk before an epileptic fit to recede totally at the moment of the fit. After recovering consciousness, the phantom reappeared only after a certain lapse of time, a possible sign of the warm-up period required by the reverberation to restart.

There is only one imaging study of ECT effects in pain patients, but SPECT studies in depressed people submitted to successful bilateral ECT show rCBF changes both in cortical and subcortical regions (ACC, basal ganglia, temporal, occipital, and parietal lobes) in various mixtures depending on patient (e.g., Scott *et al.* 1994, Elizagarate *et al.* 2001).

The minimal electrical intensity needed for a generalized seizure of a specified minimal duration appears to vary by approximately 40-fold in the population (Sackeim *et al.* 1993): this may be relevant to the onset of CP (Canavero 1994).

Efficacy

Some patients with CP have been meaningfully relieved by ECT for more than a short time (Table 15.2). Given the high rate of relapse, the need for multiple courses, possible permanent side effects (amnesia), and non-uniformity of response, ECT should be considered as a last resort in highly refractory cases. At the same time, its effects on pain are independent of its improvement of depression. Given the high prevalence of comorbid depression (up to half of all chronic pain patients) and the associated increases in pain intensity, disability, and affect, ECT may be particularly useful in this kind of patient.

Caloric vestibular stimulation

Caloric vestibular stimulation (CVS) involves irrigation of the auditory canal with water (50 mL, usually cold, iced, 4 °C) for 30–60 seconds using a syringe with a piece of soft silastic tubing attached. The patient lies supine, with the head tilted at 30 degrees, and the end of the tubing is placed close to the tympanic membrane. Nystagmus and subjective vertigo usually occur rapidly

Table 15.1. Gasserian ganglion stimulation

Author(s)	Type of pain/number of patients	Results/notes
Taub *et al.* (1997) *Tasker's group*	CPSP (7 patients) (3 brain, 3 brainstem, 1 bulbar tractotomy)	Successful pain relief: 5/7 patients (100%: 1 patient; 75%: 1 patient; 50–74%: 2 patients; 50%: 1 patient). The 2 failures had an initial success which was lost within a month (placebo effect?). 1 thalamic infarct patient relieved for 21 months, then loss of effect. Another CPSP patient no longer needed the stimulator because the pain had subsided Median follow-up: 21 months CP better relieved than PNP in this unique series

Table 15.2. Electroconvulsive therapy

Author(s)	Type of pain/number of patients	Results/notes
Von Hagen (1957)	CPSP (thalamic) with evoked pains and depression (1 patient)	Great improvement for about 10 months from 8 bilateral ECTs, then relapse (1955). Further pain control from 3 additional treatments. Previous ECT for depression
White and Sweet (1969)	CCP (post-cordotomy) (? patients)	Relief only during the confusional state
Salmon *et al.* (1988)	CPSP (thalamic) (4 patients)	Failure with *unilateral* ECT. No depressed patients
McCance *et al.* (1996)	CPSP (3 patients)	2/3 CPSP of immediate onset, 3/3 patients with allodynia, 1/3 depressed patient **(A few months CP remission in 1 patient after an epileptic fit)** A course of 6 bilateral ECT sessions over 2 weeks slightly improved CP only in 1 patient, while 2 worsened
Doi *et al.* (1999)	Brain CP (12 patients)	Abstract. *CP remission in 1 depressed patient after ECT.* Bilateral ECT (110 V for 5 min) for 6–12 sessions at 1–7 day intervals. Complete relief of both steady and evoked pain in all suprathalamic cases. Partial relief in thalamic cases. Pain recurrence relieved by a new ECT course in 9 patients
Harano *et al.* (1999)	CPSP (thalamic pain) (39 patients)	Abstract. Convulsions (plus nausea and vomiting) lasting 2–3 min induced by intracisternal (cerebellar) methylprednisolone sodium succinate 125 mg in 5 mL syringe mixed with CSF. Excellent results in 54.4%, good in 38.6%, poor in 4% Lateral position; 22G 6 cm block needle inserted at crossing point of bilateral mastoid line and sagittal halfline under fluoroscopy. 57 injections in 39 patients
Fukui *et al.* (2002a)	CPSP	Refractory to stellate ganglion blocks. IV ketamine, PO mexiletine, CBZ, nortryptiline. VAS 8–10 ECT (60 Hz PW 1 ms, 0.7 A, 2.8 s, thiopental) once a week over 8 weeks unilaterally ipsilateral to stroke Pain still occasionally felt with VAS 2–5, tolerable. Follow-up: 1.5 years relief maintained

Table 15.2. (cont.)

Author(s)	Type of pain/number of patients	Results/notes
Canavero and Bonicalzi (2003b)	Cord CP (1 patient)	No pain relief after injection of 125 mg of methylprednisolone in the lateral ventricle. No frank fit
Wasan *et al.* (2004)	CPSP (1 patient)	No detail Whole mixed group: 3 ECT weekly every other day, uni/bilateral: in total, 10–12 ECTs (PW 1 ms, 2 s, 0.8 A, 40–90 Hz). 59.8% VAS reduction

Table 15.3. Vestibular stimulation

Author(s)	Type of pain/number of patients	Results/notes
Le Chapelain *et al.* (2001)	SCI (complete) (4 patients)	2 patients had painful phantoms greatly reduced
Ramachandran *et al.* (2007b)	CPSP (2 patients) Patient 2: ACC spared, insula + parietal operculum wholly infarcted	Procedure for both: see text. Sham: water at 37 °C Patient 1: Left CVS: 30 min later, VAS from 8.5 to 5 (relapse over 30 min) Right CVS: VAS from 8 to 5.5 (at 30 min, VAS 5). 11 days later, VAS 6 (left hemiface and most of left arm VAS 0, arm numb but not painful, some reduction in leg pain) Right CVS: VAS from 6.5 to 4.5 (full relapse over next hour). Left CVS: VAS from 6 to 5. Overnight pain VAS 3. At 4 weeks: face VAS 0, left arm VAS 1, leg pain VAS 7 Patient 2: Left CVS: VAS from 7 to 2 (face), 3 (right arm), 5 (right leg). Allodynia greatly reduced. After 7 hours, pain still less than normal but relapsing. Sham: no effect. Right CVS: VAS from 4 (face)/6 (arm)/8 (leg) to 0/3/5. 5 days later, VAS 4.5. 7 weeks later, pain still reduced: allodynia in face and right arm gone, pain in these areas VAS 3 (leg 4.5). Allodynia gone
McGeoch *et al.* (2008)	CPSP (9 patients) *Patients 1 and 2: same as above*! Patient 4: right insula infarcted Patient 7: left post. insula infarcted Patient 8: infarcted post. insula	Patient 1: Left CVS: from VAS 8.5 to 5; right CVS: from 8 to 5 (face 0, hand 1, leg 7). 2 weeks of benefit post-bilateral CVS. **Data not in agreement with above**! Patient 2: VAS from 7 to 4/3 (face 2, hand 3, foot 5). Patient 3: Bilateral CVS: VAS 0! Foot pain back in 1 day, face (0.5 vs. 2.5) and hand (2 vs. 5) pain still reduced 3 weeks afterwards Patient 4: Right CVS: VAS from 6 to 3; left CVS: VAS from 4 to 2.5. Greater relief in hand than foot. Cyclical CVS: 1 month relief after bilateral CVS Patient 5 (**ineffective CVS**):

Table 15.3. (cont.)

Author(s)	Type of pain/number of patients	Results/notes
		Left CVS: tepid (sham): VAS from 8.5 to 7.5, cold from 8.5 to 8.5 (tepid more effective!). Ice pack (sham): VAS from 8.5 to 7, right cold from 7 to 5 Patient 6 (**CVS intolerable**): Left CVS: tepid (sham): from VAS 6 to 4, cold CVS: from 7.5 to 4, right cold: from 3 to 1. Patient 7 (**ineffective CVS**): Right CVS: tepid (sham): from VAS 7.5 to 2.5 (!); right cold: from 5.5 to 5; left tepid: from 7 to 6, left cold from 6.5 to 5 Patient 8 (**poorly effective**): Relief in face>hand>foot (left: VAS from 9 to 5; right: from 10 to 8) but rapid relapses (hours) Patient 9 (**poorly effective**): Right CVS, tepid: VAS from 7.5 to 6; right cold from 7 to 4.5. Left tepid from 5.5 to 4.5; left cold from 5.5 to 3. Transient response **Two responders had significant damage to right posterior insula!** **Authors' biased evaluation of results!**
McGeoch *et al.* (2008)	CCP (transverse myelitis) (1 patient)	Cold but not placebo CVS improved CP markedly for *c.* 10 days (lowest pain ever)
Canavero and Bonicalzi (unpublished, 2009)	CCP (1 patient)	No effect. Intense headache

and continue for several minutes. Infrequently a mild nausea (rarely vomiting) and a mild headache can be triggered. Generally, a cycle of therapy consists of repeated daily sessions for a few weeks.

Mechanism of action

Neuroimaging studies suggest activation of the superior temporal gyrus, inferior parietal lobe, temporoparietal junction, ACC, insula/SII/parietal operculum, and putamen and deactivation of visual and frontal area bilaterally. Cold CVS activates regions in the contralateral hemisphere, warm CVS ipsilaterally (Been *et al.* 2007). Ramachandran *et al.* (2007b) espoused the "VMpo/insular view" of CP proposed by Craig in order to explain CVS effects on CP. This theory is totally unfounded (see Appendix). Ramachandran's emphasis on greater relief in the face and hand rather than the foot as in line with insular somatotopy is equally explained by the SI homunculus (face and hand disproportionately represented).

Efficacy

Initial results do not support a meaningful therapeutic role in CP (Table 15.3). If there is one, it would be akin to TENS.

Chapter 16

Intraspinal drug infusion

There seems little doubt that neurosurgical procedures will be replaced to a large extent by drugs, at present unknown.
A. E. Walker (1950)

Drugs ineffective by the systemic route often are effective when given spinally. Unfortunately, there is only a small number of papers reporting the effect of continuous intrathecal (IT) administration of drugs on CP, and the vast majority of them deal with CP after SCI. These studies are not randomized, nor controlled, and often patients with CP are no more than one or two cases among several other pain conditions, or just single case reports. In most papers, only the outcome of the mixed group of pain patients is reported and the outcome of patients with CP remains unknown. A positive pre-implantation test does not guarantee long-term relief.

A review of the literature (Table 16.1) and of personal experience suggests the following conclusions:

(1) IT lidocaine significantly reduces pain in a proportion of SCI patients, if access to the cord cephalad to injury level is preserved; however, relief may not be obtained despite a sensory block above the level of injury. Although good relief can be obtained, the effect is only temporary, and even multiple local anesthetic blocks do not result in long-term relief of SCI pain.

(2) IT midazolam (a $GABA_A$ agonist) has significantly relieved several patients with both BCP and CCP in our experience, without side effects of any kind, although tolerance can be seen (Canavero *et al.* 2006b).

(3) IT baclofen relieves few patients of their CP in the long run, as relief is often lost (tolerance). It may even make pain worse in some patients. Although generally well tolerated, the global impression is that it has no major effects on CP (see also Slonimski *et al.* 2004).

(4) Clonidine (epidural or IT, but only poorly PO) is efficacious in some patients with both BCP and CCP. Its noradrenergic effects (α_2-agonist) may modulate pain centrally: Weber (1904) first recognized the role of α_2-adrenoceptors in spinal transmission of pain. In humans, long-term IT clonidine infusion rarely produces pain relief beyond 3 months (Ackerman *et al.* 2003).

(5) Epidural or IT morphine at a dose of 0.5–1 mg/day (or hydromorphone) is initially effective against SCI-CP in some patients (particularly those with incomplete injuries): at-level, but much less below-level, pain appears to be responsive. The general impression is that opioid efficacy in pure CP is poor, with rare patients drawing long-term benefit (similar to what is observed with oral drugs) at the price of large dosage increases (up to seven-fold!). However, in the study of IT opioids with the longest follow-up (4 years) for chronic pain, the withdrawal rate was 95% (61–73% at 3 years in others), and the evidence that IT opioids reduce pain in the long term in the relatively small proportion of patients who continue it is weak (Noble *et al.* 2008). Also, clinically relevant testosterone depletion develops in the majority of men receiving IT opioids, and these benefit from hormonal replacement (Ballantyne and Mao 2003).

(6) IT ziconotide is of little benefit, with a very narrow therapeutic index (see Black Box).

Intraspinal infusion is not risk-free: aside from generic complications (catheter dislodgement [IT > epidural], root irritation [IT > epidural], reactive arachnoiditis [IT > epidural]), infective and hemorrhagic complications are the most feared, with occasional mortality.

Analgesia with all these drugs is due to targeting of spinal above-level or supraspinal sites (e.g., Lipman and Blumenkopf 1989), **including** brainstem and **neocortex** (Taylor 2009). Concurrently, the dorsal root ganglion resides within the intrathecal space and is accessed by

Table 16.1. Intraspinal drug infusion: intrathecal (IT) or epidural (EPI)

Author(s)	Type of pain/number of patients	Drug	Results/notes
Pollock *et al.* (1951a)	SCI pain	IT tetracaine 1 mL (0.5%)	In a number (unspecified) of cases, spinal anesthesia below level: burning pain did not disappear. In 4 cases with CSF block, anesthesia above-level: in 3 distal pain gradually disappeared, then slowly returned (in 1 case, absent for 24–56 min, full relapse at 3 h)
Davis (1954)	SCI pain	IT local anesthetic	Completely relieved spontaneous, diffuse, burning, below-level pain
Waltz and Ehni (1966)	CP, thalamic (2 patients)	IT pantocaine (6 mg)	Immediate abolition of leg pain, **even before sensory block**. In one case, leg pain was abolished while arm and face pains were reduced
Namba *et al.* (1984)	CPSP (1 patient)	IT morphine	Failure
Glynn *et al.* (1986)	CCP (15 patients)	EPI clonidine (150 µg) EPI morphine (5 mg) EPI buprenorphine (0.3 mg)	Non-RCT, single-blind crossover single-dose study. EPI clonidine vs. EPI morphine. Pain relief: EPI clonidine: 7 patients (morphine-unresponsive); EPI morphine: 5 patients (3 clonidine-responsive); 3 patients unresponsive both to morphine and clonidine, 2 of them buprenorphine-responsive
Portenoy *et al.* (1990)	BCP (1 patient)	EPI lidocaine	Little effect on pain
Crisologo *et al.* (1991)	CPSP (3 patients)	IT lidocaine (0.5%, 2%, 2 mL) In all, complete or almost complete sensory block	Patient 1: thalamic stroke with left hemisoma CP; 6 months later, left stroke with right hemisoma pain. IT lidocaine: at 0.5%: 0% relief; at 2%: 100% relief in left leg for 5 h Patient 2: right hemispheric cortical stroke with CP in left arm/leg. Lidocaine at 0.5%: 0% relief; at 2%: 100% relief for 1 h, then gradual relapse at 5 h

Table 16.1. (cont.)

Author(s)	Type of pain/number of patients	Drug	Results/notes
			Patient 3: thalamic CPSP (longer duration and higher intensity than cases 1and 2): 0% relief at both concentrations, despite complete sensory block
Loubser and Donovan (1991)	SCI (21 patients)	IT lidocaine; 50–100 mg (2 injections 1 h apart)	RCT. Spontaneous burning pain and intermittent sharp pain IT lidocaine effects: (1) sensory level of anesthesia above the level of injury in patients with lumbar and thoracic injuries and to T4 in patients with cervical injuries; (2) significant reduction of pain intensity when compared with placebo (13 vs. 4); (3) analgesia lasting for a mean time of 123 min, exceeding the expected duration of action for interruption of nociceptive messages IT lidocaine effects on pain: overall: 65% relief of pain (mean) in 12/16 patients Patients with spinal canal obstruction, sensory block above SCI level: no change in 4 and 20% relief of pain in 1. Negative response in 4 patients (2 with incomplete anterior cord syndromes), despite sensory anesthesia rostral to the level of SCI (pain generator more rostral?) When spinal anesthesia proximal to SCI level was adequate, 9/11 had a positive response vs. 4/10 who did not obtain anesthesia above SCI level, because of spinal canal obstruction or high lesion level
Herman *et al.* (1992)	CCP (4 patients with MS, 1 spinal cord compression, 2 transverse myelitis) SCI (2 patients)	IT baclofen (50 μg)	CCP: RCT (crossover with placebo = vehicle) assessing the efficacy of acute IT baclofen on chronic, dysesthetic, and spasm-related pain. IT baclofen significantly suppressed

Table 16.1. (cont.)

Author(s)	Type of pain/number of patients	Drug	Results/notes
			dysesthetic pain and, after the suppression of neuropathic pain, spasm-related pain SCI: non-RCT; 1 patient with C3 SCI had leg relieved
Glynn *et al.* (1992)	CCP (6 patients)	EPI clonidine (150 μg) + IT clonidine (1 patient)	Pain relief ≥ 50%: 3 (all with spasm). IT clonidine: excellent pain relief in 1 patient. Better relief with higher clonidine concentrations in the CSF
Triggs and Beric (1992)	CCP, ASAS (1 patient)	IT morphine	Failure
Lema *et al.* (1992)	Conus/cauda myxopapillary ependymoma	Epidural (NB: dural tear, thus likely IT) T10–11 bupivacaine (30 mg), morphine sulphate (4 mg), and methylprednisolone (80 mg) all in 12 mL total volume on two occasions at 1-month interval Then: Methylprednisolone 20 mg, bupivacaine 2.5 mg, and morphine sulphate 1 mg in a total volume of 2.5 mL IT *c.* every 3 months (9 injections over 2 years) (plus oxycodone 5–10 mg/day and amitriptyline 50 mg/day)	After second injection 100% analgesia. Steroid psychosis; relief for 2 months. Bupivacaine + morphine (1 mg) gave less relief for a shorter time Another injection with methylprednisolone 20 mg again recaptured benefit without psychosis Then: Almost complete relief and no sign of endocrinological suppression. Normal lifestyle (drives, jogs, etc.)
Loubser and Clearman (1993)	SCI-CP (1 patient)	IT lidocaine (50 mg)	Dysesthetic and cramping pain in both arms and legs following a C6 incomplete injury. IT lidocaine produced a sensory block to light touch to the T8 level, with disappearance of both spasticity and pain
Reig (1993)	BCP (3 patients with thalamic CP, 1 CNS injury) CCP (1 paraplegia pain, 1 post-cordotomy pain)	IT morphine (initial dose l mg, final dose 3.4 mg/day)	Congress abstract At 3-year follow-up: never > 75% relief; none returned to work; 50–75% pain relief: some; unsatisfactory pain relief: some (numbers not clear)
Fenollosa *et al.* (1993)	SCI pain (12 patients)	IT morphine (0.3–1 mg/day, continuous infusion)	Non-RCT. Pain and spasticity improvement (> 50% relief): 8/12 patients. Minimal

Table 16.1. (cont.)

Author(s)	Type of pain/number of patients	Drug	Results/notes
			tolerance in 6/8 patients (after 3 years final dose range: 1.6–6.0 mg/day)
Taira *et al.* (1994, 1995)	CPSP (8 patients) SCI pain (6 patients)	IT baclofen (50–100 μg)	Substantial pain relief starting 1–2 h after a single injection and persisting for 10–24 h in 9/14 patients (3 SCI). Allodynia and hyperalgesia, if present, also relieved. Placebo when tried ineffective. Incomplete data on CP components Study prompted by a CPSP-suppressing effect from 25 μg of IT baclofen in 1 patient with spasticity (not relieved by baclofen) and pain
Hassenbusch *et al.* (1995)	SCI-CP (1 patient)	IT morphine (0.2 mg/h) (IT sufentanil)	NRS reduction from 9/10 to 5/10 1 month after the pump implant. At 2-year follow-up, NRS = 6/10 in spite of IT sufentanil trial and oral propoxyphene addition. At last follow-up, pain relief judged fair (25%) by the patient and a failure by the authors Positive preimplantation test
Loubser and Akman (1996)	SCI pain (12 patients) (7 at-level pain and 2 below-level CP; musculoskeletal also present in 6)	IT baclofen infusion (implanted pump)	Non-RCT. Effects on neurogenic pain at both 6- and 12-month interval: no significant change in pain severity in 7/9 patients; pain increase in 2/9 patients. Significant decrease in musculoskeletal pain (5/6 patients) **Authors' conclusions:** IT baclofen does not decrease SCI-CP. Results of other studies were possibly positive due to higher doses achieved by bolus injections and continuous infusion resulting in comparably lower CSF doses; moreover, pain relief was assessed over only 24 h

Table 16.1. (cont.)

Author(s)	Type of pain/number of patients	Drug	Results/notes
Middleton *et al.* (1996)	CCP (1 patient)	IT baclofen and IT clonidine	Anterior cord syndrome case with incomplete C5 tetraplegia. Symptoms not improved by the administration of IT baclofen through an existing programmable infusion pump. Immediate pain relief after clonidine was added to baclofen in the pump reservoir and combined IT administration started
Winkelmuller and Winkelmuller (1996)	CPSP (thalamic) (1 patient) SCI (paraplegia) (6 patients)	IT opioids (implanted pump)	Mean follow-up: 3.4 years (range 6 months to 5.7 years) 1/1 thalamic pain and 3/6 paraplegia pain patients still benefited 6 months later Initial mean morphine dosage: 2.6 mg/day; at the first follow-up: 3.6 mg/day; at the last follow-up: 5.2 mg/day No separate analysis of results for BCP/CCP
Meglio (1998)	SCI-CP (8 patients)	2 patients: IT baclofen (50 μg) 5 patients: IT morphine 1 patient: both Test: 0.5 mg IT morphine	Baclofen failure Relief in 3, then 2 (due to side effects in 1) with > 50% relief at 1 year Average morphine dosage: 3 mg/day At- and below-level pains not distinguished
Angel *et al.* (1998)	CCP (syrinx) (1 patient)	IT morphine	Initial IT morphine dosage: 0.5 mg/day; 2 years later, 3 mg/day (VAS reduction from 10 to 2)
Anderson and Burchiel (1999)	CPSP (1 patient) CCP (2 patients) (1 syrinx)	IT morphine	Outcome of CP patients (out of 30 sundry patients) not specified, but all 3 had > 50% relief at test injection
Nitescu *et al.* (1998)	CCP (5 patients with ischemic myelopathies, 2 MS, 3 post-traumatic myelopathies)	IT opioids (morphine or buprenorphine) and IT bupivacaine	Non-RCT. Drug dosage: morphine 0.5 mg/mL, buprenorphine 0.015 mg/mL, bupivacaine 4.75–5.0 mg/mL. Daily volumes tailored to give the patients satisfactory to excellent (60–100%) pain relief, with acceptable side effects

Table 16.1. (cont.)

Author(s)	Type of pain/number of patients	Drug	Results/notes
			Results: MS-related pain: effective; ischemic and post-traumatic myelopathy: ineffective in 5/8 (63%) patients (**due to pain "centralization" at higher levels**). Several refused to continue treatment
Dahm *et al.* (1998)	MS-CP (1 patient)	IT bupivacaine IT (tip at T12) infusion of 0.5% bupivacaine at 3 mL (15 mg)/day with external programmable pump; increased to 20 mg/day on the first day to (35/7; 70/21; 80/48) 95 mg/day at day 68	VAS from 7 to 1 and mean relief from 30% to 90%. Death 712 days later, not due to treatment
Belfrage *et al.* (1999)	CP (CPSP?) (2 patients)	IT adenosine	Reduction of spontaneous and evoked pain. Results not broken down according to pain type (CP vs. other pains)
Becker *et al.* (2000)	MS incomplete T5	IT baclofen (110 μg/day, continuous administration) (450 μg at each refill)	Complete pain relief for 20 months. Pain reappearance soon after baclofen discontinuation (pump explanted at patient's request after progression of MS)
Gatscher *et al.* (2002)	CP (1 patient)	IT morphine (up to 3 mg/day)	Failure
Uhle *et al.* (2000)	Conocaudal ependymoma with arachnoiditis: 3 surgeries (1 patient)	(1) IT clonidine (50 μg/day) (2) IT clonidine (60 μg/day) + buprenorphine (0.3 mg)	(1) Relief (VAS 2). After 6 months relapse (2) Recapture
Siddall *et al.* (2000)	SCI-CP (15 patients) (13 below-level, 4 at-level, 3 both types. **Figures not in agreement!**)	IT morphine (0.75 mg (mean) (IT, bolus 0.2–1.5 mg) and/or IT clonidine (50 μg (mean) (IT, bolus 50–100 μg or 300–500 μg over 6 h) Combination: half of each dose Minimum 4 injections, 1 day apart	6-day double-blind, crossover, placebo-controlled RCT. Overall pain relief (4 h after drug administration): IT morphine alone = IT clonidine = placebo IT morphine (median minimal effective dose = 0.75 mg) + IT clonidine (median dose 50 μg as bolus injection or 300–500 μg over 6 h) produced significantly more pain relief than placebo 4 h after administration

Table 16.1. (cont.)

Author(s)	Type of pain/number of patients	Drug	Results/notes
			Pain relief ≥ 50% (mixture): at-level pain: 50% of patients; below-level pain: 35% of patients (in this group of patients, IT placebo was pain-relieving in about 30% of cases) **Authors' conclusions**: at-level pain appears to be more responsive. The concentration of morphine in the cervical CSF and the degree of pain relief correlated significantly, so drugs should be administered above-level *NNT: 7.5 (combination)*
Siddall *et al.* (1994)	SCI-CP (1 patient)	IT morphine (10 mg/day) + IT clonidine (17 μg/day)	Pain unresponsive to IT morphine alone. Marked decrease in pain from IT morphine + IT clonidine combined administration
Que *et al.* (2007) (Siddall's group)	SCI-CP (1 patient)	IT hydromorphone (0.05 mg) + clonidine 25 μg, then baclofen 50 μg, then all three together	Loss of all pain and decreased spasms. Clonidine stopped due to hypotension At 18 months, VAS 2 (background pain), but VAS 5 overall
Ridgeway *et al.* (2000)	SCI-CP (2 patients)	IT ziconotide (and opioids coadministration) up to 144 μg/day	No relief at end of trial. 47% CP decrease at 14.4 μg/day. No further decrease at 28.8 μg/day. Dramatic pain increase over time, requiring an increase in concurrent opioid administration. Trial stopped and IT baclofen restarted after appearance of confusion and sedation
Penn and Paice (2000)	MS-CP (1 patient) plus 2 other chronic pain patients	IT ziconotide up to 5.3 μg/h	Ineffective. Very serious side effects. Infusion stopped. Coma. Residual memory impairment
Rogano *et al.* (2003) Plus congress abstracts	CCP (18 patients), most spinal traumas	IT morphine (1–6 mg)	VAS from 9.2 to 3.6, in both complete and incomplete lesions

Table 16.1. (cont.)

Author(s)	Type of pain/number of patients	Drug	Results/notes
			Minimum follow-up: 6 months (mean 19.1 ± 13.5 months) No details are given and data are inserted briefly in discussion. No differentiation between at- and below-level pains. Follow-up short. Nausea and vomiting frequent
Huntoon *et al.* (2004)	SCI (conus) CP (1 patient)	EPI morphine IT hydromorphone 24 mg/bupivacaine 0.75%/day	> 50% relief Catheter into spinal cord on initial placement with new pain uncontrolled by opioids PO opioids: minimal initial relief
Nuti *et al.* (2005)	CCP (1 patient)	IT morphine	Failure
Canavero *et al.* (2006b)	BCP and CCP	IT midazolam (2.5–6 mg/day)	Analgesia from IT midazolam correlates with positive propofol test. Pump implanted in a few patients. Satisfactory analgesia, although tolerance may occur. Follow-up is entering a few years. No side effects observed to date
Sadiq and Poopatana (2007)	MS-CP (9 patients) Burning/dysesthesic pain (generally in lower limb) in 7/9 patients with spastic pain	IT baclofen (implanted pump) IT baclofen + IT morphine (half the previous daily dose of baclofen + 0.5 mg morphine/day; dose ranges: baclofen: 0.005–1.2 mg; morphine: 0.8–9.5 mg)	No relief VAS from 8.6 to 1.4 sustained over a mean of 6.2 years (1–10 years) Wide dosage variations: baclofen: 5–1200 μg/day; morphine: 0.8–9.5 mg/day! Retrospective, unblinded, uncontrolled study. All patients resistant or intolerant of maximal oral antispasticity and pain medications (including narcotics). SC pump implanted after successful IT baclofen test for spasticity and spasticity-related pain. Addition of IT morphine in patients with NP unaffected by baclofen (VAS ≥ 8).

Table 16.1. (cont.)

Author(s)	Type of pain/number of patients	Drug	Results/notes
			1 patient: leg edema (due to morphine); 2 patients: constipation
Koulousakis *et al.* (2007)	Mixed group (some CP patients)	IT morphine/baclofen/ morphine	Patients with burning, cramp-like pain and associated spasticity/dystonia necessitated morphine and baclofen. Clonidine alone or with opioids used with MS, CPSP, and others Follow-up 2–36 months
Saulino (2007)	SCI (at- and below-level pain). Paraplegic 23-year-old woman (T4 traumatic lesion). At-level pain + paroxysms of shooting, electrical-like pain in the lower limbs (below-level pain, onset 1 week after the injury). No allodynia/ hyperalgesia.	IT hydromorphone (1.32 mg/day) IT ziconotide (11 μg/day) Oral oxycone (< 60 mg/day) maintained for breakthrough pain	VAS from 8.9 to 1.2 At-level pain relieved by hydromorphone but *not* ziconotide, below-level pain relieved by ziconotide but not hydromorphone. Follow-up: 15 months Below-level pain resistant to oral drugs, alternative therapies, and SCS. IT morphine-induced hyperalgesia. At-level pain: IT hydromorphone (+ baclofen, clonidine, bupivacaine) responsive but ziconotide unresponsive (VAS: 82 mm)
Bruel *et al.* (2007)	CCP (cord tumor) (1 patient)	IT morphine, bupivacaine, clonidine Ziconotide (25 μg/day)	Suboptimal relief Significant relief for whole hospital admission (!)
Saulino *et al.* (2009)	SCI (5 trauma patients, 1 transverse myelitis patient) IT catheter + SC implanted pump Titration of ziconotide based on patient's response. Mean duration of treatment: *c.* 8 months (median 6, range 2–16) Mean doses at last assessment: Group 1: IT ziconotide added to IT baclofen: ziconotide 2.2 μg/day, baclofen 266 μg/day	(1) IT baclofen + morphine / hydromorphone Baclofen (500 μg/day) + ziconotide (1.3 μg/day) (2) IT morphine + bupivacaine Baclofen (300 μg/day) + ziconotide (3.5 μg/day) (3) IT baclofen (120 μg/day) + ziconotide (2.4 μg/day) (4) IT morphine + baclofen Baclofen (190 μg/day) + ziconotide (8.1 μg/day) (5) IT baclofen + morphine Baclofen (115 μg/day) + ziconotide (1.6 μg/day)	(1) No effect VAS: −33.3% Follow-up: ? (2) Inadequate relief VAS: −45.2% Follow-up: 1 year (3) VAS: −47.8% Follow-up: 16 months (4) No effect VAS: −50% (5) Not tolerated, but VAS 4! VAS: −100% Follow-up: 8 months

Table 16.1. (cont.)

Author(s)	Type of pain/number of patients	Drug	Results/notes
	Group 2: IT baclofen added to ziconotide: ziconotide 1.6 µg/d (patient 6), 16 µg/day (patient 7); baclofen 110–115 µg/day (patient 6), 62 µg/day (patient 7) Mean age 50.2 years, mean pain duration 8.8 years, mean baseline VAS score 91 mm Group 1: 3 women, 2 men. NP and spasticity in all cases. Quadriparetic cerebral palsy, multiple spinal fusions, and scoliosis in patient 1; traumatic SCI in patients 2, 3, 4, 5 Group 2: 2 men. NP and spasticity in both cases. Transverse myelitis in patient 1; traumatic SCI in patient 2 (paraplegia)	(6) IT hydromorphone + bupivacaine + baclofen + clonidine; fentanyl + bupivacaine + clonidine Baclofen (62 µg/day) + ziconotide (14.4 µg/day)	(6) No relief VAS: –30% (PO opioids: –50%) Follow-up: > 2 years Mean VAS scores improvement (baseline vs. last assessment): 50.3%. Mean time to onset of pain relief: 15 weeks (range, 7–29 weeks) Many side effects NB: *neither diagnostic criteria for NP nor pain site (at- or below-level) reported for any patient. Cut-off VAS value for time to onset of pain relief unreported* Group 1: mean time to onset of pain relief/mean duration of treatment (weeks): 53/128 = *on average pain not relieved by ziconotide for about a half of the study period* (raw data: patient 1: 7/12; patient 2: 8/NR; patient 3: 29/52(?); patient 4: 17/64; patient 5: 13/NR) Group 2: patient 6: time to onset of pain relief 2 weeks (at 8th month NP almost completely resolved); patient 7: 1 week (length of follow-up unclear, > 2yr). *Difference in time to onset of pain relief between group 1 and group 2 patients (15 vs. 1.5 weeks) not accounted for* Ineffective oral medications and at least one previous failed IT treatment regimen in all patients. Treatment with at least 1 systemic opioid during study
Ruiz-Ortiz *et al.* (2009)	SCI (2 patients)	(1) IT morphine (8.5 mg/day), baclofen (1.05 mg/day), ziconotide (6.7 µg/day) (2) IT morphine (3.4 mg/day), baclofen (1.7 mg/day), ziconotide (4.2 µg/day)	Abstract (1) Severe refractory stabbing and burning pain in both legs. IT morphine + baclofen ineffective. IT ziconotide (2 mg) added 2 months later. 1 years later IT administration of all 3 drugs. Adequate

Table 16.1. (cont.)

Author(s)	Type of pain/number of patients	Drug	Results/notes
			control, PO painkillers down 85%. Follow-up: 1 year (2) Erratic and stabbing pain (5 years). IT morphine + baclofen. IT ziconotide added 1 month later. Pain down > 50%, PO drugs down 45%. Follow-up: 4 months. Adverse effect: somnolence
Shankar *et al.* (2008)	BCP (thalamic AVM + SAH; radiosurgery + shunt)	IT morphine (0.5 mg/day up to 0.864 mg/day)	Test dose: VAS from 9/10 to 2
Margot-Duclot *et al.* (2010) Duplicate of: Margot-Duclot *et al.* 2002	SCI (low cord + conus) (14 + 19 patients)	IT baclofen (versus placebo) (implanted pump) 50–150 μg	Low cord CP: 8 had > 60% relief; 5 implanted with pump. Effect lost in a few Cauda patients: 12 had > 60% relief and 10 implanted At long term: 33% globally still relieved **Paroxysmal component more responsive than steady pain**
Papadopoulos *et al.* (2010)	CCP (1 patient)	IT infusion of baclofen (100 μg/day), clonidine (5 μg/day), ropivacaine (5 mg/day) and morphine (0.4 mg/day) Clonidine to 30 μg/day	Pain endured (75 days). 100% relief (transient hypotension with dizziness) Follow-up: 6 months
Tsai *et al.* (2010)	SCI (2 patients)	IT morphine	Disappointing

Black Box. Ziconotide

Ziconotide (Prialt), a purported N-type voltage-gated Ca^{2+} channel blocker (the exact mechanism in humans being undetermined), is touted as a morphine-sparer, which does not depress respiration and the hormonal axis and does not induce tolerance. It is actually a paragon example of how pharmaceutical companies may bring drugs to market by manipulating the data, regulatory bodies (FDA and EMA), scientific journals, and their editors and referees. Here we review the four major trials, all most likely ghost-written. (A fifth published in *JAMA* was a duplicate, and we highlighted its weaknesses in the same journal: Bonicalzi and Canavero 2004.)

(1) A 220-patient-strong study (**Rauck *et al.* 2006**) mainly included failed back surgery syndrome patients and possibly (not clearly stated) a few CP cases. To start with, the follow-up was obscenely short: 3 weeks (!), which is an unacceptable standard in the face of pains lasting a lifetime. Secondly, the primary efficacy analysis showed a mean 14.7% VAS improvement over baseline versus 7.2% in the placebo arm, barely significant ($p = 0.036$, 0.05 being the standard cut-off for significance). Blatantly, the proportion of

responders (> 30% VAS relief) did not differ significantly between the drug and placebo arms at week 3 (16.1% vs. 12%). There were *no* significant changes on the Categorical Pain Relief Scale, *no* impact on quality of life (as assessed using the TOPS questionnaire), *no* change on the Brief Pain Inventory subscales for sleep, relations, work, mood and walking, and only marginally significant opioid utilization at completion ($p = 0.044$). Yet the "spin" process highlighted a few positive statistics: at week 3, 28.4% reported "a lot/complete" satisfaction with therapy (placebo: 12.1%). On the Clinical Global Impression Overall Pain Control subscale, 11.9% of ziconotide-treated patients reported "very good/excellent" relief (placebo: 0.9%) and also a favorable change on the enjoyment of life subscale (42.2% vs. 27.4% for placebo). Despite the low doses and slow titration employed (from 0.1 μg/h up to 0.29 μg/h over 3 weeks with a mean final dose of 6.96 μg/day), almost all patients (92.9%) reported at least one side effect (dizziness, confusion, ataxia, abnormal gait, memory impairment), with 1–2 weeks necessary for resolution after discontinuation. Uric acid, LDH, and CK were all increased.

(2) Another pivotal study included 169 patients allocated to ziconotide and 87 to placebo (**Wallace *et al.* 2006**). The number of CP cases enrolled is unclear. As evinced from Table 2, CP should have included 67 drug and 36 placebo patients, but in another table the authors labeled as "neuropathic" only 29 drug and 13 placebo cases, only to state in the main text that neuropathic patients amounted to 124! Moreover, what they considered central also included phantom pain and similar. Again the trial duration was ridiculous: 6-day titration plus 5-day-long maintenance (!). That said, the mean VAS reduction was 31.2% for ziconotide versus 6% for placebo, and at the end of the initial titration phase 15 patients (8.9%) had complete pain relief (0% placebo); including reliefs described as "moderate" and "a lot", these figures were 43.8% versus 17.5%. Yet placebo-exposed patients reported a significantly greater improvement in walking ability than ziconotide-exposed ones, and mean change of opiate use for both groups at study end was 0%! Adverse effects were universal (dizziness, nausea, nystagmus, hypotension, somnolence, urinary retention, asthenia, amblyopia, nystagmus, abnormal gait, and confusion) and 60% of these led to dose reduction or treatment interruption, even during titration; 42% of all adverse effects were rated as severe. CK increased threefold in nine cases.

(3) A safety study included 644 patients, with 119 (18.5%!) who received ziconotide for at least 1 year (**Wallace *et al.* 2008**): 101 patients were described as central neuropathic pain (15.7%) without specifications. 99.7% of all patients experienced at least one adverse effect, 99.1% during the first 2 weeks of the study. These included dizziness (> 50% of all patients), headache (40.1%), confusion (35.1%), pain (32%), somnolence (29.3%), and memory impairment (27.8%), and a greater than threefold elevation of CK in 3.4% of cases. Adverse effects were labeled as serious in 233 patients (36.2%), but only in 56 patients were they related to ziconotide (!): they included stupor and delirium (*c.* 1% each) and also hallucinations. These led to temporary or permanent discontinuation of ziconotide in 12.1% and 48.9% of all patients respectively. The authors reported 23 deaths (!), five more than 30 days after discontinuation, including three suicides: the authors offered no valid explanation, except stating that they were unrelated to ziconotide. One of these occurred one day after discontinuation, and writing it off as unrelated is a clear misrepresentation of the truth! Serious meningitis was "experienced" by 19 patients, likely due to the infusion pump being external. One patient who died had serious end-stage cardiac disease and one can only wonder why he was implanted in the first place. Interestingly, the median VAS at baseline was 76 mm, at 1 month 68 mm, but at the **last available observation (up to the second month)** 73 mm! **Also, the median duration of ziconotide therapy was 67.5 days**, which means that half of the patients received ziconotide for less than that.

(4) In a fourth study (**Ellis *et al.* 2008**), 31 patients out of 155 (103 non-cancer) stayed on ziconotide infusion for at least 1 year. At the termination of the trial, only 10 patients (6.5%) were still participating and 39.4% had dropped out due to side effects.

(5) In an open-label extension of these studies (**Webster *et al.* 2009**), the number of patients (78: 66 labeled as neuropathic and no further details) still on ziconotide fell to 23% at 2.8 years. Six patients died during the study (7.6%) and the final ziconotide dose (57 μg/day) was three times the maximum recommended dose (19.2 μg/day).

In conclusion, according to the independent journal *La Revue Prescrire* (April 2008, no. 294), following failure of IT morphine therapy, ziconotide is *not* advised, as it has *no* proven pain-relieving effects and many adverse effects.

intrathecal drugs, and some authors have suggested the existence of a GABAergic pain control system ascending from the spinal cord to the pons, unassociated with opioids (Taira and Hori 2007).

Drug combinations may be more effective. Tolerance to a combination of morphine and clonidine develops more slowly than with morphine alone, but side effects are not reduced, even with reduced doses of clonidine (hypotension, sedation). While intermittent bolus and continuous infusion may not differ in efficacy, infusion with a totally implanted pump is preferred to lower the infection rate, even if initially more expensive. The pharmacodynamics of IT-injected drugs differs considerably with type of administration: a bolus dose produces much higher concentrations of CSF baclofen compared to continuous infusion, particularly at cervical and higher levels, and a positive response to a bolus may not be duplicated during continuous infusion. Also, spasticity and analgesia may require different receptor subsets (Herman *et al.* 1992). An important caveat is that an excess of free GABA may cause postsynaptic receptor changes, leading over time to desensitization.

It has been suggested that infusion of intraspinal drugs (baclofen, clonidine) can turn SCS-unresponsive PNP patients into responders (Schechtmann *et al.* 2010), but, costs aside, no experience has accrued for CP.

Chapter 17

Complementary and alternative approaches

Trials of complementary and alternative medicine (CAM) must be considered in the light of their quality (as for any other therapy). Potpourris of several treatments such as EMG biofeedback, behavioral coping training, cognitive behavioral therapy (CBT), and progressive muscle relaxation may be moderately effective for a short time (Edwards *et al.* 2000). On the other hand, several CP patients are poorly compliant with their drug regimens (explaining some apparent failures) and it may happen that, being under the "doctor's eye," as is common in these approaches, the patient feels compelled to take drugs on a regular basis and thus obtain drug-related benefit.

Complementary invasive techniques

Peripheral/regional and epidural neurolytic blocks (phenol, alcohol, anesthetics) are basically useless in the long-term management of CP, and some may be harmful: results are short-lived or disappointing (Table 17.1). However, abolition of normal afferent stimuli can sometimes secure temporary relief, and repeated or prolonged blocks can dampen at least temporarily a patient's suffering, sometimes for longer periods of time than the duration of the block (Tasker *et al.* 1991). Since permanent surgical neural interruption at the site of successful block usually fails to relieve the pain, anesthetics likely act as pain modulators (Condouris 1976).

Complementary non-invasive techniques

Riddoch (1938) noted that CP could sometimes be diminished by **concomitant stimulation** (e.g., pinching, induced itching, fractures); also, pushing into the muscle tendons or bellies may relieve cramping pain for up to a few hours (Dr. McHenry's website: www.painonline.org). Counter-irritation (pain inhibits pain) is known to allay pain. **Topical menthol** (1 mL of a 40% solution of L-menthol dissolved in 90% ethanol on a 3 cm × 3 cm gauze pad applied to the skin for 15 minutes) – used as a local anesthetic in the past (Wright 1870) – had no effect on dynamic mechanical allodynia, but showed a trend towards reduction of cold allodynia in painful areas (but induced it in non-painful ones) (Wasner *et al.* 2008a: two CPSP patients). Some patients exhibit a marked (> 30%) reduction in the size of an allodynic area after 10 **brush strokes** (over 1 minute) with a cottonwool bud for over 1 hour: in a study, this maneuver had no effect in one CPSP patient, but did in an MS case (Love-Jones *et al.* 2009).

No reports exist on **biofeedback** techniques alone (surface EMG, temperature/thermal, EEG-based) in the CP setting. A small controlled study found that people can learn to suppress acute pain when shown the activity of the rostral ACC in real time from fMRI represented on a computer screen (**fMRI neurofeedback**) as, for example, a flame of varying size in just three 13-minute sessions, with some after-effect (DeCharms *et al.* 2005). In this case, it would be important to define neurometabolic markers of CP for possible image-guided feedback therapy.

Autogenic and/or progressive muscle relaxation training, physical and massage therapy may have some benefit. A majority of SCI patients use CAM, above all relaxation and massage therapy (Norrbrink Budh and Lundeberg 2004). These may help in treating secondary or associated musculoskeletal and other nociceptive components. Musculoskeletal pain arising from, for example, abnormal posture must be specifically addressed in all cases. On the other hand, physical activity may either increase or decrease CP in individual patients. Pain can be momentarily soothed by changing body position.

Sauna may either exacerbate or improve CP. In one study seven CPSP, two traumatic and two tumoral CCP, and one MS-CP patients were interviewed (Nurmikko and Hietaharju 1992). All had a cautious

Table 17.1. Nerve blocks for central pain (since 1980)

Author(s)	Type of pain/ number of patients	Type of block	Outcome
Kennemore (1977)	SCI pain (3 patients)	Percutaneous radiofrequency spinal rhizotomy	Failures
Tasker *et al.* (1992)	SCI pains, conocaudal (5 patients)	Rhizotomies	Transiently effective for steady pain, then worsening
Burchiel (1993)	CPSP (facial)	Glycerol injection	No effect
Dahm *et al.* (1998)	MS-CP (1 patient)	Phenol neurolysis of the obturator nerves and left lumbar plexus; IT phenol neurolysis of L4–S3 nerve roots with 1.5 mL of 50% phenol in glycerol 6 times	No enduring benefit
Ramachandran *et al.* (2007a)	CPSP (2 patients)	Cervical epidural injections of local anesthetic	0% relief
Lee *et al.* (2009)	CCP (1 patient)	Intercostal blocks	No benefit
Kim *et al.* (2010)	CCP (1 patient)	Nerve block	Unsatisfactory

approach to Finnish sauna, which reaches hot pain threshold. Exposure to sauna had no effect on eight patients, worsened CP markedly in one and moderately in another, and moderately alleviated it in three (including a patient with phantom pain). Immediate cooling (snow, shower, swimming) had no effect in 11 but moderately alleviated CP in two. There were no after-effects of sauna in 10 patients but one and two were worsened, markedly and moderately respectively.

Mirror therapy (MT) may be attempted, with the proviso that it may also worsen CP in some patients. This approach targets the mismatch between proprioceptive feedback and motor action: visual feedback substitutes for inappropriate proprioceptive feedback, and this may reduce pain. However, robust trials are needed before MT can be integrated into standard therapeutic protocols (Moseley *et al.* 2008). Moreover, in phantom pain patients, only the clenching spasm and cramping, not the burning or lancinating pains, are reduced. There is also evidence that movement (rather than visual feedback) attenuates phantom and PNP pains in "mirror box" training (Brodie *et al.* 2009).

It must be added that any factors that work to the detriment of general health will often worsen or contribute to the severity of pain, and any form of stimulation below injury level may worsen the pain (urinary tract infection, bladder stones, decubitus ulceration, paronychia, stress, bowel dysfunction, psychological factors, etc.).

Complementary mind–body techniques

CP is life-long, and a durable **rapport with the treating doctors** is vital, particularly to rein in moments of despair: thus, a "placebo approach" is warranted in all cases. For instance, excellent interpersonal relationships, demonstration of caring by the therapist, and enthusiasm, spending time with the patient, supplying accurate, rational information on the effects/results to be obtained, a predicted positive course, belief in treatment efficacy and charisma (the "*surgical look*") all affect placebo circuits. Patients with strong dependency needs and desire to please will respond positively, while those with more explicit conversion of negative affect and somatic preoccupation respond negatively (Nicholson *et al.* 2002). All this is lessened by informed consent, decreased physician paternalism/authority, and so on. When both context and expectations are completely eliminated (hidden therapy), pain relief is less than when therapy is in full view of the patient (Benedetti 2009). Anticipation of pain relief is closely tied to the **placebo response** and actual pain reduction. Since a high level of activity at prefrontal levels marks patients with high expectations and high levels of actual pain relief, prediction of response to medication may become possible by looking at the "expectation component" in patients' brain scans. Also, the same sets of neurons activated both by experienced and

Table 17.2. Complementary treatment studies of central pain

Author/date	Type of pain/ number of patients	Specific treatment	Outcome/notes
Portenoy *et al.* (1988)	MS-CP (1 patient)	Cognitive behavioral therapy	Failure
Craig *et al.* (1997)	SCI (28 patients) Consecutive admission series (+ 41 SCI controls)	Non-randomized controlled trial; measures taken before, immediately after, and 12 months after treatment. Anxiety, depressive mood, and self-esteem assessed Group cognitive behavioral therapy (CBT) during rehabilitation	No overall group differences on anxiety, depressive mood, and self-esteem; trend towards improvement for depression Highly depressed patients in treatment arm significantly less depressed 1 year after injury, vs. controls
Defrin *et al.* (2001)	CCP (15 patients)		Ameliorating factors in 30% of patients • warming the room or limb: 61% • evacuation of the bladder or stomach: 46% • sport activity or work: 30% • alcohol consumption: 23% • posture change: 15% • medication (CBZ, clonazepam, baclofen, and dypirone): 84%
Widerström-Noga and Turk (2003)	SCI	Physical therapies	50% receiving these treatments indicated that their pain was "considerably reduced" or that they were "pain free" CCP not explored
Norrbrink Budh and Lundeberg (2004)	SCI pains (90 patients)	(1) Massage (2) Heat (3) Cold (4) Mental training (5) Physical training	(1) 87% success (out of 31 patients, 24 with neuropathic pain alone or with other pains) (2) 77% success (out of 22 patients, 17 with neuropathic pain alone or with other pains) (3) 32% success (out of 9 patients, 7 with neuropathic pain alone or with other pains) (4) 60% success (out of 5 patients, 4 with neuropathic pain alone or with other pains) (5) 100% success (out of 4 patients, all with neuropathic pain and other pains) NB: Higher percentage of very good results: heat (28%), then physical training, then massage (more effective in younger patients), then cold CAM improves mood and sleep

Table 17.2. (cont.)

Author/date	Type of pain/ number of patients	Specific treatment	Outcome/notes
Norrbrink Budh *et al.* (2006)	SCI neuropathic pain (27 patients) (+ 11 controls)	Educational sessions, behavioral therapy, relaxation, stretching, light exercise, and body awareness training Parallel study 20 sessions over a 10-week period	All patients followed up 3, 6, and 12 months after completion of the program. At the 12-month follow-up: levels of anxiety and depression in the treatment group decreased compared with baseline values + tendency towards better quality of sleep seen. Better sense of coherence and improved depression in treatment arm versus controls
Svendsen *et al.* (2005)	MS-CP (50 patients)		Alleviating factors • physiotherapy/massage/ extension: 12 patients • analgesics: 11 patients • rest: 5 patients • warmth: 4 patients • cold: 4 patients • change of position: 4 patients • body movements: 3 patients
Cardenas and Jensen (2006) (updates Warms *et al.* (2002)	Severe CCP (117 patients)	(1) Strengthening exercises (2) Physical therapy (3) Heat (likely used for musculoskeletal pain) (4) Mobility/ROM exercises (5) Ice (6) Counseling/psychotherapy (7) Nerve blocks (8) Massage (9) Marijuana (10) Chiropractor (11) Biofeedback/relaxation training (12) Magnets (13) Hypnosis (14) Other treatments (all reducing pain by at least 5 points: self-hypnosis, clonazepam, staying busy with a good attitude, healer, body energy work, sex, epidural catheter, lying down, SCS, yoga)	(1) 4.21 VAS points mean relief (24 used, 16 still use) (2) 4.09 VAS points mean relief (26 used, 2 still use) (3) 4.29 VAS points mean relief (19 used, 8 still use) (4) 4.04 VAS points mean relief (15 used, 10 still use) (5) 3.44 VAS points mean relief (13 used, 2 still use) (6) 2.83 VAS points mean relief (7 used, 1 still uses) (7) 3.85 VAS points mean relief (8 used, 1 still uses) (8) **6.05** VAS points mean relief (64 used, 28 still use) (9) **6.62** VAS points mean relief (37 used, 23 still use) (10) 5 VAS points mean relief (31 used, 14 still use) (11) 4.07 VAS points mean relief (27 used, 5 still use) (12) 2.43 VAS points mean relief (20 used, 4 still use) (13) 2.9 VAS points mean relief (11 used, 3 still use) (14) **6.06** VAS points mean relief (19 used, 14 still use)

Table 17.2. (cont.)

Author/date	Type of pain/ number of patients	Specific treatment	Outcome/notes
			Best relief according to the length of relief: • weeks: TENS + chiropractor (and hypnosis) **• months: nerve blocks + biofeedback/relaxation training** • years: counselling/psychotherapy + marijuana (and chiropractor) *The type of pain that was experienced and relieved by each treatment was not studied!*
Moseley (2007)	CCP (1 patient) (+4 with cauda equina lesions =PNP).	Virtual walking	Unlike PNP, the CCP patient had pain and distress *increased*
Gustin *et al.* (2008)	SCI CCP (complete T1–T7, mean T4) (7 patients)	Movement imagery (MI). Imagining right ankle plantar-flexion and dorsiflexion for 8 minutes tid for 7 consecutive days	MI in a region of *absent* sensation in SCI patients, but not increased attention towards these regions, increased the intensity of CCP + non-painful sensations. In 2 SCI patients without CCP or non-painful sensations, movement imagery initiated unpleasant sensations in the region of sensory loss. All increases transient. MI of arm movement: no effects. 1 CCP patient with incomplete SCI (pain in flanks) : no change with MI
De Blasis *et al.* (2009)	Non-thalamic stroke patients with CRPS (not CPSP!) (24 patients; 19 ischemic)	Active mirror group vs. covered-mirror group vs. mental imagery group Randomized, sham-controlled	After 4 weeks, 7/8 patients in the active mirror group reported reduced pain (–51 mm mean) and brush-evoked allodynia versus 1/8 patients in the covered-mirror group (*5 had increased pain!*). In the mental imagery group, 2/8 reported reduced pain (*6 had increased pain!*). 11/12 patients crossing over to active mirror therapy had pain reduced
Lee *et al.* (2009)	CCP (1 patient)	Behavioral therapy	No benefit
Perry *et al.* (2010)	SCI (18 patients)	Group-based multidisciplinary cognitive-behavioral pain management (spinal-ADAPT)	Improvements significant, but some of the initial benefits not maintained 9 months later
Soler MD *et al.* (2010b)	CCP (case series)	Movement imagery, mirror therapy, virtual mirror therapy	Visual illusion did not show marked improvement of CCP: perhaps a longer time (3–8 weeks) needed

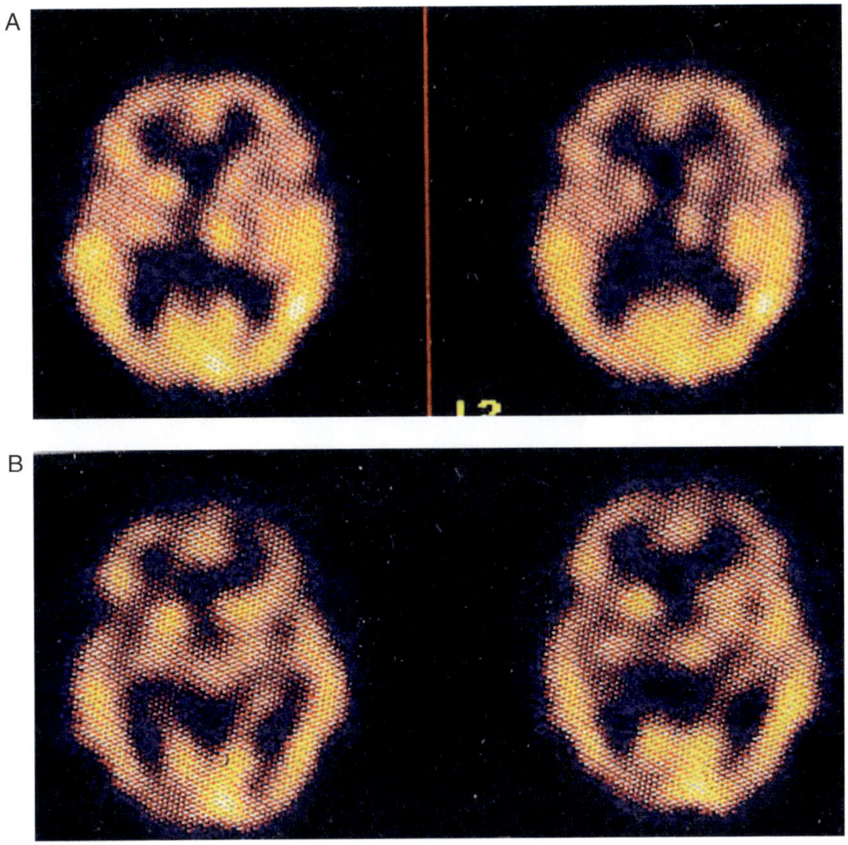

Figure 11.2. High-resolution SPECT scans showing (A) thalamic hypoperfusion in a patient with CPSP. (B) Motor cortex stimulation renormalized it, alongside analgesia.

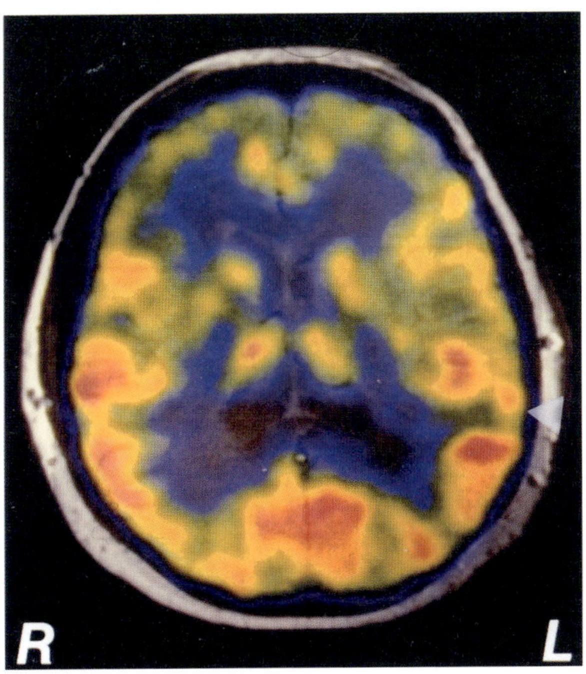

Figure 23.2. PET scan showing both SI and thalamic hypometabolism (right side of figure) in a case of BCP.

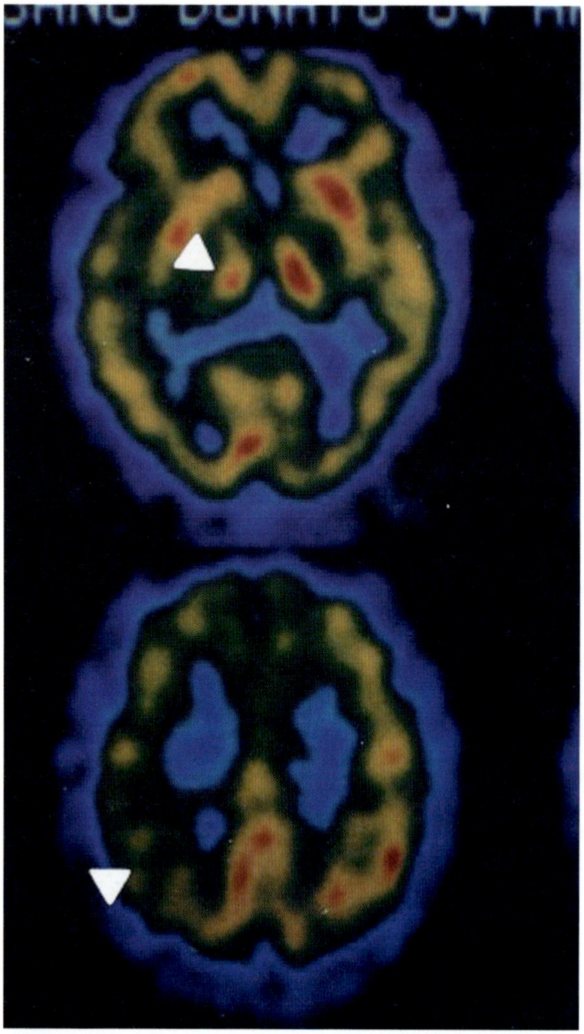

Figure 23.3. High-resolution SPECT (double-head camera) images of post-cordotomy CP. Note both thalamic (upper scan, arrowhead) and parietal hypoperfusion (lower scan, arrowhead).

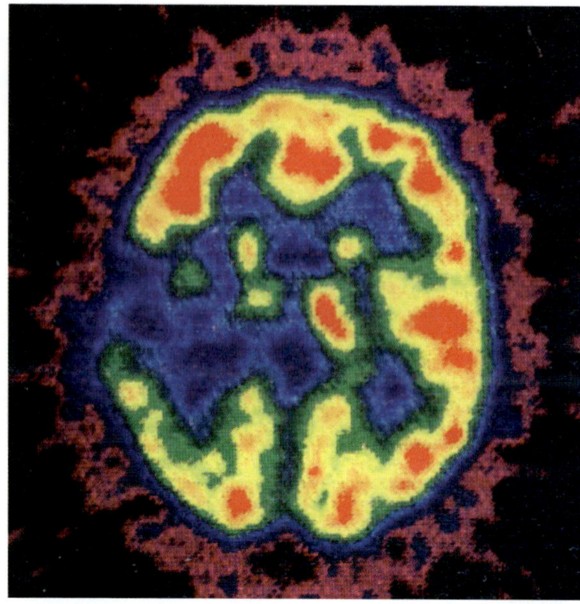

Figure 23.4. PET scan (1992) of a patient who developed central pain immediately after resection of a parietal oligodendroglioma (1987): the ipsilateral thalamus and remaining parietal cortex are both hypoactive.

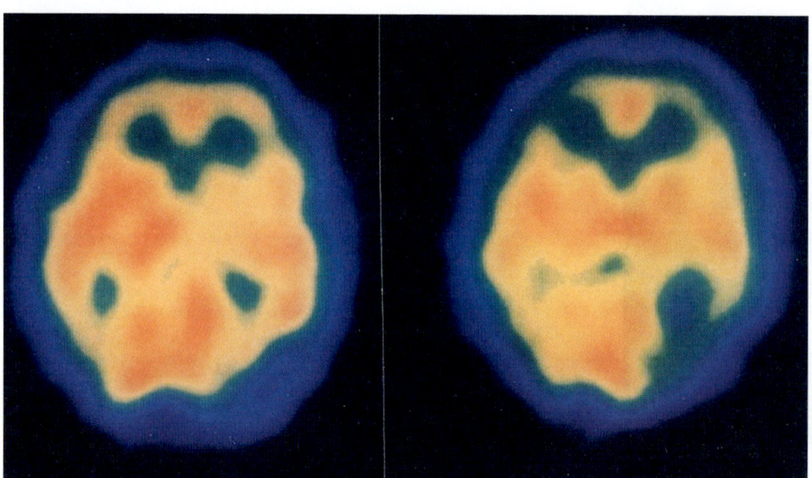

Figure 24.1. SPECT scan showing thalamic hypoperfusion in a case of central pain of thalamic origin. Propofol (0.2 mg/kg IV bolus) renormalized the asymmetry and allayed the pain.

Table 17.3. Acupuncture studies of central pain

Author/date	Type of pain/number of patients	Specific treatment	Outcome/notes
Li (2000)	"Central pain after head injury" (20 patients) **1990–1998**	Bi Tong Tang (a decoction of several herbs taken daily in divided doses for 14 days) + acupuncture in some patients for 7 days + infrared radiation (20 min/day) for 7 days	Pain disappeared in 18 patients after 2–12 weeks of therapy, and in 2 was reduced Follow-up: not available Rationale: "invigorating blood circulation"
Nayak *et al.* (2001a)	SCI (22 patients)	15 acupuncture treatments over 7.5 weeks **No control, no placebo**	Immediately post treatment: 18% reported significant improvement (> 3 points on NRS) in pain intensity, 27% moderate improvement (2–3 points): authors say 45% (*NB: it should be 44%!*). (36% 0–1.9 points and 18% an increase: *they say 54.5%!*) At 3 months: 18% significant, 14% moderate (32%) (*NB: it should be 41%, authors say 35%!*) (27% minimal, 27% increase, 5% no relief: *59% or 13 patients!* (*numbers unclear!*) At 3 months, only 6/10 responders still had at least 2 points improvement. The 3 patients who had above-level pain responded, **the 12 patients with below-level pain did not respond** Incomplete injuries responded more than complete (60% vs. 33%), musculoskeletal pain responded better than CP (80% vs. 42%) (*? Above they say below-level did not respond!*) Responders had moderate pain at onset compared to non-responders at 3 months! In sum: **patients with above-level pain are the ones who may get relief**
Nayak *et al.* (2001b)	SCI (77 patients)	Acupuncture Retrospective study	Acupuncture most tried CAM but deemed **least effective** of CAM
Rapson *et al.* (2003)	SCI (31 patients)	Electro-acupuncture Retrospective study	24 improved (especially those with bilateral/symmetrical pain), 12 *not* improved **Isolated burning pain most likely to improve**

Table 17.3. (cont.)

Author/date	Type of pain/number of patients	Specific treatment	Outcome/notes
Norrbrink Budh and Lundeberg (2004)	SCI (32 patients: 26 with neuropathic pain alone or with other pains)	Acupuncture	Relief: 28% (very good results in *c.* 3%). Best response on cutting/ stabbing and radicular pain (i.e., peripheral pains). *True CP likely unresponsive* Acupuncture more effective in younger patients **Efficacy of acupuncture in the range of gabapentin and amitriptyline!**
Donnellan (2006)	"Central pain affecting the ribcage following traumatic brain injury and rib fractures" (1 patient)	Single course of acupuncture	Rapid and significant improvement in pain and mood after a single course of acupuncture. However, changes in outcome scales were at odds with subjective improvement
Cardenas and Jensen (2006)	SCI (33 patients)	Acupuncture	Currently used by 3 patients only (average pain relief: 3.48 VAS points) Type of pain experienced and relieved not studied
Burkey and Abla-Yao (2010)	MS CCP (1 patient)	Acupuncture	No relief
Liu *et al.* (2010)	SCI pain (13 patients)	Auricular acupressure. Continuous massage for 30 seconds on each point tid for 14 days	Significant relief of pain especially on the first day of treatment. Sham: ineffective Follow-up: 14 days
Yun and Sun (2010)	(1) CPSP (thalamic hemorrhage) (1 patient) (2) CPSP (MCA) (1 patient)	Bee venom diluted in distilled water to 0.005%, 0.01%, 0.02%, 0.04% and intradermally administered into acupoints LI4, TE5, LI10, LI11 affected side, G20 both sides, GV15, GV16, GV20. Apipuncture 3 times weekly. 0.05 mL injected into each acupoint with ultrafine insulin syringe (total no more than 0.5 mL). 0.005, 0.01, and 0.02% apipuncture for the first, second, and third week and 0.04% from the fourth onwards	(1) Within 2 months, VAS from 8 to 3, could touch water again. Continues apipuncture 0.04% once a week (2) Reduction in intensity (1) Gabapentin 900 mg/day: failure. Nortriptyline 20 mg/day: failure and stopped (2) Amitriptyline 30 mg/day for 2 months: failure Slight relief of freezing pain from hot pack applied all time
Zhang *et al.* (2010)	CP (11 patients)	Crossover trial, randomized (mini-unbalance-index method) to acupuncture first and then CBZ	A: 63.6% VAS reduction, CBZ: 36.4% down **No significant difference between groups**

Table 17.3. (cont.)

Author/date	Type of pain/number of patients	Specific treatment	Outcome/notes
		(6 patients) or CBZ first, then acupuncture (5 patients) Ximen (PC4), Yinxi (HT 6), Xuehai (SP10), Zhaohai (KI6). Washout for both A and CBZ: 10 days. VAS/ ACC-MDPE	Rationale: "clearing away the heart fire, regulating the spirit, activating blood and relieving pain"
Santos and Gozzani (2011)	CPSP (1 patient)	Case report	Electroacupuncture of points in the scalp Pain controlled after 11th session, with 100% relief of hand and hemiface pain and abatement of the remaining hemisoma CP

imagined (empathy) pain (ACC and other areas, but not SI) are also set in motion by the anticipation of pain (Holden 2004 and references therein). Cortical stimulation (1 Hz [900 + 900 pulses] TMS) applied to right or left DLPFC (F3/4) can totally block expectation-induced placebo responses (Krummenacher *et al.* 2010). This forebodes a time when non-invasive cortical stimulation will be used to facilitate prefrontal cortex excitability, which may result in an amplification of expectations and consequently enhance the placebo response.

Pain is a highly intrusive event that is extremely effective at capturing attention. **Distraction** from pain through attractive and pleasant hobbies is indicated, as these compete for attention. A distracting task can reduce pain by reducing activity in sensory and affective brain areas. **Hypnosis** acts similarly. **Orgasm** too can temporarily decrease (but at times also increase) CP. **Psychologic support/therapy** may be useful in selected patients as a corollary measure, not to produce significant analgesia (very unlikely), but to improve mood and sleep (Bruguerolle and Labrecque 2007). **Mental imagery** appears to be without effect in most patients.

A review of the literature (Table 17.2) and our extensive experience show that such strategies never provide substantial relief to CP patients. Psychotherapy helps patients control depression, which may profoundly affect the perception of pain and improve sleep. It has been suggested that using a control placebo group leads to overestimation of the effects of psychological pain therapy (Thieme *et al.* 2007).

Alternative techniques

In 1892, Sir William Osler wrote in his section on treatment of neuralgia (pp. 962–3) "acupuncture may be used." However, acupuncture has never relieved our CP patients (as also experienced by Bowsher 1994). A review of the literature supports this conclusion (Table 17.3). Importantly, controlled trials used the wrong comparator (e.g., underdosed and sub-effective Western drugs!). However, acupuncture may allay at-level pain. In imaging studies (Napadow *et al.* 2009 and references), acupuncture evoked real fMRI changes as compared to sham, enhancing the same cognitive network engaged by placebo, but to a stronger degree. Acting as a distracter stimulus, acupuncture may function as a somatosensory-guided mind–body therapy.

Acupuncture is not risk-free: the risk of pneumothorax, infection, and other complications (e.g., autonomic dysreflexia) must not be underestimated, since several cases have been reported (and likely many more have not) (Ernst *et al.* 2007).

Chapter 18

Conclusions on therapy

On the basis of all the studies reviewed in previous chapters, it is possible to make recommendations for treatment (Tables 18.1 and 18.2). Strict adherence will ensure that only a minority of patients will not be helped. On the other hand, patients with good initial relief may later find that they can no longer tolerate even modest degrees of pain. There are no known ways to preempt the development of CP, nor are there markers for identifying pain-prone patients. However, non-invasive cortical stimulation should be explored in this context.

Experimental approaches include a combination of CS with DBS or SCS and any of these with intrathecal pump infusion. The efficacy and cost thereof have yet to be ascertained. The intrathalamic or intracortical infusion of drugs (e.g., $GABA_A$ agonists: Levy *et al.* 2001, or anesthetics: Mark and Tsutsumi 1974) represent interesting experimental options.

High hopes have been raised by current neuro-regeneration/transplantation studies, which include stem cells, encapsulated genetically engineered analgesic compound (e.g., GABA)-secreting cells (e.g., Wirth *et al.* 2002, Bang *et al.* 2005, Jain 2008). Promising initial clinical results have been reported with different kinds of stem cells for spinal cord reconstruction (Cristante *et al.* 2009, Moviglia *et al.* 2009, Sahni and Kessler 2010) and multiple sclerosis (Karussis *et al.* 2010). A word of caution is in order, though. A study of 44 spinally injured patients submitted to monthly infusions of autologous mesenchymal stem cells for 6 months found no differences with a group of controls; worse, 24 (*c.* 55%) developed neuropathic pain (Kishk *et al.* 2010).

Another actively pursued field is nanotechnology for drug delivery to improve solubilization of drugs, eliminating the need for injections, improving absorption, and providing sustained-release profiles, with direct coupling to targets. No application has been reported for CP. Similarly, genetic approaches in human patients (e.g., with RNA interference – siRNA) (Goss *et al.* 2007) have not as yet been pursued for CP.

In the end, it will be our contention that CP can be abolished, immediately and permanently, by a small focal lesion in the internal capsule (Chapter 26). We will try to prove that this is the only ablative technique with a place in the therapeutic armamentarium of CP. Because of the surgical risk, however, this technique should be reserved for highly refractory cases.

Table 18.1. Treatment of central pain: the TANG guidelines (revised)

(A) For continuous, spontaneous pain

(1) Amitriptyline (slow titration up to effective dose, 150 mg, or side effects)
Timeline: 3 months
If ineffective/not tolerated
⇓

(2) Mexiletine (if available) (slow titration up to effective dose, 1000 mg, or side effects)
Timeline: 1 month
If ineffective/not tolerated
⇓

(3) Lamotrigine (slow titration up to effective dose, 600–800 mg, or side effects)
Timeline: 3 months
Add-on therapy only to above drugs: **gabapentin** *or* **pregabalin** (see Chapter 9 for doses and Black Box)
Add-on: CAM

(B) For paroxysmal and shooting pains
Carbamazepine/oxcarbazepine, lamotrigine, levetiracetam
Add-on therapy only to above drugs: **gabapentin** *or* **pregabalin** (see Chapter 9 for doses and Black Box)
Add-on: CAM

If control is still unsatisfactory
⇓
Add-on: **TENS**

If control is still unsatisfactory
⇓
Add-on: **tDCS**

If control is still unsatisfactory
⇓

(A) BCP and CCP without preserved lemniscal conduction

(propofol and/or TMS responsive)

Extradural cortical stimulation (1–2 paddles)*

or (if hemisoma or diffuse pain)
IT midazolam/clonidine or IT baclofen/clonidine (+/ – bupivacaine)
[*opioids added only in still refractory cases*]
**If ECS is unavailable, try SCS, warning the patient of very low probability of meaningful, long-term relief. DBS tried only after explaining inferiority to ECS and with patient's full understanding*

(B) CCP with preserved lemniscal conduction

SCS
If control is still unsatisfactory
⇓
Extradural cortical stimulation

If control is still unsatisfactory (BCP and CCP)

⇓
Convulsive therapy
OR
Experimental approaches (Chapter 26 and Table 18.2)

Table 18.2. Drug dissection and urgent treatment of CP

All tests and infusions in intensive care environment *Each drug tried on different day*
(1) Propofol: 0.2 mg/kg IV bolus over 30 seconds (versus placebo: lipid emulsion); if effective, infusion at 0.3 mg/kg/h over several days *No specific contraindications known. During multi-day infusion, check liver enzymes and lipid levels*
(2) Lidocaine: 0.5/5 mg/kg IV over 20 minutes to 5 hours (repeat daily if necessary) *See contraindications in Chapter 9. Warning: may worsen multiple sclerosis*
(3) Ketamine: 0.1 mg/kg IV slowly (infusion *c.* 5 μg/kg/min) *See contraindications in Chapter 9*
(4) Fentanyl: 50 μg slow IV push (repeated up to 4 times) *Naloxone at hand*
(5) Adenosine: 3 mg IV (further boluses possible) *NOT in cardiac disease and arrhythmia* (see manufacturer's indications)
(6) Midazolam or propofol ± ketamine: full sedation and intubation for 1 week (experimental)

Section 4

Pathophysiology

We should not give up our own freedom of thought when enquiring into the facts of medical science . . . it is incumbent on us to arrange these facts aright, to trace out their position in the general plan of things, and to put them in their proper place.
René Leriche, The Surgery of Pain *(1939)*

Chapter 19

Introduction to pathophysiology

In biology, the findings of analysis achieve scientific meaning only when they are synthesized into principles of functional operation
Sir John Eccles (1977)

The best way to weigh the worth of a scientific theory in biomedicine is rather straightforward: Does it cure the disease it deals with? In this sense, all past and present theories of CP failed; all elucubrations spun out ot animal studies have been blind alleys (see Appendix). Lumping of CP with peripheral neuropathic pain has been fruitless too, given the many differences.

It is our contention that CP is the end result of an attractor-driven decorrelation of information processing along the sensory corticothalamocortical loop. The only permanent cure, barring complete neural restoration, is a lesion of the descending arm of this loop.

The evidence supporting this theory comes from several sources:

(1) reports of sudden disappearance of CP
(2) results of neuroablation for CP
(3) neurophysiologic studies
(4) functional imaging studies
(5) pharmacological dissection data

These will be reviewed in detail in Chapters 20–24, in order of decreasing importance.

No reference to psychological theories of CP will be made, not because of a dearth of such theories, but for the simple reason that CP is somatic pain that cannot in any way be understood in terms of a psychological (e.g., cognitive or psychodynamic) framework.

Several studies indicate that CP is not part of a psychiatric disorder. Andersen *et al.* (1995) found no statistical evidence of an association between depression, social factors, or major life events and CPSP. Mukherjee *et al.* (1999) found depression/dysthymia in 41% of CPSP versus 40% of non-CP stroke patients. Naess *et al.* (2010) found no evidence of an association between depression and CPSP. Likewise, Stenager *et al.* (1991) found no differences between MS patients with and without pain with respect to depression. Thus, the presence of depression/dysthymia does not correlate with CP. Even suicidal ideation is proportional to severity of pain and hostility, and not depression. On the other hand, like all pains (and medical conditions), the experience of CP may be *influenced* by so-called psychological and psychosocial factors (Summers *et al.* 1991, Widerström-Noga *et al.* 2009, Heutink *et al.* 2010), including catastrophizing and coping skills. Interestingly, spinal cord injured patients develop abnormalities in brain regions implicated in emotional control and depressive vulnerability and a more general impairment in emotion-related generation of autonomic bodily responses as a result of sensory deprivation: these findings would argue for early psychological support to prevent the occurrence of emotional dysfunction (Summers *et al.* 1991, Nicotra *et al.* 2006).

Chapter 20

Sudden disappearances of central pain

Vis medicatrix naturae

A handful of patients are on record whose CP *suddenly* vanished after long-standing disease. Nature is teaching us a clear-cut lesson.

CASE 1 (Spiegel *et al.* 1954, Hassler 1970). They observed sudden disappearance of thalamic hyperpathia due to a lesion of the posterior portion of the thalamus after a new larger lesion in the posterior ventral nucleus of the thalamus.

CASE 2 (Gybels and Sweet 1989, p. 342). These authors treated one patient with pain in the right leg of 12 years' duration after a left cerebral stroke. Several neurosurgical operations (not specified) had no effect, but morphine (0.05 mg) administered via a ventricular catheter was followed by a 1–2-day-long complete pain relief and severe paraparesis; 0.025 mg relieved the pain for 12 hours without motor deficits. Satisfactory relief continued for 7 months, at which time "a major left cerebral infarct produced a right hemiplegia and complete relief of her pain."

CASE 3 (Michel *et al.* 1990). Their patient 2 developed "*douleur fulgurante en coup de couteau*" (searing knife-like pain) to the left hand, plus brachial paresis and tactile and pinprick hypoesthesia. CPSP worsened, but 3 weeks later it disappeared with onset of brachiofacial left hemiplegia, only to be replaced by cheiro-oral paresthesias. A CT scan showed a superficial cortical hypodensity straddling right SI/MI.

CASE 4 (Soria and Fine 1991). Their 62-year-old patient developed an acute stroke with a right hemisensorimotor syndrome, including pain and temperature hypoesthesia. Typical CPSP with allodynia developed over 12 months. The threshold for pain, temperature, and light touch was increased, but, when exceeded, the pain resulting was intolerable. One year following the stroke, a CT revealed a small lacunar infarct of the left thalamus. Somatosensory evoked potentials revealed absent N18, N20, and P27 components. Several drugs and other kinds of treatment had no enduring, satisfactory effect. However, 7 years after the original episode, a second stroke produced sudden right hemiplegia, motor aphasia, and complete disappearance of both the pain and the allodynia. At follow-up, 5 months later, there was pain and temperature hypoesthesia in the right half of the body. A late CT scan revealed a well-demarcated, low-density lesion in the left parietal lobe, deep in the centrum semiovale, adjacent to the body of the lateral ventricle. Pain was still *absent 1 year later*.

CASE 5 (Hirato *et al.* 1993). These authors reported a patient with CP after a putaminal lesion, in whom many irregular burst discharges were encountered in the thalamus (Vim-Vc). PET revealed thalamic hypoactivity and cortical hyperactivity. CP disappeared after a small subcortical hemorrhage accidentally occurred near the cerebral cortex around the central sulcus during surgery.

CASE 6 (Canavero *et al.* 2001). This woman developed disabling left hemisoma (C4 sensory level) CP following surgery for a C4–5 herniation, with prominent thermomechanical allodynia in involved regions. She was refractory to multiple drug therapy. During MCS, a microdialysis catheter was inserted into the right SI arm area. Within 48 hours of surgery, the patient started to complain of a "dead flesh" sensation to the left arm distal to the deltoid. A CT scan showed a right SI infarction and the catheter was removed. *For 20 days*, the patient complained of her previous pain, *except for the left arm*. Thereafter, her CP returned with the same intensity and characteristics as before the stroke. During those 20 days there was complete dense anesthesia of the limb with no sign of allodynia (mechanical and thermal). Burning pain was absent (VAS/NRS: 0). MRI 8 months later showed a normal-appearing SI with only a serpiginous area inside.

CASE 7 (Helmchen *et al.* 2002). In June 1999 this 58-year-old man experienced sudden stroke with left-sided sensorimotor symptoms (bar face and neck), with both lemniscal and spinothalamic deficits. CT showed a hemorrhage in right thalamic Vc. Three months later, he noticed the gradual onset of a throbbing, burning, aching, dysesthetic pain on his left side (maximal in the arm) (VAS 8), which became

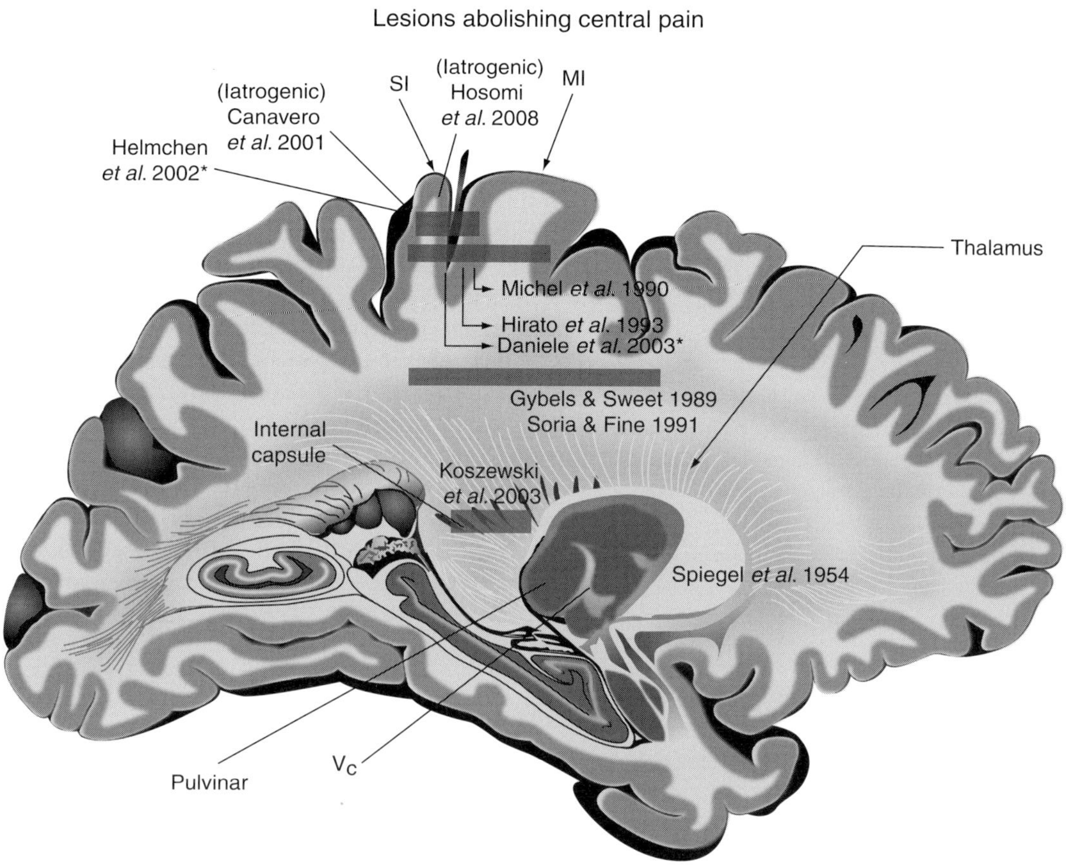

Figure 20.1. Lesions abolishing CP: drawing showing the level of all reviewed lesions described in the text (cases 1–9) plus Koszewski *et al.* (Chapter 26). *Contralateral to original stroke.

disabling and was aggravated by movements and cold stimuli. Ten months later, hemihypoesthesia and hypalgesia were unchanged (movement was improved), but there was mechanical and thermal (cold and warm) allodynia. On CT, a circumscribed hypodense lesion was seen in the posterior right thalamus. MRI also showed a few subcortical parietal and frontal infarctions in the centrum semiovale not involving the ACC. Drugs were ineffective. In April 2001, while washing his hands, he could no longer appreciate warm temperature on his right hand, although he was able to differentiate between warm and cold water on his left arm; allodynia on the left was *gone* and the spontaneous aching CP on his left side *disappeared*. He presented sensory deficits on the right side, particularly severe thermoalgesic hypoesthesia. On the left, he could differentiate warm and cold stimuli in his hand, without a trace of allodynia. There was still hemidysthesia and hypoesthesia, particularly in the arm. Simultaneous tactile but not thermal stimulation was localized to the right arm. There was no thermal or algesic sensation in his right hand, while in his left it was practically normal. Over the following 2 months, sensory deficits largely improved on the right side, bar position sense. Concomitantly, spontaneous CP and – to a smaller degree – cold thermal allodynia returned on the left side and still increased over the following months. *Almost 1 year later*, left CP still persisted, but *without warm thermomechanical allodynia*. No CP had yet developed on the right side. On SSEPs there was prolonged P40 latency on right tibial nerve stimulation. MRI showed *left* hemispheric postcentral parietal ischemic infarction (5 × 4 × 5 cm) that involved *SI*, *supramarginal gyrus*, *SII*, external capsule, and a very small portion of the posterior insula, sparing the anterior insula, internal capsule, and left thalamus.

CASE 8 (Daniele *et al.* 2003). A hypertensive 68-year-old woman developed acute left hemiparesis with mild to moderate motor impairment, hypoesthesia, and tingling sensation which increased over the days. CT showed a *right* thalamic hemorrhage. Several days after discharge, she began to complain of spontaneous pain in her left limbs, sometimes described as burning and excruciating, and tactile allodynia. Carbamazepine at 800 mg was only partially effective. Three years later, the pain was unabated, with partial reduction of hypoesthesia. Then, she suddenly developed acute aphasia. A CT showed a *left* frontoparietal ischemic lesion plus bilateral lacunar infarcts. For the next 3 years (until death) her pain and allodynia were completely gone.

CASE 9 (Hosomi *et al.* 2008). A 64-year-old man developed right thalamic infarction and subsequently complained of central pain in the left arm for 2 years. A stimulating paddle was surgically slipped subdurally in the central sulcus between MI and SI. Pain disappeared *suddenly* and completely (100%) for several months, and then gradually relapsed. Simple surgical dissection silenced the CP generator. The paddle was removed 11 months after implant.

Thus very focal strokes can selectively abolish CP, sectorially (case 6). These strokes can be spontaneous or iatrogenic. Similar cases of disappearance without pathologic confirmation are on record. For instance, White and Sweet (1955) reported a woman suffering from thalamic CPSP. Two-staged bilateral orbital gyrectomy gave no relief of pain. However, 4 months after operation the pains *inexplicably disappeared* and the patient was well. Young and Rinaldi (1997) state that in one patient, who experienced a right-sided thalamic hemorrhage, neglect of the left side of the body developed that relieved the patient of her pain, but they do not state if it was CP. Franzini *et al.* (2003) reported disappearance of CPSP partially relieved by MCS after an undetailed "brainstem stroke."

In sum, by plotting these nine cases (Fig. 20.1) we see that CP of both brain and cord origin disappeared after very focal lesion of the primary sensorimotor cortex, of the underlying corona radiata, and of the thalamus.

Chapter 21

Results of neuroablation

Current ablative techniques have no or only a limited role in the management of CP. On the other hand, they provide invaluable insight into the mechanisms subserving CP. Results of surgical procedures on the cord are reviewed in Chapter 25, while frontal and "sympathetic" surgeries are discussed in the Appendix.

Pre- and postcentral gyrectomies

Limited cortectomies relieved some cases for years, although others were failures (Table 21.1). In the CP case reported by Lende *et al.* (1971), cortical removal extended up to the border of the motor and sensory representation of the hand area and down to the sylvian fissure, with excision of the operculi of the pre- and postcentral gyri, and exposing the insula. Thus, effective cortectomies should likely include both SI and MI: sensory responses can be evoked both behind the classic SI strip (2.2 cm posterior) up to 6.8 cm forward, i.e., well beyond MI (Nii *et al.* 1996, Branco *et al.* 2003; see also Canavero 2009). An *et al.* (2008) reported on a case of transient mild thermoalgesic hypoesthesia of the contralateral thumb after right midfrontal gyrus ischemia.

At least some failures can be explained away by the wide variability in somatotopy in individuals, and by somatotopic differences not only between individuals but also between hemispheres within an individual (Penfield and Jasper 1954). Many studies point to individual variability and mosaicism in human SI. In a study (Tanriverdi *et al.* 2009), the sensory hand area could be found 1–7 cm from the sylvian sulcus and leg sensation within 3 cm of the sylvian fissure, with significant intermixing of differently coded sensory neurons, some also in MI. A single stimulus of a specific point of SI may give rise to combined responses simultaneously in the same and different parts of the body.

Anyway, SI cortectomies have a better track record than, for instance, frontal operations, including cingulectomy/cingulotomy (67% short-term relief versus 47%: Tables 21.1–21.4) and focal lesions of SI can indeed abolish CP in a somatotopographical fashion (Chapter 20). Importantly, CP never followed parietal cortectomy or hemispherectomies (Canavero and Bonicalzi 2007a, p. 103). As suggested by electrophysiologic data (Chapter 22), cortical stimulation studies (Chapter 11), and sudden disappearances of CP following lesions ipsilateral to pain (Chapter 20), *some failures of cortectomies and thalamotomies to relieve CP – but also cases of CP with apparent total destruction of SI – can simply be chalked up to lesioning the wrong side, as the corticothalamic loop posited as the generator of CP has shifted ipsilaterally to pain* (Chapter 26). After SI damage, input may also be rechanneled to *surviving areas of SI* or other sensory zones (e.g., SII) (Bittar *et al.* 2000). In sum, SI is involved in the mechanism of CP (Box 21.1).

The posterior parietal cortex (PPC, BA5–7) is connected, among others, to SI, SII/insula, MI, thalamus, ACC, while the DLPFC and the PPC are the most densely connected areas of the association cortex (Baars and Gage 2010). Lesions of the PPC produce multisensory (body schema) neglect syndromes. As such, PPC (especially BA40) is thought to be involved in conscious experience, including pain (Nakata *et al.* 2008)

Nonetheless, a role in CP is questioned by Hoogenraad *et al.* (1994), who described a 46-year-old man with ischemic infarction of the right parietal cortex following carotid dissection and, among others, left hemianesthesia with almost complete loss of all sensory modalities. MRI disclosed an infarction involving the *posterior part of the postcentral (SI)*, supramarginal and angular gyri plus inferior and superior parietal lobe. Over the next month the patient was unaware of his left arm, had no feeling in the arm, could not use it, but when he saw the arm being approached by someone it would suddenly move sideways as if it had been stung; simultaneously, he experienced a burning pain. The involuntary withdrawal movements of his left arm

Table 21.1. Pre- and postcentral gyrectomies (first proposed by Leriche 1937)

Author(s)	Type of central pain	Target/procedure	Efficacy/ (follow-up)	Notes
Dimitri and Balado (quoted by David *et al.* 1947)	Thalamic lesion (juxtainsular lesion affecting the corona radiata) (1 patient)	Cortectomy SI + large parts of superior and inferior parietal gyri Corpus-callosectomy of parietal associative fibers	0% 0%	At autopsy, juxtainsular lesion in corona radiata
Horrax (1946)	CP, glioma of the left hemisphere (1 patient) CP, rolandoparietal glioma (1 patient) SCI (bony spur at C6) (1 patient)	Tumor excision SI gyrectomy SI gyrectomy SI gyrectomy	0% Relief at 14 months, except arm/hand pain relapsed after 5 months Relief until death months later 0%	
Leriche (1949)	Thalamic lesion (1 patient)	Procaine injection into SI	Relief for 2 months	
Stone (1950)	CPSP (1 patient)	Subpial section of the postcentral gyrus	Relief for at least 14 months	No benefit from previous cervical cordotomy
Penfield and Welch (1951)	Thalamic lesion (1 patient)	SI gyrectomy MI (atrophied) gyrectomy	Relief for 18 months, then relapse Relief, then relapse	**SI stimulation triggered patient's pain**
Lewin and Phillips (1952)	CP, brain injury (1 patient)	Excision of the cerebrodural scar + underlying subcortical cyst	Relief for 4 years	Convulsive seizures preceded by an aura including torturing, deep, gnawing pain in the wrist and hand, spreading to the left limbs and left side of the face
Erickson *et al.* (1952)	CP, thalamic (2 patients)	SI in toto gyrectomy	Relief for 2 years in both	
Spiegel *et al.* (1952)	CP (1 patient)	SI gyrectomy	No relief	
White and Sweet (1955)	CPSP (1 patient)	SI gyrectomy	Relief for 18 months, then relapse	No benefit from previous cervical cordotomy
Biemond (1956)	CPSP (1 patient)	Limited (2 cm) SI cortectomy + insulectomy	Relief for months until relapse	At autopsy: softening in the parietal and insular cortex, degenerated fiber bundle tracing to thalamus (VPM) through the internal capsule, cell loss in VPM

Table 21.1. (cont.)

Author(s)	Type of central pain	Target/procedure	Efficacy/ (follow-up)	Notes
Hamby (1961)	Pure cortical CP (1 patient)	Transpial incision 5 mm deeper than the gutters of the gyri along the posterior edge of SI and over three contiguous parietal gyri. Removal of the cortex and adjacent U-fiber areas of the white matter	Relief for 10 years	**Painful, prickling sensations in the arm and hand elicited from stimulation of SI**
White and Sweet (1969)	CP, postcordotomy	SI gyrectomy (bar face sector) down to the sulcus cinguli	0%	**Pain evoked by SI stimulation**
Lende *et al.* (1971)	CPSP, brainstem (1 patient)	Cortectomy of SI-SII and MI	Relief for 20 months	Pain not relieved by previous complete trigeminal rhizotomy

Box 21.1. The primary somatosensory cortex (SI, a.k.a. SmI) and pain

SI is the principal cortical target of the Vc nucleus. There is a parallel projection to SII but this is not agreed to by all recent investigators, mainly because of differences in the manner in which the cortex of the peri-insular regions has been subdivided and because of failure to take into account the differential projections of the core and matrix cells of the Vc complex (Lenz *et al.* 2010). SI is traditionally divided into four cytoarchitectonic fields: from anterior to posterior these are areas 3a (primarily responsive to stimuli applied to deep tissues, especially muscle), 3b/1 (both responsive to low-threshold cutaneous stimuli), and 2 (responsive to deep stimuli, mainly movements of joints), each with a more or less complete representation of the contralateral half of the body in each field. Different parts of the Vc complex project to the separate fields of SI. The central core (Vcpe) has its predominant subcortical input from low-threshold cutaneous mechanoreceptors and projects to areas 3b and 1: central and peripheral parts of the core project to one or both of these areas. An anterodorsal shell region (Vcae) is dominated by low-threshold inputs from muscle and joint receptors and projects to areas 3a and 2; the anterior part of this shell is the thalamic relay for group IA afferents and projects specifically to area 3a, while the dorsal part receives less well-defined muscle and joint inputs and projects to areas 3a and 2.

The area-specific projections of Vc are formed by the axons of parvalbumin-positive neurons located in the core regions of Vcpe/Vcae and Vcai (VPL/VPM) and terminate in middle layers of SI in a highly ordered topographic array, and their terminations do not extend over the cytoarchitectonic borders of the area to which they project. The calbindin neurons of the matrix regions of Vcpe/Vcae/Vcai, by contrast, send their axons to terminate in superficial layers (LI, LII, and upper LIII) of SI, and these axons can spread over the borders of the architectonic fields. BA2 additionally receives a significant input from the calbindin cells of the enriched matrix of the anterior pulvinar nucleus, which also projects to wider areas of the parietal and parietoinsular cortex (Lenz *et al.* 2010). *Nociceptive neuron clusters are found in the intermediate layers (LIII/IV) of BA1 and/or BA3a, but also in MI.* Pain processing in SI appears to be less hierarchical than touch (Lenz *et al.* 2010).

There is strong evidence for the role of SI in pain detection and discrimination, with spatial information of nociceptive stimuli independent of the tactile system. Further evidence comes from clinical observations that patients with SI surgically removed or injured show impaired pain localization ability (Marshall 1951, Penfield and Jasper 1954). In a particularly representative case, a patient with an SI lesion reported no pain sensation, but only pain affect, which is processed elsewhere (Ploner *et al.* 1999). Data indicate that the encoding of pain intensity is more accurate and extends over a wider stimulus range over SI (Lenz *et al.* 2010).

SI may not be imaged in functional studies, leading some investigators to downplay its role in favor of an insulo-opercular view (see Appendix). Actually, several factors account for this discrepancy, including, among others, failure to resolve small somatotopically appropriate activations in SI, particularly of the deeper located BA3a within the central sulcus, insufficient amount of body surface stimulated (i.e., insufficient spatial summation considering the small receptive fields of most SI nociceptive neurons compared to SII/insular and ACC), insufficient stimulus duration, mixed inhibitory/excitatory intracortical effects (a portion of SI nociceptive neurons can be inhibited by continuous prolonged noxious stimulation). Also, direct intraoperative stimulation of SI almost never elicits painful responses, further evidence for the "negationists" that SI is not essential for pain processing. However, "biphasic square wave is not a 'meaningful' signal ... Cortical organization is such that it responds, when at all, with an organized pattern which is normally evoked by much more elaborate spatial and temporal programming ... change in distribution of subjective sensation with changing frequency, suggesting that even locus is to some extent coded temporally as well as spatially in the central nervous system" (Ervin and Mark 1960). Importantly, in light of the well-known prominent differences in RF properties among neighboring minicolumns of SI, even the simplest sensory stimulus should evoke a patchwork of active and inactive minicolumns (Tommerdahl *et al.* 2010), which might balance out in "negative" fMRI studies.

Anyway, several imaging studies using purely (laser) nociceptive stimuli confirmed the role of SI in pain processing irrespective of concomitant tactile stimulation (e.g., Kanda *et al.* 2000, Inui *et al.* 2003, Nakata *et al.* 2008). A brain electromagnetic tomography (sLORETA) study revealed significant activations of the bilateral SI and ACC and of the contralateral operculoinsular and DLPFC cortices following an acute thermode-delivered nociceptive input. Activity of these regions, excluding DLPFC, correlated with subjective numerical pain scores. However, a multivariate regression analysis distinguished the contralateral SI as the *only region* whose activation magnitude significantly predicted the subjective perception (intensity coding) of noxious stimuli and correlated with subjective pain ratings (Nir *et al.* 2008). When SI is inhibited by cortical stimulation, the activity of the pain-related cortical network decreases due to the widespread cortical connections between SI and other cortical areas (Poreisz *et al.* 2008). An MEG study of SI found that selective nociceptive stimuli induced first pain (Aδ)-related γ (60–95 Hz) oscillations (latency 200 ms) in the contralateral SI. These oscillations were particularly related to the subjective perception of pain, as their amplitudes varied with objective stimulus intensity and subjective pain intensity (Gross *et al.* 2007). Subdural recordings of laser evoked potentials in human patients found a significant LEP generator in SI (plus MI and BA5/7) outside the tactile homunculus; SI received input arising from nociceptors simultaneously with parasylvian and medial frontal cortex. This study provided "strong, new evidence for the importance of SI in pain processing" (Ohara *et al.* 2004).

SI is the *only cortical area with a clear-cut fine somatotopic organization* on neuroimaging studies, an essential pathophysiologic consideration (see also Umesaki *et al.* 2009). Actually, *SI does not truthfully map the body surface (somatotopic homunculus) on all occasions* but, depending on the stimulus, may represent an internal brain image that is linked to subjective perception, rather than to objective sensory input, being activated in a manner that corresponds to the perceived stimulus. Thus, representations on SI may reflect both integrated higher brain functions and simple topographic representations of physical stimuli detected by the periphery. The degree of SI activation enabling emergence of a perceived image is related to the type of information that generates the illusion. In many cases, the image of the world within the brain is congruent with neither the "real" nor the perceived world (Eysel 2003). In fact, SI processes not only somatic but also complex cognitive functions, e.g. extracting somatic features from social interactions (Bufalari *et al.* 2007) or contributing to memory processes in associative learning of noxious stimuli (Diesch and Flor 2007). A case of tactile agnosia with a pure SI lesion (sparing PPC) is on record (Estanol *et al.* 2008). There are also hints of multisensory processing in SI (Kayser 2010).

SI may act as an information-processing network that responds to skin stimulation by selecting a subset among all of its neurons initially activated by the skin contact with the stimulating object. This stimulus-directed dynamic selection process depends on the participation of *afferent connections* (these feed-forward connections give SI neurons their RFs and feature tuning properties but in the absence of other influences would not enable fine discriminative somesthetic perceptual performance, because they trigger stimulus-evoked activation of an excessively large SI population), *intracortical lateral connections* (these promote competitive interactions within SI that reduce the size of the responding SI neuronal population by dynamic constriction of the initial SI topographic map that most closely reflects stimulus location on the skin and by dynamic fractionation of the spatial pattern of response within that cortical region), and *feedback projections* (these can either bias SI neuron responsivity in anticipation of afferent drive or under ambiguous stimulus conditions help in the selection of neurons that will represent the stimulus). When stimulus conditions are simple and well defined, the initial SI response very rapidly is transformed by influences contributed by corticocortical and feedback connections to a response that accurately reflects stimulus attributes. Under complex and less well-defined conditions of skin stimulation, the SI response must undergo a temporally extended period of transformation before a response emerges that adequately represents stimulus attributes (Tommerdahl *et al.* 2010). It is the "unbalancing" of this transformation that accounts for the generation of CP.

were so embarrassing that he tied it to his belt. Eight months later, with eyes closed, he showed loss of superficial sensation (pain and touch) in the left side of his body, more severely in the arm than in the leg, trunk, and face, the distal parts of the extremities being affected most. No delayed pain reaction occurred. There was also complete loss of postural sense, which resulted in sensory ataxia and pseudo-athetoid movements. Vibration was not perceived. There was lack of awareness of the left half of his body and inability to move his left hand and fingers without visual control. With his eyes open and his gaze directed at his left hand, the patient was able to open and close the hand very slowly. There were no sensory abnormalities on the right side of his body. On seeing that the left part of his body was approached for sensory testing, the patient invariably made a brisk withdrawal movement; at the same time he felt a burning pain that was accompanied by grimacing. On moving about, an incidental contact that was *not anticipated* did not result in pain and withdrawal. When the patient himself approached his left arm with his right hand there was neither pain nor withdrawal. In this case, attention can engage the CP generator.

Thalamotomies

The spinothalamic (STT) and the spinotrigeminothalamic (STrT) tracts have widespread terminations in the thalamus, besides Vc, with a predilection for ending in relation to the calbindin-positive cells of the thalamic matrix, which tend to have more diffuse cortical projections than the parvalbumin-positive neurons on which lemniscal terminations are focused. VPI (Vcpce) is largely invaded by large cells of VPL. In humans, core (Vcpe) and shell (Vcae) of Vc are separate subnuclei. A diffuse matrix of small calbindin-positive cells transfers STT and STrT influences to superficial layers of SI/MI and adjacent areas; a second channel formed by a core of larger topographically organized parvalbumin-positive cells transfers lemniscal influences specifically to middle layers of SI. The intralaminar nuclei and their extensions, the limitans-suprageniculate and magnocellular medial geniculate nuclei, give rise to the greater part of the extensive thalamostriatal projection and receive STT/STrT fibers. CL (of the anterior intralaminar group), which receives STT input, projects mainly to SI and anterior parietal areas: the projection to SI is weaker than to MI and much weaker than that to anterior parietal areas (Lenz *et al.* 2010).

Although the concept of a "nucleus" in the thalamus has proved useful in the past, its limitations must be recognized. Any one nucleus or nuclear subdivision can house a variety of intermingled, functionally (and structurally) distinct relay cell types. There are many shared features across most, possibly all, thalamic nuclei. There are also differences, e.g., in the cortical layers of termination or the number of interneurons (ranging from almost 0% up to 20%) of thalamic cells serving as interneurons (Sherman and Guillery 2006). Also, thalamic nuclei can "recode" from mode to mode, e.g., motor VL may come to play a major role in sensory processing (Ro *et al.* 2007).

Thalamotomies for CP, aimed at lesioning the entrance point into the thalamus of quinto- and spinothalamic pain fibers, limitans nucleus, Vc or nonspecific nuclei (CM-Pf, CL, DM, pulvinar, and anterior nuclei), were believed to involve the spinoreticulothalamic (polysynaptic) pain pathways or thought to modify the emotional response to pain. Paradoxically, therapeutic lesions in Vc resulted in CP (White and Sweet 1969, Siegfried and Krayenbühl 1972). Cassinari and Pagni (1969) concluded that only large thalamic lesions centered on CM-limitans-CL nuclei would completely interrupt spinoreticular pathways (partial lesions would be only temporarily effective by a temporary suppression of hyperactivity of thalamic or cortical neurons, for lack of facilitation). Lesions centered on Vc always encroached on the nuclei of the diffuse projection system of the thalamus immediately close by, and this might have either promoted or limited CP onset. Mazars *et al.* (1976, p. 141) stated that all posterior thalamotomies are followed, after a more or less long time, by CP. Basal thalamotomies, placed above the midbrain at the base of the medial thalamus, extended laterally to interrupt both specific and non-specific pain afferents, and exactly enclosed Vcpc: results have been similar to other sites. *Independently of the targeted nuclei*, initial results of thalamotomies are positive in most cases, with immediate relief of CP after Vc, CM, and pulvinar lesions in some patients. Results appear to be *modestly better* (and complications lower, with no or little sensory loss) with medial (particularly bilateral) than with Vc thalamotomies (see also Tasker 1990). Bilateral medial lesions, however, increased the risk of cognitive impairment, by interfering with attentional processes. Few CP patients appear to have benefited in the long term. The great variability of response, relapse rate of pain (up to 50%), non-negligible operative mortality, dysphasia, and severe dysesthesias make stereotactic thalamotomy a poor option for CP. Bilateral lesions produced many more complications and deaths, and bilateral extensive destruction of thalamus is incompatible with life; severe, permanent complications and deaths have been reported with all thalamotomies. Interestingly, *some unilateral lesions relieved bilateral pain.*

There do not appear to be significant differences between results obtained in older studies and newer series (Table 21.2). Jeanmonod *et al.* (1996, 2001) found 50–100% improvement in 40% of CP – by far less than for PNP – at 2 years, in line with the experience of Tasker (1990) and Young *et al.* (1995), after medial thalamotomies (see also Ohye 1998). The lesions centered in CL, where most bursting units were found, revealed themselves to be the most efficient (least efficient, in descending order, were Pf, PO, PuO/M and CM, and midline nuclei). *However, both steady pain with thermal qualities and deep (proprioceptive) pain proved particularly resistant, whereas intermittent pain/allodynia and superficial pain were more responsive.* Magnin *et al.* (2001) observed that in neurogenic pain (including CP) CL stimulation leads to paresthesia, in motor disorders to motor reactions, and in psychiatric disorders to emotional feelings, and in another similar study (which included one pure CP patient, three mixed, and 20 PNP cases), evoked responses in CL were 95% somatosensory in neuropathic pain, 47% motor in Parkinson disease, and 54% affective in neuropsychiatric patients (Jetzer *et al.* 2009). In other words, *CL is NOT specifically involved in CP*, but may act as a non-specific amplifier of thalamocortical activity. It should be noted that pulvinotomy, like medial thalamotomies, can reduce chronic, but not acute, pain (Richardson 1974). Tasker (2001a) concluded that there may be a place for medial thalamotomy for evoked intermittent pains. On the other hand, Ohye (1998, Ohye and Shibazaki 2009) found that *Vim thalamotomies can ameliorate deep pain only*. He also concluded that CM-Pf used as a target in the past may have been the wrong target (Ohye 1990; but see Weigel and Krauss 2004). This is interesting, as old series did not distinguish the various components of CP sufficiently. Excellent results for CP have been reported after pulvinotomy by some (Yoshii *et al.* 1980, Laitinen 1988a), but these are difficult to analyze (Tasker 1990). In sum, available data suggest involvement of several thalamic nuclei in the genesis of CP, but, **aside from Vc and Vim, the role of other nuclei (CL, pulvinar, CM-Pf) remains to be defined**. Also, the puzzling efficacy, at least in the short term, of lesions of different nuclei must be explained.

Stereotactic lesions (particularly radiosurgical ones) can easily encroach on nearby nuclei (e.g., Vc and Vim, Vc and CM, Vc and pulvinar). An interesting possibility comes from theoretical constructs that emphasize corticothalamocortical loops between higher-order thalamic nuclei and cortical areas as the major driver of corticocortical information transfer and processing ("the cerebral cortex without thalamus is rather like a great church organ without an organist: fascinating, but useless": Sherman and Guillery 2006). Multiple thalamic nuclei could be recruited by corticothalamic fibers returning from the first area to nuclei other than that from which that area receives its principal thalamic input by way of the specific output patterns of matrix cells and might be a key element in binding together the activities of multiple cortical columns in the generation of a sensory percept (Jones 2007). This would explain effects of thalamotomies. For instance, pulvinotomy relieves CP because pulvinar is a higher-order nucleus (i.e., no STT input) with a projection to SI. It should be stressed that neurons in separate somatosensory nuclei of the dorsal thalamus influence (excite or inhibit) one another's activity through the thalamic reticular nucleus (TRN). This can be divided into a number of sectors each concerned with a different function and topographically connected to more than one thalamic nucleus and cortical area; connections are not the same for each sector. TRN acts as a nexus where several functionally related cortical areas and thalamic nuclei interact, modifying thalamocortical transmission through the inhibitory connections that go from TRN cells to TC relay cells. In the somatosensory system,

Table 21.2. Thalamotomies

Author(s)	Type of central pain	Target/procedure	Efficacy/(follow-up)	Notes
Hécaen *et al.* (1949)	CP (4 patients)	1 center median	Yes, immediate (4 months)	Thalamic hand and clonus induced by Vc stimulation, no effect with DM stimulation
Talairach *et al.* (1949)	CP, thalamic (12 patients)			
	1 center median + Vc	Yes, immediate and complete (follow-up: 1 year)		
	2 center median + DM	Yes, immediate and for at least 4 months		
	Vc (radioactive gold)	6, 75–100% reliefs; 2, 50% reliefs; 2, 25% reliefs; 2 deaths		
Baudoin and Puech (1949)	CP, brain (1 patient)	Local novocaine injection into Vc	0%	
Spiegel *et al.* (1952)	CP, brain (3 patients)	Vc	Temporary (max. 4.5 months), in one relapse after a few weeks	
Talairach (1955)	CP, brain (12 patients)	Vc	"Favorable" relief in 50% of patients	
Laspiur (1956)	CP, brain (2 patients)	Vc	Yes (in one, 100% relief, in the other, "spectacular" relief) Follow-up?	
Obrador *et al.* (1957)	CP, thalamic (2 patients)	Vc	0%	1 suicide
Hassler and Riechert (1959)	CP, brain (1 patient)	Vc	Relief, 5 weeks	
Hassler (1960)	CP, brain (4 patients)	Vc, limitans and CM	Yes, lasting relief	
Bettag and Yoshida (1960)	CP, thalamic (4 patients)	Vc (3 patients) DM (1 patient)	In all, lasting relief	
Mark *et al.* (1960)	CP, SCI (4 limb burning dysesthesias) patients?	Vc	Yes, partial	Partial pain relief, but recurrence after 6 months
Hankinson (1962)	CP, brain (2 patients)	CM and Vc	Yes (16–24 months)	
Davis and Stokes (1966)	Neurogenic pains	Lateral plus medial nc	Yes	Immediate pain relief in 75% of patients, decreasing to 50–60% after 6–12 months

Table 21.2. (cont.)

Author(s)	Type of central pain	Target/procedure	Efficacy/(follow-up)	Notes
Bettag (1966)	Neurogenic pains	CM, DM	Persisting pain relief only in 6/31 patients Pain relief only in 1/4 patients subjected to CM lesions, with or without DM	
Spiegel *et al.* (1966)	CCP (1 patient)	Medial thalamotomy	100% relief; full relapse 1 week later; 100% relief after reop. At 1.5 years, pain reduced	
	CPSP (1 patient)	Medial thalamotomy	Partial relief. Late result: indifference to pain	
	CPSP (1 patient)	Basal thalamotomy	100% relief for 3 weeks, then partial relapse (superficial vs. deep pain) with allodynia, at 3 months	
	SCI pain (1 patient)	Bilateral basal thalamotomy	100% relief, full relapse at 4 months	
Kudo *et al.* (1968)	CPSP (6 patients) out of 17 with cancer or non-cancer pain	Pulvinar	Whole series: 8 complete reliefs, 6 remarkable, 3 slight pain remaining	
White and Sweet (1969)	CP, brain (1 patient)	Pf (unilateral)	Poor result	
	CP, MS (1 patient)	Pf (unilateral)	Good relief	
	CCP (cervical) (1 patient)	Vc	Fair relief	
	CCP (conocaudal) (1 patient)	Pf (bilateral) and anterior nucleus (unilateral)	Good relief	
	Tabes dorsalis (1 patient)	Vc and DM (unilateral)	Poor relief	
Sugita *et al.* (1972)	CP, brain (unspecified)	CM, Pf, intralaminar, MD	No effect	
Siegfried and Krayenbühl (1972)	Neurogenic pain	Vc, intralaminar system plus DM	No 1 of 9 patients with Vcpc thalamotomy relieved	Not available for review
Cooper *et al.* (1973)	Burning hypoesthesia and spastic hemiplegia (3 patients)	LP-pulvinotomy	Relief in 3. No relapse	*Acute pain sensation not affected*

Table 21.2. (cont.)

Author(s)	Type of central pain	Target/procedure	Efficacy/(follow-up)	Notes
Richardson (1974)	CPSP (2 patients)	CM	Immediate reduction of dysesthesias and hyperesthesias Spontaneous complaints reduced but still present	
Amano *et al.* (1976; cited in Amano 1998) Sano *et al.* (1966)	Thalamic CP (10 patients) Other CP (14 patients)	Thalalaminotomy (i.e., CM-Pf and CL)	Thalamic CP: follow-up 1–24 months. At discharge: 100% in 3, slight residual but tolerable pain in 6, 0% relief in 1. At follow-up: 100% in 3, tolerable pain in 4, tolerable pain with drugs in 2, 0% in 1. Other CP: at discharge: 100% in 2, slight residual but tolerable pain in 6, tolerable with drugs in 3, some relief but intolerable in 1, 0% in 2. At follow-up: 100% in 2, tolerable in 4, tolerable with drugs in 3, some relief but intolerable in 2, 0% in 2	
Mayanagi and Bouchard (1976–77)	CP (thalamic: 3 patients)	Basal: CM ± pulvinar	Follow-up: 6 months CP "difficult to control"	
Mundinger and Becker (1977)	CP	Medial nc	40% good; total relief up to 14.5 years	
Siegfried (1977)	CP + neurogenic pain (13 patients)	Pulvinar	Yes, dramatic initial relief in several. Recurrence within 1 year in several	*Some had subtle sensory alterations*
Pagni (1977)	CP, brain CP, SCI	Intralaminar nc (including CM-Pf), sometimes extending to Vc and DM	Total or partial long-term relief in 12 BCP and 3 CCP Pagni's experience with CP: 30% relief	Survey. Dysesthesia can persist unmodified. Multiple thalamic (CM-VPL/VPM-pulvinar) and mesencephalic coagulations may be necessary if lesions to a single structure are unsuccessful. Center median lesions "very effective" for thalamic

Table 21.2. (cont.)

Author(s)	Type of central pain	Target/procedure	Efficacy/(follow-up)	Notes
				pain, with long-lasting results. Basal thalamotomies for brainstem lesions. Long-term results with CM-Vc, intralaminar and DM lesions generally unsatisfactory
Yoshii *et al.* (1980)	CP (14 patients)	Pulvinar (bilateral if needed; supranucleus pulvinaris medialis nc lesion in all cases)	Yes, *immediate complete* in 6 patients, almost complete in 7 patients, good in 1 patient At 3.5–10 years: 4 pain-free, 4 almost pain-free, 3 sufficient pain relief, 3 failures Cases with follow-up > 5 years: 1 pain-free, 2 almost pain-free, 3 sufficient pain relief, 2 failures	No bearing on final outcome from bilateral lesions
Hitchcock and Teixeira (1981)	CP, brain (3 patients)	Basal (including Vcpc and n. limitans portae)	Yes (2/3 patients)	CM thalamotomies deemed superior, particularly if bilateral, to basal thalamotomies (better pain relief and fewer side effects). Very high rate of complications
	Postcordotomy/thoracotomy dysesthesias (5 patients)		Yes (5/5 patients)	
	CP, brain (6 patients)	Medial (CM), some bilateral	Yes (5/6 patients)	
	Postcordotomy dysesthesias (1 patient)		Yes	
Niizuma *et al.* (1982) Includes: Niizuma *et al.* *Appl Neurophysiol* 1980, **43**, 336	CPSP (17 patients, 1 of which cheiro-oral)	Unilateral/bilateral center median	Relief (1, 100%) in 56%, then full relapse within 7 months in all	
Barcia Salorio *et al.* (1987)	CPSP (2 patients)	**LINAC radiosurgical Vc thalamotomy**	Burning paroxysms abolished, background pain diminished Follow-up 6 months	

Table 21.2. (cont.)

Author(s)	Type of central pain	Target/procedure	Efficacy/(follow-up)	Notes
Laitinen (1988a; see also Laitinen 1977)	CPSP (2 patients)	CM thalamotomy	Yes (6–24 months)	CM-intralaminar and pulvinar lesions highly effective for CP. However, in a mixed series of cancer and neurogenic pain, only 29% were pain-free after 2.5 years
	CPSP (3 patients)	CM-intralaminar thalamotomy	Yes, *immediately* (8–18 months)	
	SCI (1 patient)	CT-guided pulvinarectomy	Good early result	
Ohye (1990, 1998, Ohye and Shibazaki 2009)	CPSP, mainly deep muscle pain (*c.* 40 patients)	Vim (a part)-Vcpc (deep portion) thalamotomy (i.e., coagulation of the isolated hyperactive area around the thalamic stroke lesion)	Deep pain of compressing, burning, or sometimes squeezing nature considerably ameliorated	*No effect on paresthesia and numbness* *Relief only of deep pain or muscle pain originating deep in the extremities or movement or compression allodynia, not superficial or dysesthetic pain*
	CPSP (9 patients)	Vim and/or CL thalamotomy	Satisfactory relief in 4/9	*Gamma knife to diminish abnormal neuronal activity in the area surrounding damaged Vc destroying hyperactive Vim (which lies just ahead of Vc and receives input from muscle spindles)*
	CP (15 patients)	**Gamma knife Vim radiosurgery**; one shot, 130 Gy, 4 mm collimator	Nearly 60% success After 6/12 months pain milder and more tolerable (10 years in 1 patient)	Negligible complications
Chodakiewitz (1991)	1 patient, post-cordotomy CCP	Medial thalamotomy (pacemaker contraindicating DBS)	100% relief for 1 month of follow up	Vc/PVG DBS: 10 years of excellent relief
Jeanmonod *et al.* (1996, 2001)	CP, parietal cortex (5 patients), thalamus (3 patients), brainstem (4 patients), spinal cord (12 patients)	Medial thalamotomies (if necessary, lesion ipsilateral to pain)	50–100% relief in 40% of BCP patients and 38% of SCI patients Relief was best for evoked and intermittent pain and superficial pain, poorer for steady pain (which lingered on in more than half the cases) and deep pain *One CCP patient referred by us: 0% relief (+ complications)*	Generally without postop. somatosensory – including pain – deficits; in several, postop. improvement of somatosensory deficits
Hirato *et al.* (1995)	CPSP (thalamic and putaminal) (2 patients)	**Radiosurgical Vim thalamotomy**	(A) Vim thalamotomy: some relief, relapse, radiosurgical Vim thalamotomy, relief (B) Vim thalamotomy: poor relief, gamma thalamotomy good	Relief seen in both after 3–6 months (!?)

Table 21.2. (cont.)

Author(s)	Type of central pain	Target/procedure	Efficacy/(follow-up)	Notes
			relief (not abolition) for 3 months	
Young *et al.* (1995)	CP (thalamic) (3 patients) SCI pain (1 patient)	**Radiosurgical medial thalamotomy (gamma knife)**	Median follow-up for whole group of 20 mixed pains patients; about 1 year relief seems to have been obtained in at least some	CM gammathalamotomized patients have greatly reduced attention to their pain. CM may contribute to suffering
Frighetto *et al.* (2004)	CPSP (MCA stroke and thalamic stroke) (2 patients)	**Radiosurgical CM-Pf thalamotomy**	(A) immediate relief, relapse at 4 months (relieved by MCS) (B) some drug reduction, allodynia improved, 3 years later drugs only twice a week	No 100% abolition; effect on pain before onset of necrosis (!); necroses 3.5 × 5 mm and 8.5 × 7 mm (too large to have exclusively targeted CM-Pf)
Keep *et al.* (2006)	CPSP (1 patient)	**Gamma knife**, 4 mm collimator helmet, single shot of 140 gray to the 100% isodose line, left centromedian region *NB: their figure shows an area that must have certainly involved more than CM: CM next to VPM*	1 month later, more comfortable, at 3 months objective improvement, allodynia to face gone, sensation intact, encephalomalacia of thalamic target Pain-free at almost 7 years of follow-up	Lesions of CM yield relief preferentially to upper body and less to lower body/leg

both first- and higher-order nuclei project to the same sector (e.g., Pom – higher order – relays to SII; Vc – first order – to SI). Thalamotomies at different levels but encroaching on TRN may lead to a similar effect.

Mesencephalotomies

These have been performed to interrupt both the STT and the reticular formation (Fig. 21.1). A slow multisynaptic spinoreticulothalamic pathway (SRT) is strongly suggested by neurosurgical evidence (King 1977, Gybels and Sweet 1989, p. 192), but also by current clinical (medial medullary infarctions: Bassetti *et al.* 1997) and neurophysiological data (Rousseaux *et al.* 1999). At rostral mesencephalic level, the medial lemniscus, neospinothalamic tract, reticulothalamic tract, and PAG lie contiguously adjacent to one another (from lateral to medial, respectively).

Since STT lesions – but not coagulation of the termination site of the paleospinothalamic path – triggered new CP (Cassinari and Pagni 1969), most surgeons treating CP attempted larger medial lesions impinging on the reticular formation, thus including the paleospino-reticulo-thalamic pathways (often combined with medial thalamotomy) (Fig. 21.1). The "larger lesions appeared more effective for relief of central dysesthesia" (Nashold *et al.* 1969). However, Tasker (1989), reviewing 92 published protocols of patients with CP/PNP, showed that only 27% gained satisfactory long-term relief from mesencephalotomy, with several complications and operative deaths. Laitinen (1988a) concluded that "mesencephalotomy

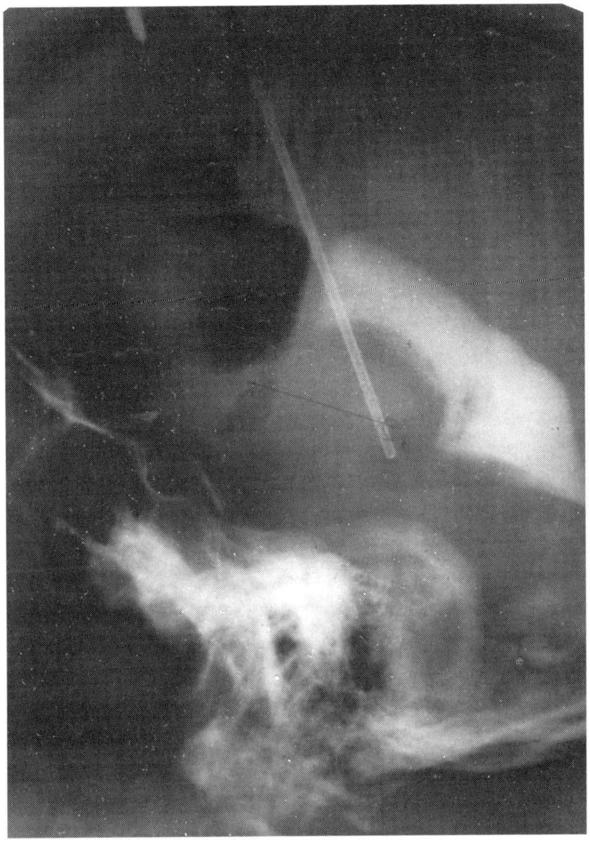

Figure 21.1. Skull radiographs illustrating the stereotactic cannula during mesencephalotomy surgery.

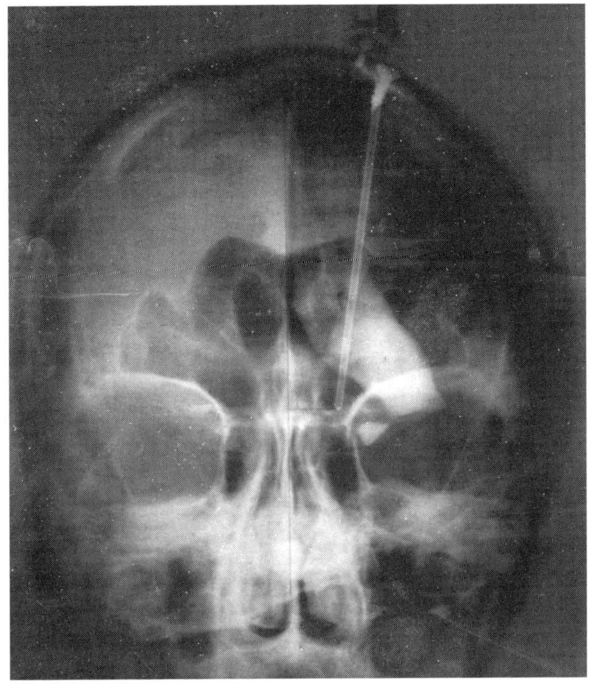

21.1. (cont)

has no place in the treatment of chronic pain. The efficacy of this approach is no better than that of nonspecific thalamotomies, but side effects are more frequent and more serious," and Bosch (1991) also concluded against the use of mesencephalotomy in CP. There are more than 70% postoperative dysesthesias after open and 15–20% after stereotactic mesencephalotomies, with 5–10% mortality in stereotactic series (Tasker 1989). However, Amano *et al.* (1980, 1986, 1992) achieved complete or near-complete long-term relief in almost two-thirds of their CP patients, with no postoperative dysesthesias or deaths, by aiming only at the reticular formation ("pure" rostral medial reticulotomy). Their target was located at the border between the PAG and the medial end of the mesencephalic reticular formation at the level between the superior colliculus and the posterior commissure (Amano *et al.* 1980). The pretectal area was avoided by burring at 30% of glabella–inion distance. Microrecording showed nociceptive neurons in the target area, characterized by large receptive fields (RFs) and delayed firing in response to pinprick stimulation. *High-frequency stimulation produced severe pain mostly contralateral to the side of stimulation in a very restricted area.* Similar results were reported by Shieff and Nashold (1988). These latter authors observed how CP resolved *gradually*, never suddenly (unlike subparietal lesions), after mesencephalotomy (Amano *et al.* did not discuss this point); also, *unilateral lesions relieved bilateral pain.* The spinoreticulothalamic system has very large and/or bilateral RFs, while CP is generally unilateral (Lenz *et al.* 2010). Kim (2007b) described a patient who developed CPSP following lateral medullary infarction with STT sensory deficits. CPSP gradually improved until the development of ipsilateral medial medullary infarct 26 months later, with mild hemiparesis and lemniscal deficits. This stroke immediately worsened CPSP to its previous level. He concluded that CP might be due to hyperexcitation of the STT pathway by the reticulothalamic system, in turn modulated by the medial lemniscal pathway.

In sum, Amano's group's results are to date the strongest evidence for a role of the reticular formation in CP: this may be involved in modulating a rostral generator and/or conscious experience of CP (Table 21.3).

Table 21.3. Mesencephalotomies (STT tractotomies and reticulotomies) and other brainstem lesions

Author(s)	Type of central pain	Target/procedure	Efficacy/(follow-up)	Notes
Walker (1942a, 1942b)	Thalamic pain (1 patient)	Open lateral	Death after 26 hours	
Torvik (1959)	CP (2 patients)		Not available for review	
Wycis and Spiegel (1962) (including patients reported in previous series)	CPSP (14 patients)	Spinothalamic tract plus reticular formation at midbrain level	11 initial pain disappearances or abatements, 3 failures, 2 deaths	3 mesencephalotomies plus thalamotomies: 1 complete relief for 10 years, 1 partial relief, 1 transient indifference
	CP due to parietal lesions (2 patients)	As per above, plus possible thalamic impingement	Follow-up: 4 full relapses (1–5 months), 2 partial relapses (1–5 months), 5 long-term good reliefs	
	1 (pontine lesion)		Pain relief (6 months)	
	1 (ACoA aneurysm)		0% relief	
	CCP (3 patients)	Mesencephalotomy	1 complete relief for 1 year, 1 transient relief, 10%	
Helfant *et al.* (1965)	CPSP (thalamic) (1 patient)	STT	0%	
Orthner and Roeder (1966) Includes Roeder and Orthner (1961)	CPSP (1 patient)	Lateral plus medial lesions	*Almost* complete relief for 26 months up to death	
Gioia *et al.* (1967)	CP + neurogenic pain (2 patients)	Medial lesion	Poor	
Turnbull (1972)	Tabes dorsalis (1 patient)	Combined mesencephalotomy-thalamotomy-cingulotomy	1 modest relief	
Schvarcz (1977)	CP (5 patients?)	Mesencephalotomy	4 pain reliefs at 6–24 months	Not available for review
Amano *et al.* (1980, 1986, 1992)	CPSP (25 patients) CP, tumor (1 patient) Postcordotomy dysesthesia (PCD) (1 patient) Tabetic pain (TB) (1 patient)	Rostral mesencephalic reticulotomy (highly selective lesion in the medialmost portion of the midbrain reticular formation, medial to the STT which is not lesioned unlike Nashold's procedure)	Group 1: 2 complete reliefs, 3 partial reliefs at 50–70 months Group 2: 6 complete reliefs, 9 almost complete reliefs, 6 partial reliefs at < 50 months PCD 0% relief	Results confirmed in 1992. 64% complete or near complete pain relief. No postop. dysesthesias One of the patients relieved 100% at 11 years noticed at year 7–8 tactile-

Table 21.3. (cont.)

Author(s)	Type of central pain	Target/procedure	Efficacy/(follow-up)	Notes
		contralateral to pain in all cases	TB almost complete relief at 57 months	thermoalgesic anesthesia of left hemisoma
Shieff and Nashold (1988) (includes all patients from Nashold's previous publications on this treatment)	CPSP, brain (20 patients) CPSP, brainstem (7 patients) **(1963–1985)**	Lesions: (1) medial lesions at superior colliculus level (2) lesions at inferior colliculus level	(1) 14 early patients: 5, 100% reliefs; 6 fair (minimal residual pain, non-opioids required); 3, 0% reliefs 12 late patients (+1 death + 1 lost to fillow-up): 7, 100% reliefs; 2 fair, 1 poor (significant residual pain), 2 0% (follow-up: 3–60 months) (2) 13 early patients: 5, 100% reliefs, 5 fair; 1 poor; 1, 0% (1 moribund) 12 late patients: 4, 100%; 3 fair; 2 poor; 3, 0%	4 patients with repeat early surgery, 6 reoperated for late relapse and 1 pain-free after 4 procedures *Unilateral lesions relieved bilateral pain* *Gradual disappearance of pain* *Lesion impinging on reticular formation*
Laitinen (1988a)	Thalamic pain (2 patients) Paraplegia pain (1 patient)	STT	?	Whole neurogenic pain group: 25% relieved at 3 years. Complications in half, including new dysesthesias
Sampson and Nashold (1992)	CPSP (brainstem) (2 patients)	Caudalis DREZ	1 complete relief, 1 partial relief (4–48 months)	Arm ataxia
Gorecki and Nashold (1995)		CPSP (4–5 patients?)	50% relief at 3 months?	
Tasker *et al.* (1991)	Brain CP (11 patients)	Mesencephalotomy with/without medial thalamotomy	Steady pain relieved in 3 (plus other 3 temporarily) and failed in 5; intermittent pain relieved in the only patient who had it; evoked pain relieved in 3 and unrelieved in 2	Evoked pain more responsive than steady pain
Bosch (1991)	Thalamic pain (2 patients)	Rostral mesencephalotomy	0% relief at 1 year	
Teixeira (1998) Teixeira *et al.* (2003)	(1) CP, Wallenberg (7 patients) (2) CP, brainstem	(1) Bulbar trigeminal stereotactic nucleotractotomy (2) Caudalis DREZ	(1) Orofacial pain <VAS 3 in 85.7% of patients immediately and at follow-up (2 years) (2) Failure	1 patient full relapse in 4 weeks and one partial relapse in 6 months. One repeat procedure

Table 21.4. Hypophysectomy–hypothalamotomy

Author(s)	Type of central pain	Target/procedure	Efficacy/(follow-up)	Notes
Laitinen (1988b)	CPSP post-SAH (1 patient)	Posteromedial hypothalmotomy	Results not stated; however, response on restlessness	
Mayanagi and Sano (1998)	CP, brain and cord (at least 2 or more BCP patients)	Posterior hypothalamotomy (medial; III ventricle gray matter)	No (0–25% in one CPSP) Max. follow-up: 17 months	Pain increased by electrical stimulation in 2 patients
Levin (1988)	CP (7 patients)	Stereotactic chemical hypophysectomy	More than 50% relief in 6, 2 still relieved 2 years later; at least 2 relapses within a few months	Significant relief immediately awaking from anesth. Within 48 hours no residual pain. 2 patients unrelieved by DBS **Complete pituitary destruction** Diabetes insipidus in all lasting 9, 5, 4 months. During the 1st postop. year, prolactin back to normal but cortisone and thyroid depressed **Periodic naloxone testing: CP not triggered**. **Hormones and endorphins** *not* **responsible for relief**
Miles (1998)	CCP (1 patient) plus another CP?	Hypophyseal stimulation	0%	
Hayashi *et al.* (2007) Includes: Hayashi *et al.* (2005)	CPSP, thalamic (27 patients) **2002–2006**	Pituitary **gamma knife radiosurgery** targeting the area connecting the pituitary gland and stalk and the lower part of the stalk into the 50% prescription isodose area; 8 mm collimator, max. irradiation 140–180 (mean 159) Gray (average dose to stalk less than half to gland).	Pain reduction marked in 17 patients (71%) usually within 2 days after treatment. Effect lasted less than 3 months in 5 and less than 6 months in another 5. At last control, marked pain reduction in 5 (21%). One patient had numbness worse, but pain improved Follow-up: 1–4 years (mean 3) in 24 patients	Pre-existing numbness unaffected. 42% of patients had treatment-related side effects (33% severe hormonal abnormalities) Neuromodulatory effect hypothesized

Hypothalamotomy and hypophysectomy

Unlike cancer pain, posteromedial hypothalamotomy is not effective for CP and other neurogenic pains (Amano 1998). Interestingly, chronic cancer pain disappears, but pain can still be induced by pinprick, a dissociation observed after medial thalamic lesions. According to Jürgens *et al.* (2009), deep brain stimulation of the posteromedial hypothalamus modulates thermal sensitivity and pain thresholds.

What remains puzzling is why pituitary lesions can temporarily allay some CP patients (Table 21.4). In an autoptic study of a CP patient relieved by pituitary radiosurgery until death (6 months), Utsuki *et al.* (2009) found the *adenohypophysis*, but not the neurohypophysis, *partially necrotic* (closest to stalk); no necrosis was observed in the hypothalamus and pituitary stalk. A hormonal effect has been excluded. A placebo effect is likely in reported studies, given the rate of relapse and discrepancy between pain relief (fast) and necrosis (slow onset).

Chapter 22

Neurophysiological studies

Recording/stimulation studies of brain central pain

(1) Obrador *et al.* (1957) failed to elicit pain by stimulating the thalamus in cases of CP.

(2) Nashold and Wilson (1970) reported on three CP patients. One (V.H., female) was affected by severe paroxysms of right lancinating facial pain plus dull, aching pain ("thalamic pain"), both worse in the cheek (which became red), due to "vascular mesencephalic lesion" associated with subarachnoid hemorrhage. During the pain paroxysms, EEG recording demonstrated "in the left dorsal mesencephalic tegmentum epileptiform spike activity grouped in trains lasting for the duration of the pain," and less striking EEG spikes coincident with dull aching pain. Electrical stimulation of this area enhanced the paroxysms, and a radiofrequency lesion eliminated both the abnormal EEG activity and the pain. Interestingly, despite gross anomalies in the anterior parietal lobe and left frontoparietal white matter (single spikes or multiple bursts at 6/s and β rhythms mixed with spike activity, with bursts every 1–3 s, minimal β activity, and slow θ), stimulation at these sites elicited no subjective responses. A second patient (P.B., male) suffered burning CP to right face, arm, and chest due to a traumatic parietal and stereotaxic midbrain lesion. Four lesions in the left dorsolateral mesencephalon, in the region in which stimulation reproduced the pain, relieved both the pain and the hyperalgesia, although an undefined discomfort in his hand lingered on. Two years later, he suddenly died from acute subdural hematoma. At autopsy, an atrophic lesion was found in the left parietal lobe. A third patient (S.M., female) suffered burning/freezing CP to the right hemisoma following thalamomesencephalic stroke. Two lesions were made in the left dorsolateral tegmentum where stimulation elicited the pain; pulvinar stimulation was silent. The patient still felt the "cold" sensation in the arm, but it was no longer unpleasant.

(3) Guecer *et al.* (1978) implanted electrodes stereotactically in (likely) Vc and nearby somatosensory nuclei and made thalamic EEG recordings (scalp EEG plus thalamograms) in seven patients with thalamic CPSP. Excessive thalamic slowing was found in four of the seven (three within range). One patient had marked rhythmical intermittent δ activity in the thalamus which was often triggered by arousing stimuli. Thalamic spindle activity was sometimes noted without concomitant spindle activity on the scalp and would occasionally occur in states of early drowsiness. All three patients with markedly abnormal scalp EEG recordings also showed excessive slowing in the thalamic leads. Marked thalamic and surface slowing of irregular (polymorphic) waveform was found to increase in the thalamic as well as the scalp leads when the patient became drowsy. In two of these three old patients, abnormal EEG scalp findings were likely due to advanced diffuse cerebrovascular disorder. Thalamic participation in the posterior α rhythm was absent or poorly developed in most patients: only two had good evidence of α rhythm, possibly depending on the electrode site (and on the degree of cortical α development). ***Marked thalamic δ activity*** likely defined a genuine pain-related abnormality (insertion trauma was ruled out by concomitant scalp EEG slowing and lack of subjective implantation complaints).

(4) Namba *et al.* (1984) reported on 11 patients with BCP. Stimulation in mesencephalic lateral tegmental fields elicited the most severe burning pain compared with Vc and internal capsule.

(5) Barcia-Salorio *et al.* (1987) studied two patients with CPSP. The preoperative EEG of patient 1 showed basal activity and marked bilateral δ waves, worse on the affected stroke side in temporal regions. The second showed slow irritative activity on scalp EEG. Deep brain recordings of scalp EEG showed ***marked δ activity in the thalamus*** of patient 1 and a cortical focus in the second case. After radiosurgical Vc thalamotomy, these findings were unchanged, despite some pain improvement.

(6) Ohye's group (Hirato *et al.* 1991), in a series of 11 patients with BCP (plus five Parkinson's disease controls), noted that "deep pain" was more marked in non-thalamic lesion (on CT) cases and "superficial pain" in cases with definite thalamic damage. Patients were submitted to microelectrode recording. In the *non-thalamic* lesion group with CP, the power amplitude voltage histogram showed a slight reduction with a mixture of various activities in and around the Vim nucleus and multiple peak configurations between 0 and 1000 Hz with a maximum at 200–300 Hz. Thalamic background neural activity in and around Vim was comparable to controls. Background neural activity in intralaminar nuclei (CL) was generally low. In *thalamic* CP, the power amplitude voltage histogram (i.e., background neural activity) showed marked decrease in and around the Vim nucleus (which shows clusters of STT fibers), suggesting damage in Vc. The background neural activity in CL was higher than in Vim, especially in its dorsal part, and was also higher than in the non-thalamic lesion group. In a case *without any CT lesion*, but a dominant superficial pain, the background neural activity in CL was relatively high. Thus, in non-thalamic CP (*deep pain* dominant), thalamic background neural activity was relatively high in Vim (where deep muscle sensation can be usually elicited), but *low in CL*, whereas in thalamic CP (*superficial pain* dominant), this was *higher in CL* than in Vim and markedly decreased in Vc. The initial small damage in Vc may have induced an abnormal state of activity in the surrounding areas in *surviving* Vc neurons and adjacent Vim neurons (and their projection areas). Ohye (1998) very often found that spontaneous activity in Vim and Vc of CP patients was considerably reduced, particularly with massive thalamic involvement. Many irregular burst discharges were encountered throughout the electrode descending in these nuclei, but he noted ***no coincidence between pain sensation and moment of burst discharge***. The topographic representation in Vim and Vc was lost. He also found more responses related, for example, to face and arm, and often convergent responses from different peripheral receptive fields (RFs). Moreover, a response to *ipsilateral* stimuli was found. Neurons of the face area (including eye movement neurons) seemed to occupy a wide area of Vim. Curiously, coagulation in this area did not change eye movements, but relieved deep pain.

(7) Fukaya *et al.* (2003) reported on cortical stimulation findings in 31 CPSP patients (28 thalamo-putamino-capsular, 3 Wallenberg's syndrome). In 23 (84%), SI stimulation at 50 Hz elicited contralateral tingling, versus 40% of non-pain patients; in 12 (39%), abnormal pain sensation or exacerbation of original CP were observed, versus 0% of non-pain patients. MI stimulation at 50 Hz had no motor effects, but evoked sensory tingling in 52% of the patients, versus 20% of non-pain patients, and very unpleasant sensations (interpreted as a sign of extensive reorganization and unfavorable prognostic sign for MCS-induced analgesia) in 6% of the patients, versus none of the non-CPSP cases. MI stimulation at 1–2 Hz evoked tingling in 25% of the patients. In these authors' experience, half of their CPSP cases submitted to Vc DBS reported more pain.

(8) Stimulation of SI at different frequencies, both invasively and non-invasively, allayed CP in some cases (see Chapter 11).

Recording/stimulation studies of cord central pain

Spinal recordings

(1) Loeser *et al.* (1968) recorded unit activity in the dorsal horn of a chronically denervated conus medullaris of a paraplegic suffering from burning rectal and thigh pain and hyperpathia following trauma: denervated cell groups (10 dorsal horn neurons *rostral to the site of injury*) had developed spontaneous high-frequency "epileptic" paroxysmal burst discharges.

(2) Evidence of high-level spontaneous activity assumed to be abnormal focal hyperactivity within

the superficial laminae of the injured cord has been recorded ***up to seven levels cephalad to injury site*** prior to computer-assisted DREZ surgery for SCI and other pains (39% of cases had hyperactivity higher than three levels above injury site) (Edgar *et al.* 1993).

(3) Falci *et al.* (2002) performed multilevel DREZ surgery on 41 CCP patients. Electrophysiological analyses of the DREZs were performed one level caudal to the injury site and *up to five DREZ levels cephalad*, exploiting an active electrode inserted free-hand 2 mm into the specific DREZ tilted 35–45° medially (the same as per coagulation). In 32 patients, additional DREZ recordings were carried out during transcutaneous C-fiber (inclusive of sympathetic fibers) stimulation in which a current perception threshold device was used (electrodes were in the distribution of a dermatome, with 5 Hz electrical stimuli activating the nerve fibers directly, but not the actual receptors in the skin due to too low current levels). The device was used for preoperative testing of dermatomal skin sensation in a C-fiber frequency band caudal to, at, and cephalad to injury level. A 5 Hz threshold above 0.35 mA was empirically assumed as significant. In general, the elevated thresholds were found in dermatomes at and cephalad to the neurological injury level in patients who were sensory-complete (occasionally also in dermatomes immediately caudal to the sensory-complete neurological level); these same skin dermatomes with elevated and *presumed* abnormal thresholds received above-threshold stimulation intraoperatively. Intramedullary recordings were then made in the DREZs corresponding to the particular skin dermatome. Data were analyzed and filtered to obtain "spindles," *presumed* to signal abnormal neural activity when exceeding 3/s. These were corroborated by higher voltage and frequencies of the activities. The same recordings were obtained after lesioning. These data were in spatial correlation with those obtained with current perception threshold. In the first nine patients, seven showed areas of DREZ neuroelectrical hyperactivity: radiofrequency microcoagulations (90 °C for 30 s) with 1 mm of separation were performed in order to silence all abnormal activity (otherwise, they were repeated). In the two cases without hyperactivity, lesioning extended at two DREZs cephalad to injury level and one below (90° for 30 s). Of the remaining 32 patients, nine, all with below-level pain, had no spontaneous DREZ hyperactivity; operative transcutaneous C-fiber stimulation of skin dermatomes with elevated C-fiber sensory thresholds resulted in evoked neuroelectrical hyperactivity in specific DREZs, *presumed* pain generators, and were used to guide lesioning: eight were totally relieved, with one failure. In the rest, both techniques guided total silencing of hyperactivity. Lack of spontaneous neuroelectrical hyperactivity in 27% of the patients was ascribed to pain being cyclical and waxing and waning in intensity: this is a poor explanation, since such a pattern would most likely be found in all other patients.

Brain recordings

(1) Lenz (1991 and references therein; Lenz *et al.* 1994) studied patients with CP following spinal cord transection. All patients experienced pain in the anesthetic part of the body; some also experienced dysesthesias in the part of the body adjacent to the area of sensory loss. They designated the area of thalamus representing the borderzone area and the anesthetic area as the borderzone/anesthetic area (BAA). Evidence of somatotopic reorganization was found. Neurons with RFs on the border of the area of sensory loss occupied more of the thalamic homunculus in Vc than in patients with controls (movement disorder patients), i.e., body parts bordering the anesthetic body part had *increased representation*. For instance, in one patient, the representation of the trunk occupied 1.2 mm of a trajectory through the part of the thalamus where the leg, anesthetic as a result of the spinal injury, is often represented. In another with clinically complete spinal transection at C6, the representation of the external ear, neck, and occiput occupied 1.5 mm of a trajectory through the forearm representation, versus 0.1–0.3 mm of neck and trunk representation in controls. Stimulation of these neurons by whatever means (e.g., touching the skin near the border of the sensory loss) could produce an abnormal sensation in the anesthetic part of the body (mislocalization). A significant increase in the number of neurons in Vc (BAA) *without RFs* was also characteristic. Unlike controls, Vc microstimulation at sites with neuronal RFs on the border of the anesthetic area of the body characteristically revealed a dissociation between the RFs and projected fields (PFs) (*RF/PF mismatch*),

with PF altered less than the somatotopic map of the inputs demonstrated by the RF. RFs were often located on the border of the anesthetic area, while PFs extended far into the anesthetic part of the body, suggesting to the authors that abnormal activity recorded in borderline regions might be reflected in sensations experienced in anesthetic areas, but also that the representation of sensory input (RFs) is much more plastic than the central representation of the part of the body (PFs). In other words, in Vc regions that would normally represent the anesthetic body part, neurons often had no RFs, although PFs were referred to the anesthetic body part, evidence that *a central representation of the anesthetic body part still exists years after total interruption of input from that part of the body*, an essential ingredient if pain is to be appreciated in that body part. Microstimulation at these Vc borderline regions often produced sensations in the anesthetic area. These regions of Vc representing parts of the body where the patient experienced pain (and possibly dysesthesias) showed *increased bursting activity*. Bursting activity was up to threefold greater for cells in the BAA without RF than for control cells (i.e., those representing body parts distant from the representation of the anesthetic part of the body). In control Vc, STT cells fired regularly at a rate of approximately 10 spikes/s, and few spike trains exhibited high-frequency bursting. In contrast, cells recorded in BAAs showed a significantly higher likelihood of a bursting pattern. Here, bursts were preceded by a period of inhibition, with the initial interspike interval being less than 6 ms in duration, becoming longer throughout the burst (i.e., decreasing number of action potentials in the burst), a pattern typical of bursts associated with Ca^{2+} spikes (as seen in sleep) and involving a low-threshold rapidly inactivating Ca^{2+} current. Moreover, cells in the BAA region without RFs had longer preburst intervals (i.e., longer periods of silence before a burst) and lower primary event rates (i.e., action potentials outside bursts). In view of their inverse correlation, these cells were believed to have tonically decreased firing rates between bursts. The most intense bursting was found in cells that appeared to be located in the posterior aspect of the Vc core and in the posteroinferior area (Lenz *et al.* 1994), where nociceptive STT terminations are most dense (Lenz and Dougherty 1997). Thermal pain-responsive cells appear to be more frequent posteroinferiorly to Vc core, with warmth and cold coded cells contiguous, but separate (see references in Hua *et al.* 2000). The increase in spontaneous thalamic activity was more pronounced with more complete interruptions of somatosensory input from a particular body part. In further microstimulation studies (Lenz *et al.* 1998) of 12 neurogenic pain patients (CPSP $n = 4$, SCI-CP $n = 4$: Lenz *et al.* 1994), and PNP ($n = 4$); controls: 10 movement disorder cases) in parts of the thalamus representing the painful area (both the core and posteroinferior areas of Vc), there was an increase in the number of sites where pain was evoked by stimulation, with a corresponding decrease in the number of sites where non-painful thermal (warm and cold) sensations were evoked. Yet the percentage of sites where pain or thermal sensations were evoked was not significantly different between parts of thalamus representing the painful and non-painful parts of the body (2%). Thus, *despite the central body image being relatively constant in the face of altered input, a reorganization occurs so that cold modalities are relabeled to signal pain in the thalamus of patients with CP*, possibly explaining cold hyperalgesia; spontaneous bursting activity at these sites may be more likely to produce the sensation of pain. In CP patients too, the number of sites where cold was evoked was significantly lower than in controls, whereas the number of sites where warmth was evoked was not different from controls (Lenz *et al.* 1994). Moreover, there was a significant increase in the number of sites where pain was evoked, but no significant difference from controls in the number of pain sites plus thermal sites.

Recording/stimulation studies in mixed series

(1) Pain and burning can be elicited in CP/PNP (but not non-pain) patients by stimulating the STT in Vc (Hassler and Riechert 1959, Levin 1966), the mesencephalon (Nashold 1974, Sano 1977, Tasker *et al.* 1983), thalamic radiations (Albe-Fessard 1973, Koszewski *et al.* 2003), and SI (Hamby 1961, Dierssen *et al.* 1969). In this latter case, the response is obtained *only* in an area related to a deafferented portion of the body, while the same stimulation in an area related to non-deafferented body parts gives

only the usual paresthesias, mimicking the patient's spontaneous pain ("in the same body part as their own pain").

(2) Epileptifom discharges related to pain paroxysms have been recorded in the lateral mesencephalic tegmentum inferior and posterior to the intralaminar nuclei in patients with PNP and CP, possibly at the site of termination of the spinomesencephalic tract (Iacono and Nashold 1982).

(3) Toth *et al.* (1984) examined neurogenic pain (including three thalamic CP cases) and non-pain patients. They studied Vc, CM, pulvinar, and mesencephalic reticular formation, with stereotactically positioned electrodes. Unlike non-pain patients, in patients with CP, the spontaneous activity in Vc and CM was strikingly dysrhythmic, containing many sharp steep waves, and the amplitude was pronounced, sometimes more than in the cortical activity. The activity contained bursts composed of sudden spike-like waves. By stimulating Vc or CM with single stimuli, 4–6 Hz waxing–waning steep potential series could be recorded. During 100 Hz/500 ms train stimulation in Vc and CM, typical electroconvulsive paroxysmal activity occurred which was strictly localized within these structures. Only slight traces appeared in the frontoparietal cortical activity (unlike Guecer *et al.* 1978). These changes were most pronounced in phantom pain (four patients), but could also be observed in CP. In CP, the spontaneous and evoked electrical activity in the specific and non-specific thalamic nuclei was characteristically paroxysmal and could be strongly enhanced from one type of nucleus to the other (Vc-medial thalamus autokindling).

(4) Tasker's group (Hirayama *et al.* 1989) performed single-unit analysis of spontaneous neuronal activity in three patients with thalamic CP and two with complete cord transection at C3 and T4, respectively (plus four PNP cases and four non-pain controls: three MS cases and one patient with dystonia following a supratentorial thrombotic stroke which produced a painless Dejerine–Roussy syndrome). They recorded three kinds of cells firing in bursts (types A–C) and one kind not firing in bursts. (1) In pain patients, 47% of the studied bursting cells were of type A, 42% of type B, and 11% of type C. Some 43% of the cells were located in Vc, 32% in Vim, 19% in Vcpc, 4% in Vop, and 2% in zona incerta. A total of 22% of bursting cells had cutaneous RFs. In other words, bursting cells typically fired at interspike intervals of 1–2 ms and interburst intervals of 50 ms. Microstimulation at sites where bursting cells were recorded usually induced no response. Bursting cells tended to be located in Vc and Vcpc (sites in pain patients believed to be in Vim could actually have been in Vc). (2) In non-pain patients, 59% of bursting cells were of type A, 23% of type B, 18% of type C. Fifty-three percent of the cells were located within Vim, 35% in centrolateralis intermedius, 6% in Vc, and 6% in Vop. None had cutaneous RFs or responded to movements. Thus, *bursting cells were rarely encountered in Vc*, and those bursting cells encountered elsewhere tended to have lower mean firing rates and longer interspike and interburst intervals. *Stimulation in Vc never induced pain.* Although it was concluded that the Vc region of pain patients (CP and PNP) contained many more bursting cells than the comparable region in non-pain patients, with different characteristics than bursting cells in non-pain patients, "***It is not possible to determine whether the bursting cells recorded in pain patients have anything to do with the pain the patient experiences.***"

The same group (Gorecki *et al.* 1989) reported thalamic exploration in 39 patients: 13 thalamic CP cases, 10 SCI pain cases, four postcordotomy pain cases, and 11 PNP cases. Macrostimulation was carried out in the first 23 cases, with microelectrode recording and microstimulation performed in the last 16 cases. In these latter cases, abnormal neuronal firing was recorded in all, as spontaneous bursts of action potentials. The interburst interval was of the order of 50 ms; 76% of bursting units did not have RFs. Stimulation at 8% of the sites where bursting units were recorded induced burning or pain, being found both in close proximity to or remote from units subserving deafferented dermatomes. The time course of appearance of these units could not be determined. Non-pain patients also demonstrated bursting cells with intervals of the order of 200 ms, burst frequency of approximately 5 Hz, usually located more anterior and dorsally with respect to Vc. Unlike normal patients, in 17 cases, 16 of whom had a clear history of hyperpathia or allodynia, stimulation in Vc elicited painful sensations, often reproducing the patient's particular pain syndrome. In 12 cases, neuronal recordings at the stimulation site indicated that the neurons had low-threshold mechanoreceptive fields corresponding to the pain location and to the dermatomes affected by sensory changes, a response most frequently obtained in Vc. *The induction of pain was thus more frequent in patients with allodynia and/or hyperpathia.*

Altered thalamic somatotopy was observed. They divided the different thalamic maps into four categories: *normal*, *empty* (when there was a general lack of response to stimulation or lack of receptive fields over a large number of trajectories or when there were only lemniscal or spinothalamic tract responses in locations at which units with receptive fields would be expected), *displaced* (thalamic units possibly shifted by atrophy or sprouting at the sites of a lesion or by altered ventricular size), and with *abnormal receptive fields*. The majority of patients with thalamic CP (8/13) had an empty thalamus. At least one patient with a thalamic infarct, but no CP, demonstrated a typical empty thalamus. In two patients, the somatotopic organization was found to have a relatively normal sequence, but individual responses were located in sagittal planes more lateral than expected. In five cases (two CCP and one thalamic CP, two PNP), somatotopic mapping demonstrated abnormal RFs. One patient with C5 clinically complete spinal cord transection had extensive RFs over the occiput and the back of the shoulders (a location where RFs have rarely been found), corresponding to the border of the deafferented region; in particular, the representation of the external ear, occiput, and neck occupied 1.5 mm of a trajectory through the part of the thalamus where the hand, anesthetic as a result of the spinal injury, would normally be represented, versus a 0.1–0.2 mm trajectory length in movement disorder cases. In this patient, there were also statistically significant differences in neuronal firing patterns in the deafferented region of the thalamus, compared with the presumably normal region of the thalamus (patient included in Lenz's series discussed above). *Two patients had wide areas of bilateral as well as ipsilateral representation with **bilateral** pain induction on stimulation.* The remainder of the patients had *"normal" maps, with a propensity for SCI patients to be in this category* (6/10). *These three types of altered thalamic somatotopy were present in patients both with and without pain states.*

In an illuminating study, this group (Parrent *et al.* 1992) reported on two patients with massive suprathalamic infarcts. Their first case, a 58-year-old woman, suffered a right hemispheric infarct following carotid endarterectomy. Shortly thereafter, she developed left hemibody CP. A cordotomy was ineffective. The pain was constant, burning, particularly significant in the shoulder. Aside from motor deficits, there was marked sensory loss on the left side, with preserved, though reduced, vibration sense in the left hand. There was no hyperpathia, barring a suggestion of cold allodynia in the left shoulder area. MRI showed parenchymal loss in the distribution of the right sylvian artery, with T1-hypointense areas in the right periventricular region. The right cerebral peduncle and thalamus were atrophic. Stereotactic exploration of the right thalamus with the patient awake and unsedated and exhaustive microrecording plus micro- and macrostimulation of Vc and medial thalamic nuclei revealed no motor or sensory responses of any kind, and no receptive fields were recorded. PVG stimulation produced no subjective sensations or effect on the patient's pain and allodynia. Their second case, a 57-year-old man, suffered a right hemispheric infarct. Almost immediately following the stroke he developed CP. Constant sharp pain was experienced in the left shoulder and hand and in the lower back and left hip (worse in the latter two), with spontaneous exacerbations occurring every 2 minutes; steady burning pain affected the medial left thigh, knee, and foot and cramping pain in the left thigh and calf. Aside from motor and other deficits, there was a diminished to absent appreciation of light touch, pinprick, and vibration in the entire left side of the body. There was allodynia to light touch and cold stimuli on the entire left side, and hyperpathia of left limbs and face. CT showed a massive infarct in the right sylvian artery distribution. Stereotactic exploration of the right thalamus with the patient awake and unsedated and microrecording plus micro- and macrostimulation obtained no motor or sensory responses. No stimulation-evoked responses were obtained in the right PVG region. Exploration of the left PVG obtained the typical stimulation responses of this region as well as acute relief of the patient's allodynia and hyperpathia. ***They concluded for a major role of the thalamus ipsilateral to pain.***

Tasker *et al.* (1994) observed bursting cells in 64% and somatotopic reorganization in all of 29 CPSP (thalamic, suprathalamic, and brainstem) patients. Recordings showed that a lesion could leave deafferented structures "*in neutral*," but capable of electrical and (therefore presumably) intrinsic stimulation to possibly produce pain. Macrostimulation of the tegmental reticulothalamic pathways (and medial thalamic nuclei), normally unresponsive to stimulation, at a threshold effective for ML/STT stimulation, induced a widespread non-somatotopographically organized burning or pain sensation (mimicking the original pain) extending beyond the involved dermatomes, often similar to that from which the patient suffered (five brainstem CPSP, one MS, one CCP). Stimulation tended to be painful in patients with evoked pain (14/16), but not without (1/4), even in the absence of contralateral functional SI (or massive hemispherectomy-like lesions); the reticular system was thus implicated in allodynia, ipsilateral structures in the mediation of constant pain (Tasker *et al.* 1983, Tasker 2001b).

Thalamic reorganization following denervation was tested by studying thalamic somatotopy (microrecording/stimulation) in 61 patients: five groups were compared according to body part in patients with pain in the deafferented body part and in controls (movement disorders). PNP and CP were considered together (Kiss *et al.* 1994). Trunk representation (RF) was significantly larger in patients with leg–foot deafferentation than in those without; however, microstimulation induced paresthesias in the face from a significantly larger thalamic area in facially denervated cases than in controls (i.e., face RFs *increased*, but maintained small discrete PFs not extending into other body parts). There were *no* significant differences in the representation of the other body parts in the five groups. In the leg-deafferented-only group, the deafferented cells responded to afferent input from an adjacent body part, yet retained their original connections to the cortical representation of the deafferented body part. In face-deafferented patients, deafferented cells ceased to respond to peripheral inputs, yet maintained their thalamocortical projections to the original body-part representation. In some patients, deafferented cells could both stop responding to peripheral input and communicate meaningfully with their cortical target.

TheVc core (*but not* other nuclei more ventroposterior to Vc) was studied in five thalamic, three suprathalamic, two internal capsule, and three cortical CP cases (versus 23 non-stroke pain and 24 movement disorder patients) with stereotactic microrecordings (Davis *et al.* 1996). Microstimulation in the *tactile core of Vc* commonly evoked paresthesias, while threshold stimulation *never* evoked pain in non-stroke patients and rarely (2%) did so in movement disorder patients. By contrast, in CP, 28% of Vc sites microstimulated evoked painful sensations at threshold (suprathreshold stimuli did so at 46% of Vc sites in CP versus 8% in other pains and 12% in movement disorder cases). There was no significant difference between the paresthesia thresholds of non-CP patients and motor patients, but these were *elevated twofold in CP patients*, except four (two patients with particularly small thalamic lesions and two patients with small cortical lesions). However, stimulation thresholds to elicit pain were similar in all patient groups. CP patients most often noted the stimulation-evoked pain as a *nondescript pain (33% of sites) or painful burning sensations (43% of sites)*, shocking (10%), or sharp (14%). In control groups, pain was elicited only with stimuli suprathreshold for paresthesias. Most common with suprathreshold stimuli was an unpleasant (or sometimes shocking) feeling in the non-CP pain group (61% of sites) and movement disorders (45%). The burning sensation so often reported by CP was never reported by the movement disorder patients and *at only two sites in the non-CP patients.* Interestingly, *qualities of evoked pain in pain patients did not necessarily relate to the quality of the patient's ongoing chronic pain.* Pain could be evoked at sites throughout tactile Vc, although most sites were located in the *ventral two-thirds.* Microstimulation within Vc almost always evoked a response, *even in the presence of suprathalamic infarcts* (and also with thalamic lesions). Vc stimulation in 62% of CP patients evoked pain: *this was not related to allodynia*, since pain was evoked in patients with (4/7) and without (3/6) it. In some CP patients, pain was evoked throughout the electrode trajectory within Vc, a clustering not seen in the other two groups. *At some Vc sites in CP patients, stimulation up to maximum current (up to 100 μA) did not evoke any sensation.* Suprathreshold stimuli in CP converted only a few responses from paresthesia to pain. In some patients with pain, there appeared to be a *decrease in cell density* in regions representing body parts whose afferents had been damaged. Although RF/PF mismatches in non-pain patients were noted for nearly half of Vc, they were minor or simple size discrepancies; stimulation at only 9% of Vc in these control patients resulted in gross mismatches. The total number of RF/PF mismatches was significantly greater *in both pain groups* compared with the motor group, due to a greater increase in gross rather than minor or size mismatches in the pain patients. *The proportion of all mismatches was the same in the non-CP and CP groups, and size mismatches were similar between CP and non-CP patients.*

In a major study, Radhakrishnan *et al.* (1999) compared the incidence of bursting in Vc of patients with neurogenic pain (including CPSP and SCI, whose numbers were not specified) and motor disorders. ***The burst indices*** (i.e., the number of bursting cells per track) ***in the pain and non-pain groups were not significantly different from each other***. Low-threshold Ca^{2+} spike-evoked bursts (with shortening of the first interspike interval, an increase in the number of interspike intervals in the burst, and progressive prolongation of successive interspike intervals) were identified in 57% of bursting cells in pain patients and 47% in non-pain patients, ***suggesting no definite rapport with pain***. Only a few cells of the bursting kind were located in Vc, the majority being anterodorsal and ventroposterior to it (see also Ohye and Narabayashi 1972).

Finally, they (Manduch *et al.* 1999) did microelectrode recordings in 40 movement disorder and 37 chronic pain patients through Vc and regions ventroposterior to it. Stimulation evoked painful or innocuous thermal sensations at 2.9% and 4.7%, respectively (5023 stimulation sites). A total of 77% were located ventroposterior to Vc, and of these 74% were located in or medial to the face/hand representation border in Vc. No significant differences were noted between controls and non-CPSP cases in the incidence of pain and temperature sites. Instead, the incidence of pain sites was higher in CPSP cases ($n = 11$) compared to the other two groups (9.5% versus 2.5% in the ventroposterior region of Vc and 15.1% versus 1.4% in Vc). In contrast, the incidence of thermal sites was lower below Vc in CPSP than in the other two groups, but *not different in Vc*.

(5) Rinaldi *et al.* (1991) observed bursting in PNP and CP (two cases), occurring in two patterns, short bursts of 2–6 spikes every 1–4 s or a long burst of 30–80 spikes, at an average rate of a burst every 1–4 s. This activity was found concentrated to the lateral aspect of MD, CL, and only a small part of CM-Pf complex.
(6) Yamashiro *et al.* (1991) made microrecordings in the Vc of two patients with SCI, one with CPSP, one with MS-associated CP, and four PNP cases. Epileptiform discharges from hyperactive neurons were recorded and two firing patterns seen. One showed regular firing which had 3–5 trains of epileptiform grouped discharges with a frequency of 4–5 Hz. The latter showed continuous firing. These hyperactive neurons were distributed in Vc, Vim, and Vop and may have received facilitation from SI/MI.
(7) Jeanmonod *et al.* (1996) recorded unit activities from the thalami of 74 fully awake patients with CP and PNP. Some 99.8% of their medial thalamic units did *not* respond to somatosensory stimulation (in contrast to a few other studies: see Lenz and Dougherty 1997). In addition to their unresponsiveness, half of the units showed a striking bursting (45.1%) activity (rhythmic: 25%; random: 30%). The rhythmic/random low-threshold Ca^{2+} spike (LTS) bursting units were considered abnormal and were found distributed throughout the posterior half of CL. The rest of their sampled units displayed unresponsive sporadic activities. Many of them exhibited occasional LTS bursts. LTS bursts displayed a θ rhythmicity, with a mean interburst discharge rate of about 4 Hz. In patients with intermittent pain without a steady component, they made recordings only during pain-free periods, and never showed a large amount of LTS bursts, as can be the case in patients with steady pain.

This group produced further highly questionable studies. In one of these (Sarnthein *et al.* 2006), they collected 17 initial patients: two were excluded due to suboptimal scalp EEG, two were not available for EEG at both 3 and 12 months, three were still awaiting follow-up EEG, and three died postoperatively due to "*unrelated causes*" (!?). The seven remaining patients were compared to 15 healthy controls (which is the incorrect choice, the correct one having been an analogous group of neurally injured patients without pain). EEG was analyzed in the eyes-closed condition because "less prone to artifacts" and because "neurogenic pain ... more easily accessed in the brain's 'idling mode'" (!?). They referred to EEG bands as θ (4–9 Hz), α (9–12 Hz), β (12–25 Hz), and γ (25–100Hz), whereas other studies used different ranges.While the initial poorly described 15 patients included two CPSP, one tumoral case with trigeminal pain, and one SCI case with leg pain (11 PNP patients), the authors did not define the pain type of the final group. Also, no data are available on the postoperative course of three CP patients, while an undetailed one appears to have been 100% relieved at 3 and 12 months. Finally, patients were assessed on antiepeileptics, which are known to alter the EEG. There was a reduction in θ power at 12 months "probably related to the surgical intervention ($p < 0.02$)," which is rather weak significance. Other frequency bands were insignificantly changed by surgery. In a duplicate, slightly expanded, study (Sarnthein and Jeanmonod 2008), they collected 28 patients with neurogenic pain in whom they microrecorded thalamic local field potentials in posterior CL and scalp EEG simultaneously. However, 18 (64%!) patients were excluded because of null finding of coherence due to "heartbeat artefacts in the LFP, uncertainties in the preparation of the LFP recording electrode and/or yet undocumented physiological factors" (!?). In the remaining 10, thalamocortical coherence exceeded 20%. Bromazepam was given 4–5 hours before recording. Although no data were given, it may be that four of these 10 cases were CP cases. In this study, the band frequency range differed from the previous one (δ: 1–4; θ: 4–9 Hz, α: 9–13 Hz, β: 13–20 Hz) for reasons unknown. The EEG power peaks were seen at 8.3 Hz, 8.3 Hz, 7.6 Hz, 7.7 Hz and the LFP power peaks at 8.3 Hz, 8.2 Hz, 7 Hz, 10.4 Hz (i.e., α and not only θ). Thalamocortical coherence peaked at 8.8, 8.5, 7.5 and 6.8 Hz, the full-width-at-half-maximum at 1.2,1.5, 2 and 1.8 Hz and the height at 68%, 27%, 36% and 26%. An α peak was also observed in hemibody pain cases. The α peak commonly found in healthy people was reduced/absent in both frontal and parietal areas. The highest thalamocortical coherence values were seen in the θ band in midfrontal electrode sites; no α thalamocortical coherence was observed. Given the serious flaws of this study, the authors'conclusion ("the basic TCD mechanism is the same for all locations where neurogenic pain is felt by the patients") is totally unwarranted.

(8) The Oxford group (Green *et al.* 2009) microrecorded in a group of four CP and eight PNP patients submitted to PAG DBS in three, Vc DBS in six, and both in another three.The most prominent finding was characteristic spindle-shaped bursts of increased amplitude at a mean of 10 Hz (slightly different in different people: 8–14 Hz) in both Vc and PAG concomitant with subjective awareness of pain. There was a significant increase in the number of bursts and increasing VAS for each patient and an increased ratio of burst-time to non-burst-time activity in the pain state. Each patient had an individual neural signature. In general, power spectra showed that there is a significant rise in the 8–12 Hz (α) activity in the PAG and a rise in the 17–30 Hz (β or γ?) activity in Vc. These spindles are rather harder to understand in PAG than in Vc. So the mechanism of this signature remains unknown and non-specific.

Evoked potentials studies

(1) Mauguière and Desmedt (1988) differentiated four types of CP of thalamic origin by somatosensory evoked potentials (SSEPs), which explore dorsal column–medial lemniscal (DC/ML) function: group 1 had no CP, but complete hemianesthesia and loss of cortical SSEPs on the affected side (analgic thalamic syndrome); group 2 had CP, severe hypoesthesia, and loss of cortical SSEPs; group 3 had CP and hypoesthesia, with cortical SSEPs present, although reduced or delayed on the affected side; group 4 had CP with preserved touch and joint sensations and normal SSEPs (pure algetic thalamic syndrome). All their 30 patients presented a thalamic lesion on CT. SSEPs did not distinguish groups 1 and 2, but separated these two groups from group 3, in whom cortical SSEPs were present.

(2) Wessel *et al.* (1994) studied 18 patients with a single ischemic thalamic lesion, who had

somatosensory disturbances and/or CP in the opposite hemibody, by correlating their clinical symptoms, SSEPs, and CT imaging findings. Patients were divided into three groups: (1) those with somatosensory deficits, CP, and abnormal SSEPs, which comprised two-thirds of the patients (classic thalamic pain syndrome); (2) those with somatosensory deficits, no CP, and abnormal SSEPs (analgetic thalamic syndrome), with a 1-year follow-up; and (3) those with almost normal sense perception, CP, and normal SSEPs (pure algetic thalamic syndrome). Six of the eight patients with the analgetic syndrome had a posterolateral thalamic stroke in the territory of the geniculothalamic artery, which includes Vc, whereas groups 1 and 3 had CT evidence of paramedian or anterolateral thalamic lesions.

(3) Misra *et al.* (2008) studied 31 consecutive CPSP patients with MRI and SSEPs (the latter in 22 cases). SSEPs were abnormal in 15 patients and normal in seven. Patients with thalamic lesions had more frequent abnormal SSEPs (10/14) compared to non-thalamic cases (5/8) ($p = 1$, non-significant). The anatomical location of stroke was unrelated to the severity of CP and SSEP abnormalities.

Scalp recording studies

(1) Stern *et al.* (2006) conducted a continuous EEG and LORETA (low-resolution tomography) study. LORETA is a brain imaging method that computes inverse solutions that approximate the cortical sources from EEG recordings and is good at detecting spreading oscillatory activations. Similarly to studies from the same group (Sarnthein *et al.*, above), this too is flawed. They again started with 18 patients submitted to CL thalamotomy: three died postoperatively, two were not available for EEG, five were still waiting (!?). In the subgroup of six remaining patients, one may have been CP, but no details whatsoever were given. For some reasons, the trigeminal group exhibited "more differential power" and "a strong involvement of midCC and the insulae" compared to leg pain cases. The relevance of this study to CP is nil.

(2) Herbert *et al.* (2007) compared the EEG (64 channels) between 10 individuals with SCI and 10 age- and sex-matched able-bodied controls. SCI participants had chronic (> 12 months) paraplegic clinically complete injuries. The 64 channels of EEG data were spread diffusely over the cortex and were compared for δ (2–4 Hz), θ (4–8 Hz), α (8–13 Hz), and β (13–30 Hz) wave components of the EEG frequency spectra. No significant magnitude or directional changes were found in the δ (2–4 Hz) or θ (4–8 Hz) wave frequency bands between these two groups. However, significant and consistent decreased α wave (8–13 Hz) and increased β wave activities (13–30 Hz) were found in the SCI participants across the cortex compared to the able-bodied control group. The same group (Boord *et al.* 2008) recorded the EEG in the eyes-open (EO) and eyes-closed (EC) conditions in 16 participants with paraplegia (eight with neuropathic pain and eight without pain) and matched able-bodied controls. Common EEG artifacts were removed using independent component analysis (ICA). Peak frequency in the θ/α band and EEG power in the δ, θ, α, and β frequency bands were compared between groups. The results show significant slowing of the EEG in people with neuropathic pain. Furthermore, people with neuropathic spinal cord injury (SCI) pain had significantly reduced EEG spectral reactivity in response to increased or decreased sensory input flowing into the thalamocortical network, as modulated by the eyes-open and eyes-closed states.

(3) Wydenkeller *et al.* (2009) studied evoked potentials following contact heat in 26 complete SCI (eight at cervical, nine at thoracic levels) patients: 17 patients suffered below-level CP (not at-level; however, they state, "in subjects with complete SCI, the location below the SCI was often situated in the border zone of the injury with some preserved function" – which is at-level!), whereas nine were pain-free. There were 26 healthy controls. CCP was symmetrically distributed on both sides, except in one case. A trend towards a higher prevalence of CCP in incomplete versus complete SCI was seen, while hyperalgesia to pinprick was equally found in both pain and non-pain patients (it should be noted that the presence of evoked pain is sufficient to make a diagnosis of CCP!). Ninety-four percent of pain SCI patients and 71% of pain-free SCI patients had STT dysfunction on CHEPs. Drugs were maintained: almost half were on strong analgesics. Time since injury was significantly shorter in CP

patients. The EEG 10–20 surface electrodes were modified to: Fz/7/8, Pz, O1/2, and A1/2 omitted; Fpz, AF1/2, F5/6, FCz/3/4, FT9/10, Cz/3/4, CPz/3/4, TP9/10, P3/4/7/8, Poz/9/10, and Iz added; Fp1'/2' 10% more laterally than Fp1/2. Their choice of frequency ranges was δ (2–6 Hz), θ (6–8 Hz), α (8–12 Hz), and β (12–30 Hz). The EEG peak frequency was significantly slower in SCI than in controls but there was no peak power difference. In patients without pain sensation below the zone of partial preservation, the EEG peak frequency showed a significant relationship to the extent of deafferentation, with slowing relating to more injured segments. Normalized EEG peak frequency was slower in CP than in non-CCP patients ($p = 0.03$, which is a rather weak significance), which remained even after excluding those on neuroactive drugs ($p = 0.034$, again weak). The EEG peak frequency of CP cases did *not* correlate with the mean pain intensity experienced in the 2 weeks before the measurement, both on and not on drugs. In contrast to the EEG peak frequency, **neither peak nor band power correlated with the extent of deafferentation and did not differ between SCI patients and controls or SCI with and without CP. The peak and band topographies did not differ statistically between these groups**. This study was limited by the heterogeneous population, which called for normalization.

(4) Churyukanov *et al.* (2010) conducted an EEG study of MS patients suffering CP and found β and θ excess in these patients as compared to pain-free MS patients.

Conclusions

Anomalous activity at several CNS levels is observed in CP patients. However, most anomalies are seen *both* in PNP and CP patients, making them *non-specific*; most importantly, they are not invariably found.

Some findings involve the thalamus in the genesis of CP: (1) an increased incidence of pain evoked at threshold in Vc (core and shell) in CP versus PNP or other controls (see also Hassler and Riechert 1959, Levin 1966, Mazars 1975); (2) a likely role of thalami ipsilateral to CP; (3) thalamic involvement in cold allodynia.

Awake human recording studies clearly show how many Vc neurons respond with activity related to conduction via Aδ/C fibers, sometimes including LTS bursts, with noxious laser responses seen in both Vc core and Vcpc (Kobayashi *et al.* 2009). Vc processes both non-noxious and noxious thermal stimuli, while more medial thalamic sites process mechanical (but not thermal) pain (Bowsher 2005b), and sensations are more likely to be referred to deep structures at stimulation sites in Vc posteroinferior areas than in the core (Lenz and Dougherty 1997). A critical volume of Vc must be involved before cool sensation is impaired, whereas perception of warm is impaired only in lesions involving nuclei posterior to Vc (Kim JH *et al.* 2007). Thus, **different participation of *Vc, Vim, and CL* and/or other nuclei may contribute to different qualities of CP**.

CP usually requires an at least partially intact thalamus, ipsi- or contralaterally, as proved by too massive a thalamic destruction being incompatible with CP (see SSEP data above and Spiegel's case of remission in Chapter 20). Lhermitte (1936) suggested that CPSP is rare in patients in whom the thalamus is completely or almost completely destroyed by a large hemorrhagic lesion. Ohye (1998) found that the initial hemorrhage or infarction in the thalamus is rather small (less than 1 cm in diameter) in cases that developed CP within 1 year; patients with massive thalamic involvement following initial stroke did not manifest CP, but only hypoesthesia in general. Similarly, in the series of Chung *et al.* (1996), large hematomas occupying the whole thalamus were accompanied by hypoesthesia, but no CPSP was observed, unlike smaller lesions involving the Vc area. Thus, the sensory thalamus is necessary for CP to arise.

Somatotopic rearrangements (such as expansion of adjacent regions into denervated) and burst firing (see Appendix) seem to be the result of denervation injury, and not a correlate of pain, since they can be observed in non-pain conditions (Jeanmonod *et al.* 1996, Tasker 2001b). Since Vc stimulation evokes tactile allodynia more commonly in CP than non-CP pains (Davis *et al.* 1996, Lenz *et al.* 1998), pain more frequently in those with hyperalgesia than in those without, and in the representation of the part of the body where the patient experienced hyperalgesia more often than in the representation of other body parts (Lenz *et al.* 1998), the findings discussed may have a special relevance to the genesis of evoked pain (see Chapter 26).

CNS injury (denervation) leads per se to slowing and other changes in EEG activity: reviewed studies do not prove that CP is truly accompanied by greater slowing, and thus add little to our neurophysiological understanding. Interestingly, acute pain is known to suppress spontaneous oscillations in right SI, MI, and BA17, and this may have an alerting function (Ploner *et al.* 2006). Also, tonic pain in healthy humans decreases α power and mostly increases β power (Chang *et al.* 2002).

The reticular formation (and related propriospinal cells and fibers in the DREZ) appears to be involved (Cassinari and Pagni 1969). Andy (1987,1989) believed that chronic pain is a reticular formation syndrome *tout court*, recruited by a low-threshold "pain oscillator" that is generated at one reticular site and subsequently permeates the rest of the multisynaptic short axon core of the reticular system. Therapeutic stimulation "jams" these low-threshold reverberating and recurring mini-discharges, which can be easily activated by a variety of sensory and cognitive inputs. According to Tasker *et al.* (1980), in "patients with deafferentation pain the medial midbrain tegmentum becomes hypersensitive to stimulation, and that along with posterior thalamus, thalamic radiations and somatosensory cortex, acquires the property, absent in somatic pain syndromes, of generating not only a painful conscious awareness but also a reasonably accurate reproduction of the patient's pain," but only in the already painful sites; "due to deafferentation, mesencephalic reticulo-thalamic-cortical circuits become sensitive not only to electrical stimulation but also to natural neural input."

Box 22.1. Rhythms of the brain: ready for prime time?

Underneath the raw EEG, there are multiple oscillatory (oscillation being an alternation between states of excitation and inhibition) streams – or waves – interacting over a wide range of frequencies (0.01–1000 Hz) along a power law (1/f) continuum (Sporns 2011). Some are locked in synchrony with each other (interlocking rhythms), some are phase locked (if there is synchrony with a lag time), many are transiently coordinated, others show cross-frequency coupling. Waves can also **interfere** with each other and degrade signaling, but might also have other roles we still do not understand. There is no perfect agreement on the boundaries between standard frequency bands (e.g., β band 13–25 Hz, γ band 26–1000 Hz) and there should probably be no rigid numbers until there is a better understanding. Very-low-frequency waves down to 0.1 Hz are also present. The α (8–12 Hz) rhythm reflects the selective suppression of task-irrelevant areas and activities in the brain, but is suggested to play a functional role in human cognition and not to be simply an idling rhythm. Different γ sub-bands routinely seem to do different tasks, and these appear to be under cholinergic control.

Some authors suggest that all brain oscillations are carried or grouped (**multiplexing**, i.e., multiple coexisting neural codes operating on different timescales, **concatenation** and **nesting**) by very slow oscillations, cycling at less than 0.5 Hz. There is direct evidence for multiplexing of γ waves on θ waves (and perhaps on α waves as well). The basic advantage of multiplexing is to lower the firing threshold of downstream neurons by reducing their membrane polarity. Thus, θ waves may spread to some target populations and make them slightly more sensitive, after which added γ waves may push them over the firing threshold. If the target neurons are able to follow the input at γ rates, they may then produce their own synchronized γ burst, thereby igniting a larger population of neurons (amplification). High levels of γ oscillations exist for sensory processing and attentional enhancement of sensory input, with both high intensity of γ activity and synchrony.

γ Synchrony allows for finer temporal resolution than the slower α. A group of interconnected neurons can strengthen each other's firing rates in the γ range by supplying synaptic inputs within the 10 ms window. At, e.g., 50 Hz it is possible to sustain an excitatory feedback loop, because converging signals can arrive within the critical 10 ms period. Below 30 Hz different spikes may arrive too late to have additive effects. Thus, a group of neurons firing in the β–γ range will exert a stronger drive on downstream neurons than lower frequencies.

Synchrony is a pervasive feature of the brain, apparently to coordinate local patches of neurons at different locations in the midst of non-synchronized populations. Synchronous activity appears to be a self-organizing feature of neurons, with multiple signaling roles (including signal boosting). Excitatory neurons can synchronize their firing when they are driven by a common inhibitory cell (coding by synchrony) (Buzsaki 2006).

Neuronal synchrony (both spike synchrony at the local level and oscillatory activity at the global level) is the most commonly suggested mechanism for population coding (i.e., neurons "work together" in coding relevant information). Oscillatory synchrony appears to be involved in coordinating long-distance neuronal communication with different frequencies of oscillatory synchrony according to a particular process (attention, memory, etc.). Locally, networks of recurring GABA neurons display extensive synchronous and oscillatory firing and pyramidal layer

V neurons have intrinsic oscillatory activity in the γ range. γ Synchrony has been implicated in **temporal binding**, i.e., the emergence of a conscious percept by synchronizing widely spaced neuronal patches. The global workspace theory of consciousness implicates brief γ phase-locking between distant parts of the cortex (Baars and Gage 2010). However, the role of γ in feature binding remains a matter of dispute and controversy, and evidence for temporal binding has proven difficult, with poorly defined and inconsistent evidence (Uhlhaas *et al.* 2009; see Velik 2010 for an overview of alternatives, including binding via isochronicity, by changing conduction velocity within the individual axons: conduction velocities slow down 10-fold upon entering the cortex). In spike synchrony too, the stimulus-dependent network properties that generate perceptually relevant synchrony are unclear (bursting? con/divergence? oscillations? chaos?) (Baars and Gage 2010). More generally, it has proved extremely difficult to demonstrate a causal relationship between oscillatory activities in the brain and overt behavior output (Panzeri *et al.* 2010).

In sum, emergent properties of neuronal networks are defined by synchrony, which can involve small local networks engaged in spike synchrony or large global networks that appear to communicate via different oscillation frequencies (i.e., independently of anatomical connectivity alone, which can be absent for a specified functional network: Mantini *et al.* 2007). Spike synchrony can code information that is independent of firing rate and can be informationally additive. However, absence of synchrony might still convey information.

Brain waves often interact with each other, with slower rhythms tending to group faster ones. Interactions are often transient and related to specific tasks. Waking rhythms may add/subtract, synchronize/desynchronize, phase lock, and multiplex. Slower waves may carry (multiplex) faster waves. Very slow oscillations (0.1–0.5 Hz), δ (0.5–3 Hz), θ (4–7 Hz), α (8–12 Hz), β (13–29 Hz), and γ (30–120 Hz) all may be multiplexed under some conditions: θ commonly carries γ activity. Although brain architecture is conducive to promoting synchrony, either globally through oscillations or locally through spike synchrony, what remains to be determined is whether the synchrony means anything functional (Jermakowicz and Casagrande 2007). Synchrony does not always seem to provide a better code than the firing rate in the somatosensory system. Thus, if information coding certainly involves some sort of population code (encoding time window, rate code, temporal latency code, temporal interspike intervals code, temporal phase of firing code, Shannon informational exchange), no general consensus exists as to exactly how this works. Given the current state of affairs, it seems premature to try to integrate this knowledge in any CP theory.

Chapter 23

Imaging studies

There are quite a few publications that are senseless and do not enhance our understanding of brain function.
N. K. Logothetis (2010)

Imaging studies are fraught with li\mitations that cast a pall on their usefulness (Canavero and Bonicalzi 2007a, pp. 250–1). This is a classic example of a technology-driven field, namely, patients with a certain condition are scanned and inferences adapted to findings. The danger is clear: without a prior well-laid-out theory, results can be interpreted differently according to results, which will most likely differ in other similar studies. This is also where the duo of bad science and bad refereeing reaches its zenith. Other fields are equally not immune. In social neuroscience, for one, fMRI studies led to implausibly high correlations between brain activation and particular forms of behavior: papers often published in high-profile journals (e.g., *Nature*) are "fundamentally flawed" ("shaky literature") (Vul *et al.* 2009).

All available techniques reveal only the presence of brain activity, but it is very difficult, if not impossible, to understand what exactly an activated region is doing (Logothetis 2010), and structural techniques, such as diffusion-based tractography of the entire human brain, are still in their infancy. Recently, it has become fashionable to statistically estimate "functional" and "effective connectivity" among spatially remote brain areas (nodes and edges) in different conditions, including chronic pain, using sophisticated techniques (e.g., Granger causality) (Sporns 2011). Similar methods:

> could produce different results that are sometimes not resolvable ... as it is practically impossible, at least in the foreseeable future, to record from every corner of the brain, these directionality estimates need to be interpreted very carefully within the limitations of biological knowledge ... The results are *meaningless without a theoretical context* ... *There should be a strong theory driven explanation for differences observed in the measurements* ... neural noise is the ultimate reason why statistical methods need to be applied carefully (Young and Eggermont 2009, emphasis added).

Similarly:

> the inappropriate representation of nodes and edges in a network and failure to consider the dynamics of the system of interest will lead to misleading conclusions and generally poor results ... (Wang *et al.* 2010) Small world topology is plausible for low frequency functional connectivity as derived from fMRI and electrophysiological data below the alpha rhythm. The evidence available so far about functional connectivity at higher frequencies is incomplete ... in all cases, even for anatomy, network descriptions are only approximations of the real systems (Ioannides 2007).

Cogently, there is no commonly agreed definition of what constitutes a functional node in the brain, and:

> it is possible that ... slow coupled fluctuations of EEG power and BOLD signal do not reflect a dynamic baseline of interareal temporal interaction but a more basic neurophysiological mechanism unrelated to functional neuronal communication (Mantini *et al.* 2007).

That said, all current imaging studies of CP are burdened by clear limitations:

(1) small numbers of patients per study;
(2) considerable differences in results between studies, likely due to a high level of heterogeneity of patients in terms of topography and etiology of the lesion, pain location, intensity, duration and quality, and associated symptoms;
(3) unstandardized inclusion criteria;
(4) frequent lack of quantitative (or even qualitative) information about the sensory deficits associated

with pain ("variations in the activation of somatosensory systems in the brain may have been due to differences in the magnitude of sensory deafferentation, independent of pain": Moisset and Bouhassira 2007);

(5) a large proportion of patients on analgesic treatments, which may have biased the results;
(6) variable proportions of patients presenting spontaneous continuous pain of variable intensity, which may have masked the effects of allodynia;
(7) the contralateral side used as a "control" in almost all studies, even though bilateral alterations follow unilateral neurological lesions;
(8) psychological variables, such as attention, anticipation, emotional state, former experiences, anxiety, depression, and catastrophizing, not assessed in many studies: these may strongly affect pain and imaging results (Moisset and Bouhassira 2007).

Also, trial averaging techniques remove noise which actually may convey important, especially rapidly transmitted, information (Ioannides *et al.* 2002, Logothetis 2010). This suggests that single case studies may provide better insights than group studies, and between-group (patients vs. controls) comparisons that find BOLD group differences could be explained by GABA concentrations regardless of the actual experimental paradigm (Muthukumaraswamy *et al.* 2009).

Interpreting fMRI data relies on the assumption that hemodynamic responses reflect neuronal activity. This assumption may be less robust than generally assumed. The coupling may depend on the specific circumstances and the task. Importantly, inhibitory and excitatory neurons may be coupled differently to hemodynamics, and the relative weight of excitatory and inhibitory neurons may even be different in each trial (Vanzetta and Slovin 2010). fMRI does not differentiate between function-specific processing and neuromodulation, or between bottom-up and top-down signals; volume transmission may affect hemodynamic responses and often makes it difficult to deduce the exact role of the area in the task at hand; the BOLD signal is slow and data points are obtained about every 1.5–2 seconds, so that fMRI-based connectivity measures underestimate the degree of interregional exchange in the brain; inter- and intra-areal synchronization and oscillatory processes may not be necessarily associated with an increase in metabolism and a change in BOLD signal, limiting fMRI utility in investigating functional connectivity (Logothetis 2010). Arterial spin labeling MRI allows continuous acquisition and becomes increasingly more sensitive than BOLD to changes in neural activation as the stimulus duration exceeds 1 minute. However, it has a poor signal-to-noise ratio, differences can only be detected using a cluster-size threshold to correct for multiple comparisons, it does not provide whole brain coverage, and spatial resolution is limited compared to BOLD fMRI.

In sum, the results of human functional neuroimaging studies must be approached cautiously and abundantly supplemented by complementary data, as reviewed in other chapters.

Not all neuroimaging studies provide the same degree of information. Some refer to the spontaneous component of CP, others assess the brain response to allodynic conditions. A few address receptor anomalies, others structural anomalies. We will review them separately. fMRI studies of the spinal cord (Lawrence *et al.* 2008) have not yet been published that addressed cord CP.

Studies assessing the spontaneous resting component

See also Box 11.1.

(1) Laterre *et al.* (1988) used fluorodeoxyglucose (FDG)-PET in the resting state (twice, with a 2-month interval) to study a woman who developed CPSP due to a small right infarct at the level of the posterior putamen and posterior limb of the internal capsule, with no visible extension into the thalamus on MRI. There was right thalamic and putaminal hypoperfusion (17% asymmetry), particularly at the level of the posterior thalamic complex as well as in the putamen. No metabolic alterations were found in the cerebral cortex.
(2) Lee *et al.* (1989) studied six CPSP patients with ^{99}mTc-HMPAO SPECT: four infarctions in the thalamus and internal capsule and two hemorrhages in internal capsule-putamen (four left, two right). Three patients showed thalamic lesions and these had decreased rCBF in ipsilateral parietal (one bilaterally) and temporal cortex and one in frontal areas. Extrathalamic lesions showed no cortical anomaly.
(3) Hirato *et al.* (1993) submitted to PET studies with ^{18}FDG and a steady-state method with $C^{15}O_2$–$^{15}O_2$ nine CP patients. MRI and CT revealed definite

thalamic (3), putaminal (3), thalamoputaminal (1), and cortical parietal (2) damage. Superficial pain was more marked in cases with definite thalamic damage. In patients with a thalamic lesion, there were many irregular burst discharges in the Vop-Vim area at stereotactic microrecording. The relative value of regional cerebral glucose metabolism (rCMRGlu) decreased in the lesioned thalamus, but increased in the cerebral cortex around the central sulcus on the lesioned side. However, the relative value of regional cerebral oxygen metabolism ($rCMRO_2$) did not increase (dissociated glucose/oxygen metabolism of the same area). In patients studied with both techniques, OGMUR (oxygen–glucose molar utilization ratios) in the premotor area and SI/MI decreased more in cases with a thalamic lesion than in those with a putaminal lesion. In a patient with a combined putaminothalamic lesion, neural activity was reduced in the Vim-Vc area, with peripheral receptive fields to electrical thalamic stimulation being predominantly in the face, hand, and sometimes the foot area. In this case, the regional oxygen extraction fraction (rOEF) was markedly increased in the cerebral cortex around the central sulcus on the side of the lesion, despite the chronic stage of cerebrovascular disease. In two patients with cortical lesions, who showed mild superficial pain with or without deep pain, rCMRGlu was decreased in the lesioned cerebral cortex. Though no ischemic lesion could be demonstrated by CT, rCMRGlu was reduced in the lesioned Vc. In patients with a subcortical lesion, rCMRGlu commonly decreased in this area. Therefore, rCMRGlu in this area was decreased in all cases with CP, including cortical cases. This study then showed that OGMUR in the cerebral cortex around the central sulcus was markedly decreased on the damaged side in cases with thalamic lesions. However, in patients with a putaminal lesion, it was only moderately decreased, particularly rostrally. In patients with subcortical lesions, the more severe the superficial pain, the higher was the relative value of glucose metabolism compared to that of oxygen (which was a reciprocal value of OGMUR) in the cerebral cortex around the central sulcus on the involved side. In the patient with combined lesions, rOEF was increased in the same area. Sensory thalamic hypoactivity (decreased rCMRGlu) was seen in all cases. In sum, in the thalamic lesion group with pain (superficial pain dominant), regional oxygen (rO_2) consumption was maintained in most brain structures, except in the lesioned thalamus, while in the cortical central sulcus this was normal, but the rO_2 extraction ratio was increased and so was the relative value of regional glucose utilization compared to rO_2 consumption. In the patients with thalamic lesions and pain (deep pain dominant), both rO_2 consumption and O_2 extraction ratio were reduced in all brain structures, and so was glucose metabolism. They concluded that **increased activity in SI/MI combined with a decreased activity in Vc appeared to be a marker of CP** (Fig. 23.1), with character of pain (superficial versus deep) depending on different processing at thalamocortical levels. The same group (Hirato *et al.* 1995) reported that in one putaminal hemorrhage case (included in the above analysis) PET renormalized after successful radiosurgical Vim thalamotomy.

(4) De Salles and Bittar (1994) studied a thalamic pain patient using FDG-PET. CP appeared 2 weeks following a stereotactic biopsy for a midbrain lesion and worsened over 1 month. The patient complained of an annoying sensation of needles and at times a burning sensation on the right hemiface and hand, with hyperesthesia to pinprick and light touch on the right face and hypoesthesia

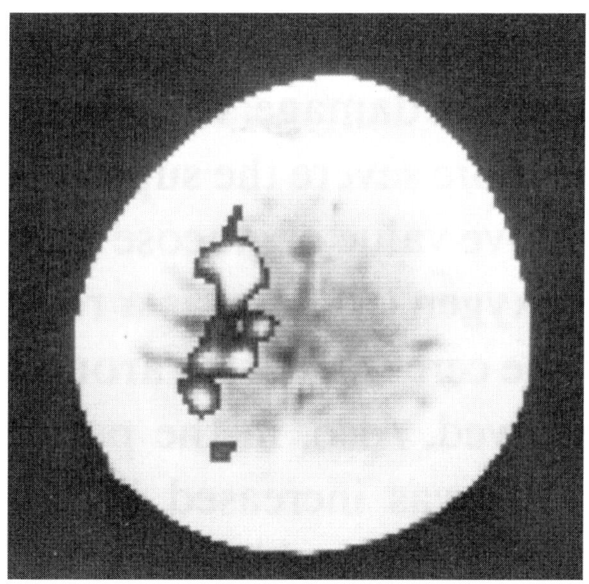

Figure 23.1. Superposition of PET and CT scans of CPSP patients showing increased activity in SI/MI (from Hirato *et al.* 1993).

to pinprick on the right fingertips. MRI disclosed that the needle had passed precisely in Vc, plus the mesencephalon (where the medial lemnicus, which courses just caudal to Vc, could have been damaged). Two months after the biopsy, PET showed marked hypo/ametabolism of the left thalamic region, right cerebellar diaschisis, and left parietal cortex hypometabolism. Ten months later, allodynia with cold intolerance persisted in the right hand and face. At this time PET showed enduring thalamic hypometabolism, with recovery of the parietal cortex anomaly (which, however, might be interpreted as a sign of hyperactivity) and the cerebellar cortex.

(5) We (Canavero *et al.* 1993, 1995a, 1999, Canavero and Bonicalzi 1995, Pagni and Canavero 1995, and unpublished observations) showed that patients with CPSP, CCP (intramedullary cyst, syringomyelia), and other CPs show basal parietal (SI) and/or frontal MI/PM/PFC (in a few cases also temporal), plus thalamic hypoperfusion on PET, HMPAO, and ECD-SPECT. These flow changes are promptly renormalized following successful treatment (propofol, evacuation, cortical stimulation) (Figs. 23.2–23.4).

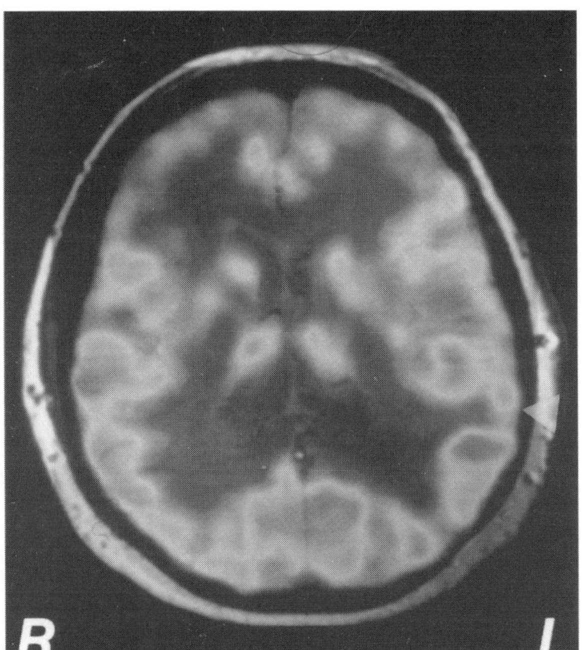

Figure 23.2. PET scan showing both SI and thalamic hypometabolism (right side of figure) in a case of BCP. *See color plate section.*

(6) Ness *et al.* (1998) studied a patient with paraplegia who, for many years, experienced rapidly fluctuating, severe, highly aversive (VAS 10), unilateral pain below the level of the lesion. The searing attacks lasted up to 10 seconds. SPECT was done in pain and non-pain conditions (threshold of significance: 10%). When experiencing pain, there was increased CBF to ACC (cingulate), increased thalamic CBF bilaterally and increased SI CBF contralaterally, plus decreased CBF in caudates bilaterally. The patient responded to gabapentin, which reduced the anomalies (and also induced mirror pain).

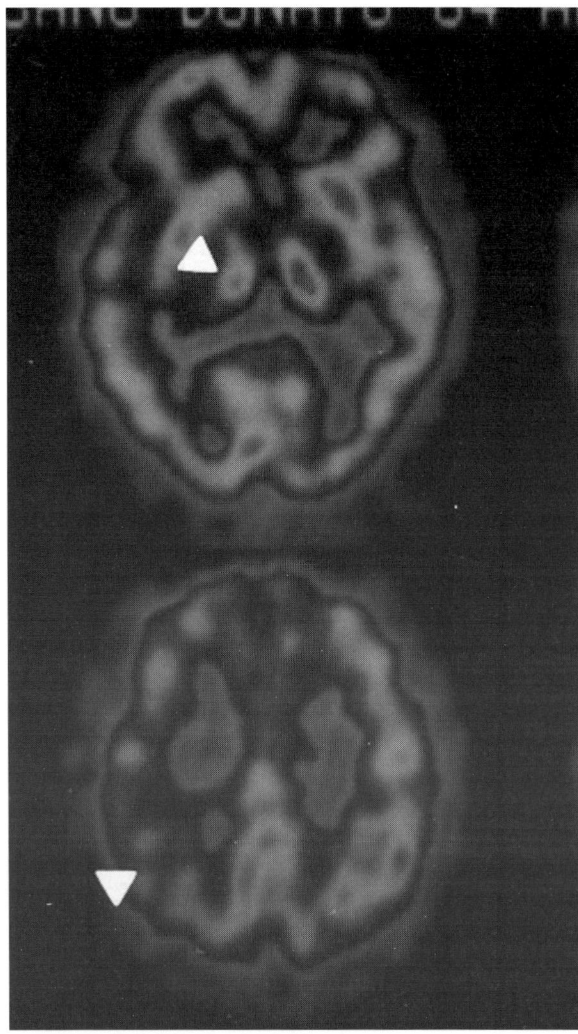

Figure 23.3. High-resolution SPECT (double-head camera) images of post-cordotomy CP. Note both thalamic (upper scan, arrowhead) and parietal hypoperfusion (lower scan, arrowhead). *See color plate section.*

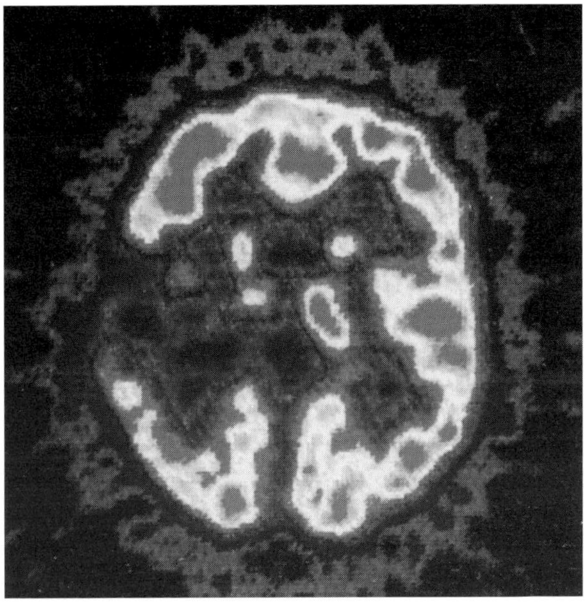

Figure 23.4. PET scan (1992) of a patient who developed central pain immediately after resection of a parietal oligodendroglioma (1987): the ipsilateral thalamus and remaining parietal cortex are both hypoactive. *See color plate section.*

(7) Doi *et al.* (1999) showed renormalization of thalamic SPECT hypoperfusion after successful convulsive therapy in five suprathalamic CP patients.

(8) Fukui *et al.* (2002b) reported on a thalamic CPSP patient with hemisoma pain. Xenon-CT was conducted before and 1 week after bilateral electroconvulsive treatment. Before ECT, the left/right thalamic CBF ratio was 61%; it rose to 85% after ECT. The left thalamic CBF after ECT increased 46%.

(9) Cahana *et al.* (2004) studied a patient with encephalitis and CP, who showed basal left thalamic (Vc region) hypoperfusion. The patient complained of "hot" left-sided paresthesias and burning pain, particularly in the chin and left palm, plus evoked pains. SSEPs were normal. Lidocaine infusions relieved the pain and the anomaly.

(10) Kishi *et al.* (2009) reported on a CPSP patient who presented with sudden mild tingling and heat anesthesia to the right hemisoma, slight pinprick hypoesthesia, but totally preserved cold sensation and no cold allodynia. MRI disclosed a small infarction in Vc with slight encroachment on the pulvinar. ECD-SPECT on the eighth day after stroke showed hypoperfusion in the left mid-CC and adjacent SMA (SI/SII CBF unchanged), ipsilateral thalamus, cerebellum, precuneus, bilateral posterior parietal cortex and dorsal midbrain. SSEPs (arm) were normal bilaterally. By the tenth day, heat anesthesia had almost disappeared, except in the face. One month and a half after stroke the patient developed full-blown CP; tingling in the right hemisoma worsened and became dysesthetic. SPECT 5 months after discharge found almost no change from the previous one. This study adds nothing, since the same CBF changes were observed with and without CP.

Studies assessing the evoked components

(1) Cesaro *et al.* (1991) studied four CPSP patients with ^{123}I-*N*-isopropyliodoamphetamine brain SPECT, with and without allodynic stimulation. In the two patients with hyperpathia (with the lesions involving the parietal subcortical white matter and the thalamocapsular area), there was hyperactivity (+20–26%) in the central thalamic region opposite the painful side. Amitriptyline relieved both the SPECT anomaly and the pain, and thermoalgesic deficits renormalized. The two patients without SPECT anomalies had subcortical or subcortical plus thalamic lesions.

(2) We (Canavero *et al.* 1993, 1995a) showed in CP patients that basal SPECT hypoperfusion of SI increases under allodynic conditions and that this anomaly spreads anteriorly to MI and other frontal areas.

(3) The Lyon group (Peyron *et al.* 1998) studied nine patients with acute unilateral CPSP after a lateral medullary infarct (Wallenberg's syndrome) with PET (resolution: 7 mm). They did *not* study spontaneous pain (present in four at a VAS value of 3–5), nor did they discuss baseline anomalies; brainstem and cerebellum were not studied. All patients showed cold allodynia (assessed with frozen water in a moving flat plastic container). During cold allodynia, statistically significant increases of rCBF were seen contralaterally to stimuli in the lateral half of the thalamus, SI, anterior insula, and inferior frontal gyrus. rCBF was increased *bilaterally* in SII and inferior (opercular) parietal areas (BA39–40) and

significantly decreased contralaterally in BA10, ipsilaterally in BA24–32, and sub-significantly in ipsilateral BA23–31. **No rCBF change was observed in BA24 (ACC).** A significant decrease was also seen bilaterally in BA18–19. During electrically (high-frequency) elicited pain to the normal side, rCBF increased significantly bilaterally in BA39–40 and SII, contralaterally in BA6 (anterior insula), ipsilaterally in BA44–45–47. rCBF decreased ipsilaterally to stimulation in BA10. Again, **no rCBF change was seen in BA24.** rCBF was significantly decreased bilaterally in BA18–19. Cold stimuli to the normal side induced significant increases in contralateral SII and BA39–40, without extending into SI, and ipsilaterally in BA46. No significant modification was detected in the thalamus and ipsilateral parietal cortex. rCBF was significantly decreased bilaterally in BA18–19 and ipsilaterally to stimulation in the caudate head. There was a sub-significant decrease in contralateral BA24–32 and ipsilateral BA10.

The same group (Peyron *et al.* 1999) studied with PET eight patients with CP (one CCP, three brainstem CP, one thalamic CP, three corticosubcortical CP). They compared rest, cold moving allodynia, and thermal heat pain. They also studied four additional patients with fMRI. Cold allodynia was associated with rCBF increases in contralateral insula-SII and SI and bilaterally in posterior parietal cortex and ACC (plus ipsilateral cerebellum). Thermal pain induced increased CBF bilaterally in insula-SII, posterior parietal, ACC, and right prefrontal cortex (plus bilateral cerebellum), but *not SI*. MR analysis showed *individual variations* in the allodynic response, except for the contralateral insular-SII activity. Compared to thermal pain, allodynic pain induced a greater activity in contralateral SI (ascribed to moving stimulus). Allodynic pain compared to control stimulation of the non-painful side showed higher activity in contralateral SI and ACC.

Peyron *et al.* (2000) also reported on a CPSP patient who complained of spontaneous paroxysmal pain, mechanical and thermal allodynia, and pinprick hyperpathia. She had severe thermal hypoesthesia of the left hand and foot. SSEPs were diminished, but not absent. This patient developed CP and allodynia in her left side after a bifocal embolic infarct following vascular surgery involving both the right parietal cortex (SI and SII) and the right rostral ACC (BA 24 and 32) plus a small anterior and inferior part of the inferior parietal lobule (BA40), plus BA6, 8, 9, and 10. Judging from the images, SI could have been still partially active, with reorganization posteriorly. SII was considered anterior to BA40 in the upper bank of the sylvian fissure. This patient was studied with both PET and fMRI, under basal (PET only), control, and allodynic stimulation. No rCBF increase was found in any part of the residual cingulate cortices, neither in the basal state (which included spontaneous pain and extensive hypoperfusion around the infarct) nor during left cold allodynic pain (see previous study). No abnormality was observed in the left cingulate cortex. PET at rest (VAS 1) showed a wide hypoperfusion including the infarct and widely extended around within the frontal and parietal cortices. Left parietal cortex, in the depth of SI, showed a significant increase of rCBF in the control condition, which remained below the statistical threshold for the allodynic condition. In the allodynic condition only, rCBF was significantly increased in the right anterior insula-SII, immediately forward to the right parietal lesion (at the boundaries of the insular-SII infarct); there were also prominent responses in the hemisphere *ipsilateral* to allodynic (but not control) stimulation: insula-SII and lateral thalamus and (sub-significantly) SI. Sub-significant rCBF increases were observed in the head of the right caudate during the control condition and in the right lateral thalamus during allodynia. **No rCBF increases, even at a sub-significant threshold, were observed in ACC on either side.** No intracerebral significant rCBF decrease was observed. Results remained unchanged even on non-normalized PET images.

Finally, these authors (Peyron *et al.* 2004) studied the brain responses of 27 patients with peripheral (5), spinal (3), brainstem (4), thalamic (5), lenticular (5), or cortical (5) lesions with fMRI as innocuous mechanical stimuli were addressed to either the allodynic territory or the homologous contralateral region. When applied to the normal side, brush and cold rubbing (which combines tactile and thermal) stimuli activated contralateral primary (SI) and secondary (SII) somatosensory cortices and insular regions. The same stimuli became severely painful when applied to the allodynic side and activated contralateral SI/SII and insular cortices with, however, lesser activation of the SII and insula. Increased activation volumes were found in contralateral SI and primary motor cortex (MI). Whereas ipsilateral responses appeared very small and restricted after control stimuli, they represented the most salient effect of allodynia and were observed mainly in the ipsilateral parietal operculum (SII), SI, and insula. Allodynic stimuli also recruited additional responses in motor/premotor areas (MI, SMA), in regions involved in spatial attention (posterior parietal cortices), and in regions linking attention and motor control (mid-ACC).

(4) Lorenz *et al.* (1998) studied a single patient who suffered Wallenberg's syndrome with selectively abolished pain and temperature sensitivity in the right leg. One year later, CP had developed in the leg, with touch and cold allodynia. P40m dipoles calculated from MEG fields after electrical stimulation of both tibial nerves were localized in SI; however, stimulation of the affected side caused deep pain sensations and elicited a large N80m component best explained by an additionally co-active dipole in the cingulate cortex. Cingulate activation was in the medial part *slightly more posterior than BA24*. Electrophysiologically, the affected limb was characterized by larger components P40 and N80 of the tibial nerve SSEP compared with the unaffected left limb. In particular, the enhanced N80 amplitude augmented in parallel with the enhancement of CPSP severity in the patient. The same group (Kohlhoff *et al.* 1999) used MEG to study four patients with Wallenberg's syndrome and CP. They found that the component around 80 ms after tibialis stimulation showed side asymmetries in the patients that exceeded the normal interindividual variability and were also reflected in the equivalent current dipole parameters. The degree of asymmetry seemed to be related to the *severity of allodynia*. They concluded that CP possibly reflected functional disorganization in SI.

(5) Jensen *et al.* (1999) studied 10 CPSP women with $H_2{}^{15}O$ PET under resting conditions and following stimulation of the painful body part and the corresponding non-painful body part with phasic heat stimuli. They observed hypoperfusion of the affected thalamic region versus non-affected thalamus under resting conditions.

(6) Olausson *et al.* (2001a) studied a hemispherectomized patient with touch-evoked pricking and burning pain, plus a robust allodynia to brush stroking (enhanced at a cold ambient temperature) in her paretic hand. Psychophysical examination showed that, on her paretic side, she confused cool and warm temperatures. On fMRI, brush-evoked allodynia activated posterior ACC, SII, and prefrontal cortex.

(7) Morrow and Casey (2002) studied a man with CPSP using $H_2{}^{15}O$ PET. He had sudden onset of constant persistent painful dysesthesias of the left hemisoma. Sensory examination was normal, barring deep pressure allodynia on the left and elevated but symmetrical cutaneous heat pain thresholds. MRI disclosed a lacunar infarction ($2 \times 4 \times 7.5$ mm) in Vc. At rest, rCBF was markedly reduced in the right Vc (as compared to left Vc) and insula. Heat stimulation (49–55 °C) of either side showed exaggerated rCBF increases relative to rest on the right (Vc and insula). They then studied four other CP (CPSP, CCP) male patients (age: 40–68), all with clinically detectable impairment of heat and/or mechanical pain sensibility on the side of CP. Each patient had abnormal, contralateral to pain, thalamic (three hemithalamic hypoactivity, one hemithalamic hyperactivity) and/or cortical asymmetry at rest and increased thalamic and/or cortical responsiveness to contralateral stimulation following contact heat stimuli.

(8) Seghier *et al.* (2005) studied a CPSP patient who suffered deep and superficial burning cold-like constant and paroxysmal pain in the left hemisoma, worse in the pectoral region, hand, and foot. The pain was triggered by cold objects and cool temperatures. He displayed a prominent mechanical allodynia. There was severe left hypoesthesia for heat, warm, and cold temperatures, selective cold allodynia, and pinprick hyperpathia. On MRI, there was an infarct of Vc and adjacent internal capsule (IC) along the STT. Under fMRI conditions, the hand was stimulated with a plastic object filled with water at 22, 15, and 5 °C (only 5 °C painful). Touch activated bilateral SI, right SII, and SMA. Increasing temperature activated the right middle insula and right medial SI. Hyperpathia activated BA24/32, BA5/7, and the left anterior putamen. The activation in the putamen and BA5/7 was *ipsilateral* to the stimulated hand. ACC activation

was not correlated with the simple cold quality of the pain-eliciting stimulus, as innocuous cold correlated with activity in, for example, right insula and right SI.

(9) Villemure *et al.* (2006) reported on a patient with typical iatrogenic cervical myelopathic CCP. The odor of cat litter, newspaper, or popcorn triggered electric shock/shooting paroxysms and also slowly increased spontaneous pain after repeated challenge. Upon moving away from the odors, pain abated. fMRI under odor challenge showed larger activations after the termination of the unpleasant odor than after the termination of pleasant ones in the contralateral thalamus, amygdala, insular cortex (bilaterally), and ACC, with similar trends in contralateral SI. Odors triggered pain only on days they were judged unpleasant.

(10) Ducreux *et al.* (2006) submitted six patients with syringomyelia and suffering CP to fMRI. Cold allodynia (felt like deep, freezing sensation, sometimes burning, with a tingling sensation) under static conditions activated the mid-posterior insula, ACC, SII, inferior parietal areas, frontal areas (BA8,9,45,46), mostly ipsilaterally, and contralateral SMA. In 2–3 patients, activation in the lenticular nucleus, hippocampus, and cerebellar lobes was also observed. Brush allodynia (felt like burning in four and electric shocks in two) activated ipsilateral and contralateral SI-SII, inferior and superior parietal cortex, ipsilateral and contralateral middle frontal gyri (including BA 45–46), contralateral thalamus, caudate, and SMA. **No activation was observed in BA24–32 or insula.**

(11) Lenz's group (Kim SH *et al.* 2007) submitted a CPSP patient with cold allodynia to a single-subject protocol of 15O-PET (voxel 2 × 2 × 2 mm) / MRI study measuring the responses to immersion of either hand in a 20 °C waterbath. The patient was scanned during rest, stimulation on the affected side, and stimulation on the unaffected side. Allodynia produced strong contralateral activation and ipsilateral inhibition around the central sulcus. There was less pronounced activation both of the inferior frontal gyrus and bilateral PFC. There was also activation of contralateral SII and increased CBF in contralateral insula/retroinsula and decreased CBF in the ipsilateral insula/retroinsula. On the unaffected side, a similar pattern was seen. Direct statistical comparisons showed that stimulation of the affected side produced significantly greater activation of the contralateral SI than did stimulation of the unaffected side. A two-way repeated-measures ANOVA confirmed that rCBF in SI was higher ipsilateral to the lesion both at rest and on stimulation, was elevated bilaterally during stimulation, and increased significantly more in the presence of stimulation ipsilaterally to lesion than contralaterally. Thus, **cold allodynia produced significantly increased activation in the contralateral sensorimotor cortex when compared with stimulation of the other hand.**

(12) McGeoch *et al.* (2009) reported on a thalamic CPSP patient who developed hemisoma (except face) pain and marked tactile hand allodynia within 24 hours of stroke. She was studied with MEG (VESTAL analysis). Tactile allodynia was elicited in the scanner at rest, and 1 and 24 hours after cold caloric vestibular stimulation (CVS). Light tapping of the unaffected hand activated SI at 70 ms with subsequent SII engagement. Identical stimulation of the allodynic left little finger produced strong hand-area MI (not SI) activation at 60 ms followed by post-stimulation strong ACC activation at 200–250 ms. One hour later, spontaneous pain lessened from VAS 9 to VAS 5, allodynia being much improved. At this point, touching the allodynic finger simultaneously activated both MI and SI at 60 ms, with a reduced area of ACC activation at 200 ms; 24 hours later (VAS 5, no allodynia), there was strong SI and much reduced MI activation at 60 ms, with no ACC activation up to 850 ms post-stimulation. SII was never activated following finger stimulation. Pain remained abated for 4 days.

(13) Gustin *et al.* (2010a) submitted 19 healthy controls and 11 complete thoracic (T1–T10) SCI patients, all with below-level pain, to a motionless movement imagery task (right ankle plantar flexion/dorsiflexion in a standardized order plus co-listening to a recording of a car accelerator regularly increasing and decreasing in power) inside a 3T MRI scanner. Nine patients said that movement imagery evoked pain ("cognitive allodynia") in the area of their usual ongoing pain (legs and feet) immediately upon practicing (in six receding during rest, in three going on for

20–40 minutes after the end of movement imagery); two reported no change. The increase in pain was restricted in most cases to the feet (and not the remaining spontaneously painful areas – unlike e.g., postherpetic neuralgia-associated allodynia). In three, the painful area also encompassed areas that were previously pain-free. In no patient did movement imagery of the wrist or attention towards the right ankle make pain worse. There was a significant negative correlation between the ongoing pain and the percentage change of pain during movement imagery, i.e., the greater the ongoing pain, the harder it was for movement imagery to evoke pain. Left MI (leg area) activated significantly only in patients versus controls, and so did a discrete region of the right superior cerebellar cortex. Significant correlations with both percent and absolute changes in pain intensity occurred in right (ipsilateral) DLPFC and perigenual ACC; other areas correlating with percent change, i.e., not linearly with absolute pain intensity (possibly those with lower ongoing pain), were SMA, bilateral anterior insula, right BA6. Since controls were healthy, and not SCI patients without pain, the significance of this study is questionable. More relevant, patients 1–7 had already been published in an unacknowledged 2008 paper: the patients' age, time since injury, and LOI differ in these two papers, and pre-imagery pain (VAS) values are very different in five cases (unexplained reason).

(14) Kalita *et al.* (2011) studied 23 consecutive CPSP patients with MRI and ^{99}Tc ECD-SPECT. MRI revealed infarction in 14 and hematoma in nine patients. Hypoperfusion was observed in the corresponding thalamus in nine, and parietal cortex in 11 patients. Semiquantative analysis revealed hyperperfusion of thalamus in four and parietal cortex in five patients. MRI and SPECT findings did not differ in CPSP patients with and without allodynia.

The study by Bowsher *et al.* (2004) has no longer been included. After closer examination, it appears that fMRI data in two patients with moderate CPSP of insular origin were not acquired under tactile allodynic conditions (which the patients complained of), but under thermal stimulation in the absence of thermal allodynia in one.

Studies assessing neurochemical changes

(1) Willoch *et al.* (2004) reported on five right-handed CP patients (aged 54–77). In three cases, CP arose following an ischemic stroke also involving the thalamus, in two after a hemorrhagic stroke (pons; parietal angioma). Both spontaneous and evoked components were present in all and involved the hemibody, barring the face in one. CP never started immediately after the insult. They assessed diprenorphine (DPN) binding with PET. Arterial sampling necessary for quantitative modeling could not be performed in three patients. Results were compared with 12 healthy controls with a mean age of 39 years. Given low opioid receptor (OR) binding, *SI* was *excluded* from the analysis. This disclosed a hemispheric asymmetry with significant relative reductions in OR binding in prefrontal BA44, parietal BA40, SII and insula (BA14), and Vc contralateral to symptoms. The insular cluster was adjacent to SII and probabilistically extended into SII. While Vc showed maximal peak difference, there was reduced binding also in anteromedial thalamic nuclei. A bilateral relative reduction in OR binding was shown along the midline in the ACC (BA24 and 32), PCC (BA7 and 31), and PVG. The ACC revealed maximal reduction posteriorly, but stretched to BA24 and 32. Non-significant reduced OR binding was observed in BA6/8 and BA21/22/38. There were only reductions compared to controls, and no increases. Actually, infarcts in the thalamus and parietal cortex could have been the basis of the observed reductions. All three patients with thalamic lesions demonstrated binding levels below the control group, but the two patients with cortical or pontine lesions revealed reductions in the lowest range of the patient group. The global mean value of DPN binding for two patients was within normal range as compared to the control group. This study is meaningless, as proper control, i.e., non-CP patients with similar lesions to study patients and homogeneous age (not a group of younger healthy people!) was lacking. Most importantly, they erroneously compared their resting findings with imaging studies of CP during allodynic stimulation, two very different situations.

(2) Jones *et al.* (2004) reported on four patients with purported "CP." The first had sudden onset of burning pain in the left hemisoma (except the face),

plus allodynia. No lesion was apparent on both CT and MRI. The pain subsided spontaneously after 1 year. PET showed right thalamic hypoperfusion increasing during allodynic stimulation. Eighteen months later, the patient reported sudden pain in the right leg and allodynia in both legs. Again, CT and MRI were negative (!). Both amitriptyline and naloxone (2 mg/kg/24 h for 10 days) were ineffective. Patient 2 had a history of "possible" stroke with right hemisoma pain and allodynia. Carbamazepine was ineffective, but amitriptyline and valproate helped. CT was negative, and the authors speculated about "a high brainstem stroke." Patient 3 suffered pain in the right limbs and mouth. CT was normal and MRI disclosed a few bilateral lesions in the basal ganglia, best defined on the left. Opiates and naloxone were both ineffective. Patient 4, a diabetic, had pain of undefined origin, either due to two separate ischemic lesions to the cord or perhaps neurosarcoidosis. MRI showed increased signal in both lentiform nuclei and no spinal lesion (!). Amitriptyline, carbamazepine, and sublingual buprenorphine were ineffective. No neurophysiological exploration was carried out in any patient. These four patients were submitted to ^{11}C-diprenorphine (which binds to μ/δ/κ opioid sites) PET (FWHM: 8.5 × 8.5 × 4.3 mm) normalized to Talairach space. Reduced opioid receptor binding was seen in bilateral BA10 (−28%), bilateral BA24, and portions of BA24/32 and BA23 (−32%), right BA40 (−18%), right insula (−25%), BA22 (−15%), and bilateral thalamus (−15%). Given the moot nature of these patients' pains, this study is useless.

(3) Maarrawi *et al.* (2007b) studied eight CPSP patients (two capsulo-thalamic, two capsulo-lenticular, one juxta-thalamic, one thalamic, two brainstem) and seven PNP patients with two PET scans at 2-week intervals. There were no differences between data from the two sessions. All patients were titrated to oral morphine. The control group consisted of 15 healthy controls matched for age and sex. In the CPSP group, there was a clearly asymmetrical opioid receptor (OR) binding decrease, with predominance in contralateral (to pain) lateral PFC (mean −32%), insula (−16%), posteromedial thalamus (−20%), posterior temporal cortex (−13%), and PAG (−20%). *The only region with strictly bilateral decrease was the perigenual ACC.* In PNP patients, there were bilateral and symmetrical decreases in insula, medial thalamus, CC, posterior temporal cortex, OFC, posterior midbrain, and striatum. No region had increased binding. All interhemispheric changes in CPSP patients corresponded to relative reductions of OR binding in the hemisphere contralateral to pain. "Contralateral minus ipsilateral" analysis showed no relative increases. No significant rCBF differences existed between the two hemispheres. Voxel-wise comparisons between CP and PNP showed between-group differences in opioid binding restricted exclusively to the hemisphere contralateral to pain. OR binding decreases in CP versus PNP comprised the insular cortex (mean −18%), posterior temporal cortex (−16%), and lateral PFC (−30%). "CPSP minus PNP" analysis showed no increase in CP versus PNP. Again, this study's conclusions collapse on a lack of appropriate controls, i.e., stroke patients without pain (and, equally, patients with peripheral damage without pain), not healthy controls (!). It is also unclear why only insula, posterior temporal cortex, and lateral PFC should display an opioid binding decrease, and not others which are equally interconnected.

(4) By means of iodine-123-labeled iomazenil SPECT, we (Canavero and Bonicalzi 2007a, p. 248) assessed the regional distribution of benzodiazepine-GABA$_A$ receptors in the cortex in five patients with CP (three women and two men; aged 41–65; time from onset: at least 3 years; three patients with a neuroradiologically confirmed thalamic and/or capsular previous stroke, ischemic or hemorrhagic, and two with pure spinal cord damage due to previous myelitis and no end-zone pain). Four patients showed reduced uptake at parietal and, in two cases, frontal cortical levels on the side opposite the painful syndrome (R/L 117, 116, 113, 114). In the fifth patient (a thalamocapsular hemorrhage), the ratio approached significance (R/L 0.91). Both brain and cord cases displayed similar binding anomalies, with reductions in CCP contralateral to worse pain, excluding direct brain damage of GABA receptors as a mechanism of such reduction.

Studies assessing structural changes

(1) Pattany *et al.* (2002) compared seven SCI (plus one tumor) (one C8, six T9–L3) pain patients with nine SCI (plus one ischemia) (four C4–8, five T7–L3)

non-pain patients and 10 controls in a magnetic resonance spectroscopy (MRS) study. A total of 74% of pain patients had complete injuries (versus 67% without pain). Pain was described as sharp, burning, aching, or electric. Pain was generally above VAS 5 (86%). Mean *N*-acetyl-aspartic acid (NAA, a neuronal marker) (nmol) was 6.305 in controls, 6.566 in painless SCI, and 6.052 in pain SCI; mean myo-inositol (Ins, a glial marker) (nmol) was 2.659 in controls, 2.263 in painless SCI, and 2.886 in pain SCI; and NAA/Ins ratios were 2.474 in controls, 2.957 in painless SCI, and 2.182 in pain SCI. Statistical analysis showed no significant differences in metabolite concentrations between the two thalami. However, NAA correlated negatively with average pain intensity and myo-inositol positively. NAA also showed a significant difference between SCI patients with pain and those without. Other trends toward significance were of moot significance. Limits of the study are inhomogeneity of ages between patient groups, exclusion of females, scanning without drug washout, and no differentiation between diffuse versus end-zone pains. Lowest values of NAA were found in the pain group, but there is no explanation why normal controls ranked next, rather than non-pain SCI patients; a similar reasoning applies for myo-inositol. All in all, the authors' statement "the NA/Ins ratio may be sensitive in predicting the early effectiveness of new therapeutic strategies for managing pain in SCI patients" is totally unsupported.

(2) Fukui *et al.* (2002b) submitted to ECT a thalamic CPSP patient. ^{1}H-MRS ($2 \times 2 \times 2$ cm voxel in the thalamus bilaterally) was performed before and after a single course of ECT. The NAA/creatine ratio was calculated. Before ECT, the L/R thalamic ratio was 62.3%: after ECT (and during analgesia), the NAA/creatine ratio of the left thalamus increased by 32%. These same authors (Fukui *et al.* 2006) found the NAA concentration in the thalamus to be decreased in a group of peripheral neuropathic pain patients, making this a non-specific finding.

(3) Gustin *et al.* (2010b) assessed 23 complete thoracic SCI patients (12 with below-level pain and 11 without) and 45 non-SCI controls with whole-brain diffusion tensor imaging (DTI) and voxel-by-voxel calculation of mean diffusivity, which measures the average degree of water diffusion and thus cell integrity (an increase in signaling cell proliferation and a decrease in cell death). CP SCI patients (versus non-CP patients) displayed increased mean diffusivity values in right PPC, right DLPFC, left anterior insula, medial OFC, and BA6, and decreased mean diffusivity in ventral pons/midbrain, left amygdala, right Vc. Apart from the brainstem cluster, all significant clusters were located completely or also within gray matter (never totally in white matter). In SCI patients, pain intensity (but not pain duration) and mean diffusivity values were positively correlated in DLPFC, PPC, anterior insula, and BA6 and negatively correlated in the amygdala and Vc. CP SCI and non-CP SCI patients' values lay *well within the range of mean diffusivity values of controls*, except for the amygdala and Vc, which displayed values well below the lowest value in controls in 80% and 90% of the cases respectively. Tractography showed the PPC cluster projecting to the DLPFC and ventral brainstem (51 patients each), thalamus (43 patients), and medial OFC (38 patients). Despite significant differences in the mean diffusivity values of the clusters from which these tracks were derived, comparisons of the fractional anisotropy (which describes the degree of directional diffusivity, or anisotropy, of the water, 0 signaling free water diffusion and 1 unidirectional diffusion, with intermediate values) values of the fiber bundles (tractography) revealed *no significant difference* in the fiber tract properties between controls and SCI pain groups. The only significant difference between controls and non-CP SCI patients was in a fiber bundle connecting PPC to the ventral brainstem. In this study, the mean age of controls was significantly lower than SCI patients and the authors admit that "results [are] not conclusive", with thalamic and amygdala *changes ensuing from injury itself.*

The same group (Stanwell *et al.* 2010) conducted a 3T brain MRS study and processed the data using "wavelet-based feature extraction and classification algorithms." The results from 10 control patients were compared to those from 10 with SCI. The SCI cohort was made up of five people with below-level pain (two on pregabalin, one on morphine, one on tramadol) and five without chronic pain. Data were collected for the left thalamus, left ACC, and left PFC. The spectroscopy data from the thalamus (but not PFC and ACC) best distinguished control patients without SCI from those with SCI with a sensitivity and specificity of 0.9 (percentage of correct classification). The spectroscopy data obtained from the PFC and ACC both distinguished between SCI patients with CP and those without CP with a sensitivity and specificity of 1.0. The thalamic changes appeared to be linked more strongly to SCI, with the ACC/PFC changes linked specifically to the presence of pain. This study did not assess SI or SII/insula, and the PFC area was rather small. The method used is highly complicated and as such open to errors, but most cogently, "these [spectral] regions may or may not be the most important biochemical changes in the disease process . . . thus *the use of these spectral regions to interpret the biomarkers of the disease process is both unwise and could be misleading. There is, however, the clear temptation to try*!"(!). Moreover, "it is likely that in this present study the magnitude of biochemical change due to deafferentation following SCI overwhelms those biochemical changes (in the thalamus) [but not PFC and ACC] *due to chronic pain*." This is another meaningless study.

Conclusions

In view of the many limits of these studies, only general conclusions are possible regarding the genesis of CP:

(1) The thalamus appears to be implicated.
(2) Somatosensory areas (including SI) appear to be involved.
(3) rCBF changes in ACC are also reported in PNP and other chronic pains, making it a non-specific finding, and an ACC lesion neither prevents nor is necessarily involved in the generation of CP. Allodynia does not necessarily activate ACC.
(4) Bilateral activation of brain areas in CP is possible simultaneously: normal inhibitory mechanisms cannot rein in incoming impulses, with spread of (de)activations.
(5) All CBF changes are functional and rapidly reversible (see Appendix).
(6) Evoked pain involves different changes from spontaneous pain and different findings according to the type of stimulus (heat versus cold versus mechanical, static versus dynamic). Spread to frontal areas (ACC, PFC) and insula may signal emotional activation (Kraemer *et al.* 2008b) and engagement of avoidance networks, as the degree of unpleasantness increases. However, similar brain areas are activated by evoked pain in both PNP and CP, making these findings non-specific.

The focus on endo-opioids as part of the mechanism of CP is ill-founded and is another example of technology-driven speculation:

(1) "The underlying mechanisms for regulation of changes to the availability of opioid receptors are . . . unclear . . . The current major obstacle in the field is presented by the inherent limitations of the currently available tracers in reporting dynamic changes in the availability of a single OR subclass in the CNS . . . The presence of specific binding in a reference region may underestimate the calculated specific binding . . . the mechanisms regulating receptor expression and binding status are complex, and a PET-study alone does not reveal the underlying mechanisms responsible for a change in the specific binding of a tracer. A derivation of cellular and subcellular processes directly from a PET-image is *speculative and data from complementary methods are required for validation of the PET data* . . . the interpretation of the receptor affinity-dependent bindings are complex . . . influenced by endogenous release of opioid peptides and/or administration of opioid receptor modulating drugs" (Henriksen and Willoch 2008). Humans may all have significant different regional OR binding at baseline; μ-OR increases with age in the cortex and striatum; women show a higher binding than men in thalamus, amygdala, and cerebellum; high concentrations of OR are found in basal ganglia and thalamus, intermediate concentrations in frontal and parietal cortices, and low ones in the cerebellum and occipital cortex. Also, endo-opioids may be involved in modulation of non-painful somatosensory stimuli (Mueller *et al.* 2010). These may all bias results if not properly accounted for.
(2) Increased occupation of binding sites (i.e., reduced tracer binding) "would require substantial local release of endogenous opioid peptides in response to CNP [central neuropathic pain] with an associated analgesic effect" (Jones *et al.* 2004). Also in light of the general refractoriness of CP to opioids in the vast majority of patients, and the negative results of a controlled trial of naloxone, a

clinically relevant endogenous opioid hypertonus as proposed by some groups as an attempt to quench pain is excluded, although opioids are involved in placebo analgesia. Also, it is not clear what mechanism would drive endo-opioid release following CNS injury (unlike chronic nociceptive pain: Bruehl *et al.* 2010). Internalization and/or receptor downregulation after prolonged stimulation has been proposed as a justification for opioid unresponsiveness, but there are more cogent reasons. Opioid tracer binding is highest in the thalamus, high in the cingulum, insula/SII, basal ganglia, and amygdala, and *lowest in the SI/MI strip*, i.e., less than one-fourth of thalamus (Baumgaertner *et al.* 2006).

(3) Findings similar to those reported in CP studies are described for other pain syndromes, namely complex regional pain syndrome, and for experimental pain in healthy people (Klega *et al.* 2010), making these non-specific, and also related to depression and anxiety, which often accompany chronic pains.

Other neurotransmitters and neuromodulators may be much more important: "activation of the endogenous opioid system ... clearly cannot be the sole pathway of pain modulation in humans," as convincingly demonstrated on neuropharmacological dissection of placebo analgesia; "more emphasis on other neurotransmitter systems" is required (Bingel *et al.* 2007). A significant $GABA_A$ downregulation, in the course of long-standing CP, at fronto (MI/premotor/PFC)-parietal (SI) level (and not diffusely) is suggested by our data, and should be pursued further. Cortical 5-HT (2A) receptors co-determine responses to tonic pain, namely in the orbitofrontal, medial inferior frontal, *primary sensorimotor*, posterior cingulate cortices, insula – but also the hypothalamus (Kupers *et al.* 2009a, 2011) – and we predict that anomalies will be reported for CP (and other chronic pains). Other transmitter/modulator systems of interest include acetylcholine and norepinephrine, among others.

The explanation for the reported deactivations at both thalamic and cortical levels remains elusive (see Canavero and Bonicalzi 2007a, pp. 252–4, plus the Appendix for a critique of the default mode hypothesis). Thalamic hypoperfusion, for one, has been reported not only in CP, but also in PNP and cancer pain, making it a non-specific finding. Data suggest that negative BOLD responses *in the primary somatosensory cortex (SI)* as a result of acute pain reflect a *functionally effective inhibition* (Kastrup *et al.* 2008), perhaps due to antagonistic lateral inhibition (Tommerdahl *et al.* 2010).

Reviewed structural studies did not meaningfully contribute to the picture (see also Appendix).

Chapter 24

Drug dissection

Ideally, drugs with clear-cut pharmacodynamic profiles could dissect neurochemical mechanisms of CP and provide crucial pathophysiologic information: that is, on the basis of drug efficacy profiles, it should be possible to "reverse engineer" the neurochemistry of CP. Unfortunately, our understanding of drug mechanisms of action is still lacking, with the possible exception of some parenteral agents. We will now review what can be safely extrapolated from such data (see also further discussion in Canavero and Bonicalzi 2007a, pp. 176–82).

GABA agonists

GABA receptors are pentameric hetero-oligomers. At least 19 distinct $GABA_A$ receptor subunit genes exist, classified into eight classes (α1–6, β1–3, γ1–3, δ, ε, θ, π, and ρ1–3) (Mirza and Munro 2010). $GABA_A$ receptor assembly can be derived from a permutation and combination of two, three, four, or even five different subunits, with the majority of subtypes in the brain composed of assemblies of α, β, and γ subunits. Distribution of the major subunits in various regions of the brain varies: e.g., the cerebral cortex has intermediate levels of α1–4 subunits and low levels of α5 subunit, whereas the thalamus contains high levels of α4 subunit and intermediate levels of δ subunit. More than 60% of all $GABA_A$ receptors in the brain are α1/β2/γ2 (including pro-oscillatory TRN-to-Vc output), 15% α2/β3/γ2, and 10–15% α3/β*n*/γ2 (α3/β3/γ2 mediating antioscillatory/desynchronizing TRN-to-Vc output); α4/β2/γ*n*, α4/β*n*/δ, α5/β1–3/γ2, α6/β2–3/γ2, and α6/β*n*/δ each account for less than 5%.

The number of synaptic $GABA_A$ receptors can be dynamically modulated, and the modulation of 5-HT and dopamine receptor function also hinges on modification of $GABA_A$ receptor activity (Canavero and Bonicalzi 2007a, p. 322). Importantly, GABA neurotransmission can be recoded to become excitatory under certain conditions (Canavero and Bonicalzi 2007a, p. 323).

The most important drug with predominantly GABA agonism assessed in a formal RCT is IV **propofol** (Canavero and Bonicalzi 2004a). Tasker (2001b, and references therein) previously reported that IV infusions of 136 mg (mean) of sodium pentothal, another agent with GABAergic properties, reduced brain CP in 73% of his patients (versus none with 15–18 mg of morphine). In our studies, propofol effectively controlled CP at 0.2 mg/kg (one-tenth of the narcotic ED95 in humans), five times as effectively as pentothal at equipotent doses for CP (Canavero *et al.* 1995a). Convergent evidence shows a specific effect of propofol for CP, but not PNP, migraine, or nociceptive pains, at the doses reported above (Canavero *et al.* 1995a, Canavero and Bonicalzi 2004a). Unlike morphine and lidocaine, which are effective in allaying mechanical allodynia–hyperalgesia, but not cold allodynia–hyperalgesia (Chapter 9), our data suggest that, in CP, GABA modulation can allay both. Propofol analgesia shows a clear-cut post-effect: after several hours of infusion, analgesia can last for up to 24 hours (or more with longer duration of infusion). Propofol modulates GABA neurotransmission in different ways from barbiturates and benzodiazepines, although IT midazolam reduces CP in propofol-responsive patients (Canavero and Bonicalzi 1998a, 2004, Canavero *et al.* 2006b). Most importantly, propofol at doses effective for CP appears to have an exclusive $GABA_A$ action, without appreciable effects on other transmitters/modulators and ion channels as seen at anesthetic doses (Canavero and Bonicalzi 2004a). Its effects have been ascribed to a specific action on $GABA_A$ receptors containing β2 subunits (Campagna-Slater and Weaver 2007, Watt *et al.* 2008) (animal models of supposed chronic pain implicate α2/3 subunits: Mirza and Munro 2010). PET studies in healthy humans show that propofol at increasing doses *first targets cortical areas* and only thereafter subcortical regions, especially the thalamus

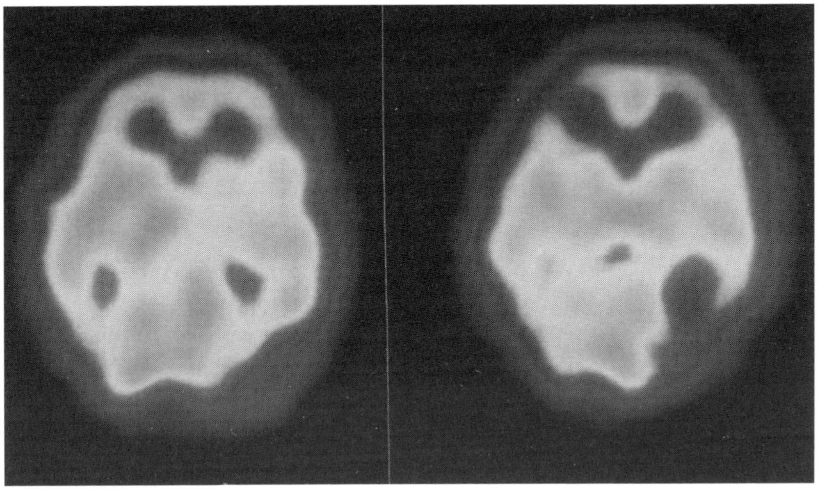

Figure 24.1. SPECT scan showing thalamic hypoperfusion in a case of central pain of thalamic origin. Propofol (0.2 mg/kg IV bolus) renormalized the asymmetry and allayed the pain. *See color plate section.*

(Sun *et al.* 2008); subhypnotic propofol renormalizes brain deactivations seen in CP patients, even at thalamic levels (Fig. 24.1). During propofol sedation, evoked responses are attenuated in SI only, while at hypnotic doses both thalamic and cortical responses cease (Rudolph and Antkowiak 2004).

Barbiturates can reduce CP, but their pharmacodynamic profile goes beyond simple GABA agonism and may induce sedation along with analgesia; also, frontal cortex deactivation is more marked with propofol than with thiopenthal (Veselis *et al.* 2004). Thiopental is administered IV at 50 mg boluses up to 225 mg and thiamylal at 50 mg IV every 5 minutes up to 250 mg: when effective, relief appears after 5–8 minutes and lasts several minutes (Migita *et al.* 1995, Mailis *et al.* 1997, Yamamoto *et al.* 1997, Koyama *et al.* 1998).

Benzodiazepines PO generally have no clinically significant effect on CP: they are believed to bind at the interface between α and γ subunits (Charney *et al.* 2006). Benzodiazepines are regarded as positive allosteric modulators of $GABA_A$ receptors; they show no affinity for receptors containing α4 or α6 subunits (Mirza and Munro 2010).

Baclofen, a $GABA_B$ agonist, has relieved CP via the IT route (Chapter 16), but no meaningful analgesia is generally seen at orally tolerated doses (< 60 mg/day).

Gabapentin and **pregabalin** may also increase GABA levels at cortical levels (Errante *et al.* 2002), but their utility is limited and "it is not immediately clear which of these various sites of action of gabapentin and pregabalin are the most important for their clinical use in chronic pain" (Taylor 2009). Also, they act differentially, as gabapentin, but not pregabalin, seems to have some antispastic action and pregabalin has six times greater α2δ1 binding affinity than gabapentin.

Other drugs with at least partial GABA agonism include **vigabatrin**, **tiagabine**, **topiramate**, **valproate**, and **levetiracetam**, but data are too sparse and generally negative.

Glutamate antagonists

Oral NMDA antagonists (**dextrometorphan**, **amantadine**, **memantine**) have little or no place in the long-term treatment of CP: their side-effect profile is unfavorable and the achieved benefit, infrequently seen, is no greater than that of other better-tolerated drugs. Also, there are data that do not support the paradigm of NMDA-mediated sensitization as a universal mechanism of neuropathic pain (Rabben *et al.* 1999). Controlled studies do not find **ketamine**, however administered, particularly effective for CP. Nonetheless, some patients report pain abatement during IV challenge. Ketamine does not depress the sensory information flow through the thalamus, and there is a suggestion that, parenterally, it may improve the cortically mediated affective component of pain (Sprenger *et al.* 2006). **Riluzole** has not been assessed; results in PNP have been disappointing. IV **traxoprodil**, a selective antagonist of the NR2B subunit of the NMDA receptor heterotetramer, found in the cortex and thalamus, reportedly relieved CCP (abstract referenced in Childers and Baudy 2007), but dizziness, depression, and hypoesthesia were seen; full details of such a study have not been published.

Sodium channel blockers

Controlled trials unequivocally prove that sodium channel blockers relieve CP (see Chapter 9) and thus implicate abnormal electrical activity in its genesis, but the anatomical location of critical sodium channel blockade has been difficult to localize. The first recorded treatment of neuropathic pain with a sodium channel blocker is probably Sigmund Freud's treatment of Ernst Von Fleischl, who suffered from trigeminal neuralgia, with cocaine injections (Bhattacharya *et al.* 2009). Voltage-gated sodium channels (VGSCs) consist of a highly processed subunit that is associated with auxiliary β subunits. The pore-forming α subunit is sufficient for channel function, but the kinetics and voltage dependence of channel gating are in part modified by the β subunits. There are 10 different α subunits (NaV1.1–1.9 and NaVX: 1.1–1.4, 1.6, 1.7 tetrodotoxin-sensitive, and 1.5, 1.8, 1.9 tetrodotoxin-resistant) and four β subunits (Bhattacharya *et al.* 2009, Zuliani *et al.* 2010). The NaV1.5 and NaV1.6 subunits are expressed in the brain.

IV **lidocaine** (and its oral congener **mexiletine**) act in an activity-dependent manner, i.e., they block channels at high-frequency depolarizations. Although a peripheral action has been established at doses below those achieving conduction block, *a central action is also likely* (Boas *et al.* 1982). Lidocaine may have a specific action on brush-evoked and mechanical allodynia, unrelated to general analgesic effects (Attal *et al.* 2000). Although the lidocaine test may predict analgesia from mexiletine in several patients, this is not generally indicated. **Lamotrigine** has been found "*moderately effective*" for brain CP and CCP associated with incomplete SCI and may have an effect on heat, but not cold and brush allodynia (Scrivani *et al.* 2010).

Not all drugs with a sodium channel blocking profile have been found effective for CP: **carbamazepine**, **phenytoin**, **topiramate** and **valproate** generally have no effect on the spontaneous component, although they may relieve paroxysmal pains in MS and SCI. Either sodium blockade is not strong enough or it engages a different mechanism. For instance, different sodium channel subtypes vary in the voltage range over which they activate and inactivate as well as in their activation/inactivation kinetics and tissue distribution, and these may be targeted differentially by available drugs, although differences of action on various subtypes among all available drugs are not large (Cummins and Rush 2007). Sodium blockade also leads to reduced glutamate release, and the differential potency of these agents may hinge on this factor. **Zonisamide**, **ralfinamide** and **lacosamide** have not yet been adequately studied.

This class of drugs has a narrow therapeutic margin with CNS liabilities (e.g., many patients drop out of an adequate trial of mexiletine or carbamazepine, because of ataxia, confusion, and sedation, among several other side effects). Due to the omnipresent role of sodium channels in vital physiological functions in addition to nociception, some form of selectivity of blockade is a safety requirement. Adult CNS neurons can express combinations of 1.1, 1.2, and 1.6 subtypes, adult DRG neurons 1.1 and 1.6–1.9; NaV1.6 channels are predominantly expressed at the nodes of Ranvier in myelinated nerve fibers (Cummins and Rush 2007). To the extent that currently marketed sodium channel blockers are selective, it is on the basis of use(frequency)-dependent inhibition of rapidly cycling channels, i.e., they prevent sodium channels rapidly cycling between resting, open, and inactivated states (e.g., in tissues, firing action potentials at high frequency), thus inhibiting the generation and propagation of action potentials. The degree of selectivity attainable with this strategy is limited because the channel motif targeted is common to all subtypes. Data implicating the 1.3/1.7/1.8/1.9 α subunits in neuropathic pain come from animal studies and are of no utility. For instance, since carbamazepine is poorly effective on the spontaneous component of CP and interacts with a slow inactivation state of NaV1.8 (Cardenas *et al.* 2006), this subtype may be excluded as a further target for CP. Equally, phenothiazines inhibit NaV1.7 (Cummins and Rush 2007): given their complete inefficacy on CP, this subtype can be ruled out too. However, so-called NaV1.7 channelopathic pain syndromes exist and are unusual in having a spatially restricted pattern of pain in the presence of a mutation at sodium channel level that is expressed widely (Waxman 2010). Study of regional expressions of sodium channel subtypes should be pursued in CP patients.

Calcium channel blockers

Voltage-gated calcium channels (VGCCs) include low-voltage-activated T type and high-voltage-activated L, N, P/Q, and R types, depending on the channel-forming CaV α subunits, and most neurons express multiple types of VGCCs (Perret and Luo 2009). The N type is the target for descending norepinephrine fibers and opioid inhibition (Perret and Luo 2009). Levetiracetam, an N-type VGCC blocker, has been found ineffective for CCP in a controlled trial (Chapter 9). Ziconotide, another N-type VGCC blocker, is of little clinical utility (Chapter 16). Ethosuximide, the only T-type blocker for clinical use, is not known to allay CP. The advertised target of gabapentin, the α2δ1 complex, is also of no significance (see also above), as this drug has a low responder rate for CP (Chapter 9).

Aminergics and allied drugs

Amitriptyline is effective on the continuous, lancinating, and thermally (but less so mechanically) evoked pains of CP (Chapter 9) and actually appears to be the most effective of all antidepressants. For a long time, it was believed that the mechanism of action was related to a potentiation of ascending and descending aminergic (norepinephrine, serotonin, etc.) brainstem control, but the exact contribution thereof, if any, is unclear (see discussion in Canavero and Bonicalzi 2004a). The range of action of amitriptyline and congeners is bewildering (discussed in Jasmin *et al.* 2003), and no hard and fast conclusions are possible. Moreover, amitriptyline has clear-cut sodium channel blocking properties at clinically effective doses (Dick *et al.* 2007), and in this regard it is more potent than all its congeners (imipramine, nortryptiline, desipramine, maprotiline, etc.), while the SSRIs (fluoxetine and congeners) have none and do not relieve CP.

Nonetheless, amines and congeners play an important role in regulating the overall setpoint of the thalamocortical system (Shepherd 2004). Thus, there is a high concentration of serotonin/histamine input to CL and related nuclei, while thalamic reticular nucleus (TRN) cells are excited by norepinephrine and serotonin (inhibiting TC output) and inhibited by acetylcholine (M_2) from Meynert's nucleus (during novelty or danger) and GABA (e.g., from basal ganglia or other TRN or inhibitory interneurons) (facilitating TC output): the process can be highly selective, creating foci of inhibition or disinhibition, e.g., in Vc. The GABAergic projection from basal forebrain may target TRN, but not Vc. The transition from burst to tonic mode in TC cells results from serotonin, norepinephrine, acetylcholine, histamine, nitric oxide, and glutamate input, vice versa only from glutamate input. Norepinephrine/dopamine fibers modulate corticothalamic rhythmicity, by acting on layers V (thalamoreceptive) and I (where dendrodendritic synapses between TC projections from CL and those from bursting pyramidal cells in layer V exist). What emerges from drug dissection studies, though, is that their modulation does not appear to be particularly effective.

Opioids/cannabinoids

The first patient in history to be diagnosed with CP was opioid-unresponsive (Edinger 1891). In 1892, Sir William Osler wrote in his highly acclaimed textbook's section on treatment of neuralgia (pp. 962–3) "morphia should be given with great caution, and only after other remedies have been tried in vain," and Davis and Martin (1947), among others, found opioids ineffective for CCP.

From a pathophysiological standpoint, opioid unresponsiveness likely depends on *low opioid receptor binding in the human SI* (Canavero and Bonicalzi 2007a, p. 181; see also Chapter 23): the "medial pain system" brain areas (i.e., thalamus, ACC, PFC, insula, temporal cortex, and others) have a high density of opioid receptors, and this would point to a critical role of the sensory cortex in CP mechanisms. However, morphine may have some effect on non-thermal allodynia, a likely sensitization-driven event. Interestingly, opioids inhibit GABA interneurons, and, in light of the high efficacy of GABA agonists, this would be further reason to limit their use. Opioid unresponsiveness of CP speaks against a functional impairment of the CNS opiate system.

Cannabinoids are of limited utility for CP, and the data argue against a role of this system in the generation of the spontaneous component of CP. Cannabinoids have an anticytokine profile (Schaefers and Sommer 2007), but, given their questionable efficacy, they do not support cytokines in the mechanism of CP.

Conclusions

The bulk of the evidence points to a dysfunction at the level of the $GABA_A$ receptors and sodium channels. We distinguish two classes of CP: GABA-responsive (class A) and GABA-refractory (class B) (Canavero and Bonicalzi 2004a). GABA responsiveness (class A) marks patients who stand the best chance of relief from cortical stimulation (Chapter 11). MRS studies should address GABA neurotransmission in CP (for healthy individuals, see Kupers *et al.* 2009b). Studies have *not* confirmed loss of GABA interneurons or receptors after nerve injury (Mirza and Munro 2010), and GABA dysfunction must involve other mechanisms, such as genetic reshuffling.There are genetic forms of idiopathic epilepsy associated with impairment of $GABA_A$ receptor function ($\alpha 1/\gamma 2/\delta$) and a similar mechanism may be active in CP: this deserves further study. A similar argument can be made for sodium channels.

Importantly, the cortex is the initial target of IV propofol, which effectively relieves CP. Lack of opioid efficacy is likely due to a dearth of opioid receptors in SI.

These drug dissection data point to a *deficit of inhibition*, followed by an *unchecked glutametergic hypertonus*, as the basis of CP (Canavero *et al.* 1996, Canavero and Bonicalzi 1998a).

Chapter 25

Is there a spinal generator of central pain?

Cord neuroablation

Anterolateral cordotomies (spinothalamic tractotomies)

Davis and Martin (1947) found cordotomies ineffective in several cases of CCP. Botterell *et al.* (1954) stated: "in complete lesions ... burning pain has proved a problem difficult of solution in cases of injury to the ... spinal cord," but "by contrast, jabbing, shooting, crampy, gripping, colicky and vice-like pains have been regularly relieved by satisfactory bilateral tractotomy" (i.e., open cordotomy). Porter *et al.* (1966) wrote: "cordotomy in relieving the symptoms of sharp, lancinating pains in the lower extremities in patients with cauda equina lesions ... had no effect, however, on the frequently encountered burning pain in the lower extremities [in traumatic paraplegia]." White and Sweet (1969) reported that, despite an initial 56% incidence of pain relief in paraplegics, only 33% remained pain-free in the long term. Low cordotomies were much less successful than higher ones, all at the expense of significant sensory loss. They concluded: "Cordotomy is very useful in paraplegia for relief of pain of radicular origin ... Provided the injury involves the cauda equina and does not extend rostrally beyond the conus medullaris to involve the cord, we believe that relief can be obtained in a high proportion of cases by anterolateral cordotomy," and White (1963) emphasized that "when the spinal cord is involved rather than its sensory roots, spinothalamic tractotomy, or even a complete myelotomy, is not likely to eliminate pain in the back and legs." Rosomoff (1969) considered cordotomies futile for CCP and found a high incidence of associated dysesthesias in this group. According to Lipton (1989), cordotomies "should not be used [for denervation pains] because when pain returns it may have dysaesthetic qualities and the patient is worse off than previously." Tasker *et al.* (1992) relieved spontaneous pain in 27%, intermittent spontaneous pain in 86%, and evoked pain in 75% of his SCI-CP cases. Tasker and North (1997) operated on 23 CCP patients with percutaneous, plus eight with open cordotomy. Pain recurred in eight after 1–21 years with gradual fading of analgesia. Repetition of cordotomy in six restored the level of analgesia in all, but pain relief was recaptured in only three. Long-surviving cord CP patients often relapse, contralaterally, ipsilaterally, or bilaterally, or new pains emerge and/or the analgesic levels achieved by cordotomy fade with time. By interrupting the spinothalamic fibers, this obviously sets the stage for further later different pains (although it was suggested that bilateral cordotomies may lessen this risk). In sum, CPSP, MS CCP, postcordotomy CCP, and pain due to scarring of the upper thoracic spinal cord are poorly responsive to anterolateral cordotomies (but also cordectomies and traditional DREZ lesions), with some exceptions, including CPSP cases (single cases of, e.g., Botterell *et al.* 1954, Davis and Martin 1947, Pollock *et al.* 1951b; see Table 7.1 in Canavero and Bonicalzi 2007a).

Dorsal root entry zone (DREZ) lesions and cordectomies

The DREZ operation in the paraplegic is generally done bilaterally (unilaterally in the case of one-sided pains), beginning at the level of the traumatic transection of the spinal cord and extending rostrally over the next three dorsal roots and caudad over two levels; laminae I through V are ablated. In the series of Falci *et al.* (2002), in 2.3% of patients a temporary pain developed at the new postoperative level of sensation. A permanent pain (VAS 1–3) developed in 4.7% of the patients at their new level of sensation at a follow-up of up to 7 years.

In Nashold's series (Nashold and Pearlstein 1996), long-term relief (pain-free) of chronic pain from SCIs was obtained in 35% of patients, with burning pain and electrical shocks being most responsive. Favorable categories included patients with incomplete neurological deficit, blunt trauma and conocaudal lesions with predominant leg pains. Approximately 70% of the paraplegic patients reported good pain relief immediately after the procedure, although half experienced some recurrence of the pain postoperatively, usually within the first year. In these patients the recurrent pain was usually described as less debilitating than the original pain. Pain in dermatomes at or just below injury (burning, shooting, or electrical), radiating down into the legs and activated by stroking/touching the skin over the adjacent dermatomes, and unilateral pains *usually responded* to surgery, but *sacrococcygeal and vague diffuse burning pains did not, or did so poorly* (Nashold and Pearlstein 1996). Another favorable group were those who proved to have nerve root avulsions at operative exposure. Sindou *et al.* (2001) came to similar conclusions. Radicellotomies performed for pain associated with below-T10 spinal cord lesions are effective only in patients whose pain has a radiculometameric distribution, i.e., the pain corresponding to the level and extent of the spinal cord lesion (end-zone pain). *Pain in the territory below the lesion, especially in the perineosacral area, is not favorably influenced* (while leg pain after caudal lesions is). Nashold also noted that in 18 cases with an intramedullary cyst (syrinx), drainage of the cyst alone did not suffice, whereas in 18 in whom this was combined with DREZ lesions, 12 good and two fair results were achieved.

Cordectomies relieved the same types of pain that respond to cordotomy and DREZ surgery (Tables 25.1 and 25.2).

Table 25.1. Cordectomies

Author(s)	Type of pain/ number of patients	Procedure	Outcome	Notes
Armour (1927)	SCI pain	Cordectomy at the lower end of the cord and adjacent cauda equina (T12–L2)	Complete pain relief in thighs and lower abdomen	War conocaudal injury
Davis and Martin (1947)	CP (cord) (1 patient)	Cordectomy	0%	
Freeman and Heimburger (1947)	CP (cord)	Removal of a 2–3 cm cord segment at T3–4	Unsuccessful	Leg pain
McCarty (1954)	Traumatic T7 total transverse lesion; pain at T5–6 (1 patient)	Removal of the lower 21 cm of the cord from T5 down to the conus	Narcotics stopped. Follow-up: 6 months Annoying girdle pains relieved 6 months later and occasional root pain at T5	
Botterell *et al.* (1954)	SCI (thoracic gunshot) pain (1 patient)	Excision of the damaged cord up to grossly normal cord + T4–5 rhizotomy	Girdle pain at lesion level totally relieved for 8 years Burning pain in the feet arising after cordectomy	
Smolik *et al.* (1960)	SCI pain (4 patients), including 1 patient with anterior spinal artery syndrome (ASAS)	Cord removal from the T10 level down through conus medullaris and upper cauda equina	Pain and spasm relief in 2 patients Unsuccessful in ASAS patient despite flaccidity	

Table 25.1. (cont.)

Author(s)	Type of pain/ number of patients	Procedure	Outcome	Notes
Werner (1961)	SCI pain (1 patient)	Cordectomy	Pain persistence after first myelectomy. Pain relief after a 2nd myelectomy	End-zone pain. First resection left the scarred proximal cord stump adhering to the dura
Druckman and Lende (1965)	SCI pain (1 patient)	Cordectomy just above trauma level (T11 vertebra) Second higher cordectomy 3 cm above previous one in normal tissue	No pain relief Complete pain relief. Follow-up: 18 months. Persistence of mild burning in legs	Conocaudal injury. Pain in lower abdominal and inguinal areas + mild burning in legs + girdle pain. No pain relief from a previous bilateral T11–12 rhizotomy
Druckman (1966; in White and Sweet 1969)	SCI pain (1 patient)	Cordectomy above injury through normal cord	Pain relief. Follow-up: 12 months	
White and Sweet (1969)	SCI pain (2 patients)	Limited cordectomy Cordectomy up to T11	No pain relief Pain relief. Follow-up 4 years	Severe burning pains in legs
Melzack and Loeser (1978)	SCI pain (5 patients) with complete transection	Cordectomy at various levels	2 unsuccessful (burning pain in legs, abdomen, buttocks) 1 partial (1st cordectomy at T9–12 abolished part of the pain for 2 years with worsening at 3rd year; 2nd cordectomy at T4–5 ineffective) 2 pain reliefs (paroxysmal shooting pains in legs abolished for 11.5 years with full relapse; thoracoabdominal pain abolished by T8–9 operation with gradual full relapse by 5 years)	Sympathetic blocks ineffective
Nashold and Bullitt (1981)	SCI pain (2 patients)	Cordectomy of tethered cord	Pain abolished	T4 fracture; severe pain in legs only upon head flexion

Table 25.1. (cont.)

Author(s)	Type of pain/ number of patients	Procedure	Outcome	Notes
		1 cm long low thoracic cordectomy	Pain relief. Follow-up: 12 years	T12–L1 fracture; pain in both legs
Durward *et al.* (1982)	SCI pain (6 patients), in 5 also post-traumatic syringomyelia	Cordectomy somewhat above the area of trauma at T6–8 (upper level of transection below the upper level of the syrinx) in 3 (1–4 years after CP onset) Cordectomy at various thoracic levels (T2 for a C6 lesion, T4–5 for major injury at T7 plus syrinx, T10–12 for same level injury)	Pain relief of arm pain in 3 No relief of leg/buttock pain in 3	
Jefferson (1983; 1987 in Gybels and Sweet 1989)	SCI pain (19 patients), diffuse to legs in 15	(1) Cordectomy at T11 and/or below (2) Cordectomy at T10–11 and T3–7 (+ limited rhizotomy)	(1) Pain relief: 70–100% in 14/15 patients (100% in 7/14 patients) Partial (leg pain abolished, abdominal/genitals/ buttock pain unrelieved) in 1 (2) 0–25% relief	Lesions at/below T11 with episodic, electric shock/spasm *non-burning* pain more likely to respond to cordectomy immediately, completely, and permanently In some cases *cured* of their pains, there was still severe widespread cord damage at the upper incision level
Tasker *et al.* (1992)	CP (cord) (12 patients)	Cordectomy	Steady pain relief: none in 70% of cases, 25–50% in 30% of cases Intermittent pain relief at 1 year: >50% in 60% of cases, 25–50% in 40% of cases Evoked pain relief (>1 year): >50% in 80% of cases, 25–50% in 20% of cases	
Pagni and Canavero (1995)	CP (cord) (2 patients)	Cordomyelotomy (T5–SI myelomeres)	Shooting pain/spasms abolished; moderate burning to legs and perineum lessened	Long-lasting (10 years) pain relief

Table 25.1. (cont.)

Author(s)	Type of pain/ number of patients	Procedure	Outcome	Notes
Raza *et al.* (2005)	CCP (post-thoracic meningioma resections) (1 patient)	T2–8 cordectomy	2 months later, no further deterioration, but bilateral arm hyperesthesia	Follow-up: not available
Ewelt *et al.* (2010a)	CCP (T12/L1 astrocytoma) (1 patient)	Cordectomy below T9 just caudal to the root entry zones with clear separation from neoplastic areas	Complete pain relief under analgesic PO-only medication	Follow-up: not available
Ewelt *et al.* (2010b)	CCP (traumatic and non-traumatic syringomyelia) (13 patients traumatic, 1 spinal ependymoma, 1 iatrogenic)	Cordectomies all at upper thoracic level	"*No change in pain*" in 11 patients (pains not characterized). In 1 patient phantom pain appeared in both legs after 6 months, in another "*paresthesias regressive*". In another, clearly described as having "*ongoing progressive burning pain in lower trunk & both legs*," who received cord transection below T3, more pain appeared in left leg, with burning in both feet. In another, with "*progressive dysesthesias*," there was "*no change in pain*." Another who also had C6/T5 and T7/conus syrinxes had "*no change in pain*" and new "*mild dysesthesias in digits 3–5 of right hand*." The final patient with "*progressive pain syndrome*" had his VAS score from 10 to 4/5	Cordectomy poorly effective

Table 25.2. DREZ surgery

Author(s)	Type of pain/ number of patients	Procedure	Outcome	Notes
Samii and Moringlane (1984)	SCI pain (5 patients)	DREZ lesions	Pain relief: 70–100% in 2/5, 50–70% in 2/5, <50% in 1/5	Pain at T2–3; burning pain in 1, burning and needles in 1, in 3 unspecified

Table 25.2. (cont.)

Author(s)	Type of pain/ number of patients	Procedure	Outcome	Notes
Dieckmann and Veras (1984)	SCI pain (2 patients)	DREZ lesions	0%	
Richter and Seitz (1984)	SCI pain (2 patients)	DREZ lesions	0% benefit	
Thomas and Jones (1984)	SCI-CP (1 patient) Tumor CCP (1 patient)	DREZ lesions	Poor relief Good relief	
Wiegand and Winkelmueller (1985)	SCI pain (20 patients)	DREZ lesions	Pain relief (5–34 months): 100% in 9, 80% in 1	At follow-up, 10 had maintained their early postoperative relief and moved from 80% to 100% relief
Pagni *et al.* (1987) IASP congress 1987 S127, poster 241	SCI CCP (1 patient)	DREZ lesions	Relief of paroxysmal, superficial pains but not deep visceral pains and dysesthesias	
Friedman and Bullitt (1988)	SCI pain (56 patients): end-zone pain (31 patients); burning dysesthesic pain (25 patients)	DREZ lesions (lesions from a few segments above to a few segments below)	Pain relief, end-zone pain: 74% good (100% relief and/or no analgesics needed or residual discomfort not interfering with daily living activities), 6% fair (still requiring some analgesics), 20% no result Pain relief, diffuse dysesthetic pains: 20% good, 12% fair, 68% no result	Bilateral pain resistant, but 9/10 with unilateral pain had good relief
Powers *et al.* (1988) Includes: Powers *et al.*, *J Neurosurg* 1984, **61**, 841–7	CCP (9 patients) SCI pain (cauda) (2 patients)	DREZ lesions, laser	5 successes, 4 failures 0% Follow-up: 4–63 months	End-zone pain in 4: all relieved Below-level pain: relief in 2/8 Midline (perineal, scrotum) pain: relief in 0/3
Sweet and Poletti (1989)	SCI pain (trauma) (1 patient)	DREZ lesions at T3–5 + posterior poliotomy (LX ablation)	Complete relief of thoracic end-zone pain and coccygeal/foot pain for 3 months. At 13 months, >50% relief	

Table 25.2. (cont.)

Author(s)	Type of pain/ number of patients	Procedure	Outcome	Notes
	CP (T12 AVM) (1 patient)	Extensive DREZ lesions	0% of diffuse bilateral pain from lower abdomen downwards	
Kumagai *et al.* (1990)	SCI pain (4 patients)	DREZ	50% relief at 11–30 months	Not available for review
Young (1990)	SCI pain (26 patients)	DREZ lesions (standard and laser)	55% of patients relieved Follow-up: up to 5 years 83% of patients with cauda equina lesions relieved	*Midline pain, especially in mid-lumbar area or genitalia, unrelieved*; end-zone pain benefited
Tasker *et al.* (1992)	SCI pain (4 patients)	DREZ lesions	No effect on steady pain 25–50% relief on evoked pain present in 2 patients (>1 year)	
Edgar *et al.* (1993)	SCI pain and other pains (120 patients)	Computer-assisted DREZ lesions	End-zone pain relieved in 92% of patients; follow-up: 2–96 months	93% had diffuse pains and/or sacral pain
		Standard DREZ lesions	End-zone pain relieved in 58% of patients	
Rath *et al.* (1996)	Paraplegia pain (22 patients)	Junctional DREZotomy	Diffuse burning: 5 failures of 6 Spinal cord cyst: 5 failures of 7 End-zone pain relieved in most who had it Follow-up: mean 54 months	
Nashold and Pearlstein (1996) (includes all previous papers of the Duke's group on this procedure)	Conocaudal pain (39 patients)	DREZ lesions	Pain relief at a mean of 3 years: good (no analgesics required) in 54% of patients; fair (non-narcotics still necessary but pain not interfering) in 20% of patients 100% relief in 35% of patients at 10 years	Narcotics down from 90% of patients to 12%. Conocaudal pain relieved in 60% *Best results in electric shock pain and end-zone pain* Facial pains abolished in 40% at 10 years
Sampson and Nashold (1992)	Pontine CPSP (1 patient)	Caudalis DREZ	100% relief *2 days later* over 4 yrs	
	CP, mesencephalic AVM (1 patient)		50% relief *8 days later* (death 4 months later during surgery)	

Table 25.2. (cont.)

Author(s)	Type of pain/ number of patients	Procedure	Outcome	Notes
Sindou *et al.* (2001) (includes all previous papers of Sindou on this procedure)	SCI (44 patients)	Radicellotomy	>50% pain relief in 14/16 patients (6 months – 7 years) Long-term good results in 68% of patients	Below-lesion pain not favorably influenced, particularly perineosacral-radiculometameric pain responsive
Prestor (2001)	SCI-CP (1 patient) Syrinx CP (6 patients)	Junctional DREZ	0%	Excellent relief (83.3%) Good (16.7%) at 6–48 months
Falci *et al.* (2002)	SCI pain (41 patients), generally at T10–L1 but 6 cases at T4–9	DREZ lesions guided by multiple electrophysiological techniques	Group A (9 patients): 100% relief in 56% of patients (50–100% relief in 78%); follow-up: 6–7 years Group B (32 patients): 100% relief in 84% (50–100% relief in 88%); follow-up: 1–6 years *End-zone pain* (present in 6/32): 100% relief in all *below-level pain* (present in 26/32 patients): 100% relief in 81% of patients (50–100% relief in 85%)	15% of repeat surgeries 4.7% of patients developed a new permanent pain of low intensity (VAS 1–3) Evaluation: telephone interview and/or outpatient evaluation (VAS/ verbal scales)
Spaic *et al.* (2002)	SCI pain (T9–L4) (26) patients	DREZ lesions	Thermal pain (burning and similar), steady pain and diffuse infralesional pains: 0% long-term relief Shooting, cutting, stabbing, sharp, cramping, constriction, throbbing end-zone pains: 100% relief in 70% of patients and >50% relief in 20% at 13–50 months	
Rogano *et al.* (2003)	SCI patients (complete/ incomplete) (11 patients)	DREZ lesions	VAS from 9.7 to 1.9: end-zone pain only	
Tsai *et al.* (2010)	SCI CCP (2 patients)	DREZ lesions and spinal tractotomy	Disappointing	
Ruiz-Juretschke *et al.* (2011)	CCP (1 patient)	DREZ lesions T10–L1 bilateral	Failure (from VAS 10 to 8 at long term)	

Spinal rhizotomies are unsuccessful (see Table 7.1 in Canavero and Bonicalzi 2007a) and can trigger anesthesia dolorosa (Pagni *et al.* 1993).

General comments

Traumatic cord injury

The pain that responds to surgical ablation of the cord is not the steady pain.

Results of cordectomies have been less rewarding with lesions and sections at levels higher than T10. Jefferson (1983), noting that diffuse, steady pain, particularly in a "bathing trunks" distribution, was relieved poorly by cordectomy, stated: "One of the very interesting, and perhaps characteristic features of the pain which is likely to respond ... is that it is episodic." According to Tasker *et al.* (1992), "destructive surgery is selectively successful in relieving the spontaneous intermittent, often shooting radicular pain that tends to project down the legs ... present in 30% of ... patients with cord central pain ... particularly associated with thoracolumbar lesions ... evoked pain, present in 47% of ... patients, responds similarly to destructive surgery," while spontaneous pain is poorly relieved. Globally, intermittent shooting (89%) and allodynia–hyperpathia (84%) respond to cordotomy–cordectomy–DREZ, whereas steady, causalgic, dysesthetic, aching pains respond only in 26%. Intermittent and evoked, but not steady, pains should be dependent upon transmission in somatosensory (probably spinothalamic) pathways, intermittent shooting pain perhaps being the result of ectopic impulses instituted at, or proximal to, injury sites (e.g., through ephapses or peripheral ectopic pacemakers) and then transmitted centrally. Pagni and Canavero (1995) also noted that the paroxysmal components, often associated with spasms, usually due to lesions at T9–T12 vertebral level, are satisfactorily relieved by cordomyelotomy.

In sum, steady burning pain referred to the lower abdomen, and burning or dysesthetic pain diffused to the legs or localized to the retroperitoneal region, buttocks, or feet, is usually not relieved by cord neuroablation, unlike shooting, paroxysmal pain (and spasms), even though referred to apparently totally anesthetic and paralyzed limbs, girdle pains, and pain worsened by bowel or bladder distension. Thus, **evoked pains appear to depend on a local cord generator, whereas diffuse steady pains depend on more rostrad stations.**

Pain relief in paraplegics after cordectomy appears to be directly related to the extent of the removal, with better results occurring when long rostral segments of the cord are resected, that is, 2–3 cm (three spinal segments) (e.g., Druckman and Lende 1965). Loeser *et al.* (1968) pointed to the cord segments rostral to injury playing an important role in the genesis of pain. Jefferson (1983) noted that, although abnormal tissue was left above the level of his resections, without apparently influencing pain relief, sometimes extension of cordectomy to apparently normal tissue was necessary.

Bilateral DREZ lesions that involve 2–3 spinal cord segments above the spinal injury, and extend into *normal cord*, achieve a better pain relief (coagulation includes laminae I–IV, but may involve up to lamina VI and adjacent white columns), as damage extends for several segments well above the injury site (Nashold 1991), whereas extension of DREZ lesions *caudad* into the sacral segments of the cord does not improve the results (only one patient with diffuse sacral pain improved in the series of Friedman and Bullitt 1988). Edgar *et al.* (1993) and Falci *et al.* (2002) found that DREZ surgery can indeed relieve diffuse pains, if lesions are extended sufficiently. In the latter paper, in 62% of patients with below-level pain, spontaneous DREZ hyperactivity was found 3–5 levels cephalad to injury level (seven in the series of Edgar *et al.*). Their findings contradicted traditional dermatomal mapping and thus they hypothesized that *below-level pain was mediated significantly by interneuronal pathways*, while *at-level pain was assumed to be mediated through more traditional pain pathways (e.g., STT) corresponding to the DREZ at injury level.* Spinal block studies (Chapter 16) also found that block above lesion level was necessary for analgesia; failure in two patients (both with below-level pain) despite anesthesia two levels cephalad to injury supports even more rostral mechanisms. Davis and Martin (1947) wrote: "If the distal end of the proximal segment of the injured spinal cord was anesthetized by spinal anesthesia, the pain disappeared", and "this suggests that the origin of the pain was the end of the proximal segment of the injured spinal cord ... operations upon the sympathetic nervous system [being] ineffective."

Studies by Finnerup *et al.* (2003a, 2003b) found a significant correlation between intensity of brush-evoked dysesthesia at lesion level and spontaneous below-level pain. In a further study (Finnerup *et al.* 2007b), touch, punctuate stimuli, cold stimuli, and topical capsaicin was applied above, at, and below injury level in 10 SCI patients with CP below a thoracic injury, in 10 SCI patients with a thoracic injury but without neuropathic pain, and in corresponding areas in 10 healthy controls. The study found increased responses to repetitive punctuate stimuli above (indicating a spread of hyperexcitability rostral to injury) and at injury level compared to controls and pain-free SCI patients, but not an increased response (secondary hyperalgesia) to capsaicin in patients with CP at, above, or below level (suggesting that peripheral input from Aδ/C fibers does not play a role in CCP). The correlation of evoked pain at injury level to the intensity of spontaneous below-level pain was weak: if dorsal horn hyperexcitability and central sensitization is present following SCI in CCP, it is not generalized to all afferent input, but mainly to Aβ input. Wydenkeller *et al.* (2009) studied evoked potentials following contact heat in 26 complete SCI patients (eight at cervical, nine at thoracic levels): 17 patients suffered below-level CP, whereas nine were pain-free. Hyperalgesia to pinprick was equally found in both pain and non-pain patients.

Finnerup *et al.* (2003c) scanned 23 SCI patients above T10 (14 with CP and nine without CP). MRI showed, at the level of maximal cord injury, lesions involving the entire cord on axial images except for a small border of lower signal intensity in 21 patients, whereas two had central lesions. Rostral to the main injury, the first image with an incomplete lesion showed significantly more involvement of gray matter in pain than in pain-free patients, suggesting a possible role as a spinal generator. However, in a later study of 10 CCP patients versus 11 without CCP (at or below level) (Finnerup *et al.* 2007a), no differences were observed in the rostrocaudal extent of the lesion between the two groups on 1.5T MRI, but only a trend towards larger lesions of the dorsal gray matter and the dorsal column in the CP cases. In this study the area of allodynia overshot the area of spontaneous CP, and was reportedly painful even in patients without spontaneous pain.

CCP appears to be much more frequent in incomplete cord injuries. Actually, **a majority of seemingly clinically complete transection injuries are subclinically incomplete and retain significant communication between segments above and below the cord injury zone even many years after the original trauma**, as shown both anatomically and electrophysiologically (Dimitrijevic 1987, Beric 1999) – so-called **dyscomplete lesions**. Also, some sensory cortical evoked responses may still be detected in SCI patients with no clinically appreciable sensory function below the lesion site; prolonged, repeated, or continuous application of different stimuli may be transmitted from below lesion level to the brain and produce the awareness that something is happening in seemingly anesthetic areas (this is the case of peripheral or central pathways still transmitting across the traumatic lesion on fast or slow conducting fibers which are, however, functionally useless (Donovan *et al.* 1982). Finnerup *et al.* (2004) compared 24 SCI patients (11 with CP and 13 without) with a clinically complete SCI (ASIA grade A), and found that painful or repetitive pinprick stimuli elicited vague localized sensations in 50% of cases. SSEPs and MRI found no difference between groups. Thus, sensory communication was retained across injury level (*sensory dyscomplete SCI*). Wasner *et al.* (2008b) studied a series of 12 clinically complete SCI CCP patients: heat applied post-capsaicin sensitization (but not mechanical or cold stimuli) *partially* rekindled pain in four SCI pain cases and induced non-noxious warm sensations in another two; thermal stimuli (0–50 °C) *partially* rekindled the pain in two subjects prior to sensitization.

Kakulas *et al.* (1990) observed that, out of 197 SCI cases, only 22 reported pain and five burning sensations. Of these, 18 had clinically incomplete and four a complete cord transection syndrome; in 10 cases the lesion was cervical, in six thoracic, and in six lumbar. They concluded that: "there is a larger proportion of patients with pain and abnormal sensations with anatomically incomplete injuries." They also noted that an extensive regeneration of nerve roots at the level of injury is more frequently observed in patients suffering from pain, and studies show a significant increase in CGRP immunoreactivity in the dorsal horns of individuals with chronic SCI (Ackery *et al.* 2007). Kakulas *et al.* also observed that most seemingly clinically complete cord transection syndromes (63/88) show, on pathological examination, continuity of nervous tracts across the lesion, with a variable residuum of descending and ascending central nervous fibers running in the wall of the lesion. They also found spinal cord lesions spreading over many segments below and above the level of the bony lesion, with lesions at times extending well above the injury site (Durward *et al.* 1982). At these levels, loss of myelinated fibers and neurons of the gray substance and gliosis intermingle. In traumatic spinal cord damage, surviving axons in injured spinal cord (MS, cervical spondylosis: Hughes 1976; extramedullary tumors: McAlhany and Netsky 1955) have neurophysiological features typical of demyelinated axons (Rasminsky 1980). Then, sensory loss would be due not so much to loss of axons (both during trauma and in MS), but rather to loss of their ability to transmit properly encoded information, conducting more slowly and ineffectively. Demyelination may involve cord tracts under the compressing lesion or on the opposite side of the cord.

Pathological afferent discharges may spontaneously originate in the surviving central stumps of divided central nerve fibers and damaged demyelinated fibers of both anterior and posterior cord quadrants, with impulses arising ectopically (Smith and McDonald 1982), in both incomplete and dyscomplete spinal cord traumatic transections. Demyelinated axons may be responsible for pain paroxysms (Pagni and Canavero 1993); minimal mechanical deformation of the cord at the lesion site increases the level of previous spontaneous activity, inducing spontaneous activity in silent fibers. Lissauer's tracts, which lie outside the area included in anterolateral cordotomies, might support the rostral spread of hyperactivity. Denny-Brown *et al.* (1973) found that the medial division of Lissauer's tract seems to exert a facilitatory effect, and the lateral division a suppressor effect on transmission of afferent impulses at the first synapse. Lesion of the lateral part gives rise to hyperesthesia extending both above and below the lesion level on the section side, while "section of the whole Lissauer's tract at any one level had prolonged release effect on the next headward dermatome." Involvement of Lissauer's tract may explain the at-level hyperesthesia noted on the lesion side after cord hemisection, Lissauer's tract section, and section of the posterior columns impinging on the dorsal horn, as well as girdle pains in spinal tumors.

However, **lesions that interrupt central pathways will result in wallerian degeneration of the axons**, and thus "**there is no way for interrupted central axons to become a source of ectopic nerve impulses, as can happen with peripheral axons, for example, in neuromas,**" as neuronal hyperexcitability requires preserved neuronal function (Willis 1991). On the other hand, Hari *et al.* (2009), in a study comparing eight below-level CP patients and eight pain-free SCI patients, concluded that the recovery of STT (pinprick) function and not the dysfunction per se may underlie CCP, suggesting that STT may be the source of a pain generator. However, the statistical significance was marginal ($p = 0.045$) and the scores of neither the early nor the later examination were significantly different. Most cogently, a few patients exhibited a decline in STT function (and not a recovery), and half of these developed CCP (!). In the study by Wasner *et al.* (2008b) of 12 clinically complete SCI CCP patients, small fiber activation and sensitization by sequentially applying L-menthol, histamine, or capsaicin to the painful area elicited *no sensation*, painful or not, *in four patients*, nixing their conclusion that partially preserved STT "could" be the site of the CP generator after SCI.

We note how previously unreported burning sensations developed after cordectomy (Botterell *et al.* 1954), and even Falci *et al.* (2002), who believed that the higher temperature they used had markedly decreased the development of new "squeezing, pressure" pains, possibly because of a more complete destruction in deeper laminas, triggered new CP sensations; moreover, not all the patients were relieved of below-level CP, implying even more rostral hyperactivity. Beric (1993) pointed out that the anterior spinal artery syndrome (ASAS) is characterized by severe, practically complete interruption of the STT at the spinal level: here, the hypothesis of dorsal horn nociceptive cell hyperactivity at the level of the lesion becomes inconceivable, and useless in explaining the painful symptoms of this syndrome.

Syringomyelia

In contrast to other types of pain that usually respond well to surgical treatment of the syrinx, dysesthetic CP can persist or even increase postoperatively, despite collapse of the syrinx, and in fact new CP can appear ex novo after surgical treatment (Tator and Agbi 1991). In the series of Milhorat *et al.* (1996), surgical treatment of syrinx resulted in total relief in only 7/37 patients (19%), with another 15 improved in respect of their dysesthetic pain. Fifteen patients (41%) reported no improvement or even worsening of pain, despite MR-confirmed collapse of syrinx. Postoperative dysesthetic pain was often disabling and poorly responsive to drugs. One year after surgery, all these 15 patients continued to complain of dysesthesias and pain, although at a lesser level in nine, and most even did so 2–6 years postoperatively. Syrinxes often encroached on the dorsolateral quadrant of the cord, but no comparison between pain and non-pain patients was attempted in order to define a possible role of the descending dorsolateral funiculus; similar arguments apply to increase of substance P staining in the dorsal horns below-level and marked reduction or absence at-level (references in Milhorat *et al.* 1997). However, Hida *et al.* (1994) found that the syrinx cavity in post-traumatic syrinx patients was more central at the caudal than at the rostral end. Sudden onset of pain immediately above the original injury level is the most common presenting complaint from patients with syrinx and often occurs in conjunction with a sudden increase in thoracic pressure (e.g., during a sneeze). Milhorat *et al.* (1997) noted that patients with syrinx pressures greater than 7.7 cm H_2O tended to have more rapidly progressive symptoms, exhibited greater improvement after shunting, and had a higher incidence of postoperative dysesthetic pain, than patients with normal or almost normal pressures (*30% vs. 0%*). Postoperative dysesthetic pain was not found to be due to injury of dorsal roots or posterior columns during myelotomy and chronic irritation of cord by shunt catheter, but only to sudden decompression of hypertensive syrinxes. Such pains resolved spontaneously in two, were less severe in another two, but persisted in a fifth at 1 year: these may have been segmental dysesthetic pains, however. In 75% of patients with pre-drainage SSEP abnormalities, decompression produced a consistent reduction of N20 latencies and a similar, but less consistent, increase in N20 amplitude. However, all comparisons between high- and low-pressure groups were not statistically significant. Prestor and Benedicic (2008) found that 9/14 patients had distressing para/dysesthetic dermatomal pain on the side with worst sensory deficit, and noted that pain location could be an additional sign of asymmetrical spinal cord damage and that syringes are mainly positioned asymmetrically with their thinnest part at the DREZ. Milhorat *et al.* (1997) cautioned against the use of the DREZ myelotomy for syrinxes that do not lateralize to that region of the spinal cord because of the risk for injury to second-order afferents that play a role in CP.

Attal *et al.* (2004a) found that shunting of syrinx significantly improved proprioceptive deficits, but not the magnitude of thermoalgesic deficits, in 15 patients, despite collapse of the cavity in 80% of the cases: only pain evoked by effort–cough–movement, *but not pain at rest*, was reduced at 2 years. Moreover, only patients operated within less than 2 years of symptom onset were improved or stabilized, including three patients whose spontaneous pain improved by at least 70%. Not finding a correlation between pain and thermoalgesic deficits, they suggested that pain might result from irritation of the cord at the rostral end of the cyst. This group further studied 37 patients with syringomyelia, 27 with neuropathic pain, and 21 controls with 3D DTI (at level C3–C4) (Hatem *et al.* 2010). Patients with and without neuropathic pain were indistinguishable on the basis of quantitative sensory testing, laser-evoked and somatosensory-evoked potentials, and three-dimensional fiber tracking analyses. However, in patients with neuropathic pain, higher average daily pain intensity was correlated with greater structural damage to the spinal cord, while the number of reconstructed nerve fibers was negatively correlated with "deep spontaneous pain" and "paresthesia/dysesthesia" (i.e., pins and needles/tingling). Significance levels were all weak ($p = 0.02–0.04$). Nonetheless, patients with spontaneous pain only had more severe spinal cord damage, with a strongly significant correlation between average daily pain intensity and fractional anisotropy of the full spinal cord ($p = 0.008$), implicating supraspinal mechanisms. By contrast, patients with both spontaneous and evoked pain had not only less structural spinal cord damage, but also better preserved spinothalamic and lemniscal tracts on quantitative sensory testing and electrophysiological testing, implying pathological activity in preserved STT (spinal cord generators), which, however, does not exclude the possibility that brush-evoked allodynia may have also been due to supraspinal alterations.

Kasai *et al.* (2008) and Laxton and Perrin (2006) found cordectomy effective for at-level pain caused by post-traumatic syrinx.

Wirth *et al.* (2002) drained and filled with fetal neural grafts a series of syringomyelias. Despite clear MRI evidence of at least partial cyst obliteration in seven patients, complete disappearance of one or more pain symptoms was noted only if collapse of the most rostral portion of the cyst was achieved and no previous or new shunt tube was present in the cyst, suggesting that **syringomyelia pain may result from or be exacerbated by irritation of the cord levels immediately rostral to the cyst**. Irritation may be due to either a mass effect secondary to increased cyst pressure and/or inflammation from tissue damage. In one patient, reopening of a collapsed cyst seemed to cause return of pain. One patient noted a delayed increase of pain after surgery, due to a delayed expansion of a second cyst distant from the transplant site. Pain intensity reports often varied substantially in time, with distribution of dysesthesias more stable. However, *complete disappearance of a dysesthesia was seen in only 2/8 patients.* In one patient, the burning sensation in the dermatomes associated with an upper C6–T3 cyst *disappeared immediately after grafting without shunting* (follow-up 2 years), with complete collapse of the cyst. Nonetheless, he developed stabbing pain in the T6–9 dermatomes 3 months after surgery due to expansion of the lower T6–9 cyst, both gradually increasing over 18 months; 27 months after the first surgery, a second graft was placed in this lower cyst, with unsatisfactory results at 1 year, despite 50% collapse of the cyst. Patient 5 had the previous stabbing pain in her legs limited to below knees at 6 weeks and complete disappearance at 9 months (complete obliteration of cyst at 9 months), but full relapse at 18 months (slight reopening at 12 months and persistence through 2 years). In the other six unrelieved patients, five had substantial collapse of the cyst at the graft site, but also a persistent cyst above the graft site or shunt tubes at or above the graft site. In the ninth, no collapse was seen.

However, Durward *et al.* (1982) reported that, although the syrinx continued upward for many segments above the level of cordectomy and the upper ends of the specimens of the cord showed pathological changes in three of their patients, they were all relieved of their arm pain, indicating that this type of abnormality may not be a generator of pain. On the other hand, in none of the other three cases where cordectomy failed was the rostral incision into histologically normal cord. In two of them with a post-traumatic syringomyelia, earlier drainage of the cyst had improved the syndrome, with the exception of the continuing pain. *The pain in these latter three failures was all referred well below the level of the lesion in the cord, and these lesions were all at levels at which Jefferson's cordectomies had also failed.*

Conclusions

According to Finnerup *et al.* (2007a), "neuronal hyperexcitability underlying this gain in sensitivity is not sufficient to cause spontaneous neuropathic pain below injury level ... the nature of such neuronal hyperexcitability and its possible location are not known ... it is conceivable that spinothalamic tract dysfunction ... but not lesion ... is necessary for central pain," thus suggesting some kind of threshold of hyperexcitability or genetic factors. These conclusions sound obvious in light of the evidence reviewed in the first edition of this book and again here. Hyperexcitability is known to follow neural injury (Stavraky 1961). While segmental pains engage local processes, below-level diffuse pains, even in the best series, are not uniformly relieved (unlike end-zone pains), so that we may conclude that cord foci of hyperactivity play a boosting role only. This diffuse, likely bilateral, network of multisynaptic reticular propriospinal systems in and around the lesioned gray matter may feed the thalamocorticothalamic loop and spread upward towards the brainstem reticular formation by way of intersegmental cross-talking interneurons. In thoracolumbar lesions, further excitatory input may derive from peripheral (root/nerve) mechanisms. This "hyperactive core" may have variable extent, depending on the person. Reduction of this bottom-up barrage in some patients (obtained by cordotomy, cordectomy, and DREZ lesions) may at least transitorily interfere with supraspinal mechanisms. Loss of STT function thus is not enough for CP: although this may be particularly susceptible to injury, it has not been possible to link the occurrence of CCP to the extent of STT dysfunction (Wydenkeller *et al.* 2009).

The notion that both a critical level of structural damage (central gray loss being related to at-level pain and axonal white matter loss to below-level pain) and a state of hyperresponsivity are necessary for CCP to arise (Defrin *et al.* 2001, Hatem *et al.* 2010) can be refuted, as this hyperexcitability is useless without STT-induced changes at corticothalamic levels, which is the first step needed for CP to arise.

Chapter 26

Attractor-driven dynamic reverberation

In the light of knowledge finally achieved, deductions seem almost obvious and can be understood by any intelligent student; but the experience of research, gropingly in the darkness, with its profound anxiety to succeed and its alternating character between certainty and discouragement, can only be understood by him who has experienced it.
Albert Einstein (1935)

The evidence reviewed makes a strong case for central pain being the result of a localized reverberating loop between the parietal cortex (SI, as discussed in Box 21.1) and the sensory thalamus (Vc, core and shell, and Vim; CL, CM, and pulvinar have a supportive role only) (Canavero *et al.* 1993, 1996, Canavero 1994). This is the only mechanism that explains CP disappearance following the lesions described in Chapter 20 (Fig. 20.1). This dipole is exquisitely adjusted to explain somatotopographical pain distribution in CP (Canavero 1994). In those cases with complete SI or thalamic destruction, the reverberant loop is activated in the opposite hemisphere. Cortical stimulation-induced analgesia is due to a direct action on SI.

In people with (presumed) defective $GABA_A$ receptors, STT injury is followed by the establishment of an "attractor state" in SI. This **locked SI** is no longer capable of correct data estimation, being less flexible (efficient) in sampling inputs and evaluating information from both evoked and spontaneous sensory stimuli (flexibility implying the capacity to occupy different bands of discharge frequencies): in this way, information processing decorrelates. Simultaneously, the outflow down the facilitatory cortico (SI)-thalamic fiber system, no longer held in check, feeds continuously into the thalamus and caudal regions, thereby engaging an out-of-balance "pain loop" (Fig. 26.1).

This construct is akin to Edelman and Tononi's proposal that conscious experience is equivalent to a functional cluster in the thalamocorticothalamic system within which reentrant neuronal interactions yield a succession of unitary states (Baars and Gage 2010).

The reticular formation and the propriospinal system become hyperactive after CNS injuries (Stavraky 1961) and provide bilateral bottom-up facilitation to the loop. The brainstem reticular formation might also play a role in engaging a dedicated pain-coded sensory loop contralaterally (analogously to the corpus callosum).

Different qualities of pain, but also different neurometabolic findings, may be explained by individual degrees of activation of the same cells or activation (frequency discharge/oscillatory changes) of several sets of cells, in different cortical layers and thalamic nuclei, depending on site and extent of damage. The loop would be under the influence of cognitive, emotional, and attentional networks, explaining fluctuations in time of CP. Immediate or delayed onset would hinge on the degree of inhibitory defectiveness in the single patient.

Dr. Lenz has abandoned his previous views, and has admitted that "the evidence of blood flow, stimulation, and lesion studies forcefully make the case that Vc and sensorimotor cortex are involved in CPSP" (Kim JH *et al.* 2007), and that the parietal lobe is necessary for CP to arise (Veldhuijzen *et al.* 2010). Garcia-Larrea *et al.* (2010) "speculate whether extension of the [insular] lesion toward lateral parietal networks not involved in pain processing may have 'protected' the patient from a full pain syndrome." Similarly, the conclusion of a study of tourniquet ischemia-induced heterotopic noxious conditioning stimulation in 10 CPSP patients with dynamic mechanical allodynia was that the data "indicate *disruption of corticofugal control* of nociceptive input by the brain injury. Either *increased facilitation* or

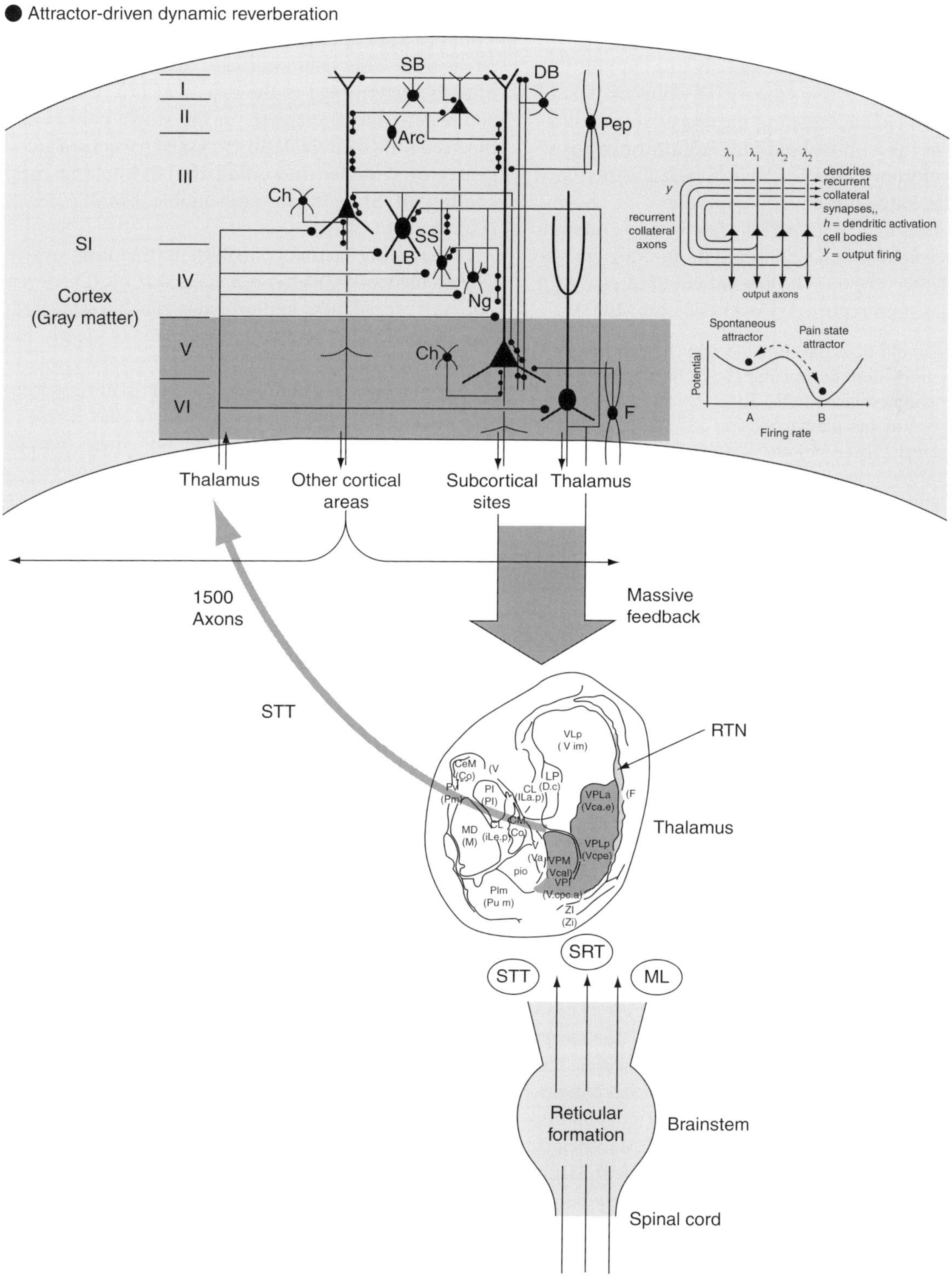

Figure 26.1. Genesis of central pain (see text for explanations).

decreased inhibition, or a combination, may be at hand" (Tuveson *et al.* 2009, emphasis added).

The theory exposed leads directly to a cure for CP: a selective lesion in the subparietal white matter, in some cases bilateral, targeting the descending facilitatory arm of the loop (**subparietal radiatotomy/posterior capsulotomy, SRPC**). Neurosurgical experience shows that, once the sensory component of chronic pain is abolished, pain affect also is renormalized (never vice versa), and this would be the case for the proposed intervention. The first patient to receive such surgery has been reported (Koszewski *et al.* 2003):

> A 72-year-old man developed a right hemispheric stroke. Immediately after the stroke he was hemiplegic and hemianesthetic. Then sensibility renormalized and his plegia became a non-disabling hemiparesis. Three months after stroke, he developed burning pain and allodynia in the left hemibody and became suicidal. MRI showed a right lesion covering most of the putamen, claustrum, external capsule, and part of the insular cortex; the internal capsule was at least partially damaged. During stereotactic surgery, 3 years after stroke, stimulation of the border between the internal pallidum and posterior limb of the internal capsule diminished, but did not fully abolish the pain. Two large lesions were done covering the whole border between the posterior limb of the internal capsule and the lentiform nucleus: in this area only, stimulation controlled the whole left side of the body. The whole CP syndrome disappeared immediately after lesioning. Right after surgery, there was motor worsening which slowly resolved to previous levels; nociceptive sensibility was fully preserved (implying that a descending input was interrupted) and no emotional change was noted. Five months later the patient was still pain-free (Fig. 26.2).

Stereotactic neurosurgery carries a small risk of mortality and permanent disabling morbidity due to the advancing of a probe inside the brain. However, this lesion can be achieved non-invasively. **Stereotactic radiosurgery** can easily mimic surgical coagulation of brain tissue, but the positioning of the stereotactic apparatus may create discomfort for the patient. **High-intensity focused ultrasound** entails no radiation, minimizes the risk of bleeding (with no risk of infection) with real-time monitoring, and avoids collateral damage. Sonications are not limited by trajectory, with several degrees of freedom. The final result is a thermal lesion up to 4 × 5 mm (Jagannathan *et al.* 2009, Martin *et al.* 2009). Targeting of the corticothalamic fibers would be achieved in both cases by DTI-guided neuronavigation. This technique has clear promise. What must be determined is the extent of this ablation to attain permanent analgesia in the single patient and the need for a bilateral lesion to quench a contralateral generator. Another interesting avenue would be **focal cooling of SI** with an implantable cooling device (Fujioka *et al.* 2010).

What other factors contribute to the onset of CP? The incidence of CP after lesions at various CNS levels does not exceed 50%, and probably much less, regardless of level. This population of patients clearly has something in common.

Gender, age, and endogenous levels of antinociceptive substances have been suggested to play a role in other chronic pain syndromes, but these remain unsubstantiated.

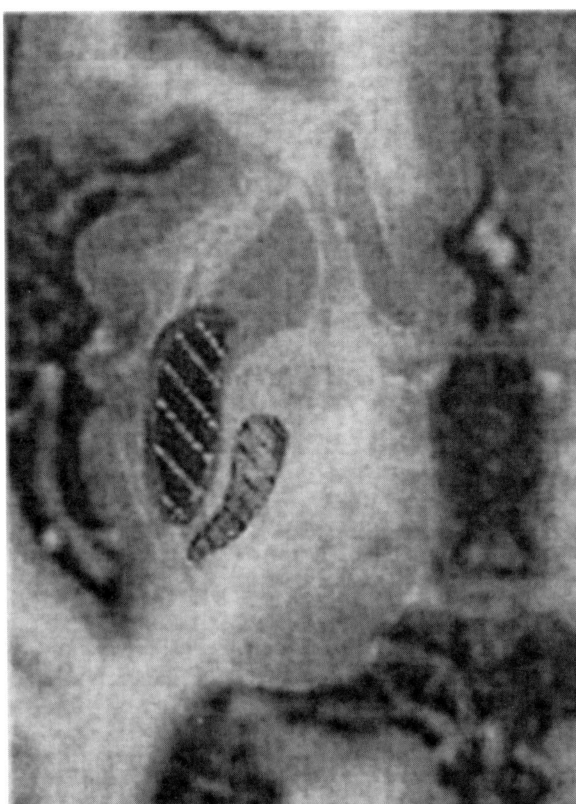

Figure 26.2. Brain MRI scan depicting surgical lesion in the posterior limb of the internal capsule abolishing central post-stroke pain. From Koszewski *et al.* 2003, with permission from VSP, an imprint of Brill Academic Publishers.

The right hemisphere is more involved than the left, with somatization symptom formation related to emotional disturbances such as migraine and other pains (Min and Lee 1997). While a damaged right hemisphere (implicated in negative affect) has been suggested as leading more frequently to CP, the evidence is still not conclusive (Canavero and Bonicalzi 1998b).

Data from human pain genetics studies are "limited and inconsistent" (Belfer and Dai 2010). These concentrated on the first few genes to be alleged as associated with pain, and were thus merely "scratching the surface of the problem in pain genetics," and "any plan to incorporate genotyping information into clinical pain practice is premature" (Mogil 2009). The β subunit (β2–3) is key to the direct actions of propofol, whereas barbiturate and benzodiazepines action hinges on α subunits (Chapter 24), and future genetic studies should focus here.

That CP needs the STT to become in some way dysfunctional is clear, but the degree of anatomical damage does not matter: CP is seen after massive (anterior spinal artery syndrome, cordotomies) or minimal (patients without sensory deficits on neurophysiological tests) impairment. CP often arises as tactile sensory (and motor) loss improves (Schott 2001), but differential engagement of the lemniscal pathway does not seem to play a significant role. However, it may be that, in predisposed people, a combination of sensory deficits is responsible (see full discussion in Canavero and Bonicalzi 2007a). Certainly, frank injury is not necessary to induce the pain state: so-called **injury discharges**, short high-frequency signals lasting several minutes at most, transmitted along nociceptive fibers, rapidly notify higher centers and prompt the pain cascade.

The central pain attractor: theoretical foundations

The question arises how neural processing can become locked in a persistent state. The exact mechanism is unknown and may vary in different contexts. Nonetheless, one such viable mechanism is the establishment of an attractor state (De Schutter 2010, Rolls and Deco 2010, Trappenberg 2010).

The flow of synaptic activity through the cortex is highly non-linear (chaotic) and only partially hierarchical (Haider and McCormick 2009, Sporns 2011). Chaotic activity (constant but variable activation of excitatory and inhibitory connections by broadly tuned spikes) maintains postsynaptic potentials just below firing threshold, allowing neurons to be more sensitive to coincident input. This ensures that the brain may switch rapidly between one neural state and another, by allowing a compromise between computational flexibility and continuity: it pays in terms of survival to be as complicated as possible without becoming totally structureless, i.e., being poised on the edge of chaos. Such "metastable" systems are poised near phase transitions (critical points) characterized by scale invariance (i.e., described by a power law) (Sporns 2011); scaling laws are parameterized by exponents and exponents vary across individuals (providing a mathematical explanation of "predisposition").

Attractors are the stable part of chaos: if the system is somehow displaced from its attractor, then it rapidly homes back in. An **attractor** is defined as some portion of the phase space such that any point which starts nearby gets closer and closer, while a **basin of attraction** (or attraction domain) of an attractor is the set of all initial conditions that lead to the attractor.

Perception depends on an underlying computation ("estimate") that is given by a probabilistic noise (fluctuation)-driven transition in a multistable neurodynamical system (i.e., multiple coexisting but competing populations of excitatory neurons). **Neural noise** comes from channel gating, fluctuations in quantal transmitter release, ion concentrations, membrane conductance, relatively random spiking times, and so on. Diffusion models postulate that the information driving the decision process is accumulated continuously over time until a decision boundary is reached.

So called **auto-association attractor systems** have two types of stable fixed points: a spontaneous state with a low firing state and one or more attractor states with high firing rates in which the positive feedback implemented by recurrent (reverberating or resonant) collateral connections maintains a high firing rate (persistent state). The firing rate is eventually stabilized by negative feedback. As a result, a stable attractor of *persistent* activity with an *elevated firing rate* is realized, which coexists with the stable spontaneous state, i.e., chaos can synchronize (Izhikevich 2007).

The attractor dynamics can be pictured by **energy landscapes** which indicate the basins of attraction by valleys and the attractor states (fixed or stable points) by the bottom of the valleys. Neural noise pushes one attractor state into another: the shallower the valley, the likelier a shift. The onset of an external sensory signal deforms the energy landscape so that only one highly excited attractor exists.

The basins in the landscape can be defined by the strengths of the synaptic weights which describe the stable operating points of the system, where the **depth of the basins** can be defined in terms of the synaptic weight space:

$$w_{ij}\ \text{(strength of the connecting synapses)} = y_i\ \text{(firing rate of the postsynaptic neuron)} \cdot y_j\ \text{(firing rate of the presynaptic neuron)} \qquad (26.1)$$

The analogy between auto-associator neural networks and physical systems with multiple attractors was drawn by Hopfield (1982), inspired by Hebb's second postulate on cell assemblies (itself extrapolated from Lorente de No's original idea that reverberating networks are a fundamental organizing principle of the brain). A stable state is obtained by lowering the network energy and combining the extended Hebb's rule with Hopfield's model energy lowering (Rolls and Deco 2010). Thus, by exploiting Hopfield's equation, we can define the energy (E) at a given time point as being a function of the synaptic weights and the current firing rates:

$$E = -1/2 \sum_{i,j} w_{ij}(y_i - \langle y \rangle)(y_j - \langle y \rangle) \qquad (26.2)$$

where y = neuron's mean firing rate.

As the depths of the basins of attraction become deeper, the attractor becomes more stable and only a sufficiently strong perturbation would drive the system from state to state (Fig. 26.1).

Part of the mechanism for the increased depth (i.e., increased stability) of the basins of attraction is **increased glutamatergic transmission**, which, as per the equation, *increases the firing rates of neurons* and the effective value of the synaptic weights between the associatively modified synapses that define an attractor (Rolls and Deco 2010). Most of the cortical excitatory drive is generated by local recurrent connections, whereas the connections that carry sensory inputs from the outside world are relatively sparse (e.g., the spinothalamic fibers reaching the cortex amount to a mere 1500 fibers!). A network integrating NMDA and GABA receptors can account for CP. Drug dissection data (Chapter 24) strongly suggest dysfunctional inhibition and unchecked excitation in CP. Both SI and sensory thalamus show a tonic inhibitory tone, modulated by sensory input: in the cortex, GABA has a particularly high density in layer IV. GABA levels in the human SI are reduced within minutes of deafferentation (Levy *et al.* 2002), and subtle reductions in GABA inhibition result in large changes in excitatory conduction and spread of activity to distant cortical sites.

An increase of NMDA or AMPA synaptic currents can increase the stability of attractor networks to the point that the intrinsic stochastic noise caused by the spiking of the neurons is much less effective in moving the system.

Stability is especially assured by the long time constant of the NMDA receptors (leading to temporal smoothing). On the other hand, increasing GABA has a large effect on the stability of the spontaneous state, making it less likely to jump to a high-firing-rate attractor state (Rolls and Deco 2010): increasing GABA currents by 10% when the NMDA currents are increased by 3% can move the persistent state away from overstability back to normal.

A local recurrent (attractor) network in SI would engage, to an undefined extent, the following layers:

Layer IV → layer II/III → layer V → layer VI → layer IV

↓ (from layer V and layer VI) Corticothalamic outflow

At the same time, long-range connections between cortical areas (corticocortical connections are present in layers II/III and V/VI) enable networks in different areas to interact in the way needed to implement an attractor single network (explaining why other brain regions are involved in imaging studies); implicit in the model, long-range inputs from MI and SII/insula and higher-order thalamic nuclei to SI layer I no longer exert a top-down control on SI.

These corticocortical intra- and interhemispheric highways follow the mathematics of a **small world network**, which consists of a power-law-described network of high-traffic highways and hubs along with numerous "small streets and alleys" for much more limited local traffic (Sporns 2011). These *highly recurrent* local networks have a strong tendency to transiently enter into stable states of enhanced excitability that dynamically interact with sensory stimulation.

In the end, this construct can explain the effect of increasing inhibition in CP (class A CP: inhibition-sensitive). On the other hand, in several patients, GABAergic drugs are not strong enough to "swamp" the glutamatergic hypertonus (Class B CP: inhibition-resistant). Thus, based on the model, the most effective way to achieve pharmacological analgesia would be to simultaneously increase inhibition and decrease excitation. At the same time, it explains why aminergic drugs may modulate CP: brain amines and other neurotransmitters/modulators may alter the "energy landscape," gating the system between states. Also, it may be postulated that different qualities of pain may be due to ever-present and fluctuating noise effects, as noise attempts to push the CP attractor out of its basin and fails.

As stated, the site of the attractor is SI, with SI locked in a hyperexcitable state. As a consequence, a pain-coded loop is engaged along the corticothalamocortical axis. The cortex controls rhythm generation in thalamic networks: by ablating its output to the thalamus, the loop is interrupted, the thalamus returns to a more normal state, and SI receives less excitatory drive, pushing it away from the attractor. This explains why patients relieved of their CP reacquire normal tactile sensations: SI is no longer locked, but has regained its flexibility in rapidly changing state.

Bilaterality of central pain

A large body of evidence proves that acute pain is processed bilaterally (reviewed in Canavero and Bonicalzi 2007a). SI is activated via a hitherto underappreciated, extensively spatially distributed, but highly organized afferent connectivity that links SI with skin regions on both sides of the body midline. Although the activity evoked by ipsilateral stimulation may seem insignificant, it does appear to have a prominent effect on the cortical response to contralateral stimulation (Tommerdahl *et al.* 2010). A somatotopic organization of purely nociceptive stimuli is represented in both contralateral and ipsilateral SI, irrespective of associated tactile stimulation (Bingel *et al.* 2004), ipsilateral SI activity resulting from uncrossed afferent or transcallosal excitatory pathways. fMRI of healthy people suggests bilateral brainstem activation when heat is applied to the face, with contralateral brainstem activity more pronounced after stimulation of V1 than V3 (Kubina *et al.* 2010). In contrast to innocuous inputs from the face, noxious information ascends *bilaterally* to the face SI through human Vc, independently of transcallosal connections (Nash *et al.* 2010) and "recordings from electrodes in the region of the [Vc] reveal similar potentials to touch and pressure stimuli both ipsi- and contralaterally" (Ervin and Mark 1960). There are reports of bilateral cheiro-oral syndrome (Chen *et al.* 1997). Tanriverdi *et al.* (2009) obtained 13.6% ipsilateral and bilateral sensory responses in SI, almost all from stimulating within 1.3 cm above the sylvian sulcus, and Lenz's group experienced two cases of unilateral CPSP with bilateral cold hypoesthesia (Greenspan *et al.* 2004, Kim JH *et al.* 2007; see also Beric *et al.* 1988, Boivie *et al.* 1989, Vestergaard *et al.* 1995). According to Stein *et al.* (1989), "when noxious stimuli are sufficiently intense, ipsilateral pathways are also recruited."

The evidence for CP bilaterality is compelling. Riddoch and Critchley (1937) reported exceptional cases of bilateral pain due to unilateral thalamic lesion. Canavero (1996) described a woman with a subparietal cavernoma and contralateral CP who, for about 10 days, complained of the same kind of pain (burning paroxysms to arm and, when severe, the whole hemisoma) on the contralateral arm. Both pains simultaneously responded to propofol. *No sensory deficits were ever observed in involved areas.* Kim (1998) described six patients with unilateral stroke who initially developed painful sensory symptoms on the side contralateral to the lesion. The patient's CPSP progressively worsened for a certain period of time when sensory symptoms also occurred on the side ipsilateral to the lesion. The delayed-onset ipsilateral sensory symptoms were mild, *unaccompanied by objective sensory deficits*, and developed in the body parts mirroring the site of the most severe CPSP. Once developed, they persisted during follow-up (new-onset PNP and strokes were excluded by appropriate exams in some patients). Silbergeld *et al.* (2011) reported on a patient who complained of bilateral vulvar tactile allodynia due to a unilateral thalamic tumor (see below). We have already seen examples of bilateral CP elicited by unilateral stimulation in Chapter 22 (Gorecki *et al.* 1989). Kim (1999) also reported on five patients with hemisensory symptoms due to unilateral strokes occurring in the left putamen, left thalamus, right putamen, right lateral medulla, and left thalamic-internal capsular area. Sensory symptoms had gradually improved or remained stable after onset. When another stroke occurred on the *contralateral* thalamic-occipital, frontoparietal, lateral medulla, temporoparietal, and pontine areas, respectively, previous sensory symptoms significantly worsened and became painful on the previously affected side. Tasker's group described cases of CP patients with "silent" thalamus, who most likely engaged the healthy contralateral hemisphere (Chapter 22). Finally, and most importantly, **two patients with sudden remission of CP following a new stroke in the unaffected hemisphere are on record** (Chapter 20).

In conclusion, one fact seems inescapable: **the mechanism that leads to CP engages both hemispheres, so that a corticothalamic pain loop can be activated on either side. Importantly, bilateral CP does not depend on structures with bilateral receptive fields (e.g., SII or ACC), or contralateral strokes would not abolish the pain.**

CP may be shifted contralaterally through the corpus callosum (30% of whose fibers are unmyelinated) or through the other structures, including spinal and brainstem commissural interneurons. Olausson *et al.* (2001b) found that cortical areas typically involved in pain processing can be activated by ipsilateral pathways directly from the periphery, but, unlike tactile information, pain activation in the hemisphere contralateral to the stimulation is dependent on transcallosal information processing. In amputees, acute hand deafferentation can elicit a focal increase in excitability in the hand motor MI representation *contralateral* to the deafferented cortex that is influenced by transcallosal interactions; $GABA_A$ agonism blocks this increased excitability (Werhahn *et al.* 2002; see also Irlbacher *et al.* 2007). Meyer *et al.* (1995) found that homotopic regions of SI are linked, so that plasticity induced in one hemisphere (in the form of RF expansion brought about by a small peripheral denervation) is *immediately* mirrored in the other hemisphere: neurons which displayed the plasticity showed no responsiveness to stimulation of the ipsilateral body surface, suggesting a specific role of maintaining integration between corresponding cortical fields (see also Fabri *et al.* 1999). SI exerts a facilitatory influence upon both SII areas, and the corpus callosum accounts for 65% of the effect (Stancak *et al.* 2002). Bilaterality of hand representation in parietal somatosensory areas is under callosal control, since it is lost after callosal section, mostly at BA2 (but much less at BA1 and almost none at BA3b) and BA5/7 levels (Iwamura *et al.* 1994). Cortical stimulation for stroke rehabilitation can modulate both hemispheres simultaneously (Canavero *et al.* 2006a). Some months after callosotomy for epilepsy control (Van Wagenen and Herren 1940), corpus callosum is replaced in discharge diffusion by other structures (brainstem, diencephalons, anterior and posterior commissures) (Papo and Quattrini 1997, Quattrini *et al.* 1997). Facilitatory interhemispheric influences are possible in patients with agenesis of the corpus callosum.

Finally, thalamic reticular nucleus cells may also project to the *contralateral dorsal thalamus* in the intrathalamic commissure, potentially influencing the cerebral cortex and basal ganglia of *both* hemispheres (Jones 2007).

The genesis of evoked pains

That evoked pains are not pivotal to CP is proved by the simple observation that, unlike steady spontaneous pain, many patients (*c.* 30%) do not complain of them. A few patients complain only of evoked pains (Chapter 3). As observed in some patients, these may follow a different time course than spontaneous pain. Greenspan *et al.* (1997) described a woman with a thalamic lesion observed over 4 years who had CP only during 3 months. Prior to spontaneous pain, there was transient but intense thermal allodynia several months earlier. Attal *et al.* (1998b) described a patient who presented uniquely with very intense brush-induced allodynia (dynamic mechanical) strictly confined to the left C2/3 dermatomes for several months. Thereafter, spontaneous pain and sensory deficits appeared and a new MRI showed an intraspinal lesion involving the C2/5 segments. Silbergeld *et al.* (2011) reported on an 18-year-old female patient who developed persistent burning at the vaginal introitus, typically lasting for 10–15 minutes after intercourse, and bilateral tactile introital allodynia that lasted 5 years, at which time an unresectable unilateral thalamic pilocytic astrocytoma was diagnosed: her disturbance had also progressed to involve first the right pelvis and subsequently the right hemisoma, being burning and tingling with "waves of cold."

Greenspan *et al.* (2004), on the basis of a study of 13 CPSP patients, concluded that *sparing of a submodality by lesions causing CP is associated with the occurrence of allodynia in that modality*, i.e., both tactile and cold/heat allodynia, even striking, were significantly associated with the presence, rather than the absence or reduction, of normal tactile and thermal sensibility. Similar observations have been reported in syringomyelia (Hatem *et al.* 2010). It was also noted how all four patients with insular (posterior) lesions had tactile allodynia, but only one had tactile sensory loss. However, both patients with insular lesions and non-insular lesions had tactile allodynia, cold allodynia, and thermotactile sensory deficits without significant differences. On the basis of microstimulation studies (Chapter 22), Greenspan *et al.* have suggested that the termination of the STT in the thalamus is reorganized to signal pain instead of cold in CP patients. Cold allodynia would be due to input from an intact cold pathway driving Vc (and not from loss of such input, disinhibiting these regions; see also Garcia-Larrea *et al.* 2002). Tactile allodynia would be due to disinhibition of Vc from loss of insula or SI/SII input.

Tasker (2001b) observed how the induction of burning and pain appears to be peculiar to patients with pain. Since all those in whom pain was induced and half those in whom burning occurred suffered from evoked pain, the phenomenon may be unrelated to the spontaneous pain ("**central allodynia**"). He also noted that allodynia and hyperpathia in CPSP appear to be suppressed by PVG DBS, as if depending on spinothalamic transmission. This central allodynia occurs at sites where normally non-painful sensations are evoked, as well as at sites where normally no sensations are evoked, being unrelated spatially to the presence of bursting or thalamic reorganization and expanded receptive fields: he ascribed it to third-order neuron sensitization. He also observed how evoked pains in SCI patients may be due to conduction through spinothalamic pathways, thus differing from steady pain (see Chapter 25).

Quantitative sensory studies and differential responses to drugs seem to indicate that evoked pains have a different genesis, e.g., thermal evoked pain (amitriptyline-responsive) versus mechanical evoked pains (lidocaine/morphine-responsive). This would argue against a generalized hyperexcitability of nociceptive neurons to any type of stimuli (Attal *et al.* 2000, 2002). Also, the effects of morphine on static mechanical allodynia suggest that static and dynamic (brush-evoked) mechano-allodynia associated with CP are sustained by different mechanisms (brush-evoked allodynia having a similar genesis as in PNP). In this regard, it should be noted that some opioids are weak NMDA, but not AMPA, blockers: hyperalgesia being a supposedly NMDA-mediated phenomenon (but see above), this might explain opioid action on hyperalgesia. Sasaki *et al.* (2009) reported on three men with severe mechanical and thermal allodynia in the forearms/hands after traumatic cervical SCI. Conservative treatment for >20 days had no effect. Mechanical allodynia in two patients totally disappeared 1 day after laminectomy, while case 3 had a marked reduction and a complete disappearance over 4 days. On the other hand, thermal allodynia decreased slowly and disappeared (VAS 0, 1, 1.5) over a few months, suggesting different mechanisms. However, our own studies (Canavero and Bonicalzi 2004a) show that both spontaneous pain and allodynia can be abolished simultaneously, although the latter to a greater extent – or even exclusively – in some cases. GABA agonism may thus affect the whole spectrum of CP. Bowsher (2005a) suggested that lesions at different sites may associate with different types of allodynia, but "the distinction is not hard and fast."

Thus, sensitization at cord, brainstem and thalamic levels may play a role in the genesis of allodynia only, but not spontaneous pain, with inappropriate activation of the STT through stimulation of receptors and fibers that normally are not involved in nociception. As we have seen in reviewing neurometabolic studies, allodynia is subserved by widespread activity particularly in frontal areas, perhaps justifying its high unpleasantness. However, sudden disappearances, as reviewed above, strongly suggest that, **once the loop sustaining spontaneous pain has been switched off, evoked pains are simultaneously abolished**.

Box 26.1. Exploring the cortical layout and its output

The interested reader is referred to Nuñez and Malmierca (2007), Briggs and Usrey (2008), Haider and McCormick (2009), Thomson (2010), and Markram (2010).

Around 86% of all synapses in a cortical column are excitatory and 14% are inhibitory. Roughly a third of the excitatory synapses are formed by the axons of neurons within that column, a third from neurons in neighboring columns, and a third from neurons in other cortical regions or the opposite hemisphere and subcortical regions. Most of the inhibitory synapses arise from neurons within the same column, some from immediately neighboring columns, and a minority from more distant columns within the same neocortical region. Neocortical synapses can display one of six types of short-term plasticity, depending on the ratio of the time constants of synaptic depression and facilitation, which yields three main classes with further subclasses with high and low probability of release. **The specific type of synaptic dynamic deployed between any two neurons is genetically determined and cannot be**

"switched" by synaptic plasticity. The axon of a neocortical neuron, and even sequential boutons on the same axon collateral, can deliver synapses that exhibit quite different dynamic properties depending on postsynaptic target. The type of synaptic dynamics expressed between pyramids and interneurons is highly predictable, due to a combinatorial identity match, a fact not applicable to inter-interneuronal synapses. Given the huge number of interneuronal types, the diversity in the mapping of the six types of dynamic synapses is enormous. Connections between cortical neurons are highly non-random, with preferred pathways and subcircuits being the rule. Nearby pyramids form highly specific connections that establish unique but flexible cortical subnetworks. In the context of such architecture, spike generation on a short timescale is determined by rapid departures (30–100 Hz) from a precise excitatory–inhibitory balance (**attractor dynamics**) which lies on top of a stable depolarization that is mediated by a broader, less temporally precise excitatory–inhibitory balance (< 10 Hz). This implies interaction of *different temporal bandwidths* and windows of opportunity in cortical processing. If nearby neurons receive relatively unique constellations of strong connections amidst a sea of weaker ones, then highly specific and sparse transmission of sensory responses can occur even if background activity levels are shared, i.e., temporary interaction of specific pathways.

Excitatory pyramids are found in layers II–VI. Layer II/III pyramids are not easily divisible into separate morphological classes. Layer IV contains classical and star pyramids. In SI, glutamatergic spiny stellate cells are a further kind and receive thalamic input. Layer V contains thin untufted pyramids that project contralaterally and thick tufted pyramids that project subcortically. **Layer VI has the greatest diversity of pyramidal morphologies**, with at least four distinct types (cortico-cortical, cortico-thalamic, cortico-callosal, and cortico-claustral). Each class has further subclasses depending on connectivity. The local arborization of a single pyramid can innervate 1–30% of neighboring pyramidal cells depending on layer and type of target. *Pyramidal interconnectivity at microcolumn level decreases from 30% in layers II/III to 20% in layer IV to 10% in layer V to 1% in layer VI*. Importantly, *there is strong interlayer connectivity, in particular from layer IV to layers II/III and thence to layers V/VI*. Target selectivity is apparent: e.g., the thick tufted pyramids innervate about 10% of other similar cells in the same layer, while hardly innervating the thin untufted cells in the same neuropil. The thin untufted pyramids are also only sparsely interconnected (around 1%), compared with 10% of the thick tufted cells. Interpyramidal synapses more typically display synaptic depression (F2). *Deploying synapses with different dynamics onto different target neurons enables differential activation thereof within a layer, across layers, across columns, and in more distant regions*.

There are four major types of inhibitory cells in layer I and nine in layers II/VI (chandelier, small and large basket cells, neurogliaform cells, double bouquet cells, and Martinotti). Each anatomical type can express up to 8–15 major types of electrical behaviors (fast spiking, regular spiking, intermediate spiking) and no fewer than 15 peptidergic phenotypes. Also considering layer differences, a neocortical column has no fewer (and probably more) than **200 morpho-electrical types of GABA interneurons**. By way of example, parvalbumin neuron (which preferentially target somata)-mediated feedforward inhibition is most effective at low frequencies, whereas somatostatin neuron (which preferentially target dendrites)-mediated inhibition is strongest at high frequencies. Interconnectivity between interneurons seems to be higher for immediately neighboring interneurons of the same type and connections, and often also involves electrical synapses. However, while some types (e.g., large basket cells) are highly interconnected, others (e.g., double bouquet cells) are much less so, if at all. GABAergic synapses display all six types of short-term plasticity, but F1/3 types are more common, i.e., there is more facilitation at GABA than glutamatergic synapses. Most importantly, GABAergic synapses, in stark contrast to glutamatergic synapses, express perfect homogeneity of synaptic dynamics onto the target population (**GABA grouping**). This allows the same synchronization effect to be imposed on a population of neurons of a given type, and a different synchronization effect on populations with different types of neurons. Synfire chains and gap junctioning are part of the mechanism. Some of these cells also make long-range connections, sending axons through white matter tracts and in the isocortex (Ascoli *et al*. 2008, Burkhalter 2008, Jinno 2009). Through fast oscillatory synchronization, distinct classes of GABA cells can help orchestrate activity in multiple brain areas by sculpting resonant columns. In other words, rapid modulation of functional connectivity across cortical areas is critically regulated by **local inhibitory subnetworks** responsible for precise spike timing in nearby pyramidal neurons and thus proper control of information flow. A basic mechanism for sensory response facilitation is a balanced mixture of excitatory and inhibitory synaptic bombardment that tonically depolarizes target neurons.

Corticothalamic axons from SI (and some from MI) leave the cortex and traverse the striatum in small bundles which split off in two streams: a dorsal one (layer VI axons) heads directly to Vc and TRN, a ventral one (layer V axons) courses down the pallidum and joins the internal capsule. At the exit from the pallidum some fibers give off branches that enter the thalamus to the posterior group. **The corticothalamic (CT) projection has been estimated to**

outnumber the TC projection by as much as 10 to 1. It is topographic and reciprocal: if a thalamic region within Vc projects to the somatotopically appropriate area in SI, that cortical area projects back to the same thalamic area. However, there is some spread beyond the borders of the zone of thalamic cells, providing input to that part of cortical representation, with a denser central core of CT projection and a thinner surrounding area. Bilateral CT projections exist, but these are small compared with the ipsilateral projection and primarily from cortical areas near the midline. Nonetheless, they can exert a synchronizing bi-hemispheric influence. Corticothalamic projections from SII are sparse (!).

The layer V corticothalamic projection (LVCT) mainly contacts association thalamic nuclei (and not Vc or TRN), being a collateral projection issued from long-range axons projecting to the brainstem and/or cord. The LVCT returns to cortex (often layer I) diffusely. Layer V displays dense firing and population rate coding (versus layer II/III's sparse firing and cell-specific temporal code). Layer V pyramidal neurons are intrinsically more depolarized than those in layer II/III and are strongly synaptically coupled to other nearby layer V pyramids in a highly recurrent excitatory microcircuit, but only weakly to layer II/III (which curbs propagation from layer V to upper layers) (Crochet and Petersen 2009). LVCT may modulate thalamic activity diffusely; this non-reciprocating projection is composed of faster conducting axons. Intracortically, LVCT cells give off an extensive system of long horizontal collaterals, mainly in layer V, but also, less uniformly, in layer III.

There are four classes of pyramidal neurons in layer VI:

(1) A minority of spiny cells that receive direct thalamocortical sensory input (like layer IV).
(2) A large group (30–50%) of corticothalamic cells. They come in two classes: one, typically found in upper layer VI, with axonal and dendritic arbors in layer IV, innervate Vc and have axon collaterals that innervate the thalamic reticular nucleus; another, typically found in deep layer VI, is made up of shorter upright pyramids with axonal and dendritic arbors that terminate in layer V (and some also ramifing in layer II/III): they innervate Vc reciprocally with modulatory synapses, but like layer V pyramids, they also innervate secondary and association regions of thalamus with large more proximal boutons; they do *not* target the thalamic reticular nucleus.
(3) Another large group of short upright pyramids and bipolar cells with axons that do not leave the cortex or, typically, ascend above layer V but extend for long distances horizontally connecting cortical columns and cortical areas, e.g., SI and MI.
(4) Claustrum projecting pyramids with a long slender apical dendrite and long horizontally oriented axons confined to the deep layers.

Layer VI pyramids are not uniform. In deep layer VI, pyramids have no spontaneous activity, no obvious receptive fields, and slower conducting axons. In superficial layer VI, cells are spontaneously active, have definable receptive fields, and are faster conducting. Only these latter can be activated orthodromically from Vc, with long latencies. Both corticocortical cells and claustrum projecting pyramids display powerful spike frequency adaptation in response to maintained depolarization. In contrast, **corticothalamic cells have a near-tonic firing pattern, with weak adaptation in response to prolonged adaptation but never ceasing firing above-threshold. Layer VI corticothalamic cells integrate already highly processed information from layer V pyramids and from layer VI corticocortical cells, with the direct input they receive from the thalamus.**

The layer VI thalamic input (LVICT), which is **much larger** than LVCT, is composed of thin slowly conducting fibers. It targets Vc in a topographical manner, but also sends collaterals to the thalamic reticular nucleus (TRN) and intrathalamic interneurons and distributes branches bearing arrays of small terminations across most of the thalamic nuclei. These CT terminals are presynaptic to the distal dendrites of thalamic relay cells. The density of CT terminations on TRN cells may be substantially less than on relay cells in the dorsal thalamus. CT synapses in primary sensory thalamic regions differ significantly from those provided by afferent sensory axons. They are smaller and more distally located on relay cell dendrites, utilize NR2B and mGluR1 receptors in addition to the AMPA receptors that dominate afferent inputs, and facilitate, rather than depress, on repetitive activation. These inputs appear to be modulatory. All thalamic relays receive a modulatory input from layer VI of cortex, but only higher-order relays (e.g., the pulvinar) receive, in addition, a driver input from layer V (which possibly provides a more powerful synaptic effect). The layer VI modulatory input is mainly feedback, whereas the layer V driver input is feed-forward (Sherman and Guillery 2006). CT inputs exhibit a slow EPSP and marked frequency-dependent facilitation that may be important in the integration of inputs, whereas EPSPs from CT synapses onto TRN are sharper and display less facilitation (i.e., greater temporal precision).

That the cortex influences the thalamus is undisputed: what is controversial is the extent of this influence and the precise conditions under which it is generated. Proposed roles (not mutually exclusive) include facilitation and augmentation of thalamic synchrony (Vc-TRN is an intrinsic oscillator) and consequently of oscillatory coherence in the corticothalamocortical network, influence on shape and strength of thalamic receptive fields (neuroplasticity), **an increase of thalamic responses to painful stimuli**, attentional filtering or generation of conductance noise within the thalamus mixing up burst and tonic firing: the final result would be a more linear transfer with enhancement of information flow between Vc and SI. This is accomplished by the distinct classes of CT neurons, which vary widely in the conduction latency of their feedback axons, each with a specific function and operating with distinct neuronal ensembles at multiple (both fast and slow) speeds (multiple time-scale modulation). One must also consider that each brain region may perform its computation in very different ways, and this adds new complexity to the picture.

Appendix: Erroneous theories of central pain

You can disprove a theory by finding even a single observation that disagrees with the predictions of the theory ... if ever a new observation is found to disagree, we have to abandon or modify the theory. At least that is what is supposed to happen.
Stephen Hawking, A Brief History of Time *(1988)*

Doubt is not a pleasant condition, but certainty is absurd.
Voltaire

A theory that accounts for all the facts is bound to be wrong, because some of the facts are bound to be wrong.
Francis Crick

In this appendix, we review theories put forth over the past 20 years or so (older ones are discussed and rejected in the first edition of this book). Each theory is first expounded and then exploded. The reader will understand how even in the imprecise field of biomedicine stringent logic can advance the field. Unfortunately, inertia (or momentum) has it that, paper after paper, current authors merely repeat authority-based mantras without pondering and often simply reading the abstracts. The vast majority of theories proposed to explain CP until now are based on incomplete "current" anatomical knowledge, selective adaptation of anatomical data (often of animal provenance) to authors' needs, scarce appreciation of the full clinical spectrum of CP and its features, exclusion of contradictory findings, or scarce familiarity with the full gamut of neurosurgical data. Some are technology-driven more than idea-driven. Dismissal of exceptions – not just single cases, but whole groups of patients – is the norm in the field. It should not come as a surprise that different authors, based on similar evidence, reached opposite conclusions. Finally, a few authors embarked on phrenological approaches, trying to paste CP to a unique brain center. Animal studies proved useless, yet not all human studies are equally useful. Most add nothing except to the publication roll for academic promotion. Hopefully this section will help dispel a few myths. Ergo, *Götterdämmerung*, the twilight of the gods!

Götterdämmerung I: Entrenched neuroplasticity

Theory

According to this view, neuropathic pain owes both its onset and its chronicity to aberrant "neuroplastic" changes at both neuronal and glial levels. Since chronic pain is so often "entrenched," the major and extensive peripheral and central somatosensory changes, including gross structural nerve damage sustained over many years (e.g., tumoral or bony compression), are envisioned as irreversible. Under this rubric, several alterations are generally discussed:

(1) **Central sensitization**. This follows prolonged or repeated noxious stimulation of STT neurons at the time of the pain-inducing lesion and consists of a spectrum of derangements which include increased **spontaneous discharge**, evoked pains, but also **denervation supersensitivity** (an enhanced response of neural cells to the transmitter lost, and then re-expressed) and **receptive field (RF) expansion**, due to loss of sensory input. It is considered to be a form of long-term potentiation. So-called **wind-up**, a progressive increase in neuronal excitability akin to sensitization, observed in a minority of spinal cells only and some, but not all, chronic pains, follows repeated stimulation of nociceptive C fibers.

(2) **Sprouting**. This is a hierarchical and lesion-specific, non-random phenomenon, which follows

injury. It includes *collateral sprouting* from uninjured neurons with variable restoration of anatomy (rapid: days, complete in days or months; extent: 40 μm), *ingrowth* from healthy, but functionally distinct neurons (1 month after injury), *pruning* (with growth of new axons from injured cell) with a more normal anatomic restoration (4 months after injury, last 2, extent up to 1 mm). Sprouting can lead to *rewiring*: e.g., intracortical sprouting can lead to generation of powerful monosynaptic excitatory feedback and intraspinally Aβ fibers may retarget STT neurons, or non-pain-relaying neurons, in lamina II, and even switch neurochemical profile and function as C fibers.

(3) **Somatotopographical rearrangements**. This is a remodeling, with expansion of RFs at all CNS levels, supposedly due to changes in synaptic efficacy, disinhibition with unmasking or strengthening of latent but ineffective excitatory and convergent synaptic inputs, changes in intracellular processes leading to altered neuronal excitability, sprouting with creation of new synaptic connections. Manipulation of sensory inputs can lead to rapid reorganization of the cerebral cortex, occurring within minutes to hours. Somatotopic rearrangements (up to 2–3 cm in cortex) have been reported in human pain states and widely believed to correlate directly with painful sensations, particularly at SI cortical levels.

(4) **Neuronal degeneration**. Injury to sensory tracts leads to degeneration of inhibitory cells, namely shrinkage, substantial dendritic atrophy, loss of dendritic spines and truncated dendrites, and/or loss of the proximal axons and perikaryo-nuclear alterations. These are followed by loss of inhibition and electrophysiological anomalies. Several (but not all) MRI studies hint that neurodegeneration ("atrophy of the thalamus," "gray matter decreases") may occur in the brain (decreases in gray matter volume and density) in cases of chronic back pain, phantom pain, migraine, tension-type headache, fibromyalgia, although with varying degree and regional distribution. On the other side, thickening in the somatosensory cortex of patients with migraine has been reported (Da Silva *et al.* 2007).

(5) **Gliopathy**. Glia have been found to be altered in models of chronic pain.

Damning evidence

(1) There are many reports of mostly *sudden* disappearance of CP after treatment of the triggering lesion, so-called **reversible CP**. Similarly, cases of years-long peripheral neuropathic pains, including trigeminal neuralgia and carpal tunnel syndrome pain, resolve immediately after pain-relieving surgery (Schott 2001); and when, e.g., phantom pain is alleviated by plexus anesthesia, the amount of cortical reorganization is also reduced. Brief anesthesia of a finger results in the expansion of the remaining fingers' SI representation, and this is reversed on removal of the block (Rossini *et al.* 1994). So-called long-term microcircuit plasticity (LTMP) drives neurons to disconnect from some neurons and connect with others within hours; spike-timing-dependent plasticity can lead to rapid redistribution of synaptic efficacy (metaplasticity). Thus, the discussed neuroplastic/degenerative changes, whether rapidly reversible (e.g., RF expansion) or not (e.g., cell loss), would be inconsequential.

(a) Michelsen (1943) reported four cases of meningiomas impinging upon the parietal cortex, in which pain and associated sensory phenomena in the involved extremities were present. In his case 4, the pain was completely relieved by removal of the lesion, and in his case 3 it was relieved for 4 years before it reappeared. His case 5, with a depressed skull fracture over the anterior and posterior central gyri with cerebral contusion, exhibited paraplegia and bilateral hyperpathia and hyperesthesia. Position sense was absent in the right leg and diminished in the left, while pain and touch were recognized and localized. After debridement, the pain gradually cleared, hyperesthesia receded, and sensation improved.

(b) Silver (1957) reported a patient who had a stroke, with hemiplegia and aphasia. Eight years later, he gradually developed very severe paroxysmal burning pain in the right arm. An arteriovenous malformation (AVM) of the left parietal area was diagnosed at angiography and completely removed in two stages. Under local anesthesia, *manipulation, traction upon, and clipping of the component blood vessels reproduced the pain*. The pain was abolished *almost immediately* and relief maintained for the 5 years of observation.

(c) Di Biagio (1959) totally and permanently relieved a CP patient with steady and intermittent paroxysmal components, but no hyperpathia or allodynia, following extirpation of a right subcortical parietal tuberculoma.

(d) Hamby (1961) reported on a young man who developed severe burning pain with allodynia in the left upper limb following a car accident. Two years later, at surgery, the parietal cortex was found to be covered by extensive pools of subarachnoid fluid. Drainage of these pools revealed yellow, atrophic, leathery-looking cortex resembling that following an old infarct. This area was sharply separable from normal cortex and extended from the sylvian fissure upward almost to the interhemispheric fissure, and apparently was limited anteriorly by the postcentral gyrus. Stimulation over the postcentral gyrus behind the motor points elicited painful prickling sensations in the upper limb. Stimulation in the normal-appearing postcentral gyrus above the arm area elicited painless prickling sensations in the foot. A transpial incision was made 5 mm deeper than the gutters of the gyri along the posterior edge of the postcentral gyrus and over three contiguous parietal gyri. The cortex and adjacent U-fiber areas of the white matter were easily removed. On the next day the patient had no subjective pain or dysesthesia or allodynia. The patient remained pain-free *10 years* after surgery.

(e) Rétif *et al.* (1967) reported on a patient (their case 3) who had an anterior parietal meningioma with purely paroxysmal fit-like pain and a jacksonian march. Removal was followed by a complete recovery. EEG showed an irritative pattern.

(f) Gonzales *et al.* (1992) reported on an AIDS patient whose CT scan showed a single ring enhancing lesion in the left lateral thalamus and adjacent posterior limb of the internal capsule. CP disappeared after anti-toxoplasmosis therapy and a 6-month treatment with amitriptyline.

(g) Stoodley *et al.* (1995) reported a 63-year-old woman who gradually (over many years) developed constant dull pain to the whole right hemisoma (worse in the face) and an unpleasant tingling sensation on being touched on those areas. There was *no* sensory deficit. Neuroradiologically, she harbored a saccular aneurysm of the bifurcation of the left internal carotid artery extending up to the left thalamus. There was complete resolution of all her sensory symptoms *immediately* following surgical clipping and for a follow-up of *18 months*.

(h) Potagas *et al.* (1997) described a patient with intermittent pain in the right arm caused by an otherwise asymptomatic low-grade glioma of the white matter of the parietal operculum whose pain stopped after excision of the tumor.

(i) Fukuhara *et al.* (1999) reported on a woman with a 9-year story of progressively worsening episodic deep aching/burning CP to the right hemisoma. *No* sensory deficit was present. Neuroimaging disclosed an AVM in the corona radiata of the parietal lobe, along the posterior horn of the lateral ventricle. Embolization achieved *complete* remission. Transient sensory hypoesthesia was seen (post-embolization subparietal ischemia?).

(j) Albe-Fessard (personal communication to Barraquer-Bordas *et al.* 1999) had a woman with CP in an anesthetic facial area. She had a huge parietal meningioma with maximal compression on the face area. Removal led to CP disappearance and renormalization of sensibility.

(k) Tasker (2001a) operated on a patient with a right parietal meningioma presenting with contralateral dysesthetic causalgic pain, which *disappeared* after removal of the tumor

(l) Amancio *et al.* (2002) reported on a woman with a meningioma affecting both parietal lobes, but contralateral pain only. After surgery, her burning sensations increased, only to clear over 2 months.

(m) We observed several cases ourselves. Pagni and Canavero (1993) reported on a woman suffering paroxysms of pain, described as "burning," "lancinating," or "electric shock-like," which increased in frequency over the months. MRI disclosed a posterior T6–7 meningioma. Extirpation resulted in total remission over 24 hours, without any further recurrence. Canavero *et al.* (1995b) described a man who developed acute Schneider's syndrome and hyperacute allodynia to the limbs (worse in the arms in C6–8 dermatomeres bilaterally) within 30 minutes of a fall. Allodynia was so intense as to make sensory examination impossible. On MRI, there was spondylotic narrowing of the vertebral canal with large osteophytes at C4–7, particularly on the posterior aspect. A voluminous spur jutted out of the right posterior aspect at C7; the C5/6 disc was posteriorly excluded, impinging upon and nicking the anterior surface of the dural sac, with greatest narrowing at C4–6. Upon reawakening from surgery (C5/6 discectomy plus stabilization), the allodynia had *completely disappeared.* Sensory examination at this time showed thermoalgesic hypoesthesia in the four limbs. Two weeks later, typical CCP involving the four limbs appeared and gradually worsened. Pagni and Canavero (1995) relieved CP involving one leg after aspiration of a benign intramedullary cyst (follow-up 15 years; unpublished observations). Canavero (1996) reported on a woman who developed burning pain in her left arm and, episodically, in the whole hemibody due to a bleeding cavernoma in the white matter deep to the inferior parietal lobe. CP totally regressed after the bleeding cleared, only to return with a new bleeding years later (unpublished observations). Canavero and Bonicalzi (2001b) reported on two patients. The first suffered from severe burning pain and allodynia to one leg which totally vanished within 24 hours of extirpation of a cystic tumor at conus level (follow-up: 3 months). The second was immediately relieved of her intermittent CP following embolization of an aneurysm at the vertebral/PICA junction impinging on the medulla (follow-up: 2 months). We relieved a 54-year-old woman of her pain to the left leg, misdiagnosed as sciatic pain, after shunting a large parieto-occipital arachnoidal cyst. Another woman with a meningioma compressing SI had painful fits to the hemibody, abolished after surgery (Canavero, unpublished observations). Lastly, a 51-year-old female doctor developed rapid-onset symptoms from a C3–T1 epidural hematoma. There was VAS 10 touch and VAS 5 ice allodynia, plus pinprick hyperalgesia in the right forearm and hand. These receded over several days after surgical evacuation.

(2) Immediate and delayed-onset CP are clinically identical. In the former, processes involving slowly developing, continually progressive neuronal changes cannot be essential for the generation of pain; likewise, loss of sensory input produces an *immediate* and *simultaneous* change in neuronal activity at multiple CNS levels – for instance, human thalamic neurons develop novel RFs within minutes (5–15 minutes) of lidocaine block (Kiss *et al.* 1995). **Such changes are observed also in cases without pain.** According to Tasker's group (Kiss *et al.* 1994), **the role of somatotopic reorganization in the genesis of CP – but also PNP – is entirely speculative.** Unlike animal models, there appear to be different patterns and degrees of somatotopic reorganization in the human, all (or none) of which may be associated with a pain syndrome. They conclude: "Although in some cases changes in somatotopic representation were observed, these changes were not consistent in all the groups and therefore unlikely to be the common cause of pain in these patients." Unlike many primate models of SI plasticity, humans display a relative preservation of the cortical sensory homunculus. Ojemann and Silbergeld (1995) found that "adult human sensory cortex retains its somatotopy even after two decades without conscious perception of that body part," after major peripheral denervation – unlike MI, whose volume decreases and NAA levels increase following SCI (Puri *et al.* 1998). Woolsey *et al.* (1979) also found maintenance of cortical sensory maps. Experience with extradural cortical stimulation in CP (Chapter 11) confirms that sensory maps (the "homunculus") are stable. Thus, in humans, *deprived but reactivated neurons do not take on new and appropriate functions, but carry out their original roles long after they have had time to adopt new ones* (Davis *et al.* 1998). In a study of 12 thoracic SCI patients, nine reported phantom sensations and two referred phantom sensations (CP was not assessed). In these two, fMRI showed a relation between SI activation and the percept of referred phantom sensations. The authors

concluded that, instead of somatotopical cortical reorganization, cortical plasticity may be the expression of co-activation of non-adjacent, even distant, representations, supported by somatotopic subcortical remapping projected to the cortex (Moore *et al.* 2000). Turner *et al.* (2003) used fMRI to examine a group of SCI patients versus healthy controls. Unlike in amputation, no evidence of expansion of the hand representation into nearby cortical areas was found, with hand sensory representation undergoing a much smaller posterior shift of hand motor representation. An MEG study of eight patients said to suffer CP (Vartiainen *et al.* 2009) found the SI digit-1-to-digit-5 distance significantly decreased in the hemisphere contralateral to the painful hand. First, the authors' description of the patients (all developing pain following herpes) does not fit CP; second, the decrease was not correlated with long-term average pain; third, there was no change in one patient. Wrigley *et al.* (2009) studied 10 complete SCI (T1–10) CCP patients versus 10 complete non-painful SCI (T3–10) patients (but one patient had allodynia!) and 21 healthy controls in a 3T MRI protocol of sensory stimulation blocks with plastic brush at 2 strokes/s. The overall pattern of brain activation and the pattern of SI activation was *similar in all three groups* and the sensory homunculus confirmed. In patients, a medial shift of the thumb and little finger occurred (i.e., the hand region shifted toward lower trunk/leg area of SI). In those with CP, the medial shift of the little finger representation (but not of the thumb and lip representations!) was statistically different to the other two groups, and correlated positively with pain intensity. The authors do not explain what might be the relevance of this single little finger shift in the face of no change in thumb and lip in patients with leg pains. Human evidence disproves the role of somatotopic rearrangement (e.g., Moore and Schady 2000, Vega-Bermudez and Johnson 2002) and referred sensations/mislocalization do not appear to be a direct perceptual correlate of cortical reorganization (Knecht *et al.* 1996). Phantom sensations can be evoked even in normal persons *without deafferentation* (Knecht *et al.* 1998), and *pain itself in chronic pain patients can lead to representational reorganization* (references in Knecht *et al.* 1996).

(3) After an extensive literature review, Tasker and Dostrovsky (1989) concluded that, if sprouting occurs, it is of very limited extent and probably limited to a subpopulation of primary afferents and/or axons of CNS neurons, playing no role in RF expansion. Denervation supersensitivity is present in both pain and non-pain cases.
(4) Transneuronal degeneration with neuronal loss is incompatible with concurrently extant central sensitization. For instance, in non-traumatic cervical ASAS, in which practically complete interruption of the STT at the spinal level is observed, STT fibers cannot be involved in any kind of transmission from the periphery, and thus maintain sensitization.
(5) Studies have *not* confirmed loss of GABA interneurons or receptors after nerve injury (Mirza and Munro 2010).
(6) "There is no satisfactory explanation for the observed relative decrease in thalamic rCBF in neuropathic pain patients . . . The reversal of this decrease . . . following various types of analgesic procedures suggests that this decrease results from functional impairment rather than degenerative processes" (Moisset and Bouhassira 2007).
(7) There is no direct evidence that central glia have a role in the pathophysiology of chronic pain in humans, and glial activation is found after neural injury with or without pain. Microglial activation occurs in the early post-injury phase, is transient, and may occur in the absence of axonal degeneration and cell death, whereas the astrocyte response occurs later, after axonal degeneration (McMahon and Malcangio 2009). "Glia are involved in all types of brain pathology . . . Astrocytes . . . may represent an integral component of the computational power of the brain. The fundamental question of whether neuroglia is involved in cognition and information processing remains . . . open" (Verkhratsky *et al.* 2011).

In sum, neuroplasticity is something intrinsic to the nervous system, independent of injury. For instance, cortical maps express experience-dependent plasticity, and SI normally reorganizes during various tasks. After injury, it serves a purpose of recovery.

Götterdämmerung II: Thermosensory disinhibition theory and the insular view

Theory

A cold signaling interoceptive Aδ STT path from spinal lamina I to thalamic nucleus VMpo to thermosensory (cold-recipient) dorsal mid/posterior insula (which then modulates brainstem thermoregulatory stations) normally inhibits a medial heat-pinch-cold (HPC) nociceptive STT path (from multimodal cells receiving input from C fibers) passing from lamina I through thalamic nucleus MDvc en route to ACC. In CP patients, a lesion of the cold path disinhibits the medial path, with cold allodynia and deep burning pain being selectively felt in the ACC, with activation of homeostatic behaviors. Cold allodynia would be due to impairment of thermal sensibility (Craig 1998). According to Craig (2009), the anterior insula "instantiates all subjective feelings from the body and feelings of emotion." This view supports strong functional specialization in the brain (neophrenology: Kanwisher 2010).

Other insular views have been advanced. According to Harris (1999), pain is the bodily response to a discrepancy. CP would thus be due to an amplification of the thalamic/posterior insular response to pain due to discrepant sensory input. Kim (2007a) concluded that "disconnection between the thalamus and SII area and subsequent reorganization process seem to be responsible for the CPSP in patients with DIPS (dominant impairment of primitive sensation)." Garcia-Larrea *et al.* (2010) emphasize how "The importance of thermal sensation deficits in central pain is the basis for the hypothesis that lesions of spinothalamic pathways, including their cortical projections, are necessary (although not sufficient) for central pain development ... In the cortex, this necessary condition appears to be present only in lesions of the posterior operculo-insular cortex, which puts patients with such lesions at higher risk of developing a painful syndrome ... Insular pain networks ... might form ... a third somatosensory area." (See also Isnard *et al.* 2011.)

Cases of CPSP following insular injury are on record (Chapter 3). Bowsher (2006a) also suggested that "it would be worthwhile ... looking to the [insular] cortex for the explanation/seat of spontaneous pain following stroke".

The emphasis on insula also stems from the clinical observation that painful sensations from direct cortical stimulation are elicited in roughly 10% of all SII and insula stimulations (both in the same amount), whereas SI stimulation never gave rise to pain reports (Ostrowski *et al.* 2002, Mazzola *et al.* 2006, 2009).

Damning evidence

(1) VMpo does not exist (it is a *myth*). In the words of thalamologist Edward G. Jones (2007, emphasis added):

> Workers ... have laid claim to the pain system on the basis of their advertised capacity to label nociceptive-specific fibers arising in lamina I of the dorsal horn, to plot them throughout the neuraxis, and to identify their terminations in the monkey and human thalamus with a specificity of immunohistochemical staining unattainable by other experimentalists. Craig *et al.* ... proposed and ... reiterated that thalamic terminations of axons arising from lamina I cells throughout the spinal and medullary dorsal horns are restricted to a very small focal area outside the confines of VPL and VPM and characterized by strong immunoreactivity for 28 kDa calbindin. This new nucleus, they christened the posterior portion of the VM and gave it the acronym VMpo. According to the authors, calbindin immunostaining specifically labels spinothalamic and spinal trigeminothalamic axons and selectively delineates VMpo. Moreover they claim that VMpo relays these inputs to cingulated and insular cortex ... rather than to primary somatosensory cortex. The authors attributed the more selective character of their immunostaining for calbindin, in comparison with other studies ..., to the use of a different monoclonal antibody obtained from a commercial source ... the simplicity of this construction has given it a certain cachet. The construction, however, does not stand up to critical examination ... *The VMpo is like one of those religious apparitions that appear to few but become believed in by many.* The VMpo is not an independent thalamic nucleus and not a specific relay nucleus in the ascending pain system (pp. 737–8) ...
>
> *This is dogma that rests upon the faith of conviction rather than upon documented evidence* (p. 752) ...
>
> A posterior region ("VMpo"), whose localization not only bears no relationship to the nuclear anatomy of the thalamus but also *seems to change with each new publication* ... Moreover, to deny the pain pathways any role in the conscious awareness of pain as a uniquely unpleasant sensation and to see them instead as part of some visceral "homeostatic" system concerned in some ill-defined way with the internal well-being of the body (Craig

2003) is to betray evidence of never having spoken to a patient with chronic pain ... to give [the thalamic terminations of the axons of superficial dorsal horn neurons] a singular terminus in the thalamus, a projection only to the peri-insular cortex, and merely a visceral function is *to fly in the face of all evidence to the contrary*. By *selectively quoting from a literature* that presents a mixed picture of the sensory deficits accruing from lesions located outside the primary somatosensory cortex (Craig 2003), it is possible to present a picture that supports an insular view of pain localization, but reference to the original works betrays a far more complicated picture in which it is difficult to separate out the relative contributions of anterior parietal and peri-insular cortex in pain localization and pain asymbolia (p. 1463).

Finally, CPSP has arisen from purely Vc-restricted lesions, outside the supposed location of VMpo (Montes *et al.* 2005, Kim SH *et al.* 2007): lesions of Vc are sufficient to impair cold and tactile sensibility.

(2) Several patients with CP do not complain of burning or thermally described pain.
(3) A minority only complain of cold allodynia, in the face of frequent (but not universal) impairment of thermal sensibility, and in one study the most extreme cold allodynia actually occurred in a patient with normal cold detection thresholds (Greenspan *et al.* 2004). Cold allodynia of CP is more likely to be mediated through activation of SI than ACC (Lenz *et al.* 2010).
(4) Disrupted thermal sensation in CPSP is not associated with a corresponding relationship between altered cold perception and spontaneous pain (Jensen *et al.* 2002); analogously, in CCP, no correlation between cold detection threshold and the intensity of burning pain is observed, with burning pain present also in cases with normal cold detection thresholds (Finnerup *et al.* 2007a).
(5) CP may be felt superficially and in depth.
(6) The theory does not explain non-thermal allodynia.
(7) Heat or increases of body temperature during exercise or fever may both allay (as suggested by this theory) or aggravate (Nurmikko and Hietaharju 1992, Romanelli and Heit 2004) CP (heat allodynia): cool air temporarily reduced the intensity of CP in at least one of our patients.
(8) No ACC activation is seen during cold allodynia in CP patients (Chapter 23).
(9) Cingulotomies are ineffective in relieving CP, but not other chronic pains (see *Götterdämmerung* IV).
(10) There is clear-cut anatomical evidence contrary to the existence and/or importance of the cold and HPC paths (see complete list in Wall 1995). Although a segregated warmth spinal path exists in humans (Iannetti *et al.* 2003, Friehs *et al.* 1995), Lahuerta *et al.* (1994) noted how surgical interruption of the STT does not abolish pain sensation completely: only 1500 STT fibers reach the cortex, and other paths are required. The peri-insular area is by no means the only terminus of the ascending pain pathway, so it is unlikely to be the sole area of the cerebral cortex concerned with pain (Lenz *et al.* 2010). As cogently observed, pain transmission is not – unlike Craig's proposal – Cartesian, whereby pain is passively transmitted along hard-wired sensory channels to the brain (Wall 1995, Bingel *et al.* 2007).
(11) Failure of elicitation of painful or unpleasant sensations by electrical stimulation, even with high currents, at sites in the ACC where pain-sensitive neurons were recorded in human patients (Hutchison *et al.* 1999), as pain-related activity in the ACC may represent descending modulation rather than perception of pain.
(12) ACC hypoactivity in chronic pain imaging studies, coupled with decreased coding for perceived pain in ACC, contradict Craig's hypothesis (Apkarian *et al.* 2005).
(13) A stroke patient with virtually complete destruction of both insulas and both ACCs, but intact SI bilaterally, and intact interoception, has been reported, showing that the insula and ACC are *not* necessary for interoceptive awareness and that the pathway involving visceral afferents projecting to the insula (and ACC) and another involving skin afferents projecting to SI (and SII) work independently (Khalsa *et al.* 2009). This patient supports the view that interoception involves "afferent information that arises from anywhere and everywhere within the body," including through the skin, via pathways that are usually considered exteroceptive.
(14) Although frequently observed in pain imaging, insular activation is not necessary for the conscious experience of pain, as clearly shown in an fMRI study of two stroke patients (Starr *et al.* 2009): both could rate the pain normally despite

absent bilateral fMR insular activation. The authors concluded that "the subjective awareness of noxious stimuli involves multiple, distinct patterns of brain activity where insular cortex is not a prerequisite."

(15) Neither insula nor SII has the same degree of fine somatotopographical representation found in SI. In a series of human stimulation studies of SI, insula, and SII, the authors concluded that insular somatotopy is **blurred** compared to SI and that insular pain somatotopy is likely to be **even fuzzier** than reported here (Mazzola *et al.* 2009). Receptive fields were large and often bilateral. Elicited pain was located in a body area restricted to face > arm > leg for 55% of stimulations and affected more than one of these regions for all others (hemisoma, trunk + limb, face + limb). The skin surface involved by painful sensations varied from 0.5% to 50% of total skin surface, **differing considerably between patients, but also for a single patient from one stimulation to another**. Pain in the limbs was mostly contralateral to the stimulated hemisphere, while facial pains were mostly ipsilateral or bilateral. Spatial resolution of the somatotopic map in SII is intermediate between SI (high) and insula (low). While evoked responses affecting the limbs were exclusively contralateral to SI stimulation, they could also be bilateral (or less often ipsilateral) during SII and insula stimulation. The highest percentage of ipsilateral or bilateral responses were observed after SII stimulation. When the sensation involved the face or trunk, they were mostly bilateral regardless of the stimulated region. SII face (47% of responses) and hand (33% of responses) were over-represented compared to other body parts, without side differences (Ostrowsky *et al.* 2002, Mazzola et al. 2006).

(16) Insula has no efferents to thalamus and thus cannot be involved in any anomalous direct loop with it.

Conclusions

Authors espousing the insular view have come to acknowledge that CP is only possible if SI is engaged (Chapter 26). *Current models of insula function fall short of explaining in detail results of lesion and imaging studies* (Jones *et al.* 2010), studies of somatosensory intensity coding properties in SII/insula produced drastically controversial results, and the location of nociceptive cortical areas around the sylvian fissure is still a matter of controversy and may differ from one person to another (Wang *et al.* 2007, Jones *et al.* 2010, Lenz *et al.* 2010). The fact that direct stimulation of SI does not elicit painful sensations only shows how SI is much more tightly regulated than SII or insula (i.e., higher levels of tonic inhibition). The view that SI is tonically inhibited by SII/insula has no support from current data. On the other hand, cross-frequency coupling is key in SI, where bottom-up feature extraction modulated by γ oscillations is equally important in top-down feedback control with θ/δ oscillations from higher sensory and/or associative regions (e.g., SII/insula): a θ network times neuronal activities between areas, (dis-)engaging each other depending on functional demands (Panzeri *et al.* 2010). After SII and insular injury, however, SI can take over their functions (Starr *et al.* 2009). Studies of hypnosis and placebo suggest that the insula may play a role in pain modulation by tuning the responsiveness of other brain areas via corticocortical interactions (Starr *et al.* 2009, Jones *et al.* 2010, Lenz *et al.* 2010). If the baseline brain activity in pACC and SII/insula is high before noxious stimulation, there is a high receptivity to pain, and stimuli may be perceived as more painful, and vice versa (Boly *et al.* 2007). Thus, the insula may simply act as a key structure in self-monitoring (Jones *et al.* 2010), explaining its activation in imaging studies.

We speculate that, in view of the dense, reciprocal interconnectivity among SI, SII, and insula, including bilateral connectivity, when SI enters into a fixed attractor state, linked areas fall into its basin of attraction (explaining imaging data).

Götterdämmerung III: Thalamocortical dysrhythmia and bursting

Theory

According to Drs. Llinas and Jeanmonod (see Chapters 21 and 22), a neural lesion leads to deafferentation of excitatory inputs on thalamic relay cells and initiates CP. A central lesion would lead to bottom-up deafferentation (i.e., decreased excitatory input to the thalamus), while a cortical lesion would lead to top-down deafferentation. The deafferentation of excitatory inputs results in disfacilitation and cell membrane hyperpolarization. In this hyperpolarized state (equated to PET hypometabolism), deinactivation of calcium T channels causes thalamic neurons to fire low-threshold Ca^{2+} spike bursts in Vc and CL at θ frequency. Such bursting Vc cells exert a rhythmic influence on thalamocortical loops in the θ frequency band. Divergent thalamocortical, corticothalamic, and reticulothalamic projections serve to diffuse low-frequency activity to an increasing number of neighboring thalamocortical loops, which may explain the delay of onset. Thalamocortical modules in θ mode (i.e., hypoactive) exert less collateral intracortical GABA inhibition on neighboring modules in a ring-like fashion, which are thereby overactivated in β/γ frequencies. The interaction between these differentially active modules has been termed the "*edge effect*." "It is the continuous and widespread overproduction of slow rhythms in the awake brain that characterizes thalamocortical dysrhythmia" (Sarnthein *et al.* 2006). In other words, it is not the abnormally bursting neurons themselves or the low-frequency oscillations in the part of the network in which they lie, but rather the heightened activity of neurons in adjacent parts of the somatosensory representation that are released from the inhibition normally imposed upon them by the focus of enhanced slow-wave activity. This would cause the unaffected cortical neurons to discharge in spontaneous, continuous high-frequency oscillations, which could lead to pain (Stern *et al.* 2006).

The three lines of evidence put forth to support the theory are: (1) relief of neurogenic pain by a lesion in the CL; (2) presence of low-threshold calcium spike bursts in Vc and in CL; (3) enhanced θ (4–9 Hz) frequency activation in EEG/MEG in patients with neurogenic pain.

Finally, this theory equally explains other neurologic and psychiatric conditions (Parkinson's disease, schizophrenia, etc.).

Damning evidence

(1) CL thalamotomies are modestly effective in 40% of CP patients, generally for evoked pains (Chapter 21).
(2) Half of all recorded CL cells do not present LTS bursting activity (Chapter 22).
(3) Neurophysiological evidence strongly suggests that EEG and related changes are due to injury, regardless of the presence of pain (Chapter 22).
(4) A cortical lesion triggering CP is associated with overexcitation, not impulse deprivation: a lesion of the corticothalamic output cancels CP (Chapters 20, 26).
(5) CP can be hyperacute, and this is not explained by the theory.
(6) Bursting is found in many different conditions, making it non-specific.
(7) There are 16 (!) basic topological types of bursting, each having different neurocomputational properties. Thus, bursts are more reliable than single spikes, overcome synaptic transmission failure, facilitate release (whereas single spikes do not), evoke long-term potentiation, have higher signal-to-noise ratio than single spikes, can be used for selective communication, can resonate with short-term synaptic plasticity, encode different features of sensory input than single spikes, and encode information in their duration or in interspike intervals (Izhikevich 2007); higher-order thalamic relays burst more than first-order relays (Ramcharan *et al.* 2005).
(8) There is no coincidence between pain sensation in CP patients and moment of burst discharge (Ohye 1998).
(9) A 1 mm increment of electrode insertion in an area of spontaneous discharge can result in an artifactual temporary increase in activation of the existing discharge patterns (Andy 1983).
(10) Bursting may be part of a robust pain-relieving mechanism (Kim *et al.* 2003).
(11) Believing that neuropathic pain, Parkinson's disease, and schizophrenia, among others, share a common basis runs counter to easily available evidence to the contrary.

For more contrary evidence, see the first edition of this book (Canavero and Bonicalzi 2007a, pp. 266–7).

Götterdämmerung IV: Emotion and chronic pain

Theory

The great French surgeon René Leriche (1939) wrote:

> The pain-malady, and the pain of the laboratory. It is of this pain – disease and not symptom – that I intend to speak to you. Frequently, it has no well-marked anatomical basis, and no organic lesion to explain it can be made out. The disease and its manifestation are concentrated in the nervous system. Apparently localized, it affects practically the whole individual . . . The pain of the laboratory . . . is tested on a healthy man . . . as soon as [the physiologist] desists, nothing remains of the

> impression it has produced . . . in this sort of pain, everything is extrinsic . . . In the suffering patient, the pain is like a storm . . . [the patient] powerless to understand, distressed in the face of this abyss into which you cannot descend . . . you will appreciate, then, that the situation is very different in the case of the physiologist and in that of the surgeon . . . Our conception of the mechanism of pain is a sort of sketch-plan . . . according to it, the whole process is concerned only with receptors, conductors, and centers, through the medium of which the pain phenomenon develops like a well-regulated film . . . adhering . . . to a lifeless or stereotyped conception . . . the pain-malady . . . has no receptors, no specific apparatus.

This (unacknowledged) line of thinking has been elaborated on, on the basis of neuroimaging evidence. Thus, neuroimaging studies "strongly support the case for dysfunctional pain processing, especially in affect regulating regions, and . . . these patterns of brain activity strongly reflect patients being in true discomfort and distress" (Tracey and Bushnell 2009). Apkarian *et al.* (2005), noting how the prefrontal cortex was the area most frequently activated in neuroimaging studies of chronic pains (81% of studies), concluded that chronic pain may entail decreased sensory processing and enhanced emotional/cognitive processing (hyperactive prefrontal cortex). Again, Apkarian (2008) emphasized how, although distinct chronic pains may have unique associated brain activity, reorganize the brain in unique ways, and also impact modulation of information processing in specific ways, nonetheless "cortical reorganization seems to impinge mainly on circuitry involved in emotional learning and memory," and May (2008) concluded that chronic pain shows strong activation and reduced gray matter density of the prefrontal cortex. This would also include CP.

Bilateral cingulotomy/capsulotomy result in decreased pain tolerance and *hyperphatic-type* responses to acute painful stimuli following frontal surgery (e.g., Davis *et al.* 1994, Talbot *et al.* 1995). In schizophrenia, affective psychosis, and psychopathic personalities (but not in controls), painful paresthesias (pathologic) and a high percentage of thermal (hot >> cold) paresthesias have been elicited by compression ischemia, pointing to abnormal paresthetic response in psychoses (Gamna *et al.* 1962). Prefrontal activity may lead to an *increased salience of pain* at the cost of other cognitive and emotional behavioral abilities, with pain constantly interfering with attention to other tasks.

Damning evidence

(1) Unlike other chronic pains (Bouckoms 1989), results of frontal surgery (lobotomy, topectomy, cingulectomy/cingulotomy, leucotomy) are generally disappointing for CP (Table A.1). In rare cases in which it was deemed effective, the pain was simply less distressing and bothersome (pain indifference), the patient less anxious or depressed by pain; spontaneous complaints about pain are diminished and a patient's ability to appreciate the meaning of the pain may be disrupted. According to Turnbull (1972), "bilateral cingulotomy alone is ineffective when pain is caused by a major organic disease," including CP. According to Freeman and Watts (1950), "the frontal lobes are important structures, not so much for the experiencing of pain as for the evaluating of the sensation, the estimation of its significance in terms of the self and of the future." The mid cingulate cortex, where cutaneous nociceptive neurons are most abundant, was also included in such lesions (see Canavero and Bonicalzi 2007a for discussion).

(2) Guiot's group is said to have temporarily relieved CP by bilateral ablation of BA6 (Garcin 1968), but stimulation in these areas never provided a benefit (one personal case plus others from a Japanese group: see Chapter 11).

(3) Lesions of the sensory corticothalamocortical loop immediately erase both sensory and affective components of CP (Chapters 20 and 21).

(4) Opioids, whose receptors are particularly dense in the prefrontal cortex, are scarcely effective on CP (Chapters 9 and 16).

(5) Studies show task-specific electrocorticographic (EcoG) synchrony between SI, the parasylvian (PS) cortex, and ACC. SI is functionally connected with PS during anticipation of the stimulus, while SI and PS are functionally connected with ACC during the response to the stimulus (Ohara *et al.* 2008, Lenz *et al.* 2010). However, "it is not clear . . . how these structures are related to each other and to pain perception" (Lenz *et al.* 2010). A functional connectivity fMRI study of tonic pain in healthy people found that, using SI as a seed region, synchronized activity was observed in bilateral SI/MI, mPFC/midCC, posterior insula/SII, and occipital cortex, but not in ACC (seed ACC also did not show a correlation with SI/SII). Using the left SII as a seed, bilateral SII, insula/operculum,

Table A.1. Results of frontal lobe surgery for central pain

Author(s)	Type of CP/ number of patients	Target/ procedure	Efficacy/follow-up	Notes
Guillaume *et al.* (1949)	Thalamic syndrome (2 patients)	Frontal lobotomy	"Indifference" towards pain, which was still present and severe (one resumed some activity after surgery)	
Wertheimer and Mansuy (1949)	CCP (1 patient)	Frontal lobotomy	0%	
Freeman and Watts (1950)	CP, thalamic (1 patient)	Prefrontal lobotomy	Relief	
Scarff (1950)	CPSP (1 patient)	Left prefrontal lobotomy	Good relief, relapse at 4 months	In other pains, unilateral lobotomy may relieve bilateral pains
Gaches (1952)	CP, brain (1 patient)	Frontal lobotomy	Improved, but not abolished	
Drake and McKenzie (1953)	Mesencephalotomy-induced CP (1 patient)	Frontal lobotomy	No	
Petit-Dutaillis *et al.* (1953)	CP, brain (1 patient)	Frontal lobotomy	Not available for review	
Le Beau *et al.* (1954)	CP (5 patients)	Bilateral BA 9–10 topectomy	Almost complete, but pain admitted on interrogation (follow-up 4 years); 0% (follow-up 6 months)	
		Unilateral BA9–10 topectomy	**Complete relief after 2nd surgery (follow-up not specified)**	
		Bilateral orbital gyrectomy	10–20% relief for 2.5 years	
		Unilateral frontal lobotomy	0% over 2 weeks	
Botterell *et al.* (1954)	CP, SCI (not available)	Prefrontal lobotomy	Gratifying (follow-up not available)	
White and Sweet (1955, 1969)	CP (2 patients)	Bilateral orbital gyrectomy (BA 11–12)	**Failure, then success at 2nd operation** 0%	
	CPSP (1 patient)	Unilateral frontal leukotomy	Pain sometimes felt, but not bothering; total disappearance over 2 years until death another 2 years later (patient had neglect)	

Table A.1. (cont.)

Author(s)	Type of CP/ number of patients	Target/ procedure	Efficacy/follow-up	Notes
	CCP, postcordotomy (4 patients)	Fractionated radiofrequency frontomedial leukotomy	Burning relieved, but PNP-associated hyperpathia 0% 100% immediate relief; total relapse at 2.5 months 0% (2 patients)	
	CCP (1 patient)	Unilateral frontal leukotomy	Not complete relief, but no longer in need of analgesics for 16 years	
Constans (1960)	CP, brain (1 patient)	Frontal operation	Unsatisfactory	
Wycis and Spiegel (1962)	Tabes dorsalis (2 patients) CP (1 patient)	Bilateral prefrontal lobotomy	0%	Transitory relief with mesencephalotomy, then relapse
Foltz and White (1966)	SCI-CP (3 patients)	Rostral cingulumotomy	1 fair at 4 years and 1 poor at 3 years (unilateral cingulumotomy); 1 excellent at 1 year, then fair at 2.5 years (bilateral)	
Porter *et al.* (1966)	CP, SCI	Prefrontal lobotomy	Gratifying	
Spiegel *et al.* (1966)	CPSP (1 patient)	Bilateral anterior capsulotomy	0%	
Nashold and Wilson (1970)	1 CPSP (brainstem)	Unilateral left frontal lobotomy	0%	
Turnbull (1972)	Tabes dorsalis (2 patients)	Bilateral cingulotomy	Relief	
Bouchard *et al.* (1977)	CP, brain (2 patients)	Ipsilateral cingulotomy Contralateral cingulotomy	No benefit Benefit	
Jefferson (1983)	CP, SCI (1 patient)	Bilateral stereotactic cingulotomy	"Reasonable relief"	Previous unsuccessful cordotomy
Ballantine and Giriunas (1988)	CP, brain (3 patients)	Bilateral stereotactic cingulotomy	No substantial relief	
Tasker (1990)	CP, SCI (1 patient)	Bilateral stereotactic cingulotomy	No relief	Followed by unsuccessful bilateral medial thalamotomy and mesencephalic tractotomy

Table A.1. (cont.)

Author(s)	Type of CP/ number of patients	Target/ procedure	Efficacy/follow-up	Notes
Pillay and Hassenbusch (1992)	CP, brain (1 patient)	Bilateral stereotactic cingulotomy	No (VAS from 9 to 8); quality of life unchanged	
Frost *et al.* (2008)	CCP (1 patient)	Bilateral cingulate gyrectomy	No relief	
Tsai *et al.* (2010)	SCI (2 patients)	Bilateral anterior stereotactic cingulotomy	Patient 1: transient exacerbation of pain for 1 week, than gradual abatement. Patient 2: marked decrease of pain the second day after surgery with improved social behavior. Follow-up: not available	

NB: dorsal ACC: cognitive (BA24b'-c', BA32'); ventral ACC (around the genu of CC): affective (BA24a-c, BA32)

left SI, and lateral PFC were correlated, but again not ACC. Instead, using the right anterior insula, bilateral anterior insula/operculum, ACC, midCC, striatum, thalamus, cerebellum and brainstem were all correlated (Kong *et al.* 2010). Thus, the cingulum does not appear to be a vital link in tonic pain processing.

In sum, the role of the prefrontal cortex may go beyond the unpleasantness, but may relate to control, namely cognitive and attentional processing of painful stimuli, and memory of past events. Loss of the frontal lobe-mediated expectancy mechanism disrupts placebo analgesia and clinical analgesia (Bingel *et al.* 2007). It may be hypothesized that the sensory attractor underlying CP engages selective attention in the frontal cortex: psychosurgery would act on this network.

Götterdämmerung V: Sympathetic pain

Theory

Historically it has been assumed that the sympathetic nervous system plays a pathogenic role in some chronic pains, largely on the grounds of physical signs commonly regarded as autonomic and of subjective symptom relief following sympatholysis. A few patients with BCP and CCP have been temporarily – and on occasion for prolonged periods – relieved by sympathetic blockade, whether complete or not, whether by local anesthetic or guanethidine.

Damning evidence

(1) The vast majority of authors report no benefit from sympathetic block and/or sympathectomy in CP (Nashold 1991, Sjölund 1991, Bowsher 1994, Tasker 2001a). Relief in a few CP patients appears to depend on hyperpathia. When relief occurs, hyperpathia, steady burning and intermittent shooting spontaneous pain, *but not usually deep pain*, disappeared. Occasionally, hyperpathia is relieved but not spontaneous pain, or hyperpathia longer than steady pain, but *spontaneous burning pain is not relieved independently of hyperpathia*. All reported studies (Table A.2) lacked a placebo control, and it is not clear why sympathetic fibers should have a role in CP with allodynia, but not without: likely, the block reduced sensory barrage *tout court*, also explaining why not all the peripheral nerves of the affected region had to have their sympathetic nerve supply blocked (cases 3–4 of Loh *et al.* 1981: see Canavero and Bonicalzi 2007a, pp. 288–90).

(2) A series of controlled studies found IV regional sympathetic (guanethidine, reserpine) blocks ineffective at reducing or abolishing "sympathetic

Table A.2. Results of sympathetic blocks for central pain (since 1990)

Author	Type of CP/ number of patients	Procedure	Outcome	Notes
Portenoy *et al.* (1990)	CP, brainstem (1 patient)	Right stellate ganglion block	Transitory moderate relief	
Tasker *et al.* (1992)	CCP (5 patients)	Rhizotomy (L4, T12–L1, L1–2 bilaterally, intercostal nerves)	No relief in 3 patients; in 2 patients (C4, T5–12) hyperpathia only relieved	
Nurmikko and Hietaharju (1992)	CP (2 patients), heat allodynia/ hyperalgesia	Sympathetic blockade	No response	1 patient reported post-sauna hyperpathia No signs of excessive sympathetic drive
D. Long (comment to Milhorat *et al.* 1996)	Syringomyelia CP	Sympathectomy	Most failures	
Milhorat *et al.* (1996, 1997)	Syringomyelia SCI-CP (2/15 patients) Syringomyelia CP (1 patient)	(1) Sympathetic block with 10 mL 0.25% bupivacaine, then stellate ganglionectomy (2) Similar blocks with sympathectomy	(1) Prolonged relief, then 100% relief at 5 months (2) Relief; 100% relief 22 months later	
Yamamoto *et al.* (1997)	CPSP, thalamic and suprathalamic (39 patients)	Stellate ganglion block with 10 mL 0.5% mepivacaine and cervical or lumbar epidural block with 5 mL 0.5% mepivacaine	Failure	
Burkey and Abla-Yao (2010)	MS-CCP (1 patient)	Four (over 6 months) left stellate ganglion blocks	No relief	No cold allodynia seen in this patient
Tanei *et al.* (2010)	MS-CP (1 patient)	Several sympathetic blocks	Only transient reliefs	

maintained pains" (e.g., Blanchard *et al.* 1990, Jadad *et al.* 1995, Ramamurthy *et al.* 1995).

(3) A microneurographic study of 24 CRPS patients was conducted with simultaneous recording from single identified sympathetic efferent fibers and C nociceptors while provoking sympathetic discharges in cutaneous nerves. No evidence of activation of nociceptors related to sympathetic discharge was found; nociceptors exhibited unrelated spontaneous pathological nerve impulse activity in six patients (Campero *et al.* 2010; see also Bonicalzi and Canavero 2000).

In sum, the vasomotor, sudomotor, and trophic disorders observed in certain cases of CP are just reflex phenomena induced by pain (Garcin 1957), secondary to change in mobility. According to the American Medical Association, "the diagnosis of CRPS has not been scientifically validated as representing a specific and discrete health condition . . . whenever this diagnosis is made, it is probably incorrect" (Rondinelli

2008). More contrary evidence is found in the first edition of this book (Canavero and Bonicalzi 2007a).

Götterdämmerung VI: The default mode network and chronic pain

Theory

This idea evolved out of an attempt to explain deactivations seen alongside activations in imaging studies (Raichle 2009). The case for a default mode comprises three related ideas: (1) the resting state (RS) of the brain as seen on neuroimaging studies constitutes an absolute, fixed baseline against which all other brain activities should be considered; (2) the level of activity in RS is substantial and thus functionally important, with changes produced by task demands just the tip of the iceberg; (3) relative to a wide range of tasks, RS is associated with higher levels of activity in a consistent set of brain regions (default mode network, DMN). This construct would thus explain the several deactivations reported in imaging studies. Chronic pain is accompanied by disruption in resting functional connectivity of widespread cortical areas (May 2008, Cauda *et al.* 2009).

Damning evidence

(1) Several technical objections have been raised by Morcom and Fletcher (2007). Here it suffices to say that the figure of about 80% of brain energy consumption attributed to ongoing neuronal activity includes a large indirect contribution from neurotransmitter recycling.

(2) Competing theories equally explain imaging results (e.g., Friston's free-energy principle of brain function: Sadaghiani *et al.* 2010).

(3) Following thermal pain stimuli, fMRI deactivations have been observed not only in core regions of the DMN (e.g., bilateral mPFC, posterior CC/precuneus), but also in non-DMN areas: lateral occipital gyri, BA6, superior frontal gyrus, and contralateral SI/MI (Kong *et al.* 2010). The voxels significantly deactivated during weak pain greatly outnumbered those significantly activated, but the opposite applied during strong pain (!). Males exhibited stronger activations than females but similar deactivations. No significant correlations were observed between pain-evoked activations and deactivations, except between the pain-activated right SI and pain-deactivated left SI/MI (plus bilateral occipital cortex during strong pain). On the basis of these data, these authors conclude against the "sentinel hypothesis" of the DMN (broad monitoring of the external environment). If the pain deactivations were due to the interruption of this monitoring, then increasing levels of pain would have to be associated with increasing deactivations. Instead, weak pain induced more deactivations in a much larger network of brain areas than strong pain. They suggest that activations and deactivations might underlie different aspects of the pain experiences: "*the mechanisms behind deactivations within and outside the default mode network might be of different nature.*"

Götterdämmerung VII: The neuromatrix and central pain

Theory

The anatomical substrate of the physical self is a network of neurons that extends throughout widespread areas of the brain (neuromatrix), whose spatial distribution and synaptic links are initially determined genetically and are later sculpted by sensory inputs. Thalamocortical and limbic loops that comprise this neuromatrix diverge to permit parallel processing in different components of the neuromatrix and converge repeatedly to permit interactions between the output products of processing. The repeated cyclical processing and synthesis of nerve impulses in the neuromatrix imparts a characteristic pattern (neurosignature) produced by the pattern of synaptic connections in the entire neuromatrix. Neuromodules of the matrix are dedicated to process specialized sensory events, which impress subsignatures on the larger one. This active neuromatrix, when deprived of modulating inputs, produces an abnormal signature pattern that subserves the different qualities of CP. To destroy the neuromatrix for the physical self is impossible. This construct stems from supposed failures of cortectomies or thalamotomies to relieve chronic pain (Melzack 1991).

Damning evidence

As seen in Chapters 20 and 21, focal lesions can abolish CP even for years. Diffuseness of the pain system is *not equivalent* to saying that chronic pain cannot be effectively abolished by selective lesions: while acute pain is necessary for survival, chronic pain is not. The impression that chronic pain cannot be abolished by focal lesions is due to poor analysis of the relevant literature and misconceptions about the exact generator of a particular chronic pain syndrome, as in the case of CP. The same neural substrates that support the bilateral distribution of nociceptive information processing during acute pain subserve bilateral spread of chronic pain. A review of imaging studies suggests that:

> Acute physiological pain and neuropathic pain have distinct although overlapping brain activation patterns, but there is no unique "pain matrix" or "allodynia network" . . . Different subtypes of allodynia may be associated with distinct patterns of brain activity, reflecting different pathophysiological mechanisms . . . The different components of neuropathic pain syndromes (spontaneous and evoked pains) probably involve different mechanisms . . . These data suggest that the different neuropathic symptoms may respond differently to treatment (Moisset and Bouhassira 2007).

Götterdämmerung VIII: Animal studies and chronic pain: "lost in translation"

Theory

Central pain, like other human disorders, can be studied in animals and effective therapies developed from these studies. There is veterinary evidence of "classical thalamic pain" following Vc lesions (e.g., Holland *et al.* 2000).

Damning evidence

(1) Several interspecies differences among mammals, such as mouse, rat, guinea pig, rabbit, and human, have been described for distinct brain areas (Henriksen and Willoch 2008). Among a myriad: (1) there are species differences in baseline neurotransmitter concentrations which are functional (Fitzgerald 2009); (2) substance P has been considered a key substance in pain transmission on the basis of animal data, but NK1 receptor antagonists failed in human trials, and so did NMDA antagonists: "advances . . . using current in vivo models . . . in virtually no instances have . . . translated into new drugs for pain control in the clinic" (Lascelles and Flecknell 2010); (3) the anatomo-functional architecture of the corpus callosum in humans and animals is definitely different (Papo and Quattrini 1997).

(2) Heat hyperalgesia, so commonly seen in animal models, is only present in a small proportion of patients suffering from CP.

(3) Even monkeys differ from humans, for instance in cognitive processing of pain (see also Pioli *et al.* 2003). In humans, the ACC is believed to play a role in detecting conflicts in information processing, but studies in monkeys have failed to find conflict-related responses. Thus, presumed anatomical homologs exhibit different functional properties (Cole *et al.* 2009).

> Humans often turn to the study of animals to understand themselves . . . monkeys . . . It has been a common belief . . . that the brains of our closest relatives have an organization and function largely similar, if not identical, to our own. Split-brain research has shown that this assumption can be spurious. Although some structures and functions are remarkably alike, differences abound. The anterior commissure provides one dramatic example . . . When this commissure is left intact in otherwise split-brain monkeys, the animals retain the ability to transfer visual information from one hemisphere to the other. People, however, do not transfer visual information in any way. Hence, the same structure carries out different functions in different species – an illustration of the limits of extrapolating from one species to another. Even extrapolating between people can be dangerous (Gazzaniga 1998).

Finally, there are differences between individual humans and between males and females; race and ethnicity also play a role.

(4) Autotomy, a "classic" sign of pain in animals, has been reported in several human patients without pain. The latest report (Frost *et al.* 2008) describes five C6 complete SCI patients. Biting first arose 3–6 years after SCI. Pain in the bitten limb/s was reported in only one patient (postoperative pain: as it resolved in 3 months, so did the biting). Two patients suffered CCP, but not in the bitten arms. Because subjective symptoms cannot be evaluated, the representation of neuropathic pain in animal models is necessarily incomplete and the human experience of pain too complex to be fully reproduced (see more cases in Canavero and Bonicalzi 2007a).

(5) Even capsaicin-evoked pain in human volunteers is not a model of neuropathic pain, as the latter is often delayed and generally permanent, whereas

capsaicin-induced hyperalgesia develops within minutes and is transient. A similar situation has been described for epilepsy. In humans, epilepsy is a chronic condition, while experimental epilepsy in animals is usually acute, and even "chronic" experiments mean a few days or weeks (Papo and Quattrini 1997). Animal models often test evoked pain, and not really pain but the presumably associated hyperactive reflexes: supposed pain in animals recedes within 8–10 weeks (Lascelles and Flecknell 2010). Animal models do not study animals with a naturally occurring disease.

(6) Despite genetic homology between humans and mice, the expression of genes may vary significantly between species (DeGraba and Pettigrew 2000).

(7) Whereas rats totally unresponsive to SCS became SCS responders after IT low-dose baclofen, no totally unresponsive PNP human was converted to responder status after a similar treatment: "these contrasting observations in basic animal studies and the clinic illustrate the difficulties to interpret animal behaviors versus human verbal reports" (Schechtmann *et al.* 2010).

(8) High-frequency stimulation of the subthalamic nuclei affects pallidal neurons, but the effect differs between rats and primates (decrease versus increase of spike activity) (Gubellini *et al.* 2009).

In all fields of medicine, animal data show profound flaws (Linazasoro 2004, Pound *et al.* 2004). Discordance between animal and human studies may be due to bias or to failure of animal models to mimic clinical disease adequately (Perel *et al.* 2007). For instance, experimental allergic encephalomyelitis is a misleading model of multiple sclerosis (Sriram and Steiner 2005). Authors concluded that "it is better not to do the experiment than to do it using the wrong model ... The FDA, and other regulatory bodics, should be concerned about the inappropriate use of animals and models which can lead to misinformation" (Alini *et al.* 2008; see also Wilke 2008). Besson (1994) stated that animal models "are limited, and most of them do not mimic chronic pain states," and Wall (1988) concluded that animal evidence "may be real science, but is not real life." Thus, it is not surprising that between 1995 and 2010, more than 200 ameliorative interventions have been reported for dementia in mice, but none translated into clinical therapies (Zahs and Ashe 2010). We urge everybody to stop inserting animal evidence into their discussions, and to stop publishing animal studies altogether. Animal studies are good for academic promotion, but have not advanced the state of pain therapy. Available drugs are either analgesics of the same class as others already in clinical use or derived from astute clinical observation in other settings.

References and bibliography

Aarabi B, Koltz M, Ibrahimi D (2008) Hyperextension cervical spine injuries and traumatic central cord syndrome. *Neurosurg Focus* **25** (5), E9.

Ackerman LL, Follett KA, Rosenquist RW (2003) Long-term outcomes during treatment of chronic pain with intracisternal clonidine or clonidine/opioid combinations. *J Pain Symptom Manage* **26**, 668–77.

Ackery AD, Norenberg MD, Krassioukov A (2007) Calcitonin gene-related peptide immunoreactivity in chronic human spinal cord injury. *Spinal Cord* **45**, 678–86.

Agnew DA, Goldberg VD (1976) A brief trial of phenytoin for thalamic pain. *Bull Los Angeles Neurol Soc* **41**, 9–12.

Ahn SH, Park HW, Lee BS, *et al.* (2003) Gabapentin effect on neuropathic pain compared among patients with spinal cord injury and different durations of symptoms. *Spine*, **28**, 341–6.

Ajmone Marsan C, Fuortes MGF, Marossero F (1951) Effects of direct currents on the electrical activity of the spinal cord. *J Phsyiol (Lond)* **113**, 316–21.

Akil H, Richardson DE, Hughes DE, Barchas JD (1978) Enkephalin-like material elevated in ventricular cerebrospinal fluid of pain patients after analgesic focal stimulation. *Science* **201**, 463–5.

Albe-Fessard D (1973) Electrophysiological methods for the identification of thalamic nuclei. *Z Neurol* **205**, 15–28.

Albert ML (1969) Treatment of pain in multiple sclerosis: preliminary report. *N Engl J Med* **280**, 1395.

Aldini G (1803) *An account of the late improvements in galvanism, with a series of curious and interesting experiments performed before the commissioners in the French national institute, and repeated lately in the anatomical theatres of London, to which is added an appendix containing experiments on the body of a malefactor executed at Newgate, and dissertations on animal electricity 1793 and 1794.* London: Cuthell & Martin and J. Murray.

Alini M, Eisenstein SM, Ito K, *et al.* (2008) Are animal models useful for studying human disc disorders/degeneration? *Eur Spine J* **17**, 2–19.

Aly MM, Saitoh Y, Hosomi K, *et al.* (2010) Spinal cord stimulation for central poststroke pain. *Neurosurgery* **67** (ONS Suppl 1), ons206–12.

Amancio EJ, Peluso CM, Santos AC, Pena-Dias AP, Debs FA (2002) [Central pain due to parietal cortex compression by cerebral tumor: report of 2 cases]. *Arq Neuropsiquiatr* **60**, 487–9.

Amano K (1998) Destructive central lesions for persistent pain: II. Outcome. In: Gildenberg PL, Tasker RR, eds., *Textbook of Stereotactic and Functional Neurosurgery.* New York, NY: McGraw-Hill, pp. 1425–9.

Amano K, Iseki H, Notani M, *et al.* (1980) Rostral mesencephalic reticulotomy for pain relief. Report of 15 cases. *Acta Neurochir Suppl* **30**, 391–3.

Amano K, Tanikawa H, Hiroshi I, *et al.* (1982) Endorphins and pain relief. Further observations on electrical stimulation of the lateral part of the periaqueductal gray matter during rostral mesencephalic reticulotomy for pain relief. *Appl Neurophysiol* **45**, 123–35.

Amano K, Kawamura H, Tanikawa T, *et al.* (1986) Long-term follow-up study of rostral mesencephalic reticulotomy for pain relief: report of 34 cases. *Appl Neurophysiol* **49**, 105–11.

Amano K, Kawamura H, Tanikawa T, *et al.* (1992) Stereotactic mesencephalotomy for pain relief: a plea for stereotactic surgery. *Stereotact Funct Neurosurg* **59**, 25–32.

Ameri D (1967) Sindrome talamico de Dejerine–Roussy en una meningitis tuberculosa de la infancia. *Arch Argent Pediatria* **65**, 173–8.

Amr YM (2010) Multi-day low dose ketamine infusion as adjuvant to oral gabapentin in spinal cord injury related chronic pain: a prospective, randomized, double blind trial. *Pain Physician* **13**, 245–9.

An JY, Song IU, Kim YI, Lee KS, Kim JS (2008) Cheiro-oral syndrome in a patient from a cortical infarction in the midfrontal gyrus. *Eur Neurol* **59**, 219–20.

Andersen G, Vestergaard K, Lauritzen L (1994) Effective treatment of post-stroke depression with the selective serotonin re-uptake inhibitor citalopram. *Stroke* **25**, 1099–104.

Andersen G, Vestergaard K, Ingeman-Nielsen M, Jensen TS (1995) Incidence of central post-stroke pain. *Pain* **61**, 187–93.

Anderson VC, Burchiel KJ (1999) A prospective study of long-term intrathecal morphine in the management of chronic nonmalignant pain. *Neurosurgery* **44**, 289–301.

André-Obadia N, Peyron R, Mertens P, *et al.* (2006) Transcranial magnetic stimulation for pain control. Double-blind study of different frequencies against placebo, and correlation with motor cortex stimulation efficacy. *Clin Neurophysiol* **117**, 1536–44.

André-Obadia N, Mertens P, Gueguen A, *et al.* (2008) Pain relief by rTMS. *Neurology* **71**, 832–40.

Andy OJ (1983) Thalamic stimulation for chronic pain. *Appl Neurophysiol* **46**, 116–23.
Andy OJ (1987) Chronic pain syndromes. *Appl Neurophysiol* **50**, 434–5.
Andy OJ (1989) Mesothalamic discharge sites. *Stereotact Funct Neurosurg* **52**, 176–82.
Angel IF, Gould HJ, Carey ME (1998) Intrathecal morphine pump as a treatment option in chronic pain of nonmalignant origin. *Surg Neurol* **49**, 92–8.
Angell M (2004) *The Truth About the Drug Companies. How They Deceive Us and What To Do About It.* New York, NY: Random House.
Antal A, Terney D, Kuehnk S, Paulus W. (2010) Anodal transcranial direct current stimulation ameliorates chronic pain and reduces short intracortical inhibition. *J Pain Symptom Manage* **39**, 890–903.
Antic B, Peric P (2009) Posterior fossa exploration in the treatment of trigeminal neuralgia associated with multiple sclerosis. *Surg Neurol* **71**, 419–23.
Apkarian AV (2008) Pain perception in relation to emotional learning. *Curr Op Neurobiol* **18**, 464–8.
Apkarian AV, Bushnell MC, Treede RD, Zubieta JK (2005) Human brain mechanisms of pain perception and regulation in health and disease. *Eur J Pain* **9**, 463–84.
Appelros P (2006) Prevalence and predictors of pain and fatigue after stroke: a population-based study. *Int J Rehabil Res* **29**, 329–33.
Arle JE, Shils JL (2008) Motor cortex stimulation for pain and movement disorders. *Neurotherapeutics* **5**, 37–49.
Arle JE, Mei LZ, Shils JL (2008) Modeling parkinsonian circuitry and the DBS electrode: I. Biophysical background and software. *Stereotact Funct Neurosurg* **134**, 1–15.
Armour D (1927) Lettsonian lecture on the surgery of the spinal cord and its membranes. *Lancet* **1**, 691–7.
Arner S, Meyerson BA (1988) Lack of analgesic effect of opioids on neuropathic and idiopathic forms of pain. *Pain* **33**, 11–23.
Arner S, Meyerson BA (1991) Genuine resistance to opioids: fact or fiction? *Pain* **47**, 116–18.
Arnett PA (2008) Cannabis bliss? *Neurology* **71**, 160–1.
Arseni G, Boetz MI (1971) *Tulburari viscero-vegetative si trofice in leziunile encefalice.* Bucharest: Editura Academiei Republicii Socialiste Romania.
Ascoli GA, Alonso-Nanclares L, Anderson SA, *et al.* (2008) Petilla terminology: nomenclature of features of GABAergic interneurons of the cerebral cortex. *Nat Rev Neurosci* **9**, 1–12.
Attal N, Brasseur B, Parker F, Chauvin M, Bouhassira D (1998a) Effects of gabapentin on the different components of peripheral and central neuropathic pain syndromes: pathophysiological considerations. *Eur Neurol* **40**, 191–200.
Attal N, Brasseur L, Chauvin M, Bouhassira D (1998b) A case of "pure" dynamic mechano-allodynia due to a lesion of the spinal cord: pathophysiological considerations. *Pain* **75**, 399–404.
Attal N, Gaudé V, Brasseur L, *et al.* (2000) Intravenous lidocaine in central pain: a double-blind, placebo-controlled, psychophysical study. *Neurology* **54**, 564–74.
Attal N, Guirimand F, Brasseur L, *et al.* (2002) Effects of IV morphine in central pain. A randomized placebo-controlled study. *Neurology* **58**, 554–63.
Attal N, Parker F, Tadiè M, Bouhassira D (2004a) Effects of surgery on central pain and sensory deficits associated with syringomyelia: a long-term prospective psychophysical study. *J Neurol Neurosurg Psychiatry* **75**, 1025–30.
Attal N, Brasseur L, Guirimand D, *et al.* (2004b) Are oral cannabinoids safe and effective in refractory neuropathic pain? *Eur J Pain* **8**, 173–7.
Attal N, Fermanian C, Fermanian J, *et al.* (2008) Neuropathic pain: are there distinct subtypes depending on the aetiology or anatomical lesion? *Pain* **138**, 343–53.
Awerbuch GI, Sandyk R (1990) Mexiletine for thalamic pain syndrome. *Int J Neurosci* **55**, 129–33.
Baars BJ, Gage NM (2010) *Cognition, Brain, and Consciousness.* San Diego, CA: Academic Press.
Backonja M, Gombar K (1992) Response of central pain syndromes to intravenous lidocaine. *J Pain Symptom Manage* **7**, 172–8.
Backonja M, Arndt G, Gombar KA, Check B, Zimmermann M (1994) Response of chronic neuropathic pain syndromes to ketamine: a preliminary study. *Pain* **56**, 51–7.
Bainton T, Fox M, Bowsher D, Wells C (1992) A double-blind trial of naloxone in central post-stroke pain. *Pain* **48**, 159–62.
Ballantine HT, Giriunas IE (1988) Treatment of intractable psychiatric illness and chronic pain by stereotactic cingulotomy. In: Schmideck W, Sweet WH, eds., *Operative Neurosurgical Techniques*, 2nd edn. New York, NY: Grune-Stratton, pp. 1069–75.
Ballantyne JC, Mao J (2003) Opioid therapy for chronic pain. *N Engl J Med* **349**, 1943–53.
Banerjee T (1974) Transcutaneous nerve stimulation for pain after spinal injury. *N Engl J Med* **291**, 796.
Banerjee TK, Kumar S (2006) Epidemiology of stroke in India. *Neurol Asia* **11**, 1–4.
Bang OY, Lee JS, Lee PH, Lee G (2005) Autologous mesenchymal stem cell transplantation in stroke patients. *Ann Neurol* **57**, 874–82.
Bannister AP (2003) Inter- and intra-laminar connections of pyramidal cells in the neocortex. *Neurosci Res* **53**, 95–103.
Barcia-Salorio JL, Roldan P, Lopez-Gomez L (1987) Radiosurgery of central pain. *Acta Neurochir (Wien) Suppl* **39**, 159–62.
Barolat G (1995) Current status of epidural spinal cord stimulation. *Neurosurg Quart* **5**, 98–124.
Barolat G, Ketcik B, He J (1998) Long-term outcome of spinal cord stimulation for chronic pain management. *Neuromodulation* **1**, 19–25.
Barone P, Antonini A, Colosimo C, *et al.* on behalf of the PRIAMO study group (2009) The Priamo study: a

multicenter assessment of nonmotor symptoms and their impact on quality of life in Parkinson's disease. *Mov Disord* **24**, 1641–9.

Barraquer-Bordas L, Molet J, Pascual-Sedano B, Català H (1999) Dolor central retardado asociado a hematoma subinsular seguido por tumor parietooccipital. Efecto favorable de la estimulacion cronica del nucleo VPL talamico. *Rev Neurologia* **29**, 1044–8.

Barrera-Chacon JM, Mendez-Suarez JL, Jauregui-Abrisqueta ML, *et al.* (2011) Oxycodone improves pain control and quality of life in anticonvulsant-pretreated spinal cord-injured patients with neuropathic pain. *Spinal Cord* **49**, 36–42.

Bassetti C, Bogousslavsky J, Mattle H, Bernasconi A (1997) Medial medullary stroke: report of seven patients and review of the literature. *Neurology* **48**, 882–90.

Bassetti RD, Bogousslavsky J, Regli F (1993) Sensory syndromes in parietal stroke. *Neurology* **43**, 1942–9.

Bates J, Nathan PW (1980) Transcutaneous electrical nerve stimulation for chronic pain. *Anesthesia* **35**, 817–22.

Baudoin A, Puech P (1949) Premiers essais d'intervention directe sur le thalamus (injection, électrocoagulation). *Rev Neurol* **81**, 78–81.

Baumgaertner U, Buchholz HG, Bellosevich A, *et al.* (2006) High opiate receptor binding potential in the human lateral pain system. *Neuroimage* **30**, 692–9.

Beatty RA (1970) Cold dysesthesia: a symptom of extramedullary tumors of the spinal cord. *J Neurosurg* **33**, 75–8.

Becker R, Uhle EI, Alberti O, Bertalanffy H (2000) Continuous intrathecal baclofen infusion in the management of central deafferentation pain. *J Pain Symptom Manage* **20**, 313–15.

Been G, Ngo TT, Miller SM, Fitzgerald PB (2007) The use of tDCS and CVS as methods of non-invasive brain stimulation. *Brain Res Rev* **56**, 346–61.

Behan RJ (1914) *Pain: Its Origin, Conduction, Perception and Diagnostic Significance.* New York, NY: Appleton.

Beiske AG, Loge JH, Rønningen A, Svensson E (2009) Pain in Parkinson's disease: prevalence and characteristics. *Pain* **141**, 173–7.

Bejjani GK, Cockerham KP (2001) Adult Chiari malformation. *Contemp Neurosurg* **23**, 1–8.

Belfer I, Dai F (2010) Phenotyping and genotyping neuropathic pain. *Curr Pain Headache Rep* **14**, 203–12.

Belfrage M, Segerdahl M, Arner S, Sollevi A (1999) The safety and efficacy of intrathecal adenosine in patients with chronic neuropathic pain. *Anesth Analg* **89**, 136–42.

Bell RF (2009) Ketamine for chronic non-cancer pain. *Pain* **141**, 210–14.

Belleville G (2010) Mortality hazard associated with anxiolytic and hypnotic drug use in the national population health survey. *Can J Psychiatry* **55**, 558–67.

Benaim C, Froger J, Cazottes C, *et al.* (2007) Use of the Faces Pain Scale by left and right hemispheric stroke patients. *Pain* **128**, 52–8.

Benedetti F (2009) *Placebo Effects: Understanding the Mechanisms in Health and Disease.* Oxford: Oxford University Press.

Beric A (1993) Central pain: "new" syndromes and their evaluation. *Muscle Nerve* **16**, 1017–24.

Beric A (1999) Spinal cord damage: injury. In: Wall PD, Melzack R, eds., *Textbook of Pain*, 4th edn. Edinburgh: Churchill-Livingstone, pp. 915–27.

Beric A, Dimitrijevć MR, Lindblom U (1988) Central dysesthesia syndrome in spinal cord injury patients. *Pain* **34**, 109–16.

Besson JM. (1994) The pharmacology of pain: 25 years of hope, despair and hope. In: Gebhart GF, Hammond DL, Jensen TS, eds., *Proceedings of the 7th World Congress on Pain.* Seattle, WA: IASP Press, pp. 23–39.

Bettag W (1966) Results of treatment of pain by interruption of the medial pain tract of the brain stem. *Excerpta Med Int Cong Ser* **110**, 771–5.

Bettag W, Yoshida T (1960) Über stereotaktischen schmerzoperationen. *Acta Neurochir* **8**, 299–317.

Bharadwaj P, Danilychev M (2006) Central post-stroke syndrome treated with parenteral lidocaine. *J Pain Symptom Manage* **32**, 400–1.

Bhattacharya A, Wickenden AD, Chaplan SR (2009) Sodium channel blockers for the treatment of neuropathic pain. *Neurotherapeutics* **6**, 663–78.

Biemond A (1956) The conduction of pain above the level of the thalamus opticus. *Arch Neurol Psychiatry* **75**, 231–44.

Biju G, Taly AB, Sinha S, *et al.* (2005) Painful gynecomastia following traumatic spinal cord injury. *Clin Neurol Neurosurg* **107**, 439–43.

Binder A, Schattschneider J, Wolff S, *et al.* (2002) Inhibition of human motor cortex by tonic cutaneous pain. A fMRI study. *IASP Congress* **2002**, 1125–P41.

Bingel U, Lorenz J, Glauche V, *et al.* (2004) Somatotopic organization of human somatosensory cortices for pain: a single trial fMRI study. *Neuroimage* **23**, 224–32.

Bingel U, Schoell E, Büchel C (2007) Imaging pain modulation in health and disease. *Curr Opin Neurol* **20**, 424–31.

Birklein F, Rolke R, Mueller-Forell W (2005) Isolated insular infarction eliminates contralateral cold, cold pain, and pinprick sensation. *Neurology* **65**, 1381.

Bitanga ES, Baroque AC, Santos-Ocampo AS, *et al.* (2002) Safety, tolerability, and efficacy of gabapentin in neuropathic pain: results of a post-marketing surveillance study in 1214 Filipino patients. *Neurol J Southeast Asia* **7**, 25–34.

Bittar RG, Ptito A, Reutens DC (2000) Somatosensory representation in patients who have undergone hemispherectomy: a functional magnetic resonance imaging study. *J Neurosurg* **92**, 45–51.

Blair RDG, Lee RG, Vanderlinden G (1975) Dorsal column stimulation. Its effect on the somatosensory evoked responses. *Arch Neurol* **32**, 826–9.

Blanchard J, Ramamurthy S, Walsh N, Hoffman J, Schoenfeld L (1990) Intravenous regional sympatholysis:

a double-blind comparison of guanethidine, reserpine, and normal saline. *J Pain Symptom Manage* **5**, 357–61.

Blond S, Touzet G, Reyns N, *et al.* (2000) Les techniques de neurostimulation dans le traitement de la douleur chronique. *Neurochirurgie* **46**, 466–82.

Boas RA, Corvino BG, Shahnarian A (1982) Analgesic responses to i.v. lignocaine. *Br J Anaesth* **54**, 501–5.

Boggio PS, Amancio EJ, Correa CF, *et al.* (2009) Transcranial DC stimulation coupled with TENS for the treatment of chronic pain. A preliminary study. *Clin J Pain* **25**, 691–5.

Bogousslavsky J, Regli F, Uske A (1988) Thalamic infarcts: clinical syndromes, etiology, and prognosis. *Neurology* **38**, 837–48. Erratum in *Neurology* 1988, **38**, 1335.

Boivie J, Leijon G, Johansson I (1989) Central post-stroke pain. A study of the mechanisms through analyses of the sensory abnormalities. *Pain* **37**, 173–85.

Boly M, Balteau E, Schnakers C, *et al.* (2007) Baseline brain activity fluctuations predict somatosensory perception in humans. *Proc Natl Acad Sci U S A* **104**, 12187–192.

Bonicalzi V, Canavero S (2000) Sympathetic pain again? *Lancet* **360**, 1426–7.

Bonicalzi V, Canavero S (2004) Intrathecal ziconotide for chronic pain. *JAMA* **292**, 1681–2.

Boord P, Siddall PJ, Tran Y, *et al.* (2008) Electroencephalographic slowing and reduced reactivity in neuropathic pain following spinal cord injury. *Spinal Cord* **46**, 118–23.

Bornstein B (1949) Sur le phénomène du membre fantôme. *Encéphale* **38**, 32–46.

Bosch DA (1991) Stereotactic rostral mesencephalotomy in cancer pain and deafferentation pain: a series of 40 cases with follow-up results. *J Neurosurg* **75**, 747–51.

Botterell EH, Callaghan JC, Jousse T (1954) Pain in paraplegia: clinical management and surgical treatment. *Proc R Soc Med* **47**, 281–8.

Bouchard G, Mayanagi Y, Martins LF (1977) Advantages and limits of intracerebral stereotactic operations for pain. In: Sweet WH, Obrador S, Martin-Rodriguez JC, eds., *Neurosurgical Treatment in Psychiatry, Pain, and Epilepsy*. Baltimore, MD: University Park Press, pp. 693–6.

Bouckoms AF (1989) Psychosurgery for pain. In: Wall PD, Melzack R, eds., *Textbook of Pain*. Edinburgh: Churchill Livingstone, pp. 868–81.

Boutron I, Dutton S, Ravaud P, Altman DG (2010) Reporting and interpretation of randomized controlled trials with statistically nonsignificant results for primary outcomes. *JAMA* **303**, 2058–64.

Bowsher D (1989) Contralateral mirror-image pain following anterolateral cordotomy. *Pain* **33**, 63–5.

Bowsher D (1994) La douleur neurogene. *Doul Analg* **2**, 65–9. (See also Bowsher D (1995) The management of central post-stroke pain. *Postgrad Med J* **71**, 599–604.)

Bowsher D (1996) Central pain: clinical and physiological characteristics. *J Neurol Neurosurg Psychiatry* **61**, 62–9.

Bowsher D (2001) Stroke and central poststroke pain in an elderly population. *J Pain* **2**, 258–61.

Bowsher D (2002) The time factor in tricyclic treatment of postherpetic neuralgia (PHN) and central post-stroke pain (CPSP). In: *10th World Congress on Pain, Book of Abstracts*. Seattle, WA: IASP Press, A890–P160.

Bowsher D (2005a) Allodynia in relation to lesion site in central post-stroke pain. *J Pain* **6**, 736–40.

Bowsher D (2005b) Representation of somatosensory modalities in pathways ascending from the spinal anterolateral funiculus to the thalamus demonstrated by lesions in man. *Eur Neurol* **54**, 14–22.

Bowsher D (2006a) Somatic sensation and the insular-opercular cortex: relationship to central pain. *Eur Neurol* **55**, 160–5.

Bowsher D (2006b) A case of visceral post-stroke pain. *J Pain Symptom Manage* **32**, 398–400.

Bowsher D, Lahuerta J (1987) A case of tabes dorsalis with tonic pupils and lightning pains relieved by sodium valproate. *J Neurol Neurosurg Psychiatry* **50**, 239–41.

Bowsher D, Leijon G, Thomas KA (1998) Central poststroke pain: correlation of MRI with clinical pain characteristics and sensory abnormalities. *Neurology* **51**, 1352–8.

Bowsher D, Brooks J, Enevoldson P (2004) Central representation of somatic sensations in the parietal operculum (SII) and insula. *Eur Neurol* **52**, 211–25.

Branco DM, Coehlo TM, Branco BM, *et al.* (2003) Functional variability of the human cortical motor map: electrical stimulation findings in perirolandic epilepsy surgery. *J Clin Neurophysiol* **20**, 17–25.

Brefel-Courbon C, Grolleau S, Thalamas C, *et al.* (2009) Comparison of chronic analgesic drugs prevalence in Parkinson's disease, other chronic diseases and the general population. *Pain* **141**, 14–18.

Breuer A, Cuervo H, Selkoe DJ (1981) Hyperpathia and sensory level due to parietal lobe arteriovenous malformation. *Arch Neurol* **38**, 722–4.

Breuer B, Pappagallo M, Knotkova H, *et al.* (2007) A randomized, double-blind, placebo-controlled, two-period, crossover, pilot trial of lamotrigine in patients with central pain due to multiple sclerosis. *Clin Ther* **29**, 2022–30.

Briggs F, Usrey WM (2008) Emerging views of corticothalamic function. *Curr Op Neurobiol* **18**, 403–7.

Brodie EE, Kane FMA, Gijsbers K, Niven CA (2009) Contralateral limb movement modulates cold pressor pain. *Acute Pain* **11**, 121–8.

Broggi G, Franzini A, Giorgi C, Servello D, Spreafico R (1984) Preliminary results of specific thalamic stimulation for deafferentation pain. *Acta Neurochir Suppl* **33**, 497–500.

Broggi G, Servello D, Dones I, Carbone G (1994) Italian multicentric study on pain treatment with epidural spinal cord stimulation (SCS). *Stereotact Funct Neurosurg* **62**, 273–8.

Bronstein JM, Tagliati M, Alterman RL, *et al.* (2011) Deep brain stimulation for Parkinson disease: an expert consensus and review of key issues. *Arch Neurol* **68**, 165.

Brown JA, Pilitsis JG (2005) Motor cortex stimulation for central and neuropathic facial pain: a prospective study of

10 patients and observations of enhanced sensory and motor function during stimulation. *Neurosurgery* **56**, 290–7.

Bruehl S, Chung OY, Chont M (2010) Chronic pain-related changes in endogenous opioid analgesia: a case report. *Pain* **148**, 167–71.

Bruel BM, Burton AW, Ting J, Mosura M (2007) Rapid titration of ziconotide for the treatment of severe intractable back pain from metastatic spinal anaplastic ependymoma. *Eur J Pain* **11**, S142–3, A321.

Bruguerolle B, Labrecque G (2007) Rhythmic pattern in pain and their chronotherapy. *Adv Drug Deliv Rev* **59**, 883–95.

Bryce TN, Norrbrink Budh C, Cardenas DD, *et al.* (2007) Pain after spinal cord injury: an evidence-based review for clinical practice and research. *J Spinal Cord Med* **30**, 421–40.

Buchhaas U, Koulousakis A, Nittner K (1989) Experience with spinal cord stimulation (SCS) in the management of chronic pain in a traumatic transverse lesion syndrome. *Neurosurg Rev* **12** (Suppl 1), 582–7.

Budd K (1985) The use of the opiate antagonist naloxone in the treatment of intractable pain. *Neuropeptides* **5**, 419–22.

Bufalari I, Aprile T, Avenanti A, Di Russo F, Aglioti SM (2007) Empathy for pain and touch in the human somatosensory cortex. *Cereb Cortex* **17**, 2553–61.

Bugnicourt JM, Garcia PY, Canaple S, Lamy C, Godefroy O (2011) Central neuropathic pain after cerebral venous thrombosis is not so uncommon: an observational study. *J Neurol*, in press.

Burchiel KJ (1993) Trigeminal neuropathic pain. *Acta Neurochir Suppl (Wien)* **58**, 145–9.

Burke DC (1973) Pain in paraplegia. *Paraplegia* **10**, 297–313.

Burkey AR, Abla-Yao S (2010) Successful treatment of central pain in a multiple sclerosis patient with epidural stimulation of the dorsal root entry zone. *Pain Med* **11**, 127–32.

Burkhalter A (2008) Many specialists for suppressing cortical excitation. *Front Neurosci* **2** (Issue 2).

Buzsaki G (2006) *Rhythms of the Brain*. Oxford: Oxford University Press.

Cabral NL, Goncalves AR, Longo AL, *et al.* (2009) Incidence of stroke subtypes, prognosis and prevalence of risk factors in Joinville, Brazil: a 2 year community based study. *J Neurol Neurosurg Psychiatry* **80**, 755–61.

Cahana A, Carota A, Montadon ML, Annoni JM (2004) The long-term effect of repeated intravenous lidocaine on central pain and possible correlation in positron emission tomography measurements. *Anesth Analg* **98**, 1581–4.

Calabrò RS, Marra A, Quattrini F, *et al.* (2010) Central neuropathic pain: an unusual case of painful ejaculation responding to topiramate. *J Sex Med*, in press.

Calmels P, Mick G, Perrouin-Verbe B, Ventura M (2009) Neuropathic pain in spinal cord injury: identification, classification, evaluation. *Ann Phys Rehabil Med* **52**, 83–102.

Cameron T (2004) Safety and efficacy of spinal cord stimulation for the treatment of chronic pain: a 20-year literature review. *J Neurosurg* **100** (Suppl 3), 254–67.

Campagna-Slater V, Weaver DF (2007) Anaesthetic binding sites for etomidate and propofol on a GABAA receptor model. *Neurosci Lett* **418**, 28–33.

Campero M, Bostock H, Baumann TK, Ochoa JL (2010) A search for activation of C nociceptors by sympathetic fibers in complex regional pain syndrome. *Clin Neurophysiol* **121**, 1072–9.

Canavero S (1994) Dynamic reverberation: a unified mechanism for central and phantom pain. *Med Hypotheses* **42**, 203–7.

Canavero S (1996) Bilateral central pain. *Acta Neurol Belg* **96**, 135–6.

Canavero S, ed. (2009) *Textbook of Therapeutic Cortical Stimulation*. New York, NY: Nova Science,

Canavero S (2011) Surface stimulation. In: Arle JE, Shils JL, eds., *Essential Neuromodulation*. New York, NY: Elsevier-Academic Press.

Canavero S, Bonicalzi V (1995) Cortical stimulation for central pain. *J Neurosurg* **83**, 1117.

Canavero S, Bonicalzi V (1996) Lamotrigine control of central pain. *Pain* **68**, 179–81.

Canavero S, Bonicalzi V (1998a) Review article. The neurochemistry of central pain: evidence from clinical studies, hypothesis and therapeutic implications. *Pain* **74**, 109–14.

Canavero S, Bonicalzi V (1998b) Pain after thalamic stroke: right diencephalic predominance and clinical features in 180 patients. *Neurology* **51**, 927–8.

Canavero S, Bonicalzi V (2001a) Electroconvulsive therapy and pain. *Pain* **89**, 301–2.

Canavero S, Bonicalzi V (2001b) Reversible central pain. *Neurol Sci* **22**, 271–3.

Canavero S, Bonicalzi V (2002) Therapeutic extradural cortical stimulation for central and neuropathic pain: a review. *Clin J Pain* **18**, 48–55.

Canavero S, Bonicalzi V (2003a) Chronic neuropathic pain. *N Engl J Med* **348**, 2688–9.

Canavero S, Bonicalzi V (2003b) Neuromodulation for central pain. *Expert Rev Neurother* **3**, 591–607.

Canavero S, Bonicalzi V (2004a) Intravenous subhypnotic propofol in central pain: a double-blind, placebo-controlled, crossover study. *Clin Neuropharmacol* **27**, 182–6.

Canavero S, Bonicalzi V (2004b) Norepinephrine and pain. *Pain* **107**, 279.

Canavero S, Bonicalzi V (2005a) Mexiletine–gabapentin for central pain: an efficacy and long-term study. In: *11th World Congress on Pain, Book of Abstracts*. Seattle, WA: IASP Press. P-218 A596 P-202.

Canavero S, Bonicalzi V (2005b) Transcranial magnetic stimulation for central pain. *Curr Pain Headache Rep* **9**, 87–9.

Canavero S, Bonicalzi V (2007a) *Central Pain Syndrome: Pathophysiology, Diagnosis and Management*. Cambridge: Cambridge University Press.

Canavero S, Bonicalzi V (2007b) Central pain syndrome: elucidation of genesis and treatment. *Exp Rev Neurother* 7, 1485–97.

Canavero S, Bonicalzi V (2007c) Extradural cortical stimulation for central pain. In: Sakas D, Simpson B, Krames E, eds., *Operative Neuromodulation*, Vol. 2. Vienna: Springer-Verlag, pp. 27–36.

Canavero S, Pagni CA, Castellano G, *et al.* (1993) The role of cortex in central pain syndromes: preliminary results of a long-term technetium-99 hexamethylpropyleneamineoxime single photon emission computed tomography study. *Neurosurgery* **32**, 185–91.

Canavero S, Pagni CA, Duca S, Bradac GB (1994) Spinal intramedullary cavernous angiomas: a literature metaanalysis. *Surg Neurol* **41**, 381–8.

Canavero S, Bonicalzi V, Pagni CA, *et al.* (1995a) Propofol analgesia in central pain: preliminary clinical observations. *J Neurol* **242**, 561–7.

Canavero S, Pagni CA, Bonicalzi V (1995b) Transient hyperacute allodynia in Schneider's syndrome: an irritative genesis? *Ital J Neurol Sci* **16**, 555–7.

Canavero S, Bonicalzi V, Castellano G (1996) Two in one: the genesis of central pain. *Pain* **64**, 394–5.

Canavero S, Bonicalzi V, Massa-Micon B (1997) Central neurogenic pruritus: a literature review. *Acta Neurol Belg* **97**, 244–7.

Canavero S, Bonicalzi V, Paolotti R, Cerutti A (1998) Extradural cortical stimulation for neurogenic pain and Parkinson's disease: the Turin experience. *Proceedings of the 4th International Congress of the International Neuromodulation Society*, Luzern, August 20–26, 1998.

Canavero S, Bonicalzi V, Castellano G, Perozzo P, Massa-Micon B (1999) Painful supernumerary phantom arm following motor cortex stimulation for central post-stroke pain. *J Neurosurg* **91**, 121–3.

Canavero S, Bonicalzi V, Lacerenza M, *et al.* (2001) Disappearance of central pain following iatrogenic stroke. *Acta Neurol Belg* **101**, 221–3.

Canavero S, Bonicalzi V, Paolotti R (2002a) Lack of effect of topiramate for central pain. *Neurology* **58**, 831–2.

Canavero S, Bonicalzi V, Paolotti R (2002b) Reboxetine for central pain: a single-blind prospective study. *Clin Neuropharmacol* **25**, 238–9.

Canavero S, Bonicalzi V, Dotta M, *et al.* (2002c) Transcranial magnetic cortical stimulation relieves central pain. *Stereotact Funct Neurosurg* **78**, 192–6.

Canavero S, Bonicalzi V, Dotta M, Vighetti S, Asteggiano G (2003) Low-rate repetitive TMS allays central pain. *Neurol Res* **25**, 151–2.

Canavero S, Bonicalzi V, Intonti S, Crasto S, Castellano G (2006a) Effects of bilateral extradural cortical stimulation for plegic stroke rehabilitation. *Neuromodulation* **9**, 28–33.

Canavero S, Bonicalzi V, Clemente M (2006b) No neurotoxicity from long-term (>5 years) intrathecal infusion of midazolam in humans. *J Pain Symptom Manage* **32**, 1–3.

Cantor F (1972) Phenytoin treatment of thalamic pain. *Br Med J* **2**, 590.

Capel ID, Dorrell HM, Spencer EP, Davis MW (2003) The amelioration of the suffering associated with spinal cord injury with subperception transcranial electrical stimulation. *Spinal Cord* **41**, 109–17.

Cardenas CA, Cardenas CG, De Armendi AJ, Scroggs RS (2006) Carbamazepine interacts with a slow inactivation state of Na-v1.8-like sodium channels. *Neurosci Lett* **408**, 129–34.

Cardenas DD, Felix ER (2009) Pain after spinal cord injury: a review of classification, treatment approaches, and treatment assessment. *PMR* **1**, 1077–90.

Cardenas DD, Jensen MP (2006) Treatments for chronic pain in persons with spinal cord injury: a survey study. *J Spinal Cord Med* **29**, 109–17 (updates Warms CA, Turner JA, Marshall HM, Cardenas DD (2002) Treatments for chronic pain associated with spinal cord injuries: many are tried, few are helpful. *Clin J Pain* **18**, 154–63.)

Cardenas DD, Warms CA, Turner JA, *et al.* (2002) Efficacy of amitriptyline for relief of pain in spinal cord injury: results of a randomised controlled trial. *Pain* **96**, 365–73.

Carlsson KC, Hoem NO, Moberg ER, Mathisen LC (2004) Analgesic effect of dextromethorphan in neuropathic pain. *Acta Anaesthesiol Scand* **48**, 328–36.

Carrieri PB, Provitera VV, Lavorgna L, Bruno R (1998) Response of thalamic pain syndrome to lamotrigine. *Eur J Neurol* **5**, 625–6.

Carroll D, Joint C, Maartens N, *et al.* (2000) Motor cortex stimulation for chronic neuropathic pain: a preliminary study of 10 cases. *Pain* **84**, 431–7.

Carroll IR, Kaplan KM, Mackey SC (2008) Mexiletine therapy for chronic pain: survival analysis identifies factors predicting clinical success. *J Pain Symptom Manage* **35**, 321–6.

Carter ML (2004) Spinal cord stimulation in chronic pain: a review of evidence. *Anaesth Intensive Care* **32**, 11–21.

Cassinari V, Pagni CA (1969) *Central Pain: a Neurosurgical Survey*. Cambridge, MA: Harvard University Press.

Cattaneo L, Chierici E, Cucurachi L, Cobelli R, Pavesi G (2007) Posterior insular stroke causing selective loss of contralateral nonpainful thermal sensation. *Neurology* **68**, 237.

Cauda F, Sacco K, Duca, S, *et al.* (2009) Altered resting state in diabetic neuropathic pain. *PLOS ONE* **4**, e4542.

Cepeda MS, Africano JM, Polo R, Alcala R, Carr DB (2003) What decline in pain intensity is meaningful to patients with acute pain? *Pain* **105**, 151–7.

Cereda C, Ghika J, Maeder P, Bogousslavsky J (2002) Strokes restricted to the insular cortex. *Neurology* **59**, 1950–5.

Cesaro P, Mann MW, Moretti JL, *et al.* (1991) Central pain and thalamic hyperactivity: a single photon emission computerized tomographic study. *Pain* **47**, 329–36.

Chang PF, Arendt-Nielsen L, Chen AC (2002) Dynamic changes and spatial correlation of EEG activities during cold pressor test in man. *Brain Res Bull* **57**, 667–75.

Chari V, Tunks E (2010) Poststroke pain – but multiple pain mechanisms. *Pain Res Manage* **15**, 24–6.

Charlesworth G, Soryal I, Smith S, Sisodiya SM (2009) Acute, localized paroxysmal pain as the initial manifestation of focal seizures: a case report and a brief review of the literature. *Pain* **141**, 300–5.

Charlton BG (2008) Figureheads, ghost-writers and pseudonymous quant bloggers: the recent evolution of authorship in science publishing. *Med Hypotheses* **71**, 475–80.

Charney DS, Mihic SJ, Harris RA (2006) Hypnotics and sedatives. In: Brunton LL, Lazo JS, Parker KL, eds., *Goodman & Gilman's The Pharmacological Basis of Therapeutics*. New York, NY: McGraw-Hill, pp. 401–28.

Chatterjee A, Almahrezi A, Ware M, Fitzcharles MA (2002) A dramatic response to inhaled cannabis in a woman with central thalamic pain and dystonia. *J Pain Symptom Manage* **24**, 4–6.

Chen B, Stitik TP, Foyc PM, Nadler SF, DeLisa JA (2002) Central post-stroke pain syndrome: yet another use for gabapentin? *Am J Phys Med Rehab* **81**, 718–20.

Chen L, Yang H, Yang T, *et al.* (2009) Effectiveness of surgical treatment for traumatic central cord syndrome. *J Neurosurg Spine* **10**, 3–8.

Chen WH, Lan MY, Chang YY, *et al.* (1997) Bilateral cheirooral syndrome. *Clin Neurol Neurosurg* **99**, 239–43.

Childers WE, Baudy RB (2007) N-methyl-D-aspartate antagonists and neuropathic pain: the search for relief. *J Med Chem* **50**, 2557–62.

Chiou-Tan FY, Tuel SM, Johnson JC, *et al.* (1996) Effect of mexiletine on spinal cord injury dysesthetic pain. *Am J Phys Med Rehab* **75**, 84–7.

Chitsaz A, Janghorbani M, Shaygannejad V, *et al.* (2009) Sensory complaints of the upper extremities in multiple sclerosis: relative efficacy of nortriptyline and Transcutaneous Electrical Nerve Stimulation. *Clin J Pain* **25**, 281–5.

Chodakiewitz JW (1991) Thalamotomy lesions. *J Neurosurg* **75**, 832–4.

Chodakiewitz JW, Rinaldi P (2007) Treatment of intractable pain with DBS. *Stereotact Funct Neurosurg* **85**, 57–8.

Chung CS, Caplan LR, Han W, *et al.* (1996) Thalamic haemorrhage. *Brain* **119**, 1873–86.

Churyukanov MV, Alexeev VV, Kukushkin ML, Krupina NA (2010) Chronic pain syndrome in multiple sclerosis. *Eur J Pain Suppl* **4**, 101, A353.

Cianchetti C, Zuddas A, Randazzo AP, Perra L, Marrosu MG (1999) Lamotrigine adjunctive therapy in painful phenomena in MS: preliminary observations. *Neurology* **53**, 433.

Cioni B, Meglio M (2007) Motor cortex stimulation for chronic non-malignant pain: current state and future prospects. *Acta Neurochir Suppl* **97**, 45–9.

Cioni B, Meglio M, Pentimalli L, Visocchi M (1995) Spinal cord stimulation in the treatment of paraplegic pain. *J Neurosurg* **82**, 35–9.

Clifford DB, Trotter JL (1984) Pain in multiple sclerosis. *Arch Neurol* **41**, 1270–2.

Coffey RJ (2001) Deep brain stimulation for chronic pain: results of two multicenter trials and a structured review. *Pain Med* **2**, 183–92.

Cohen SP, Abdi J (2002) Venous malformations associated with central pain: report of a case. *Anesth Analg* **95**, 1358–60.

Cohen SP, DeJesus M (2004) Ketamine patient-controlled analgesia for dysesthetic central pain. *Spinal Cord* **42**, 425–8.

Cole JD, Illis LS, Sedgwick EM (1987) Pain produced by spinal cord stimulation in a patient with allodynia and pseudo-tabes. *J Neurol Neurosurg Psychiatry* **50**, 1083–4.

Cole JD, Illis LS, Sedgwick EM (1991) Intractable central pain in spinal cord injury is not relieved by spinal cord stimulation. *Paraplegia* **29**, 167–72.

Cole MW, Yeung N, Freiwald WA, Botvinick M (2009) Cingulate cortex: diverging data from humans and monkeys. *Trends Neurosci* **32**, 566–74.

Condouris GA (1976) Local anesthetics as modulators of neural information. In: Bonica JJ, Albe-Fessard DG, eds., *Advances in Pain Research and Therapy*, Vol. 1. New York, NY: Raven Press, pp. 663–7.

Constans JP (1960) Chirurgie frontale de la douleur. *Acta Neurochir (Wien)* **8**, 251–81.

Cooper IS, Amin I, Candra R, Waltz JM (1973) A surgical investigation of the clinical physiology of the LP-pulvinar complex in man. *J Neurol Sci* **18**, 89–110.

Craig AD (1998) A new version of the thalamic disinhibition hypothesis of central pain. *Pain Forum* **7**, 1–14.

Craig AD (2009) How do you feel – now? The anterior insula and human awareness. *Nat Rev Neurosci* **10**, 59–70.

Craig AR, Hancock K, Dickson H, Chang E (1997) Long-term psychological outcomes in spinal cord injured persons: results of a controlled trial using cognitive behavior therapy. *Arch Phys Med Rehabil* **78**, 33–8.

Crane DA, Jaffee KM, Kundu A (2009) Intractable pruritus after traumatic spinal cord injury. *J Spinal Cord Med* **32**, 436–9.

Crisologo PA, Neal B, Brown R, McDanal J, Kissin I (1991) Lidocaine-induced spinal block can relieve central poststroke pain: role of the block in chronic pain diagnosis. *Anesthesiology* **74**, 184–5.

Cristante AF, Barros-Filho TEP, Tatsui N, *et al.* (2009) Stem cells in the treatment of chronic spinal cord injury: evaluation of somatosensory evoked potentials in 39 patients. *Spinal Cord* **47**, 733–8.

Crochet S, Petersen CCH (2009) Cortical dynamics by layer. *Neuron* **64**, 298–300.

Cruz-Almeida Y, Felix ER, Martinez-Arizala A, Widerström-Noga G (2009) Pain symptom profiles in persons with spinal cord injury. *Pain Med* **10**, 1246–59.

Cummins TR, Rush AM (2007) Voltage-gated sodium channel blockers for the treatment of neuropathic pain. *Expert Rev Neurother* **7**, 1597–612.

Dahm PO, Nitescu PV, Appelgren LK, Curelaru I (1998) Long-term intrathecal (i.t.) infusion of bupivacaine relieved intractable pain and spasticity in a patient with multiple sclerosis. *Eur J Pain* **2**, 81–5.

D'Aleo G, Sessa E, Di Bella P, *et al.* (2001) Topiramate modulation of R3 nociceptive reflex in multiple sclerosis patients suffering paroxysmal symptoms. *J Neurol* **248**, 996–9.

Daniele O, Fierro B, Brighina F, Magaudda A, Natalé E (2003) Disappearance of haemorrhagic stroke-induced thalamic (central) pain following a further (contralateral ischaemic) stroke. *Funct Neurol* **18**, 95–6.

DaSilva AFM, Granziera C, Snyder J, Hadjikhani N (2007) Thickening in the somatosensory cortex of patients with migraine. *Neurology* **69**, 1990–5.

David M, Talairach J, Hécaen H (1947) Étude critique des interventions neurochirurgicales actuellement pratiquées dans le traitement de la douleur. *Semaine des Hopitaux de Paris* **234**, 1651–65.

Davidoff G, Roth E, Guarracini M, Sliwa J, Yarkony G (1987a) Function-limiting dysesthetic pain syndrome among traumatic spinal cord injury patients: a cross-sectional study. *Pain* **29**, 39–48.

Davidoff G, Guarracini M, Roth E, Sliwa J, Yarkony G (1987b) Trazodone hydrochloride in the treatment of dysesthetic pain in traumatic myelopathy: a randomized, double-blind, placebo-controlled study. *Pain* **29**, 151–61.

Davies HTO, Crombie IK, Lonsdale M, Macrae WA (1991) Consensus and contention in the treatment of chronic nerve-damage pain. *Pain* **47**, 191–6.

Davis KD, Hutchison WD, Lozano AM, Dostrovsky JO (1994) Altered pain and temperature perception following cingulotomy and capsulotomy in a patient with schizoaffective disorder. *Pain* **59**, 189–99.

Davis KD, Kiss ZHT, Tasker RR, Dostrovsky JO (1996) Thalamic stimulation-evoked sensations in chronic pain patients and in nonpain (movement disorder) patients. *J Neurophysiol* **75**, 1026–37.

Davis KD, Kiss ZH, Luo L, *et al.* (1998) Phantom sensations generated by thalamic microstimulation. *Nature* **391**, 385–7.

Davis KD, Taub E, Duffner F, *et al.* (2000) Activation of the anterior cingulate cortex by thalamic stimulation in patients with chronic pain: a positron emission tomography study. *J Neurosurg* **92**, 64–9.

Davis L (1954) Treatment of spinal cord injuries. *AMA Arch Surg* **69**, 488–95.

Davis L, Martin J (1947) Studies upon spinal cord injuries: II. The nature and treatment of pain. *J Neurosurg* **4**, 483–91.

Davis R, Lentini R (1975) Transcutaneous nerve stimulation for treatment of pain in patients with spinal cord injury. *Surg Neurol* **4**, 100–1.

Davis RA, Stokes JW (1966) Neurosurgical attempts to relieve thalamic pain. *Surg Gynecol Obstet* **123**, 371–84.

Davison C, Schick W (1935) Spontaneous pain and other subjective sensory disturbances. A clinicopathological study. *Arch Neurol Psychiatry* **34**, 1204–37.

De Ajuriaguerra J (1937) *La douleur dans les affections du systéme nerveux central.* Paris: Doin.

De Blasis E, Necozione S, Di Orio F, Santilli V (2009) Mirror therapy for chronic complex regional pain syndrome type 1 and stroke. *N Engl J Med* **361**, 634–5.

DeCharms RC, Maeda F, Glover GH, *et al.* (2005) Control over brain activation and pain learned by using real-time functional MRI. *Proc Natl Acad Sci U S A* **102**, 18626–31.

Defazio G, Berardelli A, Fabbrini G, *et al.* (2008) Pain as a nonmotor symptom of Parkinson disease: evidence from a case–control study. *Arch Neurol* **65**, 1191–4.

Defrin R, Ohry A, Blumen N, Urca G (1999) Acute pain threshold in subjects with chronic pain following spinal cord injury. *Pain* **83**, 275–82.

Defrin R, Ohry A, Blumen N, Urca G (2001) Characterization of chronic pain and somatosensory function in spinal cord injury subjects. *Pain* **89**, 253–63.

Defrin R, Peleg S, Weingarden H, Heruti R, Urc G (2007a) Differential effect of supraspinal modulation on the nociceptive withdrawal reflex and pain sensation. *Clin Neurophysiol* **118**, 427–37.

Defrin R, Grunhaus L, Zamir D, Zeilig G (2007b) The effect of a series of repetitive transcranial magnetic stimulations of the motor cortex on central pain after spinal cord injury. *Arch Phys Med Rehabil* **88**, 1574–80.

DeGraba TJ, Pettigrew LC (2000) Why do neuroprotective drugs work in animals but not in humans? *Neurol Clinics* **19**, 475–93.

Dejerine J, Egger M (1903) Contribution à l'étude de la physiologie pathologique de l'incoordination motrice. *Rev Neurol* **11**, 397.

Dejerine J, Roussy G (1906) Le syndrome thalamique. *Rev Neurol* **14**, 521–32.

Delavallée M, Abu-Serieh B, de Tourchaninoff M, Raftopoulos C (2008) Subdural motor cortex stimulation for central and peripheral neuropathic pain: a long-term follow-up study in a series of eight patients. *Neurosurgery* **63**, 101–5.

Dellemijn PL, Vanneste JA (1997) Randomised double-blind active-placebo-controlled crossover trial of intravenous fentanyl in neuropathic pain. *Lancet* **349**, 753–8.

Demchuk N (2010) Pain as a nonmotor symptom in Parkinson's disease. *Eur J Pain Suppl* **4**, 101.

Demirel T, Braun W, Reimers CD (1984) Results of spinal cord stimulation in patients suffering from chronic pain after a two year observation period. *Neurochirurgia (Stuttg)* **27**, 47–50.

Denny-Brown D, Kirk EJ, Yanagisawa N (1973) The tract of Lissauer in relation to sensory transmission in the dorsal horn of the spinal cord in the macaque monkey. *J Comp Neurol* **151**, 175–200.

De Ridder D, De Mulder G, Verstraeten E, Sunaert S, Moller A (2007) Somatosensory cortex stimulation for deafferentation pain. *Acta Neurochir Suppl* **97**, 67–74.

De Salles AF, Bittar GT (1994) Thalamic pain syndrome: anatomic and metabolic correlations. *Surg Neurol* **41**, 147–51.

De Schutter E, ed. (2010) *Computational Modeling Methods for Neuroscientists*. Cambridge, MA: MIT Press.

Deutsch H (2010) Pain outcomes after surgery in patients with intramedullary spinal cord cavernous malformations. *Neurosurg Focus* **29**, E15.

Devulder J, Vermeulen H, De Colvenaer L, *et al.* (1991) Spinal cord stimulation in chronic pain: evaluation of results, complications, and technical considerations in sixty-nine patients. *Clin J Pain* **7**, 21–8.

Dey DD, Landrum O, Oaklander AL (2005) Central neuropathic itch from spinal-cord cavernous hemangioma: a human case, a possible animal model, and hypotheses about pathogenesis. *Pain* **113**, 233–7.

Deyo RA, Patrick DL (2005) *Hope or Hype: the Obsession With Medical Advances and the High Cost of False Promises*. New York, NY: AMACOM.

Di Biagio F (1959) Dolore centrale da lesione sopratalamica regredito con atophanyl. *Riv Neurol* **29**, 476–81.

Dick IE, Brochu RM, Purohit Y, *et al.* (2007) Sodium channel blockade may contribute to the analgesic efficacy of antidepressants. *J Pain* **8**, 315–24.

Dieckmann G, Veras G (1984) Plexus avulsion pain (neurogenic pain). High frequency coagulation of the dorsal root entry zone in patients with deafferentation pain. *Acta Neurochir (Wien) Suppl* **33**, 445–50.

Dieckmann G, Witzmann A (1982) Initial and long-term results of deep brain stimulation for chronic intractable pain. *Appl Neurophysiol* **45**, 167–72.

Dieleman JP, Kerklaan J, Huygen FJ, Bouma PA, Sturkenboom MC (2008) Incidence rates and treatment of neuropathic pain conditions in the general population. *Pain* **137**, 681–8.

Dierssen G, Odoriz B, Hernando C (1969) Sensory and motor response to stimulation of the posterior cingulate cortex in man. *J Neurosurg* **31**, 435–40.

Diesch E, Flor H (2007) Alteration in the response properties of primary somatosensory cortex related to differential aversive Pavlovian conditioning. *Pain* **131**, 171–80.

Dijkers M, Bryce T, Zanca J (2009) Prevalence of chronic pain after traumatic spinal cord injury: a systematic review. *J Rehabil Res Dev* **46**, 13–30.

Dimitrijevic MR (1987) Neurophysiology in spinal cord injury. *Paraplegia* **25**, 205–8.

Djaldetti R, Shifrin A, Rogowski Z, *et al.* (2004) Quantitative measurement of pain sensation in patients with Parkinson disease. *Neurology* **62**, 2171–5.

Djaldetti R, Yust-Katz S, Kolianov V, Melamed E, Dabby R (2007) The effect of duloxetine on primary pain symptoms in Parkinson disease. *Clin Neuropharmacol* **30**, 201–5.

Doi N, Nakamura M, Isse K, *et al.* (1999) Electroconvulsive therapy for central post-stroke pain. In: *9th World Congress on Pain, Book of Abstracts*. Seattle, WA: IASP Press, A203, p. 436.

Donnellan CP (2006) Acupuncture for central pain affecting the ribcage following traumatic brain injury and rib fractures. Case report. *Acupunct Med* **24**, 129–33.

Donovan WH, Dimitrijevic MR, Dahm L, Dimitrijevic M (1982) Neurophysiological approaches to chronic pain following spinal cord injury. *Paraplegia* **20**, 135–46.

Drake CG, McKenzie KG (1953) Mesencephalic tractotomy for pain: experience with six cases. *J Neurosurg* **10**, 457–62.

Drewes AM, Andreasen A, Poulsen LH (1994) Valproate for treatment of chronic central pain after spinal cord injury: a double-blind cross-over study. *Paraplegia* **32**, 565–9.

Drouot X, Nguyen JP, Peschanski M, Lefaucheur JP (2002) The antalgic efficacy of chronic motor cortex stimulation is related to sensory changes in the painful area. *Brain* **125**, 1660–4.

Druckman R, Lende R (1965) Central pain of spinal cord origin: pathogenesis and surgical relief in one patient. *Neurology* **15**, 518–22.

Duchenne de Boulogne G (1855) *De l'électrisation localisée et de son application à la physiologie, à la pathologie et à la thérapeutique*. Paris: Baillière.

Ducreux D, Attal N, Parker F, Bouhassira D (2006) Mechanisms of central neuropathic pain: a combined psychophysical and fMRI study in syringomyelia. *Brain* **129**, 963–76.

Duncan GH, Bushnell CM, Marchand S (1991) Deep brain stimulation: a review of basic research and clinical studies. *Pain* **45**, 49–59.

Duncan GH, Kupers RC, Marchand S, *et al.* (1998) Stimulation of human thalamus for pain relief: possible modulatory circuits revealed by positron emission tomography. *J Neurophysiol* **80**, 3326–30.

Durward QJ, Rice GP, Ball MJ, Gilbert JJ, Kaufmann JCE (1982) Selective spinal cordectomy: clinicopathological correlation. *J Neurosurg* **56**, 359–67.

Dworkin GF, Staats WE (1985) Posttraumatic syringomyelia. *Arch Phys Medic Rehab* **66**, 329–31.

Eames P (1997) Feeling cold: an unusual brain injury symptom and its treatment with vasopressin. *J Neurol Neurosurg Psychiatry* **62**, 198–9.

Eccles J (1977) My scientific odyssey. *Ann Rev Physiol* **39**, 1–20.

Edelsberg J, Oster G (2009) Summary measures of number needed to treat: how much clinical guidance do they provide in neuropathic pain? *Eur J Pain* **13**, 11–16.

Edgar RE, Best LG, Quail PA, Obert AD (1993) Computer-assisted DREZ microcoagulation: posttraumatic spinal deafferentation pain. *J Spinal Dis* **6**, 48–56.

Edinger L (1891) Giebt es central entstehende Schmerzen? *Dtsch Z Nervenheilk* **1**, 262–82.

Edmondson EA, Simpson RK, Stubler DK, Beric A (1993) Systemic lidocaine therapy for poststroke pain. *South Med J* **86**, 1093–6.

Edwards CL, Sudhakar S, Scales MT, *et al.* (2000) Electromyographic (EMG) biofeedback in the comprehensive treatment of central pain and ataxic tremor following thalamic stroke. *Appl Psychophysiol Biofeedback* **25**, 229–40.

Edwards WT, Habib F, Burney RG, Begin G (1985) Intravenous lidocaine in the management of various chronic pain states. *Reg Anaesth* **10**, 1–6.

Eide PK, Stubhaug A, Stenehjem AE (1995) Central dysesthesia pain after traumatic spinal cord injury is dependent on N-methyl-D-aspartate receptor activation. *Neurosurgery* **37**, 1080–7.

Eisenach JC, Rauck RL, Curry R (2003) Intrathecal, but not intravenous adenosine reduces allodynia in patients with neuropathic pain. *Pain* **105**, 65–70.

Eisenberg E, Brecker C (2002) Lumbar spinal cord stimulation for cervical-originated central pain: a case report. *Pain* **100**, 299–301.

Ekbom KA (1966) Tegretol, a new therapy of tabetic lightning pains. *Acta Med Scand* **179**, 251–2.

Ekbom KA, Westerberg CE, Osterman P (1968) Focal sensory motor seizures of spinal origin. *Lancet* **1**, 67.

Elizagarate E, Cortes J, Gonzalez Pinto A, *et al.* (2001) Study of the influence of electroconvulsive therapy on the regional cerebral blood flow by HMPAO-SPECT. *J Affect Disord* **65**, 55–9.

Ellis DJ, Dissanayake S, McGuire D, *et al.* (2008) Continuous intrathecal infusion of ziconotide for treatment of chronic malignant and nonmalignant pain over 12 months: a prospective, open-label study. *Neuromodulation* **11**, 40–9.

Enarson MC, Hays H, Woodroffe MA (1999) Clinical experience with oral ketamine. *J Pain Symptom Manage* **17**, 384–6.

Enggaard TP, Scherer C, Andersen C (2007) Dysaesthetic pain and burning skin sensations as adverse effects to spinal cord stimulator implantation for treatment of angina pectoris. *J Pain Symptom Manage* S183, A412.

Epstein FJ, Farmer JP, Freed D (1993) Adult intramedullary spinal cord ependymomas. The result of surgery in 38 patients. *J Neurosurg* **79**, 204–9.

Erickson TC, Bleckwenn WJ, Woolsey CN (1952) Observations on the post central gyrus in relation to pain. *Trans Am Neurol Assoc* **77**, 57–9.

Eriksson MBE, Sjölund BH, Nielzen S (1979) Long term results of peripheral conditioning stimulation as an analgesic measure in chronic pain. *Pain* **6**, 335–47.

Eriksson MBE, Sjölund BH, Sundbärg G (1984) Pain relief from peripheral conditioning stimulation in patients with chronic facial pain. *J Neurosurg* **61**, 149–55.

Ernst E, Pittler MH, Wider B (2007) *Complementary Therapies for Pain Management: an Evidence-Based Approach*. Edinburgh: Elsevier Mosby.

Ernst G, Gericke A, Berg P (2004) Central pain and complex motoric symptoms after gosarelin therapy of prostate cancer. *Sci World J* **4**, 969–73.

Errante LD, Williamson A, Spencer DD, Petroff OAC (2002) Gabapentin and vigabatrin increase GABA in the human neocortical slice. *Epilepsy Res* **49**, 203–10.

Ervin FR, Mark VH (1960) Stereotactic thalamotomy in the human. *Arch Neurol* **3**, 368–80.

Ervin FR, Brown CE, Mark VH (1966) Striatal influence on facial pain. *Confinia Neurologica* **27**, 75–86.

Espir ML, Millac P (1970) Treatment of paroxysmal disorders in multiple sclerosis with carbamazepine (Tegretol). *J Neurol Neurosurg Psychiatry* **33**, 528–31.

Estanol B, Baizabal-Carvallo JF, Senties-Madrid H (2008) A case of tactile agnosia with a lesion restricted to the post-central gyrus. *Neurol India* **56**, 471–3.

Ewelt C, Stummer W, Klink B, *et al.* (2010a) Cordectomy as final treatment option for diffuse intramedullary malignant glioma using 5-ALA fluorescence-guided resection. *Clin Neurol Neurosurg* **112**, 357–61.

Ewelt C, Stalder S, Steiger HJ, Hildebrandt G, Heilbronner R (2010b) Impact of cordectomy as a treatment option for posttraumatic and non-posttraumatic syringomyelia with tethered cord syndrome and myelopathy. *J Neurosurg Spine* **13**, 193–9.

Eysel UT (2003) Illusions and perceived images in the primate brain. *Science* **302**, 789–90.

Fabri M, Polonara G, Quattrini A, *et al.* (1999) Role of the corpus callosum in the somatosensory activation of the ipsilateral cerebral cortex: an fMRI study of callosotomized patients. *Eur J Neurosci* **11**, 3983–94.

Fagundes-Pereyra WJ, Teixeira MJ, Reyns N, *et al.* (2010) Motor cortex electric stimulation for the treatment of neuropathic pain. *Arq Neuropsiquiatr* **68**, 923–9.

Falci S, Best L, Bayles R, Lammertse D, Starnes C (2002) Dorsal root entry zone microcoagulation for spinal cord injury-related central pain: operative intramedullary electrophysiological guidance and clinical outcome. *J Neurosurg* **97**, 193–200.

Farrar JT, Young JP, LaMoreaux L, Werth JL, Poole RM (2001) Clinical importance of changes in chronic pain intensity measured on an 11-point numerical pain rating scale. *Pain* **94**, 149–58.

Felix ER, Cruz-Almeida Y, Widerström-Noga EG (2007) Chronic pain after spinal cord injury: what characteristics make some pains more disturbing than others? *J Rehabil Res Dev* **44**, 703–15.

Felix ER, Widerström-Noga EG (2009) Reliability and validity of quantitative sensory testing in persons with spinal cord injury and neuropathic pain. *J Rehabil Res Dev* **46**, 69–83.

Fenollosa P, Pallares J, Cervera J, *et al.* (1993) Chronic pain in the spinal cord injured: statistical approach and pharmacological treatment. *Paraplegia* **31**, 722–9.

Fessler RG, Brown FD, Rachlin JR, Mullan S, Fang VS (1984) Elevated beta-endorphin in cerebrospinal fluid after electrical brain stimulation: artifact of contrast infusion? *Science* **224**, 1017–19.

Fields HL, Adams JE (1974) Pain after cortical injury relieved by electrical stimulation of the internal capsule. *Brain* **97**, 169–78.

Fine W (1967) Post-hemiplegic epilepsy in the elderly. *Br Med J* **1**, 199–201.

Finet P, Raftopoulos C (2009) Interhemispheric subdural motor cortex stimulation : two cases. *Surg Neurol* **72**, 522–3.

Finnerup NB, Johannesen IL, Sindrup SH, Bach FW, Jensen TS (2001) Pain and dysesthesia in patients with spinal cord injury: a postal survey. *Spinal Cord* **39**, 256–62.
Finnerup NB, Sindrup SH, Bach FW, Johannesen IL, Jensen TS (2002) Lamotrigine in spinal cord injury pain: a randomized controlled trial. *Pain* **96**, 375–83.
Finnerup NB, Johannesen IL, Bach FW, Jensen TS (2003a) Sensory function above lesion level in spinal cord injury patients with and without pain. *Somatosens Mot Res* **20**, 71–6.
Finnerup NB, Johannesen IL, Fuglsang-Frederiksen A, Bach FW, Jensen TS (2003b) Sensory function in spinal cord injury patients with and without central pain. *Brain* **126**, 57–70.
Finnerup NB, Gyldensted C, Nielsen E, *et al.* (2003c) MRI in chronic spinal cord injury patients with and without central pain. *Neurology* **61**, 1569–75.
Finnerup NB, Gyldensted C, Fuglsang-Frederiksen A, Bach FW, Jensen TS (2004) Sensory perception in complete spinal cord injury. *Acta Neurol Scand* **109**, 194–9.
Finnerup NB, Biering-Sorensen F, Johannesen IL, *et al.* (2005) Intravenous lidocaine relieves spinal cord injury pain: a randomized controlled trial. *Anesthesiology* **102**, 1023–30.
Finnerup NB, Sørensen L, Biering-Sørensen F, Johannesen IL, Jensen TS (2007a) Segmental hypersensitivity and spinothalamic function in spinal cord injury pain. *Exp Neurol* **207**, 139–49.
Finnerup NB, Pedersen LH, Terkelsen AJ, Johannesen IL, Jensen TS (2007b) Reaction to topical capsaicin in spinal cord injury patients with and without central pain. *Exp Neurol* **205**, 190–200.
Finnerup NB, Faaborg P, Krogh K, Jensen TS (2008) Abdominal pain in long-term spinal cord injury. *Spinal Cord* **46**, 198–203.
Finnerup NB, Grydehøj J, Bing J, *et al.* (2009) Levetiracetam in spinal cord injury pain: a randomized controlled trial. *Spinal Cord* **47**, 861–7.
Fisher K, Hagen NA (1999) Analgesic effect of oral ketamine in chronic neuropathic pain of spinal origin: a case report. *J Pain Symptom Manage* **18**, 61–6.
Fishman SM, Ballantyne JC, Rathmell JP, eds. (2010) *Bonica's Management of Pain*, 4th edn. Baltimore, MD: Lippincott, Williams & Wilkins.
Fitzgerald PJ (2009) Neuromodulating mice and men: are there functional species differences in neurotransmitter concentration? *Neurosci Biobehav Rev* **33**, 1037–41.
Foltz EL, White LE (1966) Rostral cingulotomy and pain "relief". In: Knighton RS, Dumke PR, eds., *Pain. Henry Ford Hospital International Symposium*. Boston, MA: Little Brown, pp. 469–91.
Förster O (1927) *Die Leitungsbahnen des Schmerzgefühls und die chirurgische Behandlung der Schmerzzustände*. Berlin: Urban and Schwarzenberg.
Frank B, Serpell MG, Hughes J, Matthews JN, Kapur D (2008) Comparison of analgesic effects and patient tolerability of nabilone and dihydrocodeine for chronic neuropathic pain: randomised, crossover, double blind study. *BMJ* **336**, 199–201.
Frank F, Frank G, Gaist G, Fabrizi A, Sturiale C (1984) Deep brain stimulation in chronic pain syndromes. *Acta Neurochir (Wien)* Suppl **33**, 491–5.
Franzini A, Ferroli P, Dones I, Marras C, Broggi G (2003) Chronic motor cortex stimulation for movement disorders: a promising perspective. *Neurol Res* **25**, 123–6.
Franzini A, Cordella R, Nazzi V, Broggi G (2008) Long-term chronic stimulation of internal capsule in post-stroke pain and spasticity. Case report, long-term results and review of the literature. *Stereotact Funct Neurosurg* **86**, 179–83.
Freeman LW, Heimburger RF (1947) Surgical relief of pain in paraplegic patients. *Arch Surg* **55**, 433–40.
Freeman W, Watts JW (1950) *Psychosurgery in the Treatment of Mental Disorders and Intractable Pain*, 2nd edn. Springfield, IL: Thomas.
Fregni F, Boggio PS, Lima MC, *et al.* (2006) A sham-controlled, phase II trial of transcranial direct current stimulation for the treatment of central pain in traumatic spinal cord injury. *Pain* **122**, 197–209.
Friedman AH, Bullitt E (1988) Dorsal root entry zone lesions in the treatment of pain following brachial plexus avulsion, spinal cord injury and herpes zoster. *Appl Neurophysiol* **51**, 164–9.
Friehs GM, Schroettner O, Pendl G (1995) Evidence for segregated pain and temperature conduction within the spinothalamic tract. *J Neurosurg* **83**, 8–12.
Frighetto L, De Salles A, Wallace R, *et al.* (2004) Linear accelerator thalamotomy. *Surg Neurol* **62**, 106–13.
Frost FS, Mukkamala S, Covington E (2008) Self-inflicted finger injury in individuals with spinal cord injury: an analysis of 5 cases. *J Spinal Cord Med* **31**, 109–16.
Fuji M, Ohmoto Y, Kitahara T, *et al.* (1997) [Motor cortex stimulation therapy in patients with thalamic pain]. *No Shinkei Geka* **25**, 315–19.
Fujioka H, Fujii M, Koizumi H, *et al.* (2010) An implantable, focal brain cooling device suppresses nociceptive pain in rats. *Neurosc Res* **66**, 402–5.
Fukaya C, Katayama Y, Yamamoto T, *et al.* (2003) Motor cortex stimulation in patients with post-stroke pain: conscious somatosensory response and pain control. *Neurol Res* **25**, 153–6.
Fukuhara T, McKhann GMII, Santiago P, *et al.* (1999) Resolution of central pain after embolization of an arteriovenous malformation. Case report. *J Neurosurg* **90**, 575–9.
Fukui S, Shigemori S, Nosaka S (2002a) A case of central post-stroke pain with beneficial response to electroconvulsive therapy: a proton magnetic resonance spectroscopy study. *Pain Clin* **14**, 173–8.
Fukui S, Shigemori S, Nosaka S (2002b) Central pain associated with low thalamic blood flow treated by electroconvulsive therapy. *J Anaesth* **16**, 255–7.
Fukui S, Matsuno M, Inubushi T, Nosaka S (2006) N-Acetylaspartate concentrations in the thalami of neuropathic pain patients and healthy comparison

subjects measured with (1)H-MRS. *Magn Reson Imag* **24**, 75–9.
Gaches J (1952) Résultat thérapeutique des interventions corticales préfrontales limitées dans les traitment de certains syndromes douloureux dit irreductibles. *Semaine des Hopitaux de Paris* **28**, 3667–75.
Galer BS, Miller KV, Rowbotham MC (1993) Response to intravenous lidocaine infusion differs based on clinical diagnosis and site of nervous system injury. *Neurology* **43**, 1233–5.
Gamna G, Ferrio L, Della Rovere S (1962) Studio delle parestesie provocate mediante ischemia da compressione in un gruppo di malati mentali. *Ann Fren Sci Aff* **75**, 443–9.
Garcia-Larrea L, Peyron R, Mertens P, *et al.* (1997) Positron emission tomography during motor cortex stimulation for pain control. *Stereotact Funct Neurosurg* **68**, 141–8.
Garcia-Larrea L, Peyron R, Mertens P, *et al.* (1999) Electrical stimulation of motor cortex for pain control: a combined PET-scan and electrophysiological study. *Pain* **83**, 259–73.
Garcia-Larrea L, Convers P, Magnin M, *et al.* (2002) Laser-evoked potential abnormalities in central pain patients: the influence of spontaneous and provoked pain. *Brain* **125**, 2766–81.
Garcia-Larrea L, Maarrawi J, Peyron R, *et al.* (2006) On the relation between sensory deafferentation, pain and thalamic activity in Wallenberg's syndrome: a PET-scan study before and after motor cortex stimulation. *Eur J Pain* **10**, 677–88.
Garcia-Larrea L, Perchet C, Creac'h C, *et al.* (2010) Operculo-insular pain (parasylvian pain): a distinct central pain sindrome. *Brain* **133**, 2528–39.
Garcin R (1937) La douleur dans les affections organiques du système nerveux central. *Rev Neurol* **68**, 105–53.
Garcin R (1957) La douleur dans les affections du système nerveux central (thalamus, region bulbo-protuberantielle). In: Alajouanine T, ed., *La douleur et les douleurs*. Paris: Masson, pp. 199–213.
Garcin R (1968) Thalamic syndrome and pain of central origin. In: Soulairac A, Cahn J, Charpentier J, eds., *Pain*. London: Academic Press, pp. 521–39.
Gatscher S, Becker R, Uhle E, Bertalanffy H (2002) Combined intrathecal baclofen and morphine infusion for the treatment of spasticity related pain and central deafferentation pain. *Acta Neurochir* **79** (Suppl.), 75–6.
Gazzaniga MS (1998) The split brain revisited. *Sci Am* **279**, 50–5.
Gharabaghi A, Hellwig D, Rosahl SK, *et al.* (2005) Volumetric image guidance for motor cortex stimulation: integration of three-dimensional cortical anatomy and functional imaging. *Neurosurgery* **57** (ONS Suppl. 1), 114–20.
Gibson JC, White LE (1971) Denervation hyperpathia: a convulsive syndrome of the spinal cord responsive to carbamazepine therapy. *J Neurosurg* **35**, 287–90.
Gierthmuehlen J, Arning P, Binder A, *et al.* (2010) Influence of deep brain stimulation and levodopa on sensory signs in Parkinson's disease. *Mov Disord* **25**, 1195–202.
Gildenberg PL, Murthy KSK (1980) Influence of dorsal column stimulation upon human thalamic somatosensory-evoked potentials. *Appl Neurophysiol* **43**, 8–17.
Gimenez-Roldan S, Martin M (1981) Tabetic lightning pains: high-dosage intravenous penicillin versus carbamazepine therapy. *Eur Neurol* **20**, 424–8.
Gioia DF, Wallace PB, Fuste FJ, Greene M (1967) A stereotaxic method of surgery for the relief of intractable pain. *Int Surg* **48**, 409–16.
Glynn CJ, Jamous MA, Teddy PJ, Moore RA, Lloyd JW (1986) Role of spinal noradrenergic system in transmission of pain in patients with spinal cord injury. *Lancet* **ii**, 1249–50.
Glynn CJ, Jamous MA, Teddy PJ (1992) Cerebrospinal fluid kinetics of epidural clonidine in man. *Pain* **49**, 361–7.
Godlee F, Loder E (2010) Missing clinical trial data: setting the record straight. *BMJ* **341**, c5641.
Gonzales GR, Herskovitz S, Rosenblum M, *et al.* (1992) Central pain from cerebral abscess: thalamic syndrome in AIDS patients with toxoplasmosis. *Neurology* **42**, 1107–9.
Gonzales GR, Tuttle SL, Thaler HT, Manfredi PL (2003) Central pain in cancer patients. *J Pain* **4**, 351–4.
Gorecki JP, Nashold BS (1995) The Duke experience with the nucleus caudalis DREZ operation. *Acta Neurochir (Wien) Suppl* **64**, 128–31.
Gorecki J, Hirayama T, Dostrovsky JO, Tasker RR, Lenz FA (1989) Thalamic stimulation and recording in patients with deafferentation and central pain. *Stereotact Funct Neurosurg* **52**, 219–26.
Goss JR, Goins WF, Glorioso JC (2007) Gene therapy applications for the treatment of neuropathic pain. *Expert Rev Neurother* **7**, 487–506.
Goto T, Saitoh Y, Hashimoto N, *et al.* (2008) Diffusion tensor fiber tracking in patients with central post-stroke pain: correlation with efficacy of repetitive transcranial magnetic stimulation. *Pain* **140**, 509–18.
Graff-Radford NR, Damasio H, Yamada T, Eslinger PJ, Damasio AR (1985) Nonhaemorrhagic thalamic infarction: clinical, neuropsychological and electrophysiological findings in four anatomical groups defined by computerized tomography. *Brain* **108**, 485–516.
Green AL, Wang S, Stein JF, *et al.* (2009) Neural signatures in patients with neuropathic pain. *Neurology* **72**, 569–71.
Greenspan JD, Joy SE, McGillis SLB, Checkosky CM, Bolanowski SJ (1997) A longitudinal study of somesthetic perceptual disorders in an individual with a unilateral thalamic lesion. *Pain* **72**, 13–25.
Greenspan JD, Ohara S, Sarlani E, Lenz FA (2004) Allodynia in patients with post-stroke central pain (CPSP) studied by statistical quantitative sensory testing within individuals. *Pain* **109**, 357–66.

Greiff F (1883) Zur localisation der Hemichorea. *Arch Psychol Nervenkrankheit* **14**, 598.

Gross J, Schnitzler A, Timmermann L, Ploner M (2007) Gamma oscillations in human primary somatosensory cortex refelect pain perception. *PLOS Biol* **5**, e133, 1168–73.

Gubellini P, Salin P, Kerkerian-Le Goff L, Baunez C (2009) Deep brain stimulation in neurological diseases and experimental models: from molecule to complex behavior. *Progr Neurobiol* **89**, 79–123.

Guecer G, Niedermeyer E, Long MD (1978) Thalamic recordings in patients with chronic pain. *J Neurol* **219**, 47–61.

Guetti C, Angeletti C, Marinangeli F, *et al.* (2011) Transdermal buprenorphine for central neuropathic pain: clinical reports. *Pain Pract*, in press.

Guillaume J, De Seze S, Mazars G (1949) *Chirurgie cérébro-spinale de la douleur.* Paris: Presses Universitaires de France.

Gustin SM, Wrigley PJ, Gandevia SC, *et al.* (2008) Movement imagery increases pain in people with neuropathic pain following complete thoracic spinal cord injury. *Pain* **137**, 237–44.

Gustin SM, Wrigley PJ, Henderson LA, Siddall PJ (2010a) Brain circuitry underlying pain in response to imagined movement in people with spinal cord injury. *Pain* **148**, 438–45.

Gustin SM, Wrigley PJ, Siddall PJ, Henderson LA (2010b) Brain anatomy changes associated with persistent neuropathic pain following spinal cord injury. *Cereb Cortex* **20**, 1409–19.

Gybels J, Sweet WH (1989) Neurosurgical treatment of persistent pain. In: Gildenberg PL, ed., *Pain and Headache.* Basel: Karger.

Gybels J, Kupers R, Nuttin B (1993) Therapeutic stereotactic procedures on the thalamus for pain. *Acta Neurochir* **124**, 19–22.

Hachen HJ (1978) Psychological, neurophysiological and therapeutic aspects of chronic pain: preliminary results with transcutaneous electrical stimulation. *Paraplegia* **15**, 353–67.

Hagelberg NM, Peltoniemi MA, Saari TI, *et al.* (2010) Clarithromycin, a potent inhibitor of CYP3A, greatly increases exposure to oral S-ketamine. *Eur J Pain* **14**, 625–9.

Haider B, McCormick DA (2009) Rapid neocortical dynamics: cellular and network mechanisms. *Neuron* **62**, 171–89.

Haines DR, Gaines SP (1999) N-of-1 randomised controlled trials of oral ketamine in patients with chronic pain. *Pain* **83**, 283–7.

Hamamci N, Dursun E, Ural C, Cakci A (1996) Calcitonin treatment in reflex sympathetic dystrophy: a preliminary study. *Br J Clin Pract* **50**, 373–5.

Hamani C, Schwalb JM, Rezai AR, *et al.* (2006) Deep brain stimulation for chronic neuropathic pain: long-term outcome and the incidence of insertional effect. *Pain* **125**, 188–96.

Hamauchi S, Kyongsong K, Morimoto D, *et al.* (2010) [Ketamine treatment for severe neuropathic pain with cervical spondylotic myelopathy: a case report.] *No Shinkei Geka* **38**, 1121–5.

Hamby WB (1961) Reversible central pain. *Arch Neurol* **5**, 528–32.

Hampf G, Bowsher D (1989) Distigmine and amitriptyline in the treatment of chronic pain. *Anesth Progr* **36**, 58–62.

Hanagasi HA, Akat S, et al. (2010) Pain is common in Parkinson's disease. *Clin Neurol Neurosurg* **113**, 11–13.

Hanihara T, Takahashi T, Washizuka S, Ogihara T, Kobayashi M (2009) Delusion of oral parasitosis and thalamic pain syndrome. *Psychosomatics* **50**, 534–7.

Hankinson J (1962) Neurosurgical aspects of relief of pain at the cerebral level. In: Keele CA, Smith R, eds., *The Assessment of Pain in Man and Animals.* Edinburgh: Livingstone, pp. 135–43.

Hanley MA, Jensen MP, Ehde DM, *et al.* (2006) Clinically significant change in pain intensity rating in persons with spinal cord injury or amputation. *Clin J Pain* **22**, 25–31.

Hans G, Van Maldeghem K, Robert D (2007) Intravenous administration of adenosine (Adenocor) in the treatment of severe, therapy-resistant, central neuropathic pain. *Eur J Pain* **11**, S145 A326.

Hans GH, Robert DN, Van Maldeghem KN (2008) Treatment of an acute severe central neuropathic pain syndrome by topical application of lidocaine 5% patch: a case report. *Spinal Cord* **46**, 311–13.

Hansebout RR, Blight AR, Fawcett S, Reddy K (1993) 4-Aminopyridine in chronic spinal cord injury: a controlled, double-blind, cross-over study in eight patients. *J Neurotrauma* **10**, 1–18.

Hansen C, Hopf HC, Treede RD (1996) Paradoxical heat sensation in patients with multiple sclerosis: evidence for a supraspinal integration of temperature sensation. *Brain* **119**, 1729–36.

Harano K, Koga A, Takasaki M, Totoki T (1999) Intracisternal methylprednisolone administration for thalamic and other intractable pains. In: *9th World Congress on Pain, Book of Abstracts.* Seattle, WA: IASP Press, A234, p. 445.

Harden R, Brenman E, Saltz S, Houle T (2002) Topiramate in the management of spinal cord injury pain: a double-blind, randomised, placebo-controlled pilot study. *Progr Pain Res Manage* **23**, 393–407.

Harden R, Houle T, Tyburski M, *et al.* (2006) Levetiracetam in the management of neuropathic pain conditions: a double blind, randomized, crossover, placebo controlled pilot study using time series and hierarchical analysis. *J Pain* **7** (4 Suppl): S34, A727.

Hari AR, Wydenkeller S, Dokladal P, Halder P (2009) Enhanced recovery of human spinothalamic function is associated with central neuropathic pain after SCI. *Exp Neurol* **216**, 428–30.

Hariz MI, Bergenheim AT (1995) Thalamic stereotaxis for chronic pain: ablative lesion or stimulation? *Stereotact Funct Neurosurg* **64**, 47–55.

Harrington M, Bone I (1981) Spinal meningioma presenting as focal epilepsy: a case report. *Br Med J* **282**, 1984–5.

Harris AJ (1999) Cortical origin of pathological pain. *Lancet* **354**, 1464–6.

Harrop JS, Sharan A, Ratliff J (2006) Central cord injury: pathophysiology, management, and outcomes. *Spine J* **6**, 198S–206S.

Hassenbusch SJ, Stanton-Hicks M, Covington EC, Walsh JG, Guthrey DS (1995) Long-term intraspinal infusions of opioids in the treatment of neuropathic pain. *J Pain Symptom Manage* **10**, 527–43.

Hassler R (1960) Die zentrale Systeme des Schmerzes. *Acta Neurochir* **8**, 365–423.

Hassler R (1970) Dichotomy of facial pain conduction in the diencephalon. In: Hassler R, Walker AE, eds., *Trigeminal Neuralgia*. Philadelphia, PA: Saunders, pp. 123–38.

Hassler R, Riechert T (1959) Klinische und anatomische Befunde bei sterotaktischen Schmerz-operationen im Thalamus. *Arch Psychiat* **200**, 93–122.

Hatem SM, Attal N, Ducreux D, *et al.* (2010) Clinical, functional and structural determinants of central pain in syringomyelia. *Brain* **133**, 3409–22.

Hayashi M, Chernov MF, Taira T, *et al.* (2007) Outcome after pituitary radiosurgery for thalamic pain syndrome. *Int J Radiation Oncology Biol Phys* **69**, 852–7 (updates: Hayashi M, Taira T, Ochiai T, *et al.* (2005) Gamma knife surgery of the pituitary: new treatment for thalamic pain syndrome. *J Neurosurg* **102** (Suppl.), 38–41; and Hayashi *et al.* (2003) *Stereotact Funct Neurosurg* **81**, 75–83).

Hayes KC, Potter PJ, Wolfe DL, *et al.* (1994) 4-Aminopyridine-sensitive neurologic deficits in patients with spinal cord injury. *J Neurotrauma* **11**, 433–46.

Head H, Holmes G (1911) Researches into sensory disturbances from cerebral lesions. *Brain* **34**, 102–254.

Hécaen H, Talairach J, David M, Dell MB (1949) Coagulations limitées du thalamus dans les algies du syndrome thalamique. Résultats thérapeutiques et physiopathologiques. *Rev Neurol* **81**, 917–31.

Heilporn A (1978) Two therapeutic experiments on stubborn pain in spinal cord lesions: coupling melitracen-flupenthixol and the transcutaneous nerve stimulation. *Paraplegia* **15**, 368–72.

Heiskanen T, Hartel B, Dahl ML, Seppala T, Kalso E (2002) Analgesic effects of dextromethorphan and morphine in patients with chronic pain. *Pain* **96**, 261–7.

Heiss WD, Pawlik G, Herholz K, *et al.* (1986) Remote metabolic disturbances in lesions of brain stem and diencephalons: a PET study. In: Samii M, ed., *Surgery In and Around the Brain Stem and the Third Ventricle*. Berlin: Springer-Verlag, pp. 207–12.

Helfant MH, Leksell L, Strang RR (1965) Experiences with intractable pain treated by sterotaxic mesencephalotomy. *Acta Chir Scand* **129**, 573–80.

Helmchen C, Lindig M, Petersen D, Tronnier V (2002) Disappearance of central thalamic pain syndrome after contralateral parietal lobe lesion: implications for therapeutic brain stimulation. *Pain* **98**, 325–30.

Henderson JM, Boongird A, Rosenow JM, LaPresto E, Rezai AR (2004) Recovery of pain control by intensive reprogramming after loss of benefit from motor cortex stimulation for neuropathic pain. *Stereotact Funct Neurosurg* **82**, 207–13.

Henkel K, Bengel D (2005) Gekreuztes zentral-neuropatisches Schmerzsyndrom nach bakterieller Meningoenzephalitis. *Der Schmerz* **19**, 55–8.

Henriksen G, Willoch F (2008) Imaging of opioid receptors in the central nervous system. *Brain* **131**, 1171–96.

Herbert D, Tran Y, Craig A, *et al.* (2007) Altered brain wave activity in persons with chronic spinal cord injury. *Int J Neurosci* **117**, 1731–46.

Herman RM, D'Luzansky SC, Ippolito R (1992) Intrathecal baclofen suppresses central pain in patients with spinal lesions: a pilot study. *Clin J Pain* **8**, 338–45.

Herregodts P, Stadnik T, Deridder F, D'Haens J (1995) Cortical stimulation for central neuropathic pain: 3-D surface MRI for easy determination of the motor cortex. *Acta Neurochir (Wien) Suppl* **64**, 132–5.

Heutink M, Post MWM, Luthart P, *et al.* (2010) A multidisciplinary cognitive behavioural programme for coping with chronic neuropathic pain following spinal cord injury: the protocol of the CONECSI trial. *BMC Neurol* **10**, 96.

Hida K, Iwasaki Y, Imamura H, Abe H (1994) Postraumatic syringomyelia: its characteristics magnetic resonance imaging findings and surgical management. *Neurosurgery* **36**, 886–91.

Hiraga A, Sakakibara R, Mizobuchi K, *et al.* (2005) Putaminal hemorrhage disrupts thalamocortical projection to secondary somatosensory cortex: case report. *J Neurol Sci* **231**, 81–3.

Hirato M, Kawashima Y, Shibasaki T, Ohye C (1991) Pathophysiology of central (thalamic) pain: a possible role of the intralaminar nuclei in superficial pain. *Acta Neurochir (Wien) Suppl* **52**, 133–6.

Hirato M, Horikoshi S, Kawashima Y, *et al.* (1993) The possible role of the cerebral cortex adjacent to the central sulcus for the genesis of central (thalamic) pain: a metabolic study. *Acta Neurochir (Wien) Suppl* **58**, 141–4.

Hirato M, Ohye C, Shibazaki T, *et al.* (1995) Gamma knife thalamotomy for the treatment of functional disorders. *Stereotact Funct Neurosurg* **64** (Suppl 1), 164–71.

Hirayama A, Saitoh Y, Kishima H, *et al.* (2006) Reduction of intractable deafferentation pain by navigation-guided repetitive transcranial magnetic stimulation of the primary motor cortex. *Pain* **122**, 22–7.

Hirayama T, Dostrovsky JO, Gorecki J, Tasker RR, Lenz FA (1989) Recordings of abnormal activity in patients with deafferentation and central pain. *Stereotact Funct Neurosurg* **52**, 120–6.

Hitchcock ER, Teixeira MJ (1981) A comparison of results from center-median and basal thalamotomies for pain. *Surg Neurol* **15**, 341–51.

Hoffmann W (1933) Thalamussyndrom auf Grund einer Kleinen Laesion. *J Psychol Neurol* **45**, 362–74.

Holden C (2004) Imaging studies show how brain thinks about pain. *Science* **303**, 1121.

Holland CT, Charles JA, Smith SH, Cortaville PE (2000) Hemihyperaesthesia and hyperresponsiveness resembling central pain syndrome in a dog with a forebrain oligodendroglioma. *Aust Vet J* **78**, 676–80.

Holmes G (1919) Pain of central origin. In Osler W, ed., *Contributions to Medical and Biological Research*. New York, NY: Paul B Hoeber, pp. 235–46.

Holsheimer J, Lefaucheur JP, Buitenweg JR, *et al.* (2007) The role of intra-operative motor evoked potentials in the optimization of chronic cortical stimulation for the treatment of neuropathic pain. *Clin Neurophysiol* **118**, 2287–96.

Honey CR, Stoessl J, Tsui JK, Schulzer M, Calne DB (1999) Unilateral pallidotomy for reduction of parkinsonian pain. *J Neurosurg* **91**, 198–201.

Hong JH, Bai DS, Jeong JY, *et al.* (2010) Injury of the spino-thalamo-cortical pathway is necessary for central post-stroke pain. *Eur Neurol* **64**, 163–8.

Hoogenraad TU, Ramos LMP, Van Gijn J (1994) Visually induced central pain and arm withdrawal after right parietal lobe infarction. *J Neurol Neurosurg Psychiatry* **57**, 850–2.

Hopfield JJ (1982) Neural networks and physical systems with emergent collective computational abilities. *Proc Natl Acad Sci U S A* **81**, 3088–92.

Horrax G (1946) Experiences with cortical excisions for the relief of intractable pain in the extremities. *Surgery* **20**, 593–602.

Hosobuchi Y (1986) Subcortical electrical stimulation for control of intractable pain in humans. Report of 122 cases (1970–1984). *J Neurosurg* **64**, 543–53.

Hosobuchi Y (1990) Alpha-methyldopa blocks the analgesic effect of sensory thalamic stimulation in humans. *Pain* **5** (Suppl), S274.

Hosobuchi Y (1993) Motor cortical stimulation for control of central deafferentation pain. In: Devinsky O, Beric A, Dogari M, eds., *Electrical and Magnetic Stimulation of the Brain and Spinal Cord*. New York, NY: Raven Press, pp. 215–17.

Hosomi K, Saitoh Y, Kishima H, *et al.* (2008) Electrical stimulation of primary motor cortex within central sulcus for intractable neuropathic pain. *Clin Neurophysiol* **119**, 993–1001.

Houtchens MK, Richert JR, Sami A, Rose JW (1997) Open label gabapentin treatment for pain in multiple sclerosis. *Mult Scler* **3**, 250–3.

Hua SE, Garonzik IM, Lee JI, Lenz FA (2000) Microelectrode studies of normal organization and plasticity of human somatosensory thalamus. *J Clin Neurophysiol* **17**, 559–74.

Hughes JT (1976) Diseases of the spine and spinal cord. In: Blackwood W, Corsellis J, eds., *Greenfield's Neuropathology*. London: Arnold, pp. 652–87.

Hunt WE, Goodman JH, Bingham WG (1975) Stimulation of the dorsal spinal cord for treatment of intractable pain: a preliminary report. *Surg Neurol* **4**, 153–6.

Huntoon MA, Hurdle MFB, Marsh RW, Reeves RK (2004) Intrinsic spinal cord catheter placement: implications of new intractable pain in a patient with a spinal cord injury. *Anesth Analg* **99**, 1763–5.

Hutchison WD, Davis KD, Lozano AM, Tasker RR, Dostrovsky JO (1999) Pain-related neurons in the human cingulate cortex. *Nat Neurosci* **2**, 403–5.

Iacono RP, Nashold BS (1982) Mental and behavioral effects of brain stem and hypothalamic stimulation in man. *Human Neurobiol* **1**, 273–9.

Iannetti GD, Truini A, Romaniello A, *et al.* (2003) Evidence of a specific spinal pathway for the sense of warmth in humans. *J Neurophysiol* **89**, 562–70.

Ikeda A, Ohara S, Matsumoto R, *et al.* (2008) Role of primary somatosensory corticies in generating inhibitory motor response in humans. *Brain* **123**, 1710–21.

Ikei Y, Uno T (1987) Cervical epidural stimulation for the patient suffering from thalamic pain. IASP Congress, S8.

Inui K, Wang X, Qiu Y, *et al.* (2003) Pain processing within the primary somatosensory cortex in humans. *Eur J Neurosci* **18**, 2859–66.

Ioannides AA (2007) Dynamic functional connectivity. *Curr Opin Neurobiol* **17**, 161–70.

Ioannides AA, Kostopoulos GK, Laskaris NA, *et al.* (2002) Timing and connectivity in the human somatosensory cortex from single trial mass electrical activity. *Hum Brain Mapp* **15**, 231–46.

Ioannidis JPA (2005) Why most published research findings are false. *Plos Med* **2**, e124, 696–701.

Iranami H, Yamazaki A, Hatano Y (2006) Tramadol challenge for relief of intractable central poststroke pain. *Mayo Clin Proc* **81**, 566–9.

Irlbacher K, Kuhnert J, Roericht S, Meyer BU, Brandt SA. (2006) Zentrale und periphere Deafferenzierungsschmerzen: Therapie mit der repetitiven transkraniellen Magnetstimulation? *Nervenarzt* **77**, 1196–203.

Irlbacher K, Brocke J, Mechow JV, Brandt SA (2007) Effects of GABA A and GABA B agonists on interhemispheric inhibition in man. *Clin Neurophysiol* **118**, 308–16.

Isnard J, Magnin M, Jung J, Mauguière F, Garcia-Larrea L, (2011) Does the insula tell our brain that we are in pain? *Pain* **152**, 946–51.

Ito M, Kuroda S, Takano K, *et al.* (2006) [Motor cortex stimulation for post-stroke pain using neuronavigation and evoked potentials: report of 3 cases] *No Shinkei Geka* **34**, 919–34.

Iwamura Y, Iriki A, Tanaka M (1994) Bilateral hand representation in the postcentral somatosensory cortex. *Nature* **369**, 554–6.

Izhikevich EM (2007) *Dynamical Systems in Neuroscience: the Geometry of Excitability and Bursting*. Cambridge, MA: MIT Press.

Jadad AR, Carroll D, Glynn CJ, McQuay HJ (1995) Intravenous regional sympathetic blockade for pain relief in reflex sympathetic dystrophy: a systematic review and a randomized, double-blind crossover study. *J Pain Symptom Manage* **10**, 13–20.

Jagannathan J, Sanghvi NT, Crum LA, *et al.* (2009) High-intensity focused ultrasound surgery of the brain: Part 1-

A historical perspective with modern applications. *Neurosurgery* **64**, 201–11.

Jain KK (2008) Cell therapy for pain. *Exp Opin Biol Ther* **8**, 1847–53.

Jasmin L, Tien D, Janni G, Ohara PT (2003) Is noradrenaline a significant factor in the analgesic effect of antidepressants? *Pain* **106**, 3–8.

Jeanmonod D, Magnin M, Morel A (1996) Low-threshold calcium spike bursts in the human thalamus. Common physiopathology for sensory, motor and limbic positive symptoms. *Brain* **119**, 363–75.

Jeanmonod D, Magnin M, Morel A, Siegemund M (2001) Surgical control of the human thalamocortical dysrhythmia: I Central lateral thalamotomy in neurogenic pain. *Thalam Rel Syst* **1**, 71–9.

Jefferson A (1983) Cordectomy for intractable pain in paraplegia. In: Lipton S, Miles J, eds., *Persistent Pain: Modern Methods for Treatment*, Vol. 4. London: Grune and Stratton, pp. 115–32.

Jenkins K, Kaplan SE, Leahy LF, *et al.* (2002) Oxcarbazepine in central neuropathic pain with allodynia following spinal cord injury. *J Pain* **3**, 10.

Jensen TS, Gottrup H, Johansen P, *et al.* (1999) Positron emission tomography (PET) and psychophysical studies in post-stroke pain. In: *9th World Congress on Pain, Book of Abstracts.* Seattle, WA: IASP Press, A77.

Jensen TS, Gottrup H, Kristensen AD, Andersen G, Vestergaard K (2002) Cold sensation in central post-stroke pain. In: *10th World Congress on Pain, Book of Abstracts.* Seattle, WA: IASP Press, A95–P91.

Jermakowicz WJ, Casagrande VA (2007) Neural networks a century after Cajal. *Brain Res Rev* **55**, 264–84.

Jetzer AK, Morel A, Magnin M, Jeanmonod D (2009) Cross-modal plasticity in the human thalamus: evidence from intraoperative macrostimulations. *Neurosci* **164**, 1867–75.

Jiang B, Wang W, Chen H, *et al.* (2006) Incidence and trends of stroke and its subtypes in China. *Stroke* **37**, 63.

Jiang CJ, Tan YC, Yang YJ, *et al.* (2009) [Sequential drugs treatment for central pain following spinal cord injury] *Zhongguo Gu Shang* **22**, 458–9.

Jinno S (2009) Structural organization of long range GABAergic projection system in the hippocampus. *Front Neurosci* **3**, article 13.

Johnson RE, Kanigsberg ND, Jimenez CL (2000) Localized pruritus: a presenting symptom of a spinal cord tumor in a child with features of neurofibromatosis. *J Am Acad Dermatol* **43**, 958–61.

Johnson S, Summers J, Pridmore S (2006) Changes to somatosensory detection and pain thresholds following high frequency repetitive TMS of the motor cortex in individuals suffering from chronic pain. *Pain* **123**, 187–92.

Jones AKP, Watabe H, Cunningham VJ, Jones T (2004) Cerebral decreases in opioid receptor binding in patients with central neuropathic pain measured by [11C] diprenorphine binding and PET. *Eur J Pain* **8**, 479–85.

Jones CL, Ward J, Critchley HD (2010) The neuropsychological impact of insular cortex lesions. *J Neurol Neurosurg Psychiatry* **81**, 611–18.

Jones EG (2007) *The Thalamus*, 2nd edn. Cambridge: Cambridge University Press.

Jönsson AC, Lindgren I, Hallström B, Norrving B, Lindgren A (2006) Prevalence and intensity of pain after stroke: a population based study focusing on patients' perspectives. *J Neurol Neurosurg Psychiatry* **77**, 590–5.

Jürgens TP, Leone M, Proietti-Cecchini A, *et al.* (2009) Hypothalamic deep-brain stimulation modulates thermal sensitivity and pain thresholds in cluster headache. *Pain* **146**, 84–90.

Kabirov EI, Staroselseva NG (2002) Transcutaneous electrostimulation in the treatment of dysesthetic pain in syringomyelia. In: *10th World Congress on Pain, Book of Abstracts.* Seattle, WA: IASP Press, A1656–P204.

Kakulas BA, Smith E, Gaekwad U, Kaeln C, Jacobsen PF (1990) The neuropathology of pain and abnormal sensation in human spinal cord injury derived from the clinicopathological data base of the Royal Perth Hospital. In: Dimitrijevic MR, Wall PD, Lindblom U, eds., *Recent Achievements in Restorative Neurology: 3. Altered Sensation and Pain.* Basel: Karger

Kalita J, Kumar B, Misra UK, Pradhan PK (2011) Central post stroke pain: clinical, MRI, and SPECT correlation. *Pain Med* **12**, 282–8.

Kalman S, Österberg A, Sorensen J, Boivie J, Bertler A (2002) Morphine responsiveness in a group of well-defined multiple sclerosis patients: a study with i.v. morphine. *Eur J Pain* **6**, 69–80.

Kameda W, Kawanami T, Kurita K, *et al.* for the Study Group of the Association of Cerebrovascular Disease in Tohoku (2004) Lateral and medial medullary infarction. A comparative analysis of 214 patients. *Stroke* **35**, 694–9.

Kameyama M (1976–77) Vascular lesions of the thalamus on the dominant and nondominant side. *Appl Neurophysiol* **39**, 171–7.

Kanwisher N (2010) Functional specificity in the human brain: a window into the functional architecture of the mind. *Proc Natl Acad Sci U S A* **107**, 11163–70.

Karst M, Salim K, Burstein S, *et al.* (2003) Analgesic effect of the synthetic cannabinoid CT-3 on chronic neuropathic pain. A randomized controlled trial. *JAMA* **290**, 1757–62.

Karussis D, Karageorgiou C, Vaknin-Dembinsky A, *et al.* (2010) Safety and immunological effects of mesenchymal stem cell transplantation in patients with multiple sclerosis and amyotrophic lateral sclerosis. *Arch Neurol* **67**, 1187–94.

Kasai Y, Kawakita E, Morishita K, Uchida A (2008) Cordectomy for post-traumatic syringomyelia. *Acta Neurochir (Wien)* **150**, 83–6.

Kassirer JP (2005) *On the Take. How America's Complicity With Big Business Can Endanger Your Health.* NewYork, NY: Oxford University Press.

Kastrup A, Baudewig J, Schnaudigek S, *et al.* (2008) Behavioral correlates of negative BOLD signal changes in

the primary somatosensory cortex. *Neuroimage* **41**, 1364–71.
Kamano S (2003) Author's experience of lateral medullary infarction – thermal perception and muscle allodynia. *Pain* **104**, 49–53.
Kanda M, Nagamine T, Ikeda A, *et al.* (2000) Primary somatosensory cortex is actively involved in pain processing in human. *Brain Res* **853**, 282–9.
Kang BS, Shin HI, Bang MS (2009) Effect of repetitive transcranial magnetic stimulation over the hand motor cortical area on central pain after spinal cord injury. *Arch Phys Med Rehabil* **90**, 1766–71.
Kapadia NP, Harden N (2000) Gabapentin for chronic pain in spinal cord injury: a case report. *Arch Phys Med Rehabil* **81**, 1439–41.
Karakulova Y, Novikova N (2010) Central neuropathic pain, psychovegetative status and serum serotonin level in syringomyelia patients. *Eur J Pain Suppl* **4**, 102.
Katayama Y, Tsubokawa T, Yamamoto T (1994) Chronic motor cortex stimulation for central deafferentation pain: experience with bulbar pain secondary to Wallenberg syndrome. *Stereotact Funct Neurosurg* **62**, 295–9.
Katayama Y, Fukaya C, Yamamoto T (1998) Poststroke pain control by chronic motor cortex stimulation: neurological characteristics predicting a favorable response. *J Neurosurg* **89**, 585–91.
Katayama Y, Yamamoto T, Kobayashi K, *et al.* (2001) Motor cortex stimulation for post-stroke pain: comparison of spinal cord and thalamic stimulation. *Stereotact Funct Neurosurg* **77**, 183–6.
Kavak A, Dosoglu M (2002) Can a spinal cord tumor cause brachioradial pruritus? *J Am Acad Dermatol* **46**, 437–40.
Kawahara N, Sato K, Muraki M, *et al.* (1986) CT classification of small thalamic hemorrhages and their clinical implications. *Neurology* **36**, 165–72.
Kawamura M, Hirayama K, Shinohara Y, Watanabe Y, Sugishita M (1987) Alloaesthesia. *Brain* **110**, 225–36.
Kayser C (2010) The multisensory nature of unisensory cortices: a puzzle continued. *Neuron* **67**, 178–80.
Keep MF, Mastrofrancesco L, Craig AD, Ashby LS (2006) Gamma knife surgery targeting the centromedian nucleus of the thalamus for the palliative management of thalamic pain: durable response in stroke-induced thalamic pain syndrome. *J Neurosurg* **105** (Suppl), 222–8.
Kennemore DE. (1977) Percutaneous radiofrequency spinal rhizotomy for the treatment of pain. Presented at the 45th Annual Meeting of the American Association of Neurological Sugeons.
Kern KU, Kohl M, Kiefer RT (2010) Lidocain-Pflaster zur Therapie neuropatischer und nichtneuropatischer Schmerzen. Klinische Fallstudie an 87 patienten. *Nervenarzt.* **376**, 2000–8.
Khalsa SS, Rudrauf D, Feinstein JS, Tranel D (2009) The pathways of interoceptive awareness. *Nature Neuroscience* **12**, 1494–6.
Khedr EM, Korb L, Kamel NF, *et al.* (2005) Long-lasting antalgic effects of daily sessions of repetitive transcranial magnetic stimulation in central and peripheral neuropathic pain. *J Neurol Neurosurg Psychiatry* **76**, 833–8.
Kim D, Park D, Choi S, *et al.* (2003) Thalamic control of visceral nociception mediated by T-type Ca^{2+} channels. *Science* **302**, 117–19.
Kim HJ, Paek SH, Kim JY, *et al.* (2008) Chronic subthalamic deep brain stimulation improves pain in Parkinson disease. *J Neurol* **255**, 1889–94.
Kim JH, Greenspan JD, Coghill RC, Ohara S, Lenz FA (2007) Lesions limited to the human thalamic principal somatosensory nucleus (ventral caudal) are associated with loss of cold sensations and central pain. *J Neurosci* **27**, 4995–5004.
Kim JK, Hong SH, Lee JK (2010) High-level cervical spinal cord stimulation used to treat intractable pain arising from transverse myelitis caused by schistosomiasis. *J Korean Neurosurg Soc* **47**, 151–4.
Kim JS (1996) Bilateral perioral sensory symptom after unilateral stroke: does it have a localizing value? *J Neurol Sci* **140**, 123–8.
Kim JS (1998) Delayed-onset ipsilateral sensory symptoms in patients with central post-stroke pain. *Eur Neurol* **40**, 201–6.
Kim JS (1999) Aggravation of poststroke sensory symptoms after a second stroke on the opposite side. *Eur Neurol* **42**, 200–4.
Kim JS (2003) Central post-stroke pain or paresthesia in lenticulocapsular hemorrhages. *Neurology* **61**, 679–82.
Kim JS (2007a) Patterns of sensory abnormality in cortical stroke: evidence for a dichotomized sensory system. *Neurology* **68**, 174–80.
Kim JS (2007b) Medial medullary infarct aggravates central poststroke pain caused by previous lateral medullary infarct. *Eur Neurol* **58**, 41–3.
Kim JS, Bae YH (1997) Pure or predominant sensory stroke due to brain stem lesion. *Stroke* **28**, 1761–4.
Kim JS, Choi-Kwon S (1999) Sensory sequelae of medullary infarction: differences between lateral and medial medullary syndrome. *Stroke* **30**, 2697–703.
Kim JS, Bashford G, Murphy K, *et al.* (2011) Safety and efficacy of pregabalin in patients with central post-stroke pain. *Pain* **152**, 1018–23.
Kim LJ, Klopfenstein JD, Zabramski JM, Sonntag VK, Spetzler RF (2006) Analysis of pain resolution after surgical resection of intramedullary spinal cord cavernous malformations. *Neurosurgery* **58**, 106–11.
Kim SH, Tasker RR, Oh MY (2001) Spinal cord stimulation for nonspecific limb pain versus neuropathic pain and spontaneous versus evoked pain. *Neurosurgery* **48**, 1056–65.
Kim SH, Kim SH, Kim SW, Jang SH (2007) Sacral nerve and spinal cord stimulation for intractable neuropathic pain caused by spinal cord infarction. *Neuromodulation* **10**, 369–72.
Kimyai-Asadi A, Nousari HC, Kimyai-Asadi T, Dilani F (1999) Poststroke pruritus. *Stroke* **30**, 692.
King CA, Huff FJ, Jorizzo JL (1982) Unilateral neurogenic pruritus: paroxysmal itching associated with central nervous system lesions. *Ann Intern Med* **97**, 222–3.

King RB (1977) Anterior commissurotomy for intractable pain. *J Neurosurg* **47**, 7–11.

Kinnier-Wilson SA (1927) Dysesthesias and their neural correlates. *Brain* **50**, 428–61.

Kinsella LJ, Carney-Godley, Feldmann E (1992) Lichen simplex chronicus as the initial manifestation of intramedullary neoplasm and syringomyelia. *Neurosurgery* **30**, 418–21.

Kiriakopoulos ET, Tasker RR, Nicosia S, Wood ML, Mikulis DJ (1997) Functional magnetic resonance imaging: a potential tool for the evaluation of spinal cord stimulation. Technical case report. *Neurosurgery* **41**, 501–4.

Kirsch I (2009) *The Emperor's New Drugs: Exploding the Antidepressant Myth*. London: Random House.

Kishi M, Sakakibara R, Nagao T, Terada H, Ogawa E (2009) Thalamic infarction disrupts spinothalamocortical projection to the mid-cingulate cortex and supplementary motor area. *J Neurol Sci* **281**, 104–7.

Kishima H, Saitoh Y, Osaki Y, *et al.* (2007) Motor cortex stimulation in patients with deafferentation pain: activation of the posterior insula and thalamus. *J Neurosurg* **107**, 43–8.

Kishima H, Saitoh Y, Oshino S, *et al.* (2010) Modulation of neuronal activity after spinal cord stimulation for neuropathic pain: H2 15O PET study. *Neuroimage* **49**, 2564–9.

Kishk NA, Gabr H, Hamdy S, *et al.* (2010) Case control series of intrathecal autologous bone marrow mesenchymal stem cell therapy for chronic spinal cord injury. *Neurorehabil Neural Repair* **24**, 702–8.

Kiss ZHT, Dostrovsky JO, Tasker RR (1994) Plasticity in human somatosensory thalamus as a result of deafferentation. *Stereotact Funct Neurosurg* **62**, 153–63.

Kiss ZHT, Davis KD, Tasker RR, Lozano AM, Dostrovsky JO (1995) Human thalamic neurons develop novel receptive fields within minutes of deafferentation. *J Neurosurg* **82**, 373A (A841).

Klega A, Eberle T, Buchholz HG, *et al.* (2010) Central opioidergic neurotransmission in complex regional pain syndrome. *Neurology* **75**, 129–36.

Klit H, Finnerup NB, Andersen G, Jensen TS (2011) Central poststroke pain: a population-based study. *Pain* **152**, 818–24.

Knecht S, Henningsen H, Elbert T, *et al.* (1996) Reorganizational and perceptional changes after amputation. *Brain* **119**, 1214–19.

Knecht S, Soros P, Guertler S, *et al.* (1998) Phantom sensations following acute pain. *Pain* **77**, 209–13.

Kobayashi K, Winberry J, Liu CC, Treede RD, Lenz FA (2009) A painful cutaneous laser stimulus evokes responses from single neurons in the human thalamic principal somatic sensory nucleus ventral caudal (Vc). *J Neurophysiol* **101**, 2210–17.

Kohlhoff H, Lorenz J, Scharein E, *et al.* (1999) Cortical disorganization in patients with post-stroke pain studied by MEG. In: *9th World Congress on Pain, Book of Abstracts*. Seattle, WA: IASP Press, A27.

Kong J, Loggia ML, Zyloney C, *et al.* (2010) Exploring the brain in pain: activations, deactivations and their relation. *Pain* **148**, 257–67.

Kong KH, Woon VC, Yang SY (2004) Prevalence of chronic pain and its impact on health-related quality of life in stroke survivors. *Arch Phys Med Rehabil* **85**, 35–40.

Koppel BS (1986) Amitriptyline in thalamic pain. *South Med J* **79**, 759–61.

Koszewski W, Jarosz J, Pernak-De Gast J (2003) Stereotactic posterior capsulo-lentiform deafferentation as an effective treatment in central post-stroke pain. A new surgical method for intractable central pain control? *Pain Clin* **15**, 115–23.

Koulousakis A, Kuchta J, Bayarassou A, Sturm V (2007) Intrathecal opioids for intractable pain syndromes. *Acta Neurochir (Wien) Suppl* **97**, 45–8.

Koyama T, Arakawa Y, Shibata M, Mashimo T, Yoshiya I (1998) Effect of barbiturate on central pain: difference between intravenous administration and oral administration. *Clin J Pain* **14**, 86–8.

Kraemer HH, Seddigh S, Moseley GL, Birklein F (2008a) Dysinchiria is not a common feature of neuropathic pain. *Eur J Pain* **12**, 128–31.

Kraemer HH, Stenner C, Seddigh S, *et al.* (2008b) Illusion of pain: pre-existing knowledge determines brain activation of "imagined allodynia". *J Pain* **9**, 543–51.

Krainick JU, Thoden U (1989) Spinal cord stimulation. In: Wall PD, Melzack R, eds., *Textbook of Pain*, 2nd edn. Edinburgh: Churchill-Livingstone, pp. 920–4.

Kramer KM, Levine AM (1997) Posttraumatic syringomyelia. *Clin Orthoped Rel Res* **334**, 190–9.

Krauss JK, Pohle T, Weigel R, Kalbarzcyk A (2001) Somatosensory thalamic stimulation versus center-median-parafascicular complex stimulation in 11 patients with neuropathic pain. *Stereotact Funct Neurosurg* **77**, 194.

Krummenacher P, Candia V, Folkers G, Schedlowski M, Schönbächler G (2010) Prefrontal cortex modulates placebo analgesia. *Pain* **148**, 368–74.

Kubina B, Ristic D, Weber J, *et al.* (2010) Bilateral brainstem activation by thermal stimulation of the face in healthy volunteers. *J Neurol* **257**, 271–80.

Kudo T, Yoshii N, Shimizu S, *et al.* (1968) Sterotaxic thalamotomy for pain relief. *Tohoku J Exp Med* **96**, 219–34.

Kueper M, Kollia K, Kastrup O (2008) Isolated spinothalamic sensory impairment of the left arm following contralateral medullary infarction: a case report. *Eur Neurol* **59**, 216–18.

Kumagai Y, Taga K, Hokari T, *et al.* (1990) The effect of DREZ (dorsal root entry zone) lesions on intractable pain in patients with spinal cord injury. *Masui* **39**, 632–8.

Kumar K, Toth C, Nath RK (1997) Deep brain stimulation for intractable pain: a 15-year experience. *Neurosurgery* **40**, 736–47 (updates *Can J Surg* 1985, **28**, 20–2; *Neurosurgery* 1980, **26**, 774–82).

Kumar K, Hunter G, Demeria D (2006) Spinal cord stimulation in treatment of chronic benign pain: challenges in treatment planning and present status, a 22-year experience. *Neurosurgery* **58**, 481–96 (updates: *J Neurosurg* 1991, **75**, 402–7; *Surg Neurol* 1998, **50**, 110–21).

Kumral E, Celebisoy N (1996) Visually evoked hyperpathia due to thalamic hemorrhage: a variant of Dejerine–Roussy syndrome. *Stroke* **27**, 774–5.

Kumral E, Kocaer T, Ertübey N, Kumral K (1995) Thalamic hemorrhage: a prospective study of 100 patients. *Stroke* **26**, 964–70.

Kumral E, Evyapan D, Balkir K, Kutluhan S (2001) Bilateral thalamic infarction: clinical, etiological and MRI correlates. *Acta Neurol Scand* **103**, 35–42.

Kuong PG (1984) [*Practical Neuroanatomy and Neurological Syndromes*]. Beijing: People's Army Medical Publishing.

Kupers R, Konings H, Adriaensen H, Gybels JM (1991) Morphine differentially affects the sensory and affective pain ratings in a neurogenic and idiopathic forms of pain. *Pain* **47**, 5–12.

Kupers R, Frokjaer VG, Naert A, *et al.* (2009a) A PET [18F] altanserin study of 5-HT2A receptor binding in the human brain and responses to painful heat stimulation. *Neuroimage* **44**, 1001–7.

Kupers R, Danielsen ER, Kehlet H, Christensen R, Thomsen C (2009b) Painful tonic heat stimulation induces GABA accumulation in the prefrontal cortex in man. *Pain* **142**, 89–93.

Kupers R, Frokjaer VG, Erritzoe D, *et al.* (2011) Serotonin transporter binding in the hypothalamus correlates negatively with tonic heat pain ratings in healthy subjects: A [11C]DASB PET study. *Neuroimage* **54**, 1336–43.

Kuptniratsaikul V, Kovindha A, Suethanapornkul S, Manimmanakorn N, Archongka Y (2009) Complications during the rehabilitation period in Thai patients with stroke: a multicenter prospective study. *Am J Phys Med Rehabil* **88**, 92–9.

Kuroda R, Yamada Y, Kondo S, *et al.* (2000) Electrical stimulation of the second somatosensory cortex for intractable pain: a case report and experimental study. *Stereotact Funct Neurosurg* **74**, 226.

Kvarnstrom A, Karlsten R, Quiding H, Gordh T (2004) The analgesic effect of intravenous ketamine and lidocaine on pain after spinal cord injury. *Acta Anaesthesiol Scand* **48**, 498–506.

Lahuerta J, Bowsher D, Lipton S, Buxton PH (1994) Percutaneous cervical cordotomy: a review of 181 operations on 146 patients with a sudy on the location of "pain fibers" in the C-2 spinal cord segment of 29 cases. *J Neurosurg* **80**, 975–85.

Laitinen LV (1977) Anterior pulvinotomy in the treatment of intractable pain. In: Sweet WH, Obrador S, Martin-Rodriguez JG, eds., *Neurosurgical Treatment in Psychiatry, Pain, and Epilepsy*. Baltimore, MD: University Park Press, pp. 669–72.

Laitinen LV (1988a) Mesencephalotomy and thalamotomy for chronic pain. In: Lunsford LD, ed., *Modern Sterotactic Neurosurgery*. Boston, MA: Martinus Nijhoff, pp. 269–77.

Laitinen LV (1988b) Psychosurgery today. *Acta Neurochir (Wien) Suppl* **44**, 158–62.

Lampl C, Yazdi K, Roeper C (2002) Amitriptyline in the prophylaxis of central post-stroke pain. Preliminary results of 39 patients in a placebo-controlled, long-term study. *Stroke* **33**, 3030–2.

Lampl C, Schweiger C, Haider B, Lechner A (2010) Pregabalin as mono- or add-on therapy for patients with refractory chronic neuropathic pain: a post-marketing prescription-event monitoring study. *J Neurol* **257**, 1265–73.

Lampl Y, Gilad R, Eshel Y, Sarova-Pinhas I (1995) Neurological and functional outcome in patients with supratentorial hemorrhages: a prospective study. *Stroke* **26**, 2249–53.

Lance JW (1996) The red ear syndrome. *Neurology* **47**, 617–20.

Landefeld CS, Steinman MA (2009) The Neurontin legacy: marketing through misinformation and manipulation. *N Engl J Med* **360**, 103–6.

Landerholm AH, Hansson PT (2011) Mechanisms of dynamic mechanical allodynia and dysesthesia in patients with peripheral and central neuropathic pain. *Eur J Pain*, in press.

Langworthy OR, Fox HM (1937) Thalamic syndrome. Syndrome of the posterior cerebral artery: a review. *Arch Int Med* **60**, 203–24.

Larson SJ, Sances A, Riegel DH, *et al.* (1974) Neurophysiological effects of dorsal column stimulation in man and monkey. *J Neurosurg* **41**, 217–23.

Lascelles BDX, Flecknell PA (2010) Do animal models tell us about human pain? *Pain Clin Updates* **18**, issue 5.

Laspiur RD (1956) Estereotaxis. En relacion a dos casos operados de sindrome talamico vascular. *Arch Inst Neurochir* **97**, 113.

Laterre EC, De Volder AG, Goffinet AM (1988) Brain glucose metabolism in thalamic syndrome. *J Neurol Neurosurg Psychiatry* **51**, 427–8.

Laurent B, Peyron R, Garcia-Larrea L, *et al.* (1999) Inside the mechanisms of motor cortex stimulation-induced analgesia. In: *9th World Congress on Pain, Book of Abstracts*. Seattle, WA: IASP Press, A187.

Law J (2006) *Big Pharma: How the World's Biggest Drug Companies Control Illness*. New York, NY: Basic Books.

Lawrence JM, Stroman PW, Kollias SS (2008) Functional magnetic resonance imaging of the human spinal cord during vibration stimulation of different dermatomes. *Neuroradiology* **50**, 273–80.

Laxton AW, Perrin RG (2006) Cordectomy for the treatment of posttraumatic syringomyelia. Report of four cases and review of the literature. *J Neurosurg Spine* **4**, 174–8.

Lazorthes Y (1979) *European Study on Deep Brain Stimulation. Resumé, Third European Workshop on Electrical Neurostimulation*. Paris: Medtronic.

Lazorthes Y, Siegfried J, Verdie JC, Casaux J (1995) La stimulation médullaire chronique dans le traitement des douleurs neurogènes. Etude coopèrative et rètrospective sur 20 ans de suivi. *Neurochirurgie* **41**, 73–88.

Le Beau J, Choppy M, Gaches J, Rosier M (1954) *Psychochirurgie et fonctions mentales: techniques, résultats, applications physiologiques*. Paris: Masson.

Le Chapelain L, Beis JM, Paysant J, André JM (2001) Vestibular caloric stimulation evokes phantom limb illusions in patients with paraplegia. *Spinal Cord* **39**, 85–7.

Lee MG, Choi SS, Lee MK, *et al.* (2009) Thoracic spinal cord stimulation for neuropathic pain after spinal meningioma removal: a case report. *Clin J Pain* **25**, 167–9.

Lee MS, Choi IS, Chung TS (1989) Thalamic syndrome and cortical hypoperfusion on technetium-99m HM-PAO brain SPECT. *Yonsei Med J* **30**, 151–7.

Lefaucheur JP (2008) Use of repetitive transcranial magnetic stimulation in pain relief. *Expert Rev Neurother* **8**, 799–808.

Lefaucheur JP, Drouot X, Keravel Y, Nguyen JR (2001a) Pain relief induced by repetitive transcranial magnetic stimulation of precentral cortex. *Neuroreport* **12**, 2963–5.

Lefaucheur JP, Drouot X, Nguyen JP (2001b) Interventional neurophysiology for pain control: duration of pain relief following repetitive transcranial magnetic stimulation of the motor cortex. *Neurophysiol Clin* **31**, 247–52.

Lefaucheur JP, Drouot X, Menard-Lefaucheur L, *et al.* (2004a) Neurogenic pain relief by repetitive transcranial magnetic cortical stimulation depends on the origin and the site of pain. *J Neurol Neurosurg Psychiatry* **75**, 612–16.

Lefaucheur JP, Drouot X, Menard-Lefaucheur I, Nguyen JP (2004b) Neuropathic pain controlled for more than a year by monthly sessions of repetitive transcranial magnetic cortical stimulation. *Neurophysiol Clin* **34**, 91–5.

Lefaucheur JP, Drouot X, Menard-Lefaucheur I, Keravel Y, Nguyen JP (2006a) Motor cortex rTMS restores defective intracortical inhibition in patients with chronic neuropathic pain: correlation with pain relief. *Neurology* **67**, 1568–74.

Lefaucheur JP, Hatem S, Nineb A, Mènard-Lefaucheur I, Wendling S, Nguyen JP (2006b) Somatotopic organization of the analgesic effects of motor cortex rTMS in neuropathic pain. *Neurology* **67**, 1998–2004.

Lefaucheur JP, Drouot X, Menard-LeFaucheur I, Keravel Y, Nguyen JP (2008) Motor cortex rTMS in chronic neuropathic pain: pain relief is associated with thermal sensory perception improvement. *J Neurol Neurosurg Psychiatry* **79**, 1044–9.

Lefaucheur JP, Keravel Y, Nguyen JP (2011) Treatment of post-stroke pain by epidural motor cortex stimulation using a new octopolar lead. *Neurosurgery*, **68** (Suppl. 1), 180–7.

Leijon G, Boivie J (1989a) Central post-stroke pain: a controlled trial of amitriptyline and carbamazepine. *Pain* **36**, 27–36.

Leijon G, Boivie J (1989b) Central post-stroke pain: the effect of high and low frequency TENS. *Pain* **38**, 187–91.

Lema MJ, Shady JA, Zoll JG, West CR (1992) Management of intractable back pain from caudal ependymoma with spinal methylprednisolone, bupivacaine and morphine. *Pain* **48**, 245–8.

Lende RA, Kirsh WM, Druckman R (1971) Relief of facial pain after combined removal of precentral and postcentral cortex. *J Neurosurg* **34**, 537–43.

Lenz FA (1991) The thalamus and central pain syndromes: human and animal studies. In: Casey KL, ed., *Pain and Central Nervous System Disease. The Central Pain Syndromes*. New York: Raven Press, pp. 171–82.

Lenz FA, Dougherty PM (1997) Pain processing in the human thalamus. In: Steriade M, Jones EG, McCormick DA, eds., *Thalamus: II. Experimental and Clinical Aspects*. Amsterdam: Elsevier, pp. 617–52.

Lenz FA, Kwan HC, Martin R, *et al.* (1994) Characteristics of somatotopic organization and spontaneous neuronal activity in the region of the thalamic principal sensory nucleus in patients with spinal cord transections. *J Neurophysiol* **72**, 1570–87.

Lenz FA, Gracely RH, Baker FH, Richardson RT, Dougherty PM (1998) Reorganization of sensory modalities evoked by stimulation in the region of the principal sensory nucleus (ventral caudal, Vc) in patients with pain secondary to neural injury. *J Comp Neurol* **399**, 125–38.

Lenz FA, Casey KL, Jones EG, Willis WD (2010) *The Human Pain System: Experimental and Clinical Perspectives*. Cambridge: Cambridge University Press.

Leo RJ, Latif T (2007) Repetitive transcranial magnetic stimulation (rTMS) in experimentally induced and chronic neuropathic pain: a review. *J Pain* **8**, 453–59.

Leriche R (1937) *La chirurgie de la douleur*. Paris: Masson (3rd edn. 1949).

Leriche R (1939) *The Surgery of Pain*. Baltimore, MD: Williams & Wilkins.

Levendoglu F, Ogun CO, Ozerbil O, Ogun TC, Ugurlu H (2004) Gabapentin is a first line drug for the treatment of neuropathic pain in spinal cord injury. *Spine* **29**, 743–51.

Levin AB (1988) Stereotactic chemical hypophysectomy. In: Lunsford LD, ed., *Modern Stereotactic Neurosurgery*. Boston, MA: M Nijhoff, pp. 365–74 (see also *J Neurosurg* 1983, **59**, 1002–6).

Levin G (1966) Electrical stimulation of the globus pallidus and thalamus. *J Neurosurg* **24**, 415.

Levy LM, Ziemann U, Chen R, Cohen LG (2002) Rapid modulation of GABA in sensorimotor cortex induced by acute deafferentation. *Ann Neurol* **52**, 755–61.

Levy R, Lang AE, Dostrovsky JO, *et al.* (2001) Lidocaine and muscimol microinjections in subthalamic nucleus reverse Parkinsonian symptoms. *Brain* **124**, 2105–18.

Levy RM, Lamb S, Adams JE (1987) Treatment of chronic pain by deep brain stimulation: long term follow-up and review of the literature. *Neurosurgery* **21**, 885–93.

Lewin W, Philips CG (1952) Observations on partial removal of the post-central gyrus for pain. *J Neurol Neurosurg Psychiatry* **15**, 143–7.

Lhermitte J (1936) Symptomatologie de l'hémorrhagie du thalamus. *Rev Neurol* **65**, 89–93.

Li J (2000) Clinical analysis and treatment of central pain due to head injury. *Chin J Traumatol* **3**, 126–7.

Liepert J, Restemeyer C, Muenchau A, Weiller C (2005) Motor cortex excitability after thalamic infarction. *Clin Neurophysiol* **116**, 1621–7.

Lima MC, Fregni F (2008) Motor cortex stimulation for chronic pain: systematic review and meta-analysis of the literature. *Neurology* **70**, 2329–37.

Linazasoro G (2004) Recent failures of new potential symptomatic treatment for Parkinson's disease: causes and solutions. *Mov Disord* **19**, 743–54.

Lindblom U, Meyerson BA (1975) Influence on touch, vibration and cutaneous pain of dorsal column stimulation in man. *Pain* **1**, 257–70.

Lipman JL, Blumenkopf B (1989) Comparison of subjective and objective analgesic effects of intravenous and intrathecal morphine in chronic pain patients by heat beam dolorimetry. *Pain* **39**, 249–56.

Lipton S (1989) Percutaneous cordotomy. In: Wall PD, Melzack R, eds., *Textbook of Pain*, 2nd edn. Edinburgh: Churchill Livingstone, pp. 832–9.

Liu CW, Chen CH, Huang YF, Huang MH (2010) Auricular acupressure as a treatment for neuropathic pain in patients with spinal cord injury. *Eur J Pain Suppl* **4**, 132.

Loeser JD, Ward AA, White LE (1968) Chronic deafferentation of human spinal cord neurons. *J Neurosurg* **29**, 48–50.

Logothetis NK (2010) Neurovascular uncoupling: much ado about nothing. *Front Neuroenergetics* **2**, art. 4.

Logothetis NK, Augath M, Murayama Y, *et al.* (2010) The effects of electrical microstimulation on cortical signal propagation. *Nature Neurosci* **13**, 1283–91.

Loh L, Nathan PW, Schott GD (1981) Pain due to lesions of central nervous system removed by sympathetic block. *Br Med J* **282**, 1026–8.

Long DM, Erickson DE (1975) Stimulation of the posterior columns of the spinal cord for relief of intractable pain. *Surg Neurol* **4**, 134–41.

Long DM, Hagfors N (1975) Electrical stimulation in the nervous system: the current status of electrical stimulation of the nervous system for relief of pain. *Pain* **1**, 109–23.

Long DM, Campbell JN, Gucer G (1979) Transcutaneous electrical stimulation for relief of chronic pain. In: Bonica JJ, Liebeskind JC, Albe-Fessard DG, eds., *Advances in Pain Research and Therapy*. New York, NY: Raven Press, pp. 593–9.

Lorenz J, Kohlhoff H, Hansen HC, Kunze, Bromm B (1998) Abeta-fiber mediated activation of cingulate cortex as correlate of central post-stroke pain. *NeuroReport* **9**, 659–63.

Loubser PG, Akman NM (1996) Effects of intrathecal baclofen on chronic spinal cord injury pain. *J Pain Symptom Manage* **12**, 241–7.

Loubser PG, Clearman RR (1993) Evaluation of central spinal cord injury pain with diagnostic spinal anesthesia. *Anesthesiology* **79**, 376–8.

Loubser PG, Donovan WH (1991) Diagnostic spinal anaesthesia in chronic spinal cord injury pain. *Paraplegia* **29**, 25–36.

Love-Jones SJ, Besson M, Steeds CE, *et al.* (2009) Homotopic stimulation can reduce the area of allodynia in patients with neuropathic pain. *Eur J Pain* **13**, 942–8.

Lozano AM, Parrent A, Tasker RR (1992) Central pain from thalamic neoplasms. *Sterotact Funct Neurosurg* **59**, 77.

Lundstrom E, Smits A, Terent A, Borg J (2009) Risk factors for stroke-related pain 1 year after first-ever stroke. *Eur J Pain* **16**, 188–93.

Maarrawi J, Peyron R, Mertens P, *et al.* (2007a) Motor cortex stimulation for pain control induces changes in the endogenous opioid system. *Neurology* **69**, 827–34.

Maarrawi J, Peyron R, Mertens P, *et al.* (2007b) Differential brain opioid receptor availability in central and peripheral neuropathic pain. *Pain* **127**, 183–94.

Magilner D (2006) Localized cervical pruritus as the presenting symptom of a spinal cord tumor. *Ped Emerg Care* **22**, 746–7.

Magnin M, Jetzer U, Morel A, Jeanmonod D (2001) Microelectrode recording and macrostimulation in thalamic and subthalamic MRI guided stereotactic surgery. *Neurophysiol Clin* **31**, 230–8.

Maier C, Baron R, Tölle TR, *et al.* (2010) Quantitative sensory testing in the German Research Network on Neuropathic Pain (DFNS): somatosensory abnormalities in 1236 patients with different neuropathic pain syndromes. *Pain* **150**, 439–50.

Mailis A, Bennett GJ (2002) Dissociation between cutaneous and deep sensibility in central post-stroke pain (CPSP). *Pain* **98**, 331–4.

Mailis A, Amani N, Umana M, Basur R, Roe S (1997) Effect of intravenous sodium amytal on cutaneous sensory abnormalities, spontaneous pain and algometric pain pressure thresholds in neuropathic pain patients: a placebo-controlled study. *II. Pain* **70**, 69–81.

Mailis-Gagnon A, Yegneswaran B, Bharatwal B, Krassioukov AV (2009) Effects of intravenous sodium amobarbital vs. lidocaine on pain and sensory abnormalities in patients with spinal cord injury. *J Spinal Cord Med* **2**, 49–53.

Mamie C, Morabia A, Bernstein M, Klopfenstein LE, Forster A (2000) Treatment efficacy is not an index of pain intensity. *Can J Anaesth* **47**, 1166–70.

Manduch M, Davis KD, Lozano AM, Tasker RR, Dostrovsky JO (1999) Thalamic stimulation-evoked pain and temperature sites in pain and non-pain patients. In: *9th World Congress on Pain, Book of Abstracts*. Seattle, WA: IASP Press, A70-P151.

Mann L (1892) Kasuistischer Beitrag zur Lehre vom Central entstehenden Schmerze. *Berlin Klin Wochenschr* **29**, 244–5.

Mantini D, Perrucci MG, Del Gratta C, Romani GL, Corbetta M (2007) Electrophysiological signatures of resting state networks in the human brain. *Proc Natl Acad Sci U S A* **104**, 13170–5.

Marchand S, Bushnell MC, Molina-Negro P, Martinez SN, Duncan GN (1991) The effects of dorsal column stimulation on measures of clinical and experimental pain in man. *Pain* **45**, 249–57.

Marchand S, Kupers RC, Bushnell MC, Duncan GH (2003) Analgesic and placebo effects of thalamic stimulation. *Pain* **105**, 481–8.

Margot-Duclot A, Silhouette B, Thiebaut JB (2010) Intrathecal baclofen for intractable neuropathic pain-predictive study of efficacy and long term results. *Eur J Pain* Suppl **4**, 104, A364 (duplicate of: Margot-Duclot *et al.* IASP Congress 2002, A221-P217).

Mark VH, Tsutsumi H (1974) The suppression of pain by intrathalamic lidocaine. *Adv Neurol* **4**, 715–21.

Mark VH, Ervin FR, Hackett TP (1960) Clinical aspects of stereotactic thalamotomy in the human. The treatment of chronic severe pain. *Arch Neurol* **3**, 351–67.

Markram H (2010) Microcircuitry of the neocortex. In: Shepherd GM, Grillner S, eds., *Handbook of Microcircuits*. New York, NY: Oxford University Press, pp. 22–30.

Marshall J (1951) Sensory disturbances in cortical wounds with special reference to pain. *J Neurol Neurosurg Psychiatry* **14**, 187–204.

Martin E, Jeanmonod D, Morel A, Zadicario E, Werner B (2009) High-intensity focused ultrasound for noninvasive functional neurosurgery. *Ann Neurol* **66**, 858–61.

Martini E, Gualtierotti T, Marzorati A (1943) Die Rueckenmarkeelektronarkose (R.E.N.). *Pflueger's Arch* **246**, 585–96.

Martin-Sanchez E, Furukawa TA, Taylor J, Martin JLR (2009) Systematic review and meta-analysis of cannabis treatment for chronic pain. *Pain Med* **10**, 1353–68.

Massey EW (1984) Unilateral neurogenic pruritus following stroke. *Stroke* **15**, 901–3.

Masson C, Koskas P, Cambier J, Masson M (1991) Syndrome cortical pseudothalamique gauche et asymbolie à la douleur. *Rev Neurol (Paris)* **147**, 668–70.

Mauguière F, Desmedt JE (1988) Thalamic pain syndrome of Dejérine–Roussy: differentiation of four subtypes assisted by somatosensory evoked potentials data. *Arch Neurol* **45**, 1312–20.

Maurer M, Henn V, Dittrich A, Hofmann A (1990) Delta-9-tetrahydrocannabinol shows antispastic and analgesic effects in a single case double-blind trial. *Eur Arch Psychiatry Clin Neurosci* **240**, 1–4.

May A (2008) Chronic pain may change the structure of the brain. *Pain* **137**, 7–15.

Mayanagi Y, Bouchard G (1976–77) Evaluation of stereotactic thalamotomies for pain relief, with reference to pulvinar intervention. *Appl Neurophysiol* **39**, 157–9.

Mayanagi Y, Sano K (1998) Stimulation and coagulation of the posterior hypothalamus for intractable pain. In: Gildenberg PL, Tasker RR, eds., *Textbook of Stereotactic and Functional Neurosurgery*. New York, NY: McGraw-Hill, pp. 1453–4.

Mazars G (1975) Intermittent stimulation of nucleus ventralis posterolateralis for intractable pain. *Surg Neurol* **4**, 93–5 (includes Mazars *et al.*, *Neurochirurgie* 1974, **20**, 117–24).

Mazars G, Roge R, Mazars Y (1960) [Results of the stimulation of the spinothalamic fasciculus and their bearing on the physiopathology of pain] *Rev Prat* **103**, 136–8.

Mazars G, Mérienne L, Cioloca C (1976) État actuel de la chirurgie de la douleur. *Neurochirurgie* **22** (Suppl), 1–164.

Mazars G, Mérienne L, Cioloca C (1979) Comparative study of electrical stimulation of posterior thalamic nuclei, periaqueductal gray, and other midline mesencephalic stuctures in man. *Adv Pain Res Ther* **3**, 541–6.

Mazzola L, Isnard J, Mauguiere F (2006) Somatosensory and pain responses to stimulation of the second somatosensory area (SII) in humans. A comparison with SI and insular responses. *Cerebral Cortex* **16**, 960–8.

Mazzola L, Isnard J, Peyron R, Guenot M, Mauguiere F (2009) Somatotopic organization of pain responses to direct electrical stimulation of the human insular cortex. *Pain* **156**, 99–104.

McAlhany HS, Netsky MG (1955) Compression of the spinal cord by extramedullary neoplasms. *J Neuropath Exp Neurol* **14**, 276–81.

McCance S, Hawton K, Brighouse D, Glynn C (1996) Does electroconvulsive therapy (ECT) have any role in the management of intractable thalamic pain? *Pain* **68**, 129–31.

McCarty GW (1954) The treatment of spastic paraplegia by selective spinal cordectomy. *J Neurosurg* **11**, 539–45.

McCleane G (1998a) Lamotrigine can reduce neurogenic pain associated with multiple sclerosis. *Clin J Pain* **14**, 268–70.

McCleane G (1998b) A prospective audit of the use of lamotrigine in 300 chronic pain patients. *Pain Clin* **11**, 97–102.

McCormick PC, Torres R, Post KD, Stein BM (1990) Intramedullary ependymoma of the spinal cord. *J Neurosurg* **72**, 523–33.

McGeoch PD, Ramachandran VS (2008) Vestibular stimulation can relieve central pain of spinal origin. *Spinal Cord* **46**, 756–7.

McGeoch PD, Williams LE, Lee RR, Ramachandran VS (2008) Behavioural evidence for vestibular stimulation as a treatment for central post-stroke pain. *J Neurol Neurosurg Psychiatry* **79**, 1298–301.

McGeoch PD, Williams LE, Song T, *et al.* (2009) Post-stroke tactile allodynia and its modulation by vestibular stimulation: a MEG case study. *Acta Neurol Scand* **119**, 404–9.

McGowan DJL, Janal MN, Clark WC, *et al.* (1997) Central post-stroke pain and Wallenberg's lateral medullary infarction: frequency, character, and determinants in 63 patients. *Neurology* **49**, 120–5.

McMahon SB, Malcangio M (2009) Current challenges in glia-pain biology. *Neuron* **64**, 46–54.

McQuay HJ, Carroll D, Jadad AR, *et al.* (1994) Dextrometorphan for the treatment of neuropathic pain: a double-blind randomised controlled crossover trial with integral n-of-1 design. *Pain* **59**, 127–33.

Meadows J, Guarnieri M, Miller K, *et al.* (2001) Type I Chiari malformation: a review of the literature. *Neurosurg Quart* **11**, 220–9.

Meglio M (1998) Evaluation and management of central and peripheral deafferentation pain. In: Gildenberg PL, Tasker RR, eds., *Textbook of Stereotactic and Functional Neurosurgery.* New York: McGraw-Hill, pp. 1631–6.

Melzack R (1991) Central pain syndromes and theories of pain. In: Casey KL, ed., *Pain and Central Nervous System Disease. The Central Pain Syndromes.* New York: Raven Press, pp. 59–64.

Melzack R, Loeser JD (1978) Phantom body pain in paraplegics: evidence for a central pattern generating mechanism for pain. *Pain* **4**, 195–210.

Menefee LA, Cohen MJ, Anderson WR, *et al.* (2000) Sleep disturbance and nonmalignant chronic pain: a comprehensive review of the literature. *Pain Med* **1**, 156–72.

Mercadante S (1998) Gabapentin in spinal cord injury pain. *Pain Clin* **10**, 203–6.

Merren MD (1998) Gabapentin for the treatment of pain and tremor: a large case series. *South Med J* **91**, 739–44.

Meyer BU, Roericht S, Graefin von Einsiedel H, Kruggel F, Weindl A (1995) Inhibitory and excitatory interhemispheric transfers between motor cortical areas in normal humans and patients with abnormalities of the corpus callosum. *Brain* **118**, 429–40.

Meyerson BA, Lindblom U, Linderoth B, Lind B, Herregodts P (1993) Motor cortex stimulation as treatment of trigeminal neuropathic pain. *Acta Neurochir Suppl* **58**, 150–3.

Michel D, Laurent B, Convers P, *et al.* (1990) Douleurs corticales: étude clinique, électrophysiologique et topographique de 12 cas. *Rev Neurol* **146**, 405–14.

Michelsen JJ (1943) Subjective disturbances of the sense of pain from lesions of the cerebral cortex. *Ass Res Nerv M Dis Proc* **23**, 86–99.

Middleton JW, Siddall PJ, Walker S, Molloy AR, Rutkowski SB (1996) Intrathecal clonidine and baclofen in the management of spasticity and neuropathic pain following spinal cord injury: a case study. *Arch Phys Med Rehabil* **77**, 824–6.

Migita K, Uozumi T, Arita K, Monden S (1995) Transcranial magnetic coil stimulation of motor cortex in patients with central pain. *Neurosurgery* **36**, 1037–40.

Miles J (1998) The pituitary gland and pain relief. In: Gildenberg PL, Tasker RR, eds., *Textbook of Stereotactic and Functional Neurosurgery.* New York, NY: McGraw-Hill, pp. 1457–62.

Milhorat TH, Kotzen RM, Mu HTM, Capocelli AL, Milhorat RH (1996) Dysesthetic pain in patients with syringomyelia. *Neurosurgery* **38**, 940–7.

Milhorat TH, Capocelli AL, Kotzen RM, *et al.* (1997) Intramedullary pressure in syringomyelia: clinical and pathophysiological correlates of syrinx distension. *Neurosurgery* **41**, 1102–10.

Min SK, Lee BO (1997) Laterality in somatization. *Psychosom Med* **59**, 236–40.

Miró J, Garcia-Monco C, Leno C, Berciano C (1988) Pelvic pain: an undescribed paroxysmal manifestation of multiple sclerosis. *Pain* **32**, 73–5.

Mirza NR, Munro G (2010) The role of GABA A receptor subtypes as analgesic targets. *Drug News Perspect* **23**, 351–60.

Misra UK, Kalita J, Kumar B (2008) A study of clinical, magnetic resonance imaging, and somatosensory-evoked potential in central post-stroke pain. *J Pain* **9**, 1116–22.

Mittal B, Thomas DG, Walton P, Calder I (1987) Dorsal column stimulation in chronic pain: report of 31 cases. *Ann R Coll Surg Engl* **69**, 104–9.

Mladinich EK (1974) Diphenylhydantoin in the Wallenberg syndrome. *JAMA* **230**, 372–3.

Modesti LM, Waszak M (1975) Firing pattern of cells in human thalamus during dorsal column stimulation. *Appl Neurophysiol* **38**, 251–8.

Moens M, De Smedt A, D'Haese J, D'Haens J, Chaskis C (2009) Refractory neuropathic pain in tethered cord syndrome treated with spinal cord stimulation: a case report. *Surg Neurol* **72**, 522.

Mogil JS (2009) Are we getting anywhere in human pain genetics? *Pain* **146**, 231–2.

Mogilner AY, Rezai AR (2001) Epidural motor cortex stimulation with functional imaging guidance. *Neurosurg Focus* **11**, article 4.

Moisset X, Bouhassira D (2007) Brain imaging of neuropathic pain. *Neuroimage* **37**, S80–8.

Molet J, Rodriguez R, Munoz F, *et al.* (2007) Estimulacion cortical para el tratamiento del dolor cronico neuropatico. *Abstracts, Spanish Neurosurgical Society 2007 Congress*, Zaragoza, p. 20.

Mondani M, D'Auria S, Ius T, *et al.* (2008) Refractory pain in patients with thalamic involvement. Results obtained by motor cortex stimulation. *Acta Neurochir (Wien)* **150**, 968 (A09)

Montes C, Mertens P, Convers P, *et al.* (2002) Cognitive effects of precentral cortical stimulation for pain control: an ERP study. *Neurophysiol Clin* **32**, 313–25.

Montes C, Magnin M, Maarrawi J, *et al.* (2005) Thalamic thermo-algesic transmission: ventral posterior (VP) complex versus Vmpo in the light of a thalamic infarct with central pain. *Pain* **113**, 223–32.

Montgomery BM, King WW (1962) Hemiplegic migraine: a case with paroxysmal shoulder–hand syndrome. *Ann Intern Med* **57**, 450–5.

Montgomery EB (2010) *Deep Brain Stimulation Programming: Principles and Practice.* New York, NY: Oxford University Press.

Moore CEG, Schady W (2000) Investigation of the functional correlates of reorganization within the human somatosensory cortex. *Brain* **123**, 1883–95.

Moore CI, Stern CE, Dunbar C, *et al.* (2000) Referred phantom sensations and cortical reorganization after spinal cord injury in humans. *Proc Natl Acad Sci U S A* **97**, 14703–8.

Moraci A, Ambrosio D, Mignini R (1982) Spinal cord stimulation in the treatment of post-traumatic intractable pain. *Rass Int Clin Ter* **62**, 649–53.

Morcom AM, Fletcher PC (2007) Does the brain have a baseline? Why we should be resisting a rest. *Neuroimage* **37**, 1073–82.

Mori F, Codecà C, Kusayanagi H, *et al.* (2010) Effects of anodal transcranial direct current stimulation on chronic neuropathic pain in patients with multiple sclerosis. *J Pain* **11**, 436–42.

Mori S, Sadoshima S, Ibayashi S, Fujishima M, Iino K (1995) Impact of thalamic hematoma on six-month mortality and motor and cognitive functional outcome. *Stroke* **26**, 620–6.

Morley JS, Bridson J, Nash TP, *et al.* (2003) Low-dose methadone has an analgesic effect in neuropathic pain: a double-blind randomized controlled crossover trial. *Palliat Med* **17**, 576–87.

Morrow TJ, Casey KL (2002) Understanding central pain: new insights from forebrain imaging studies of patients and of animals with central lesions. *Progr Pain Res Manage* **23**, 265–79.

Moseley GL (2007) Using visual illusion to reduce at-level neuropathic pain in paraplegia. *Pain* **130**, 294–8.

Moseley GL, Gallace A, Spence C (2008) Is mirror therapy all it is cracked up to be? Current evidence and future directions. *Pain* **138**, 7–10.

Mottelay PF (1922) *Bibliographical History of Electricity and Magnetism*. London: C. Griffin.

Moulin DE, Foley KM, Ebers GC (1988) Pain syndromes in multiple sclerosis. *Neurology* **38**, 1830–4.

Moviglia GA, Varala G, Brizuela JA, *et al.* (2009) Case report on the clinical results of a combined cellular therapy for chronic spinal cord injured patients. *Spinal Cord* **47**, 499–503.

Mueller C, Klega A, Buchholz HG, *et al.* (2010) Basal opioid receptor binding is associated with differences in sensory perception in healthy human subjects: a [18F] diprenorphine PET study. *Neuroimage* **49**, 731–7.

Mukherjee CS, Sarkhel A, Banerjee TK, Sen S (1999) Community survey of central post-stroke pain (CPSP). In: *9th World Congress on Pain, Book of Abstracts*. Seattle, WA: IASP Press, A338.

Multiple Sclerosis Society UK (2008) www.mssociety.org.uk.

Mundinger F, Becker P (1977) Late results of central stereotactic interventions for pain. *Acta Neurochir Suppl* **24**, 229.

Mundinger F, Neumuller H (1982) Programmed stimulation for control of chronic pain and motor diseases. *Appl Neurophysiol* **45**, 102–11.

Mundinger F, Salomão JF (1980) Deep brain stimulation in mesencephalic lemniscus medialis for chronic pain. *Acta Neurochir Suppl* **30**, 245–58.

Murakami T, Takino R, Ozaki I, *et al.* (2010) High-frequency transcutaneous electrical nerve stimulation (TENS) differentially modulates sensorimotor cortices: an MEG study. *Clin Neurophysiol* **121**, 939–44.

Murphy T, Griesing T, Whalen E (2007a) Evaluation of safety and efficacy of pregabalin for chronic central neuropathic pain following spinal cord injury (SCI): an open-label extension study. *J Pain* **8**, S26, A703.

Murphy T, Siddall P, Griesing T (2007b) Efficacy, by baseline severity of anxiety symptoms, of pregabalin for treating central neuropathic pain in patients with spinal cord injury (SCI). *Eur J Pain* **11**, S134–5, A304.

Muthukumaraswamy SD, Edden RA, Jones DK, Swettenham JB, Singh KD (2009) Resting GABA concentration predicts peak gamma frequency and fMRI amplitude in response to visual stimulation in humans. *Proc Natl Acad Sci U S A* **106**, 8356–61.

Naess H, Lunde L, Brogger J, Waje-Andreassen U (2010) Post-stroke pain on long-term follow-up: the Bergen stroke study. *J Neurol* **257**, 1446–52.

Nagaro T, Amakawa K, Kimura S, Arai T (1993) Reference of pain following percutaneous cervical cordotomy. *Pain* **53**, 205–11.

Nagaro T, Shimizu C, Inoue H, *et al.* (1995) [The efficacy of intravenous lidocaine on various types of neuropathic pain]. *Masui* **44**, 862–7.

Nahmias F, Debes C, Ciampi De Andreade D, Mhalla A, Bouhassira D (2009) Diffuse analgesic effects of unilateral repetitive transcranial magnetic stimulation (rTMS) in healthy volunteers. *Pain* **147**, 224–32.

Nair DR, Najm I, Bulacio J, Lueders H (2001) Painful auras in focal epilepsy. *Neurology* **57**, 700–2.

Nakata H, Tamura Y, Sakamoto K, *et al.* (2008) Evoked magnetic fields following noxious laser stimulation of the thigh in humans. *Neuroimage* **42**, 858–68.

Nakazato Y, Yoshimaru K, Ohkuma A, *et al.* (2004) [Central post-stroke pain in Wallenberg syndrome]. *No To Shinkei* **56**, 385–8.

Namba S, Nakao Y, Matsumoto Y, Ohmoto T, Nishimoto A (1984) Electrical stimulation of the posterior limb of the internal capsule for treatment of thalamic pain. *Appl Neurophysiol* **47**, 137–48 (see also *J Neurosurg* 1985, **63**, 224–34).

Nandi D, Aziz TZ (2004) Deep brain stimulation in the management of neuropathic pain and multiple sclerosis tremor. *J Clin Neurophysiol* **21**, 31–9.

Nandi D, Smith H, Owen S, *et al.* (2002) Periventricular gray stimulation versus motor cortex stimulation for poststroke neuropathic pain. *J Clin Neurosci* **9**, 557–61.

Nandi D, Aziz T, Carter H, Stein J (2003) Thalamic field potentials in chronic central pain treated by periventricular gray stimulation: a series of eight cases. *Pain* **101**, 97–107.

Napadow V, Dhond RP, Kim J, *et al.* (2009) Brain encoding of acupuncture sensation: coupling on-line rating with fMRI. *Neuroimage* **47**, 1055–65.

Nash PG, Macefield VG, Klineberg IJ, *et al.* (2010) Bilateral activation of the trigeminothalamic tract by acute orofacial cutaneous and muscle pain in humans. *Pain* **151**, 384–93.

Nashold BS (1974) Central pain: its origin and treatment. *Clin Neurosurg* **21**, 311–22.

Nashold BS (1975) Dorsal column stimulation for control of pain: a three-year follow-up. *Surg Neurol* **4**, 146–7.

Nashold BS (1991) Paraplegia and pain. *Adv Pain Res Ther* **19**, 301.

Nashold BS, Bullitt E (1981) Dorsal root entry zone lesions to control central pain in paraplegics. *J Neurosurg* **55**, 414–19.

Nashold BS, Friedman H (1972) Dorsal column stimulation for control of pain. Preliminary report on 30 patients. *J Neurosurg* **30**, 590–7.

Nashold BS, Pearlstein RD, eds. (1996) *The DREZ Operation*. Park Ridge, IL: AANS Publications.

Nashold BS, Wilson WP (1970) Central pain and irritable midbrain. In: Crue B, ed., *Pain and Suffering. Selected Aspects*. Springfield, IL: CC Thomas, pp. 95–118 (also *Conf Neurol* 1966, **27**, 30–4; *Adv Neurol* 1974, 191–6).

Nashold BS, Wilson WP, Slaughter DG (1969) Stereotactic midbrain lesions for central dysesthesia and phantom pain. Preliminary report. *J Neurosurg* **30**, 116–26.

Nasreddine ZS, Saver JL (1997) Pain after thalamic stroke: right diencephalic predominance and clinical features in 180 patients. *Neurology* **48**, 1196–9.

Nathanson M (1962) Paroxysmal phenomena resembling seizures related to spinal cord and root pathology. *J Mt Sinai Hosp* **29**, 147–51.

Naver H, Blomstrand C, Ekholm S, *et al.* (1995) Autonomic and thermal sensory symptoms and dysfunction after stroke. *Stroke* **26**, 1379–85.

Nayak S, Shiflett SC, Schoenberger E, *et al.* (2001a) Is acupuncture effective in treating chronic pain after spinal cord injury? *Arch Phys Med Rehabil* **82**, 1578–86.

Nayak S, Matheis RJ, Agostinelli S, Shifleft SC (2001b) The use of complementary and alternative therapies for chronic pain following spinal cord injury: a pilot survey. *J Spinal Cord Med* **24**, 54–62.

Nègre-Pagès L, Regragui W, Bouhassira D, Grandjean H, Rascol O, on behalf of the DoPaMiP Study Group (2008) Chronic pain in Parkinson's disease: the cross-sectional French DoPaMiP survey. *Mov Disord* **23**, 1361–9.

Nepomuceno C, Fine PR, Richards JS, *et al.* (1979) Pain in patients with spinal cord injury. *Arch Phys Med Rehab* **60**, 605–9.

Ness TJ, San Pedro EC, Richards JS, *et al.* (1998) Clinical note. A case of spinal cord injury-related pain with baseline rCBF brain SPECT imaging and beneficial response to gabapentin. *Pain* **78**, 139–43.

Ness TJ, Putzke JD, Liu HG, Mountz J (2002) Examples of the use of gabapentin in the treatment of spinal cord injury pain. *Progr Pain Res Manage* **23**, 379–92.

Nguyen JP, Lefacheur JP, Decq P, *et al.* (1999) Chronic motor cortex stimulation in the treatment of central and neuropathic pain: correlations between clinical, electrophysiological and anatomical data. *Pain* **82**, 245–51.

Nguyen JP, Velasco F, Brugieres P, *et al.* (2008) Treatment of chronic neuropathic pain by motor cortex stimulation: results of a bicentric controlled crossover trial. *Brain Stimulation* **1**, 89–96.

Nguyen JP, Lefaucheur JP, Raoul S, *et al.* (2009) Motor cortex stimulation for the treatment of neuropathic pain. In: Krames E, Peckham PH, Rezai AR, eds., *Neuromodulation*. London: Academic Press, pp. 515–26.

Nicholson K, Mailis A, Taylor A (2002) Psychometric correlates of placebo and nocebo responses. In: *10th World Congress on Pain, Book of Abstracts*. Seattle, WA: IASP Press, A317–P596.

Nicotra A, Critchley HD, Mathias CJ, Dolan RJ (2006) Emotional and autonomic consequences of spinal cord injury explored using functional brain imaging. *Brain* **129**, 718–28.

Nii Y, Uematsu S, Lesser RP, Gordon B (1996) Does the central sulcus divide motor and sensory functions? Cortical mapping of human hand areas as revealed by electrical stimulation through subdural grid electrodes. *Neurology* **46**, 360–7.

Niizuma H, Kwak R, Ikeda S, *et al.* (1982) Follow-up results of centromedian thalamotomy for central pain. *Appl Neurophysiol* **45**, 324–5.

Nir RR, Lev R, Moont R, *et al.* (2008) Neurophysiolgy of the cortical pain network: revisiting the role of S1 in subjective pain perception via standardized low-resolution brain electromagnetic tomography (sLORETA). *J Pain* **9**, 1058–69.

Nitescu P, Dahm P, Appelgren L, Curelaru I (1998) Continuous infusion of opioid and bupivacaine by externalized intrathecal catheters in long-term treatment of "refractory" nonmalignant pain. *Clin J Pain* **14**, 17–28.

Noble M, Tregear SJ, Treadwell JR, Schoelles K (2008) Long-term opioid therapy for chronic noncancer pain: a systematic review and meta-analysis of efficacy and safety. *J Pain Symptom Manage* **35**, 214–28.

Norrbrink C (2009) Transcutaneous electrical nerve stimulation for the treatment of spinal cord injury neuropathic pain. *J Rehabil Res Dev* **46**, 85–94.

Norrbrink C, Lundeberg T (2009) Tramadol in neuropathic pain after spinal cord injury. A randomized, double-blind, placebo-controlled trial. *Clin J Pain* **25**, 177–84.

Norrbrink Budh C, Lundeberg T (2004) Non-pharmacological pain-relieving therapies in individuals with spinal cord injury: a patient perspective. *Complement Ther Med* **12**, 189–97.

Norrbrink Budh C, Lundeberg T (2005) Use of analgesic drugs in individuals with spinal cord injury. *J Rehabil Med* **37**, 87–94.

Norrbrink Budh C, Kowalski J, Lundeberg T (2006) A comprehensive pain management programme comprising educational, cognitive and behavioural interventions for neuropathic pain following spinal cord injury. *J Rehabil Med* **38**, 172–80.

North R, Ewend MG, Lawton MT, Piantadosi S (1991) Spinal cord stimulation for chronic, intractable pain: superiority of "multi-channel" devices. *Pain* **44**, 119–30.

North RB, Kidd DH, Zahurak M, James CS, Long DM (1993) Spinal cord stimulation for chronic,intractable pain: experience over two decades. *Neurosurgery* **32**, 384–95.

Notcutt W, Price M, Miller R, *et al.* (2004) Initial experience with medicinal extracts of cannabis for chronic pain: results from 34 "N of 1" studies. *Anaesthesia* **59**, 440.

Nuñez A, Malmierca E (2007) Corticofugal modulation of sensory information. *Adv Anat Embryol Cell Biol* **187**, 1–74.

Nurmikko T, Hietaharju A (1992) Effect of exposure to sauna heat on neuropathic and rheumatoid pain. *Pain* **49**, 43–51.

Nuti C, Peyron R, Garcia-Larrea L, *et al.* (2005) Motor cortex stimulation for refractory neuropathic pain: four year outcome and predictors of efficacy. *Pain* **118**, 43–52.

Nyquist JK, Greenhoot JH (1973) Responses evoked from the thalamic centrum medianum by painful input: suppression by dorsal funiculus conditioning. *Exp Neurol* **39**, 215–22.

Obersteiner H (1881) On allochiria: a peculiar sensory disorder. *Brain* **4**, 153–63.

Obrador S, Dierssen G, Ceballos R (1957) Consideraciones clinicas, neurologicas y anatomicas sobre el llamado dolor talamico. Con motivo de dos casos personales. *Acta Neurol Latinoamer* **3**, 58–77.

O'Connell NE, Wand BM, Marston L, Spencer S, Desouza LH (2010) Non-invasive brain stimulation techniques for chronic pain. *Cochrane Database Syst Rev* **9**, CD008208.

O'Connor AB, Schwid SR, Herrmann DN, Markman JD, Dworkin RH (2008) Pain associated with multiple sclerosis: systematic review and proposed classification. *Pain* **137**, 96–111.

Ofek H, Defrin R (2007) The characteristics of chronic central pain after traumatic brain injury. *Pain* **131**, 330–40.

Ohara S, Crone NE, Weiss N, Treede RD, Lenz FA (2004) Cutaneous painful laser stimuli evoke responses recorded directly from primary somatosensory cortex in awake humans. *J Neurophysiol* **91**, 2734–6.

Ohara S, Crone NE, Weiss N, Kim JH, Lenz FA (2008) Analysis of synchrony demonstrates that the presence of "pain networks" prior to a noxious stimulus can enable the perception of pain in response to that stimulus. *Exp Brain Res* **185**, 353–8.

Ohta Y, Akino M, Iwasaki Y, Abe H (1992) Spinal epidural stimulation for central pain caused by a cord lesion. *No Shinkei Geka* **20**, 147–52.

Ohye C (1990) Thalamus. In: Paxinos G, ed., *The Human Nervous System*. San Diego, CA: Academic Press, pp. 439–68.

Ohye C (1998) Stereotactic treatment of central pain. *Stereotact Funct Neurosurg* **70**, 71–6.

Ohye C, Narabayashi H (1972) Activity of thalamic neurons and their receptive fields in different functional states in man. In: Somjen GG, ed., *Neurophysiology Studies in Man*. Amsterdam: Excerpta Medica, pp. 79–84.

Ohye C, Shibazaki T (2009) Treatment of functional disorders with gamma knife thalamotomy. *Progr Neurol Surg* **22**, 170–81.

Ojemann JG, Silbergeld DL (1995) Cortical stimulation mapping of phantom limb rolandic cortex. Case report. *J Neurosurg* **82**, 641–4.

Olausson H, Ha B, Duncan GH, *et al.* (2001a) Cortical activation by tactile and painful stimuli in hemispherectomized patients. *Brain* **124**, 916–27.

Olausson H, Marchand S, Bittar RG, *et al.* (2001b) Central pain in a hemispherectomized patient. *Eur J Pain* **5**, 209–17.

Orthner H, Roeder F (1966) Further clinical and anatomical experiences with stereotactic operations for relief of pain. *Confin Neurol* **27**, 418–30.

Osler W (1892) *The Principles and Practice of Medicine*. New York, NY: Appleton.

Österberg A, Boivie J (2010) Central pain in multiple sclerosis: sensory abnormalities. *Eur J Pain* **14**, 104–10.

Österberg A, Boivie J, Holmgren H, Thuomas K, Johansson I (1994) The clinical characteristics and sensory abnormalities of patients with central pain caused by multiple sclerosis. In: Gebhart GF, Hammond DL, Jensen TS, eds., *Proceedings of the 7th World Congress on Pain*. Seattle, WA: IASP Press, pp. 789–96.

Österberg A, Boivie J, Thuomas KA (2005) Central pain in multiple sclerosis: prevalence and clinical characteristics. *Eur J Pain* **9**, 531–42.

Osterman PO (1976) Paroxysmal itching in multiple sclerosis. *Br J Dermatol* **95**, 555–8.

Ostrowsky K, Magnin M, Ryvlin P, *et al.* (2002) Representation of pain and somatic sensation in the human insula: a study of responses to direct electrical cortical stimulation. *Cereb Cortex* **12**, 376–85.

Owen SLF, Green AL, Stein JF, Aziz TZ (2006) Deep brain stimulation for the allevaiation of post-stroke neuropathic pain. *Pain* **120**, 202–6.

Owen SLF, Green AL, Nandi DD, *et al.* (2007) Deep brain stimulation for neuropathic pain. *Acta Neurochir (Wien)* Suppl **97**, 111–16.

Paciaroni M, Bogousslavsky J (1998) Pure sensory syndromes in thalamic stroke. *Eur Neurol* **39**, 211–17.

Pagni CA (1977) Central pain and painful anesthesia. Pathophysiology and treatment of sensory deprivation syndromes due to central and peripheral nervous system lesions. *Progr Neurol Surg* **8**, 132–257.

Pagni CA, Canavero S (1993) Paroxysmal perineal pain resembling tic douloureux, only symptom of a dorsal meningioma. *Ital J Neurol Sci* **14**, 323–4.

Pagni CA, Canavero S (1995) Functional thalamic depression in a case of reversibile central pain due to a spinal intramedullary cyst. *J Neurosurg* **83**, 163–5.

Pagni CA, Regolo P (1987) Epilessia sensitivo-motoria di origine spinale. Sintomo di esordio raro dei meningiomi spinali. *Minerva Chir* **42**, 2003–9.

Pagni CA, Lanotte M, Canavero S (1993) How frequent is anesthesia dolorosa following spinal posterior rhizotomy? A retrospective analysis of fifteen patients. *Pain* **54**, 323–7.

Panerai AE, Monza G, Movilia P, *et al.* (1990) A randomized, within-patient, cross-over, placebo-controlled trial on the efficacy and tolerability of the tricyclic antidepressants chlorimipramine and nortriptyline in central pain. *Acta Neurol Scand* **82**, 34–8.

Panzeri S, Brunel N, Logothetis NK, Kayser C (2010) Sensory neural codes using multiplexed temporal scales. *Trends Neurosci* **33**, 111–20.

Papadopoulos G, Tzimas P, Zigouris A, Voulgaris S, Karanikolas M (2010) Subarachnoid clonidine for treatment of central neuropathic pain persisting for twenty-four years after spinal cord injury. A case report. *Eur J Pain* **54**, 102, A359.

Papo I, Quattrini A (1997) The role of corpus callosum in experimental epileptogenesis: a brief survey of the literature. *J Neurosurg Sci* **41**, 27–30.

Parrent AG, Lozano AM, Dostrovsky JO, Tasker RR (1992) Central pain in the absence of functional sensory thalamus. *Stereotact Funct Neurosurg* **59**, 9–14.

Pattany PM, Yeziersky RP, Widerström-Noga EG, *et al.* (2002) Proton magnetic resonance spectroscopy of the thalamus in patients with chronic neuropathic pain after spinal cord injury. *AJNR Am J Neuroradiol* **23**, 901–5 (duplicate of: Pattany *et al.* (2002) Proton magnetic resonance spectroscopy following spinal cord injury: evaluation of patients with chronic neuropathic pain. *Progr Brain Res Manage* **23**, 301–11).

Peker S, Dincer A, Pamir N (2009) Vascular compression of the trigeminal nerve is a frequent finding in asymptomatic individuals: 3-T MR imaging of 200 trigeminal nerves using 3D CISS sequences. *Acta Neurochir* **151**, 1081–8.

Penfield W, Gage L (1933) Cerebral localization of epileptic manifestations. *Arch Neurol Psychiatry* **30**, 709–27.

Penfield W, Jasper H (1954) *Epilepsy and the Functional Anatomy of the Human Brain*. Boston, MA: Little, Brown.

Penfield W, Welch K (1951) The supplementary motor area of the cerebral cortex: a clinical and experimental study. *Arch Neurol Psychiatry* **66**, 298–317.

Penn RD, Paice JA (2000) Adverse effects associated with the intrathecal administration of ziconotide. *Pain* **85**, 291–6.

Pereira EAC, Green AL, Bradley KM, *et al.* (2007) Regional cerebral perfusion differences between periventricular grey, thalamic and dual target deep brain stimulation for chronic neuropathic pain. *Stereotact Funct Neurosurg* **85**, 175–83.

Pereira EAC, Moir L, McIntyre C, Green AL, Aziz TZ (2008) Deep brain stimulation for central post-stroke pain: relating outcomes and stimulation parameters in 21 patients. *Acta Neurochir (Wien)* **150**, 968.

Perel P, Roberts I, Sena E, *et al.* (2007) Comparison of treatment effects between animal experiments and clinical trials: systematic review. *BMJ* **334**, 197.

Perret D, Luo D (2009) Targeting voltage-gated calcium channels for neuropathic pain management. *Neurotherapeutics* **6**, 679–92.

Perry KN, Nicholas MK, Middleton JW (2010) Comparison of a pain management program with usual care in a pain management center for people with spinal cord injury-related chronic pain. *Clin J Pain* **26**, 206–16.

Peskine A, Galland A, Weill-Chounlamountry A, Pradat-diehl P (2008) L'insula, une ile oubliée? *Rev Neurol* **164S**, A19.

Petit-Dutaillis D, Messimy R, Berges L (1953) La psychochirurgie des algies irreductibles: étude basée sur 57 cas. *Semaine des Hopitaux de Paris* **29**, 3893–903.

Peyron R, Garcia-Larrea L, Deiber MP, *et al.* (1995) Electrical stimulation of precentral cortical area in the treatment of central pain: electrophysiological and PET study. *Pain* **62**, 275–86.

Peyron R, Garcia-Larrea L, Gregoire MC, *et al.* (1998) Allodynia after lateral-medullary (Wallenberg) infarct. A PET study. *Brain* **121**, 345–56.

Peyron R, Garcia-Larrea L, Costes N, *et al.* (1999) The haemodynamic pattern of central pain patients with allodynia. In: *9th World Congress on Pain, Book of Abstracts*. Seattle, WA: IASP Press, A78.

Peyron R, Garcia-Larrea L, Gregoire MC, *et al.* (2000) Parietal and cingulate processes in central pain. A combined positron emission tomography (PET) and functional magnetic resonance imaging (fMRI) study of an unusual case. *Pain* **84**, 77–87.

Peyron R, Schneider F, Faillenot I, *et al.* (2004) An fMRI study of cortical representation of mechanical allodynia in patients with neuropathic pain. *Neurology* **63**, 1838–46.

Peyron R, Faillenot I, Mertens P, Laurent B, Garcia-Larrea L (2007) Motor cortex stimulation in neuropathic pain. Correlations between analgesic effect and hemodynamic changes in the brain. A PET study. *Neuroimage* **34**, 310–21.

Phillips NI, Bhakta BB (2000) Effect of deep brain stimulation on limb paresis after stroke. *Lancet* **356**, 222–3.

Pickering AE, Thornton SR, Love-Jones SJ, Steeds C, Patel NK (2009) Analgesia in conjunction with normalization of thermal sensation following deep brain stimulation for central post-stroke pain. *Pain* **147**, 299–304.

Pillay PK, Hassenbusch SJ (1992) Bilateral MRI-guided stereotactic cingulotomy for intractable pain. *Stereotact Funct Neurosurg* **59**, 33–8.

Pioli EY, Gross CE, Meissner W, Bioulac BH, Bezard E (2003) The deafferented nonhuman primate is not a reliable model of intractable pain. *Neurol Res* **25**, 127–9.

Pirotte B, Voordecker P, Neugroschl C, *et al.* (2005) Combination of functional magnetic resonance imaging-guided neuronavigation and intraoperative cortical brain mapping improves targeting of motor cortex stimulation in neuropathic pain. *Neurosurgery* **56** (ONS Suppl 2), 344–59.

Ploner M, Freund HJ, Schnitzler A (1999) Pain affect without pain sensation in a patient with a postcentral lesion. *Pain* **81**, 211–14.

Ploner M, Gross J, Timmermann L, Pllok B, Schnitzler A (2006) Pain suppresses spontaneous brain rhythms. *Cereb cortex* **16**, 537–40.

Plotkin R (1982) Results in 60 cases of deep brain stimulation for chronic intractable pain. *Appl Neurophysiol* **45**, 173–8.

Pollock LJ, Boshes B, Finkelmann I, *et al.* (1951a) Management of residual injuries to spinal cord and cauda equina. *J Am Med Assoc* **146**, 1551–63.

Pollock LJ, Brown M, Boshes B, *et al.* (1951b) Pain below the level of injury of the spinal cord. *Arch Neurol Psychiatry* **65**, 319–22.

Poreisz C, Antal A, Boros K, *et al.* (2008) Attenuation of N2 amplitude of laser-evoked potentials by theta burst stimulation of primary somatosensory cortex. *Exp Brain Res* **185**, 611–21.

Portenoy RK, Foley KM (1986) Chronic use of opioid analgesics in-non malignant pain: report of 38 cases. *Pain* **25**, 171–86.

Portenoy RK, Yang K, Thornton D (1988) Chronic intractable pain: an atypical presentation of multiple sclerosis. *J Neurol* **235**, 226–8.

Portenoy RK, Foley KM, Inturrisi CE (1990) The nature of opioid responsiveness and its implications for neuropathic pain: new hypotheses derived from studies of opioid infusions. *Pain* **43**, 273–86.

Porter RW, Hohmann GW, Bors E, French JD (1966) Cordotomy for pain following cauda equina injury. *Arch Surg* **92**, 765–70.

Potagas C, Avdelidis D, Singounas E, Missir O, Aessopos A (1997) Episodic pain associated with a tumor in the parietal operculum: a case report and literature review. *Pain* **72**, 201–8.

Potter PJ, Hayes KC, Hsieh JT, Delaney GA, Segal JL (1998) Sustained improvements in neurological function in spinal cord injured patients treated with oral 4-aminopyridine: three cases. *Spinal Cord* **36**, 147–55.

Pound P, Ebrahim S, Sandercock P, Bracken MB, Roberts I (2004) Where is the evidence that animal research benefits humans? Reviewing Animal Trials Systematically (RATS) Group. *BMJ* **328**, 514–17.

Powers SK, Barbaro NM, Levy RM (1988) Pain control with laser-produced dorsal root entry zone lesions. *Appl Neurophysiol* **51**, 243–54 (see also *J Neurosurg* 1984, **61**, 841–7).

Prestor B (2001) Microsurgical junctional DREZ coagulation for treatment of deafferentation pain syndromes. *Surg Neurol* **56**, 259–65.

Prestor B, Benedicic M (2008) Electrophysiological and clinical data support the use of dorsal root entry zone myelotomy in syringosubarachnoid shunting for syringomyelia. *Surg Neurol* **69**, 466–73.

Price CIM, Curless RH, Rodgers H (1999) Can stroke patients use visual analogue scales? *Stroke* **30**, 1357–61.

Procacci P, Maresca M (1991) Central pruritus: case report. *Pain* **47**, 369–70.

Puri BK, Smith HC, Cox IJ, *et al.* (1998) The human motor cortex after incomplete spinal cord injury: an investigation using proton magnetic resonance spectroscopy. *J Neurol Neurosurg Psychiatry* **65**, 748–54.

Putzke JD, Richards JS, Kezar L, Hicken BL, Ness TJ (2002) Long-term use of gabapentin for treatment of pain after traumatic spinal cord injury. *Clin J Pain* **18**, 116–21.

Quattrini A, Papo I, Cesarano R, *et al.* (1997) EEG patterns after callosotomy. *J Neurosurg Sci* **41**, 85–92.

Que JC, Siddall PJ, Cousins MJ (2007) Pain management in a patient with intractable spinal cord injury pain: a case report and literature review. *Anesth Analg* **105**, 1462–73.

Quigley DG, Arnold J, Eldridge PR, *et al.* (2003) Long-term outcome of spinal cord stimulation and hardware complications. *Stereotact Funct Neurosurg* **81**, 50–6.

Rabben T, Skjelbred P, Oye I (1999) Prolonged analgesic effect of ketamine, an N-methyl-D-aspartate receptor inhibitor, in patients with chronic pain. *J Pharmacol Exp Ther* **289**, 1060–6.

Radhakrishnan V, Tsoukatos J, Davis KD, *et al.* (1999) A comparison of the burst activity of lateral thalamic neurons in chronic pain and non-pain patients. *Pain* **80**, 567–75.

Raichle M (2009) Two views of brain function. In: Gazzaniga MS, ed., *The Cognitive Neurosciences*, 4th edn. Cambridge, MA: MIT Press, pp. 1067–74.

Ramachandran VS, McGeoch PD, Williams L (2007a) Can vestibular caloric stimulation be used to treat Dejerine–Roussy Syndrome? *Med Hypotheses* **69**, 486–8.

Ramachandran VS, McGeoch PD, Williams L, Arcilla G (2007b) Rapid relief of thalamic pain syndrome induced by vestibular caloric stimulation. *Neurocase* **13**, 185–8.

Ramadan A, Demierre B, Berney J, *et al.* (1987). Cordotomy for non-malignant pain. IASP Congress, Poster 244.

Ramamurthy S, Hoffman J (1995) Intravenous regional guanethidine in the treatment of reflex sympathetic dystrophy/causalgia: a randomized, double-blind study. Guanethidine Study Group. *Anesth Analg* **81**, 718–23.

Ramcharan EJ, Gnadt JW, Sherman SM (2005) Higher-order thalamic relays burst more than first-order relays. *Proc Natl Acad Sci U S A* **102**, 12236–41.

Ramsaransing G, Zwanikken C, De Keyser J (2000) Worsening of symptoms of multiple sclerosis associated with carbamazepine. *BMJ* **320**, 1113.

Rapson LM, Wells N, Pepper J, Majid N, Boon H (2003) Acupuncture as a promising treatment for below-level central neuropathic pain: a retrospective study. *J Spinal Cord Med* **26**, 21–6.

Rasche D, Siebert S, Stippich C, *et al.* (2005) [Spinal cord stimulation in Failed Back Surgery Syndrome. Preliminary study for the evaluation of therapy by

functional magnetic resonance imaging (fMRI). *Schmerz* **19**, 497–500, 502–5.
Rasche D, Ruppolt M, Stippich C, Unterberg A, Tronnier VM (2006a) Motor cortex stimulation for long-term relief of chronic neuropathic pain: a 10 year experience. *Pain* **121**, 43–52.
Rasche D, Rinaldi P, Young RF, Tronnier VM (2006b) Deep brain stimulation for the treatment of various chronic pain syndromes. *Neurosurg Focus* **21**, E8.
Rasminsky M (1980) Physiology of conduction in demyelinated axons. In: Waxman, ed., *Physiology and Pathobiology of Axons*. New York, NY: Raven Press, pp. 361–76.
Rasmussen PV, Sindrup SH, Jensen TS, Bach FW (2004) Therapeutic outcome in neuropathic pain: relationship to evidence of nervous system lesion. *Eur J Neurol* **11**, 545–53.
Rath SA, Braun V, Soliman N, Antoniadis G, Richter MP (1996) Results of DREZ coagulations for pain related to plexus lesions, spinal cord injuries and postherpetic neuralgia. *Acta Neurochir (Wien)* **138**, 364–9.
Rauck RL, Wallace MS, Leong MS, *et al.* (2006) A randomized, double-blind, placebo-controlled study of intrathecal ziconotide in adults with severe chronic pain. *J Pain Symptom Manage* **31**, 393–406.
Ravenscroft A, Ahmed YS, Burnside IG (1999) Chronic pain after spinal cord injury: a survey of practice in UK spinal injury units. *Spinal Cord* **37**, 25–8.
Ray CD, Burton CV (1980) Deep brain stimulation for severe chronic pain. *Acta Neurochir (Wien) Suppl* **30**, 289–93.
Ray DA, Tai YM (1988) Increasing doses of naloxone hydrochloride by infusion to treat pain due to the thalamic syndrome. *Br Med J* **296**, 969–70.
Ray WA, Meredith S, Thapa PB, Hall K, Murray KT (2004) Cyclic antidepressants and the risk of sudden cardiac death. *Clin Pharmacol Ther* **75**, 234–41.
Raza SM, Anderson WS, Eberhart CG, Wolinsky JP, Gokaslan ZL (2005) The application of surgical cordectomy in the management of an intramedullary-extramedullary atypical meningioma. *J Spinal Disord Tech* **18**, 449–54.
Reboiledo PE, Gonzalez X, Valenzuela P, Larraguibel F, Mujica A (2002) Study of gabapentin and clomipramine use for chronic pain management in spinal cord injury. In: *10th World Congress on Pain, Book of Abstracts*. Seattle, WA: IASP Press, A925–P195.
Reig E (1993) Spinal infusion of morphine for the treatment of neuropathic pain. Medtronic Conference on Advances in Chronic Pain Treatment, Padova, November 27, 1993.
Rennefeld C, Wiech K, Schoell ED, Lorenz J, Bingel U (2010) Habituation to pain: further support for a central component. *Pain* **148**, 503–8.
Rétif J (1963) Douleur centrale et lesion suprathalamique. Méningiome temporo-pariétal se manifestant par un syndrome algique paroxystique à caractère pseudo-radiculaire du membre inférieur controlateral. *Acta Neurol Psychiat Belg* **63**, 955–69.
Rétif J, Brihaye J, Vanderhaegen JJ (1967) Syndrome douloureux "thalamique" et lesion parietale. À propos de trois observations de tumeur à localisation pariétale, s'étant accompagnées de douleurs spontanées de l'hemicorps contralatéral. *Neurochirurgie* **13**, 375–84.
Reyns N, Houdayer E, Bourriez JL, *et al.* (2008) Motor cortex stimulation-induced modulation of central beta rhythms and somatosensory evoked potentials. A correlation with its analgesic effect. *Acta Neurochir (Wien)* **150**, 970–1.
Rezai AR, Lozano AM, Crawley AP, *et al.* (1999) Thalamic stimulation and functional magnetic resonance imaging: localization of cortical and subcortical activation with implanted electrodes. Technical note. *J Neurosurg* **90**, 583–90.
Richardson DE (1974) Thalamotomy for control of chronic pain. *Acta Neurochir (Wien) Suppl* **21**, 77–88.
Richardson DE, Akil H (1977a) Pain reduction by electrical brain stimulation in man: 1. Acute administration in periaqueductal and periventricular sites; 2. Chronic self-administration in the periventricular gray matter. *J Neurosurg* **47**, 178–83; 184–94.
Richardson DE, Akil H (1977b) Long-term results of periventricular gray self-stimulation. *Neurosurgery* **1**, 199–202.
Richardson RR, Meyer PR, Cerullo LJ (1980) Neurostimulation in the modulation of intractable paraplegic and traumatic neuroma pains. *Pain* **8**, 76–84.
Richter HP, Seitz K (1984) Dorsal root entry zone lesions for the control of deafferentation pain: experiences in ten patients. *Neurosurgery* **15**, 956–9.
Riddoch G (1938) The clinical features of central pain. Lumleian lecture. *Lancet* **234**, 1093–8; 1150–6; 1205–9.
Riddoch G, Critchley M (1937) La physiopathologie de la douleur d'origine centrale. *Rev Neurol* **68**, 77–104.
Ridgeway B, Wallace M, Gerayli A (2000) Ziconotide for the treatment of severe spasticity after spinal cord injury. *Pain* **85**, 287–9.
Rinaldi PC, Young RF, Albe-Fessard D, Chodakiewitz J (1991) Spontaneous neuronal hyperactivity in the medial and intralaminar thalamic nuclei of patients with deafferentation pain. *J Neurosurg* **74**, 415–21.
Rintala DH, Holmes SA, Courtade D, *et al.* (2007) Comparison of the effectiveness of amitriptyline and gabapentin on chronic neuropathic pain in persons with spinal cord injury. *Arch Phys Med Rehabil* **88**, 1547–60.
Rintala DH, Fiess RN, Tan G, Holmes SA, Bruel BM (2010) Effect of dronabinol on central neuropathic pain after spinal cord injury. *Am J Phys Med Rehab* **89**, 840–8.
Ro T, Farnè A, Johnson RM, *et al.* (2007) Feeling sounds after a thalamic lesion. *Ann Neurol* **62**, 433–41.
Rodriguez RF, Contreras N (2002) Bilateral motor cortex stimulation for the relief of central dysesthetic pain and intentional tremor secondary to spinal cord surgery: a case report. *Neuromodulation* **5**, 189–95.
Roebling R, Lerche H (2009) Painful seizures associated with a lesion in the midcingulate cortex. *J Neurol* **256**, 1012–14.

Roeder F, Orthner H (1961) Erfahrungen mit sterotaktischen Eingriffen. III Mitteilung. Über zerebrale Schmerzoperationen, insbesondere mediale Mesencephalotomie bei thalamischer Hyperpathie und bei Anaesthesia Dolorosa. *Confin Neurol* **21**, 51–97.

Rog DJ, Nurmikko TJ, Friede T, Young CA (2005) Randomized, controlled trial of cannabis based medicine in central pain in multiple sclerosis. *Neurology* **65**, 812–19.

Rog DJ, Nurmikko TJ, Young CA (2007) Oromucosal delta9-tetrahydrocannabinol/cannabidiol for neuropathic pain associated with multiple sclerosis: an uncontrolled, open-label, 2-year extension trial. *Clin Ther* **29**, 2068–79.

Rogano L, Teixeira MJ, Lepski G (2003) Chronic pain after spinal cord injury: clinical characteristics. *Stereotact Funct Neurosurg* **81**, 65–9.

Rollnik JD, Wustefeld S, Dauper J, *et al.* (2002) Repetitive transcranial magnetic stimulation for the treatment of chronic pain: a pilot study. *Eur Neurol* **48**, 6–10.

Rolls ET, Deco G (2010) *The Noisy Brain: Stochastic Dynamics as a Principle of Brain function*. Oxford: Oxford University Press.

Romanelli P, Heit G (2004) Patient-controlled deep brain stimulation can overcome analgesic tolerance. *Stereotact Funct Neurosurg* **82**, 77–9.

Romano J, Merritt HH (1941) The singular affection of Gaspard Viesseux. Nearly description of the lateral medullary syndrome. *Bull Hist Med* **9**, 72–9.

Rondinelli RD, ed. (2008) *Guides to the Evaluation of Permanent Impairment*, 6th edn. Chicago, IL: American Medical Association, pp. 450–1.

Roosink M, Renzenbrink GJ, Buitenweg JR, *et al.* (2011) Somatosensory symptoms and signs and conditioned pain modulation in chronic post-stroke shoulder pain. *J Pain*, **12**, 476–85.

Rosen JA, Barsoum AH (1979) Failure of chronic dorsal column stimulation in multiple sclerosis. *Ann Neurol* **6**, 66–7.

Rosenberg JM, Harrell C, Ristic H, Werner RA, de Rosayro AM (1997) The effect of gabapentin on neuropathic pain. *Clin J Pain* **13**, 251–5.

Roser F, Ebner FH, Sixt C, Hagen JM, Tatagiba MS (2010) Defining the line between hydromyelia and syringomyelia. A differentiation is possible based on electrophysiological and magnetic resonance imaging studies. *Acta Neurochir (Wien)* **152**, 213–19.

Rosner H, Rubin L, Kestenbaum A (1996) Gabapentin adjunctive therapy in neuropathic pain states. *Clin J Pain* **12**, 56–8.

Rosomoff HL (1969) Bilateral percutaneous cervical radiofrequency cordotomy. *J Neurosurg* **31**, 41–6.

Rossi S, Mataluni G, Codecà C, *et al.* (2009) Effects of levetiracetam on chronic pain in multiple sclerosis: results of a pilot, randomized, placebo-controlled study. *Eur J Neurol* **16**, 360–6.

Rossini PM, Martino G, Narici L, *et al.* (1994) Short-term brain "plasticity" in humans: transient finger representation changes in sensory cortex somatotopy following ischemic anesthesia. *Brain Res* **642**, 169–77.

Rousseaux M, Cassim F, Bayle B, Laureau E (1999) Analysis of the perception of and reactivity to pain and heat in patients with Wallenberg syndrome and severe spinothalamic tract dysfunction. *Stroke* **30**, 2223–9.

Roussy G (1907) Les couches optiques: étude anatomique, physiologique et clinique. Thèse de Paris.

Roux FE, Ibarrola D, Lazorthes Y, Berry I (2001) Chronic motor cortex stimulation for phantom limb pain: a functional magnetic resonance imaging study: technical case report. *Neurosurgery* **48**, 681–7.

Rowbotham MC, Twilling L, Davies PS, *et al.* (2003) Oral opioid therapy for chronic peripheral and central neuropathic pain. *N Engl J Med* **348**, 1223–32.

Rudolph U, Antkowiak B (2004) Molecular and neuronal substrates for general anaesthetics. *Nat Rev Neurosci* **5**, 709–20.

Ruiz-Juretschke F, García-Salazar F, García-Leal R, *et al.* (2011) Tratamiento del dolor neuropático por desaferentización mediante lesión DREZ: resultados a largo plazo. *Neurologia* **26**, 26–31.

Ruiz-Ortiz S, Galvez R, Romero Cotelo J, *et al.* (2009) Intrathecal ziconotide combined with other two drugs in two cases of refractory spinal cord injury pain. *Eur J Pain* **13**, S260, A917.

Sackeim HA, Prudic J, Devanand DP, *et al.* (1993) Effects of stimulus intensity and electrode placement on the efficacy and cognitive effects of electroconvulsive therapy. *N Engl J Med* **328**, 839–46.

Sadaghiani S, Hesselmann G, Friston KJ, Kleinschmidt A (2010) The relation of ongoing brain activity, evoked neural responses, and cognition. *Front Systems Neurosci* **4**, art.20.

Sadiq SA, Poopatana CA (2007) Intrathecal baclofen and morphine in multiple sclerosis patients with severe pain and spasticity. *J Neurol* **254**, 1464–5.

Sadosky A, Dukes E (2007) Pain severity, management and patient functioning in central neuropathic pain: results from a cross-sectional survey in six European countries. *Eur J Pain* **11**, S136–7.

Sahni V, Kessler JA (2010) Stem cell therapies for spinal cord injury. *Nat Rev Neurol* **6**, 363–72.

Saitoh Y, Kato A, Ninomiya H, *et al.* (2000) Primary motor cortex stimulation within the central sulcus for treating deafferentation pain. *Acta Neurochir Suppl* **87**, 149–52.

Saitoh Y, Osaki Y, Nishimura H, *et al.* (2004) Increased regional cerebral blood flow in the contralateral thalamus after successful motor cortex stimulation in a patient with poststroke pain. *J Neurosurg* **100**, 935–9.

Saitoh Y, Hirayama A, Kishima H, *et al.* (2007) Reduction of intractable deafferentation pain due to spinal cord or peripheral lesion by high-frequency repetitive transcranial magnetic stimulation of the primary motor cortex. *J Neurosurg* **107**, 555–9.

Sakai T, Tomiyasu S, Ono T, Yamada H, Sumikawa K (2004) Multiple sclerosis with severe pain and allodynia alleviated by oral ketamine. *Clin J Pain* **20**, 375–6.

Sakas DE, Flaskas TN, Panourias IG, Georgakoulias N (2011) Bifocal cortical electrical stimulation for pain by interdural implantation of the electrodes. *J Neurosurg* **114**, 180–5.

Sakurai M, Kanazawa I (1999) Positive symptoms in multiple sclerosis: their treatment with sodium channel blockers, lidocaine and mexiletine. *J Neurol Sci* **162**, 1628.

Salmon JB, Hanna MH, Williams M, Toone B, Wheeler M (1988) Thalamic pain: the effect of electroconvulsive therapy. *Pain* **33**, 67–71.

Samii M, Moringlane JR (1984) Thermocoagulation of the dorsal root entry zone for the treatment of intractable pain. *Neurosurgery* **15**, 953–5.

Samkoff LM, Daras M, Tuchman AJ, Koppel BS (1997) Amelioration of refractory dysesthetic limb pain in multiple sclerosis by gabapentin. *Neurology* **49**, 304–5.

Sampson JH, Nashold BS (1992) Facial pain due to vascular lesions of the brain stem relieved by dorsal root entry zone lesions in the nucleus caudalis. Report of two cases. *J Neurosurg* **77**, 473–5.

Samuelsson M, Samuelsson L, Lindell D (1994) Sensory symptoms and signs and results of quantitative sensory thermal testing in patients with lacunar infarct syndromes. *Stroke* **25**, 2165–70.

Sandroni P (2002) Central neuropathic itch: a new treatment option? *Neurology* **59**, 778–9.

Sandyk R (1985) Spontaneous pain, hyperpathia and wasting of the hand due to parietal lobe haemorrhage. *Eur Neurol* **24**, 1–3.

Sanford PR, Lindblom LB, Haddox JD (1992) Amitriptyline and carbamazepine in the treatment of dysesthesia pain in spinal cord injury. *Arch Phys Medic Rehab* **73**, 300–1.

Sang C, Jenkins K, Wang K, Sarin A, Coccoli S (2006) Fosphenytoin relieves central neuropathic pain following spinal cord injury. *J Pain* **7** (Suppl 1), 2 A312/692.

Sano K (1977) Intralaminar thalamotomy (thalamolaminotomy) and posteromedial hypothalamotomy in the treatment of intractable pain. In: Krayenbühl H, Maspes PE, Sweet WH, eds., *Progress in Neurological Surgery. Pain – Its Neurosurgical Management: II. Central Procedures*. Basel: Karger, pp. 50–103.

Sano K, Yoshioka M, Ogashiwa M, Ishijima B, Ohye C (1966) Thalamolaminotomy: a new operation for relief of intractable pain. *Conf Neurol* **27**, 63–6.

Santos AB, Gozzani JL (2011) Acupuncture as adjuvant therapy in thalamic syndrome: case report. *Rev Bras Anestesiol* **61**, 88–94.

Sarnthein J, Jeanmonod D (2008) High thalamocortical theta coherence in patients with neurogenic pain. *Neuroimage* **39**, 1910–17.

Sarnthein J, Stern J, Aufenberg C, Rousson V, Jeanmonod D (2006) Increased EEG power and slowed dominant frequency in patients with neurogenic pain. *Brain* **129**, 55–64.

Sasaki M, Akebura M, Morris S, *et al.* (2009) Allodynia corresponding to the levels of cervical cord injury treated by surgical decompression: a report of 3 cases. *Surg Neurol* **72**, 281–5.

Saulino M (2007) Successful reduction of neuropathic pain associated with spinal cord injury via a combination of intrathecal hydromorphone and ziconotide: a case report. *Spinal Cord* **45**, 749–52.

Saulino M, Burton AW, Danyo DA, *et al.* (2009) Intrathecal ziconotide and baclofen provide pain relief in seven patients with neuropathic pain and spasticity: case reports. *Eur J Phys Rehabil Med* **45**, 61–7.

Savas A, Kanpolat Y (2005) Comment. *Neurosurgery* **56**, 296.

Scarff JE (1950) Unilateral prefrontal lobotomy for the relief of intractable pain. Report of 58 cases with special consideration of failures. *J Neurosurg* **7**, 330–6.

Schaefers M, Sommer C (2007) Anticytokine therapy in neuropathic pain management. *Expert Rev Neurother* **7**, 1613–27.

Schechtmann G, Lind G, Winter J, Meyerson B, Linderoth B (2010) Intrathecal clonidine and baclofen enhance the pain-relieving effect of spinal cord stimulation: a comparative placebo-controlled, randomized trial. *Neurosurgery* **67**, 173–81 (includes Lind *et al.*, *Eur J Pain* 2008, **12**, 132–6).

Schestatsky P, Kumru H, Valls-Solé J, *et al.* (2007) Neurophysiologic study of central pain in patients with Parkinson disease. *Neurology* **69**, 2162–9.

Schlaier JR, Eichhammer P, Langguth B, *et al.* (2007) Effects of spinal cord stimulation on cortical excitability in patients with chronic neuropathic pain: a pilot study. *Eur J Pain* **11**, 863–8.

Schmahmann JD, Leifer D (1992) Parietal pseudothalamic pain syndrome. Clinical features and anatomic correlates. *Arch Neurol* **49**, 1032–7.

Schoenen J, Grant G (2004) Spinal cord: connections. In: Paxinos G, Mai JK, eds., *The Human Nervous System*, 2nd edn. Amsterdam: Elsevier Academic Press, pp. 233–50.

Scholz J, Vieregge P, Moser A (1999) Central pain as a manifestation of partial epileptic seizures. *Pain* **80**, 445–50.

Schott B, Laurent B, Mauguire F (1986) Les douleurs thalamiques: étude critique de 43 cas. *Rev Neurol* **142**, 308–15.

Schott GD (1996) From thalamic syndrome to central poststroke pain. *J Neurol Neurosurg Psychiatry* **61**, 560–4.

Schott GD (2001) Delayed onset and resolution of pain: some observations and implications. *Brain* **124**, 1067–76.

Schott GD, Loh L (1984) Anticholinesterase drugs in the treatment of chronic pain. *Pain* **20**, 201–6.

Schvarcz JR (1977) Periaqueductal mesencephalotomy for facial central pain. In: Sweet WH, Obrador S, Martin-Rodriguez JG, eds., *Neurosurgical Treatment in*

Psychiatry, Pain and Epilepsy. Baltimore, MD: University Park Press, pp. 661–7.

Schvarcz JR (1980) Chronic self-stimulation of the medial posterior inferior thalamus for the alleviation of deafferentation pain. *Acta Neurochir Suppl* **20**, 295–301.

Schyns F, Coutts F (2007) Does TENS have an effect on neuropathic pain? A pilot study in MS. *J Pain Symptom Manage* **S189–90**, A428.

Scott AIF, Dougall N, Ross M, *et al.* (1994) Short-term effects of electroconvulsive treatment on the uptake of 99mTc-Exametazime into brain in major depression shown with single photon emission tomography. *J Affect Disord* **30**, 27–34.

Scrivani S, Wallin D, Moulton EA, *et al.* (2010) A fMRI evaluation of lamotrigine for the treatment of trigeminal neuropathic pain: pilot study. *Pain Med* **11**, 920–41.

Sedan R, Lazorthes Y (1978) La neurostimulation électrique thérapeutique. Soc. Neurochir. Langue Franc. XXVIII Congres Annuel Neurochirurgie, pp. 1–138.

Seghier ML, Lazayras F, Vuilleumier P, Schnider A, Carota A (2005) Functional magnetic resonance imaging and diffusion tensor imaging in a case of central poststroke pain. *J Pain* **6**, 208–12.

Semple DM, McIntosh AM, Lawrie SM (2005) Cannabis as a risk factor for psychosis: systematic review. *J Psychopharmacol* **19**, 187–94.

Seo WK, Kwon DY, Seo SH, Park MH, Park KW (2009) Neuropathic pruritus following Wallenberg syndrome. *Neurology* **72**, 676.

Serpell MG (2002) Gabapentin in neuropathic pain syndromes: a randomised, double-blind, placebo-controlled trial. Neuropathic Pain Study Group. *Pain* **99**, 557–66.

Seyal M, Shatzel AJ, Richardson SP (2005) Crossed inhibition of sensory cortex by 0.3 Hz transcranial magnetic stimulation of motor cortex. *J Clin Neurophysiol* **22**, 418–41.

Shabalov VA, Isagulyan ED, Tomskiy AA (2008) Motor cortex stimulation in the treatment of central pain syndromes. *Acta Neurochir (Wien)* **150**, 968 A11.

Shankar V, Kabazie A, Boyle A (2008) Use of an implantable intrathecal morphine pump in the treatment of refractory pain caused by thalamic syndrome. *J Pain* **9** (Suppl 2), 41, A261.

Shapiro PE, Braun CW (1987) Unilateral pruritus after a stroke. *Arch Dermatol* **123**, 1527–30.

Shepherd GM (2004) *The Synaptic Organization of the Brain*. Oxford: Oxford University Press.

Sherman SM, Guillery RW (2006) *Exploring the Thalamus and Its Role in Cortical function*. Cambridge, MA: MIT Press.

Shieff C (1991) Treatment of central deafferentation syndromes: thalamic syndrome. In: Nashold BS, Ovelmen-Levitt J, eds., *Deafferentation Pain Syndromes: Pathophysiology and Treatment*, New York, NY: Raven Press, pp. 285–90.

Shieff C, Nashold BS (1988) Thalamic pain and stereotactic mesencephalotomy. *Acta Neurochir (Wien) Suppl* **42**, 239–42 (same series appearing in *Br J Neurosurg* 1987, **1**, 305–10 and *Neurol Res* 1987, **9**, 101–4).

Shimodozono M, Kawahira K, Kamishita T, *et al.* (2002) Reduction of central poststroke pain with the selective serotonin reuptake inhibitor fluvoxamine. *Int J Neurosci* **112**, 1173–81.

Shimoji K, Higashi H, Kano T, *et al.* (1971) Electrical management of intractable pain. *Jpn J Anesthesiol* **20**, 444–7.

Shimoji K, Hokari T, Kano T, *et al.* (1993) Management of intractable pain with percutaneous epidural spinal cord stimulation: differences in pain-relieving effects among diseases and sites of pain. *Anesth Analg* **77**, 110–16.

Shulman R, Turnbull IM, Diewold P (1982) Psychiatric aspects of thalamic stimulation for neuropathic pain. *Pain* **13**, 127–35.

Siddall PJ, Gray M, Rutkowski S, Cousins MJ (1994) Intrathecal morphine and clonidine in the management of spinal cord injury pain: a case report. *Pain* **59**, 147–8.

Siddall PJ, Molloy AR, Walker S, *et al.* (2000) The efficacy of intrathecal morphine and clonidine in the treatment of pain after spinal cord injury. *Anesth Analg* **9**, 1493–8.

Siddall PJ, Cousins MJ, Otte A, *et al.* (2006) Pregabalin in central neuropathic pain associated with spinal cord injury: a placebo-controlled trial. *Neurology* **67**, 1792–800. (*see comment*: Kruszewski SP, Shane JA (2007) *Neurology* **68**, 2158–9)

Siegfried J (1977) Stereotactic pulvinarotomy in the treatment of intractable pain. *Progr Neurol Surg* **8**, 101–13.

Siegfried J (1991) Therapeutical neurostimulation: indications reconsidered. *Acta Neurochir (Wien) Suppl* **52**, 112–17.

Siegfried J, Krayenbühl H (1972) Clinical experience in the treatment of intractable pain. In: Janzen R, Keidel WD, Herz A, Steichele C, eds., *Pain: Basic Principles – Pharamacology – Therapy*. Stuttgart: Georg Thieme, pp. 202–4.

Silbergeld DL, Hebb AO, Loeser JD (2011) Vaginal allodynia as the presentation of a thalamic tumor. *Pain* **152**, 698–702.

Silver M, Blum D, Grainger D, Hammer AE, Quessy S (2007) Double-blind, placebo-controlled trial of lamotrigine in combination with other medications for neuropathic pain. *J Pain Symptom Manage* **34**, 446–54.

Silver ML (1957) "Central pain" from cerebral arteriovenous aneurysm. *J Neurosurg* **14**, 92–6.

Simpson BA (1991) Spinal cord stimulation in 60 cases of intractable pain. *J Neurol Neurosurg Psychiatry* **54**, 196–9.

Simpson BA (1999) Spinal cord stimulation. *Pain Rev* **1**, 199–230.

Sindou M, Keravel Y (1980) Analgésie par la méthode d'électrostimulation transcutanée. Résultats dans les douleurs d'origine neurologique. A propos de 180 cas. *Neurochirurgie* **26**, 153–7.

Sindou M, Mertens P, Garcia-Larrea L (2001) Surgical procedures for neuropathic pain. *Neurosurg Quart* **11**, 45–65.

Sindou M, Mertens P, Bendavid U, Garcia-Larrea L, Mauguiere F (2003) Predictive value of somatosensory evoked potentials for long-lasting pain relief after spinal cord stimulation: practical use for patient selection. *Neurosurgery* **52**, 1374–84.

Sist TC, Filadora VA, Miner M, Lema M (1997) Experience with gabapentin for neuropathic pain in the head and neck: report of ten cases. *Reg Anesth* **22**, 473–8.

Sitzmann L, Silhouette B, Margot-Duclot A, Andrianasolo H, Thiebaut JB (2007) Spinal cord stimulation in allodynic spinal cord injury (SCI) pain. *J Pain Symptom Manage* **S191**, A431.

Sjölund BH (1991) Role of transcutaneous electrical nerve stimulation, central nervous system stimulation, and ablative procedures in central pain syndromes. In: Casey KL, ed. *Pain and Central Nervous System Disease: the Central Pain Syndromes*. New York, NY: Raven Press, pp. 267–75.

Sjöqvist O (1950) La section chirurgicale des cordons et des voies de la douleur dans la moelle et le tronc cérébral. *Rev Neurol* **83**, 38–40.

Slawek J, Reclowicz D, Zielinski P, Sloniewski P, Nguyen JP (2005) [Motor cortex stimulation in the central pain syndrome] *Neurol Neurochir Pol* **39**, 237–40.

Slonimski M, Abram SE, Zuniga RE (2004) Intrathecal baclofen in pain management. *Reg Anesth Pain Med* **29**, 269–76.

Smith E, Joint C, Nandi D, Stein JF, Aziz TZ (2000) Motor cortex stimulation for neuropathic pain. *Neurosurg Focus* **11**, E2.

Smith KJ, McDonald WI (1982) Spontaneous and evoked electrical discharges from a central demyelinating lesion. *J Neurol Sci* **55**, 39–47.

Smith R (2006) *The Trouble With Medical Journals*. London: Royal Society of Medicine.

Smolik FA, Nash FP, Machek O (1960) Spinal cordectomy in the management of spastic paraplegia. *Am Surg* **26**, 639–45.

Sokal P, Harat M, Gryz J, Ackerman D (2006) [Motor cortex stimulation in the treatment of the central pain: a case report] *Neurol Neurochir Pol* **40**, 253–7.

Sol JC, Casaux J, Roux FE, *et al.* (2001) Chronic motor cortex stimulation for phantom limb pain: correlations between pain relief and functional imaging studies. *Stereotact Funct Neurosurg* **77**, 172–6.

Solaro C, Brichetto G, Amato MP, *et al.* and the PaIMS Study Group (2004) The prevalence of pain in multiple sclerosis: a multicenter cross-sectional study. *Neurology* **63**, 919–21.

Solaro C, Brichetto G, Battaglia MA, Messmer Uccelli M, Mancardi GL (2005) Antiepileptic medications in multiple sclerosis: adverse effects in a three-yer follow-up study. *Neurol Sci* **25**, 307–10.

Solaro C, Restivo D, Mancardi GL, Tanganelli P (2007) Oxcarbazepine for treating paroxysmal painful symptoms in multiple sclerosis: a pilot study. *Neurol Sci* **28**, 156–8.

Solaro C, Boehmker M, Tanganelli P (2009) Pregabalin for treating paroxysmal painful symptoms in multiple sclerosis: a pilot study. *J Neurol* **256**, 1773–4.

Soler D, Kumru H, Vidal J, *et al.* (2010) Transcranial direct current stimulation (tDCS) and virtual reality (VR) techniques for treatment of neuropathic central pain in spinal cord injury (NP-SCI). *Eur J Pain Suppl* **4**, 105, A370.

Soler MD, Kumru H, Vidal J, *et al.* (2010a) Referred sensations and neuropathic pain following spinal cord injury. *Pain* **150**, 192–8.

Soler MD, Kumru H, Pelayo R, *et al.* (2010b) Effectiveness of transcranial direct current stimulation and visual illusion on neuropathic pain in spinal cord injury. *Brain* **133**, 2565–77.

Son BC, Lee SW, Choi ES, *et al.* (2006) Motor cortex stimulation for central pain following a traumatic brain injury. *Pain* **123**, 210–16.

Sonnenberg A (2007) Why is academic medicine run by former C-students? *Med Hypotheses* **69**, 218–20.

Soria ED, Fine EJ (1991) Disappearance of thalamic pain after parietal subcortical stroke. *Pain* **44**, 285–8.

Spaic M, Markovic N, Tadic R (2002) Microsurgical DREZotomy for pain of spinal cord and cauda equina injury origin: clinical characteristics of pain and implications for surgery in a series of 26 patients. *Acta Neurochir (Wien)* **144**, 453–62.

Spiegel EA, Wycis HT, Freed H (1952) Stereoencephalotomy. Thalamotomy and related procedures. *J Am Med Assoc* **148**, 446–51.

Spiegel EA, Kletzkin M, Szekely EG, Wycis HT (1954) Role of hypothalamic mechanisms in thalamic pain. *Neurology* **4**, 735–51.

Spiegel EA, Wycis HT, Szekely EG, Gildenberg PL (1966) Medial and basal thalamotomy in so-called intractable pain. In: Knighton RS, Dumke PR, eds., *Pain*. Boston, MA: Little Brown, pp. 503–17.

Spiegelmann R, Friedman WA (1991) Spinal cord stimulation: a contemporary series. *Neurosurgery* **28**, 65–71.

Spooner J, Yu H, Kao C, Sillay K, Konrad P (2007) Neuromodulation of the cingulum for neuropathic pain after spinal cord injury: case report. *J Neurosurg* **107**, 169–72.

Sporns O (2011) *Networks of the Brain*. Cambridge, MA: MIT Press.

Sprenger T, Valet T, Woltmann R, *et al.* (2006) Imaging pain modulation by subanesthetic S-(+)-ketamine. *Anesth Analg* **103**, 729–37.

Sriram S, Steiner I (2005) Experimental allergic encephalomyelitis: a misleading model of multiple sclerosis. *Ann Neurol* **58**, 939–45.

Stancak A, Hoechstetter K, Tintera J, *et al.* (2002) Source activity in the human secondary somatosensory cortex

depends on the size of corpus callosum. *Brain Res* **936**, 47–57.
Stancak A, Kozak J, Vrba I, *et al.* (2008) Functional magnetic resonance imaging of cerebral activation during spinal cord stimulation in failed back surgery syndrome patients. *Eur J Pain* **12**, 137–48.
Stanwell P, Siddall P, Keshava N, *et al.* (2010) Neuro magnetic resonance spectroscopy using wavelet decomposition and statistical testing identifies biochemical changes in people with spinal cord injury and pain. *Neuroimage* **53**, 544–52.
Starr CJ, Sawaki L, Wittenberg GF, *et al.* (2009) Roles of the insular cortex in the modulation of pain: insights from brain lesions. *J Neurosci* **29**, 2684–94.
Stavraky GW (1961) *Supersensitivity Following Lesions of the Nervous System.* Toronto: University of Toronto Press.
Stein BE, Price DD, Gazzaniga MS (1989) Pain perception in a man with total corpus callosum transection. *Pain* **38**, 51–6.
Stenager E, Knudsen L, Jensen K (1991) Acute and chronic pain syndromes in multiple sclerosis. *Acta Neurol Scand* **84**, 197–200.
Stern J, Jeanmonod D, Sarnthein J (2006) Persistent EEG overactivation in the cortical pain matrix of neurogenic pain patients. *Neuroimage* **31**, 721–31.
Stone TT (1950) Phantom limb pain and central pain. Relief by ablation of portion of posterior central cerebral convolution. *Arch Neurol Psychiatry* **63**, 739–48.
Stoodley MA, Warren JD, Oatey PE (1995) Thalamic syndrome caused by unruptured cerbral aneurysm. Case report. *J Neurosurg* **82**, 291–3.
Strong K, Mathers C, Bonita R (2007) Preventing stroke: saving lives around the world. *Lancet Neurol* **6**, 182–7.
Sugita K, Mutsuga N, Rakaoka T, Doi T (1972) Results of stereotaxic thalamotomy for pain. *Conf Neurol* **34**, 265–74.
Sullivan MJ, Drake ME. (1984) Unilateral pruritus and nocardia brain abscess. *Neurology* **34**, 828–9.
Summers CG, MacDonald JT (1988) Paroxysmal facial itch: a presenting sign of childhood brainstem glioma. *J Child Neurol* **3**, 189–92.
Summers JD, Rapoff MA, Varghese G, Porter K, Palmer RE (1991) Psychosocial factors in chronic spinal cord injury. *Pain* **47**, 183–9.
Sun X, Zhang H, Gao C, *et al.* (2008) Imaging the effects of propofol on human cerebral glucose metabolism using positron emission tomography. *J Int Med Res* **36**, 1305–10.
Suzuki M, Davis C, Symon L, Gentili F (1985) Syringoperitoneal shunt for treatment of cord cavitation. *J Neurol Neurosurg Psychiatry* **48**, 620–7.
Svendsen KB, Jensen TS, Bach FW (2004) Does the cannabinoid dronabinol reduce central pain in multiple sclerosis? Randomised double blind placebo controlled crossover trial. *BMJ* **329**, 253.
Svendsen KB, Jensen TS, Hansen HJ, Bach FW (2005) Sensory function and quality of life in patients with multiple sclerosis and pain. *Pain* **114**, 473–81.
Svendsen KB, Sørensen L, Jensen TS, Hansen HJ, Bach FW (2011) MRI of the central nervous system in MS patients with and without pain. *Eur J Pain* **15**, 395–401.
Sweet WH, Poletti CE (1989) Operations in the brain stem and cord, with an appendix on open cordotomy. In: Wall PD, Melzack R, eds., *Textbook of Pain*, 2nd edn. Edinburgh: Churchill Livingstone, pp. 811–31.
Sweet WH, Wepsic JG (1974) Stimulation of pain suppressor mechanisms. A critique of some current methods. *Adv Neurol* **4**, 734–46.
Sweet WH, Wepsic J (1975) Stimulation of the posterior columns of the spinal cord for pain control. *Surg Neurol* **4**, 133.
Swenson JR, Doucette S, Fergusson D (2006) Adverse cardiovascular events in antidepressant trials involving high-risk patients: a systematic review of randomized trials. *Can J Psychiatry* **51**, 923–9.
Tai Q, Kirschblum S, Chen B, *et al.* (2002) Gabapentin in the treatment of neuropathic pain after spinal cord injury: a prospective, randomized, double-blind, crossover trial. *J Spinal Cord Med* **25**, 100–5.
Taira T, Hori T (2007) Intrathecal baclofen in the treatment of post-stroke central pain, dystonia, and persistent vegetative state. *Acta Neurochir Suppl* **97**, 227–9.
Taira T, Tanikawa T, Kawamura H, Iseki H, Takakura K (1994) Spinal intrathecal baclofen suppresses central pain after a stroke. *J Neurol Neurosurg Psychiatry* **57**, 381–2.
Taira T, Kawamura H, Tanikawa T, *et al.* (1995) A new approach to control central deafferentation pain: spinal intrathecal baclofen. *Stereotact Funct Neurosurg* **65**, 101–5 (see also Taira T, *Pain* 1998, **78**, 221–6).
Takahashi Y, Hashimoto K, Tsuji S (2004) Successful use of zonisamide for central poststroke pain. *J Pain* **5**, 192–4.
Takano M, Takano Y, Sato I (1999) The effect of oral amantadine in chronic pain patients with positive ketamine challenge test. In: *9th World Congress on Pain, Book of Abstracts.* Seattle, WA: IASP Press, Abst. 220–P68.
Talairach J (1955) Chirurgie stéréotaxique du thalamus. Bases anatomiques et techniques. Indications et résultats thérapeutiques. VI Congr Lat Am Neurocir (Montevideo), pp. 865–925.
Talairach J, Hecaen H, David M, Monnier M, De Ajuraguerra J (1949) Recherches sur la coagulation thérapeutique des structures souscorticales chez l'homme. *Rev Neurol* **81**, 4–24.
Talbot JD, Villemure JG, Bushnell MC, Duncan GH (1995) Evaluation of pain perception after anterior capsulotomy: a case report. *Somatosens Mot Res* **12**, 115–26.
Tan G, Rintala DH, Thornby JI, *et al.* (2006) Using cranial electrotherapy stimulation to treat pain associated with spinal cord injury. *J Rehabil Res Dev* **43**, 461–74.
Tanaka E, Tobita T, Murai Y, *et al.* (2009) Thiamylal antagonizes the inhibitory effects of dorsal column stimulation on dorsal horn activities in humans. *Neurosci Res* **64**, 391–6.
Tanei T, Kajita Y, Wakabayashi T (2010) Motor cortex stimulation for intractable neuropathic facial pain related to multiple sclerosis. *Neurol Med Chir (Tokyo)* **50**, 604–7.

Tanei T, Kajita Y, Noda H, *et al.* (2011) Efficacy of motor cortex stimulation for intractable central neuropathic pain : comparison of stimulation parameters between post-stroke pain and other central pain. *Neurol Med Chir (Tokyo)* **51**, 8–14.

Tani N, Saitoh Y, Hirata M, *et al.* (2004) Bilateral cortical stimulation for deafferentation pain after spinal cord injury. *J Neurosurg* **101**, 687–9.

Tanriverdi T, Al-Jehani H, Poulin N, Olivier A (2009) Functional results of electrical cortical stimulation of the lower sensory strip. *J Clin Neurosci* **16**, 1188–94.

Tasker RR (1989) Stereotactic surgery. In: Wall PD, Melzack R, eds., *Textbook of Pain*, 2nd edn. Edinburgh: Churchill Livingstone, pp. 840–55.

Tasker RR (1990) Thalamotomy. *Neurosurg Clin N Am* **1**, 84–6.

Tasker RR (2001a) Central pain states. In: Loeser JD, ed., *Bonica's Management of Pain*, 3rd edn. Philadelphia, PA: Lippincott Williams & Wilkins, pp. 433–57 (see also previous edn, 1990).

Tasker RR (2001b) Microelectrode findings in the thalamus in chronic pain and other conditions. *Stereotact Funct Neurosurg* **77**, 166–8.

Tasker RR, Dostrovsky J (1989) Deafferentation and central pain. In: Wall PD, Melzack R, eds., *Textbook of Pain*. London: Churchill-Livingstone, pp. 154–80.

Tasker RR, North RB (1997) Cordotomy and myelotomy. In: North RB, Levy RM, eds., *Neurosurgical Management of Pain*. New York, NY: Springer, pp. 191–220.

Tasker RR, Organ LW, Hawrylyshyn P (1980) Deafferentation and causalgia. In: Bonica JJ, ed., *Pain*. New York: Raven Press, pp. 305–30.

Tasker RR, Tsuda T, Hawrylyshyn P (1983) Clinical neurophysiological investigation of deafferentation pain. *Adv Pain Res Ther* **5**, 713–38.

Tasker RR, DeCarvalho G, Dostrovsky JO (1991) The history of central pain syndromes, with observations concerning the pathophysiology and treatment. In: Casey KL, ed., *Pain and Central Nervous System Disease. The Central Pain Syndromes*. New York, NY: Raven Press, pp. 31–58.

Tasker RR, DeCarvalho GTC, Dolan EJ (1992) Intractable pain of spinal cord origin: clinical features and implications for surgery. *J Neurosurg* **77**, 373–8.

Tasker RR, Parrent AG, Kiss Z, Davis K, Dostrovsky JO (1994) Surgical treatment of stroke-induced pain. *Stereotact Funct Neurosurg* **62**, 311–12.

Tator CH, Agbi CB (1991) Complications in the management of syringomyelia. *Perspect Neurol Surg* **2**, 143–50.

Taub E, Munz M, Tasker RR (1997) Chronic electrical stimulation of the gasserian ganglion for the relief of pain in a series of 34 patients. *J Neurosurg* **86**, 197–202.

Taylor C (2009) Reply to: Devor M. How does gabapentin relieve neuropathic pain? *Pain* **145**, 259–61.

Teixeira MJ (1998) Various functional procedures for pain: II. Facial pain. In: Gildenberg PL, Tasker RR, eds., *Textbook of Stereotactic and Functional Neurosurgery*. New York, NY: McGraw-Hill, pp. 1389–402.

Teixeira MJ, Lepski G, Aguiar PHP, *et al.* (2003) Bulbar trigeminal stereotactic nucleotractotomy for treatment of facial pain. *Stereotact Funct Neurosurg* **81**, 37–42.

Terney D, Bergmann I, Poreisz C, *et al.* (2008) Pergolide increases the efficacy of cathodal direct current stimulation to reduce the amplitude of laser-evoked potential in humans. *J Pain Symptom Manage* **36**, 79–91.

Thieme K, Turk DC, Flor H (2007) Responder criteria for operant and cognitive-behavioral treatment in fibromyalgia. *Arthritis Rheum* **15**, 830–6.

Thomas DGT, Jones SJ (1984) Dorsal root entry zone lesions (Nashold's procedure) in brachial plexus avulsion. *Neurosurgery* **15**, 966–8.

Thomas-Anterion C, Creac'h C, Dionet E, *et al.* (2010) De novo artistic activity following insular-SII ischemia. *Pain* **150**, 121–7.

Thompson SC (1981) Will it hurt less if I can control it? A complex answer to a simple question. *Psychol Bull* **90**, 89–101.

Thomson AM (2010) Neocortical layer 6, a review. *Front Neuroanat* **4**, art. 13.

Tirakotai W, Riegel T, Sure U, *et al.* (2004) Image-guided motor cortex stimulation in patients with central pain. *Minim Invas Neurosurg* **47**, 273–7.

To TP, Lim TC, Hill ST, *et al.* (2002) Gabapentin for neuropathic pain following spinal cord injury. *Spinal Cord* **40**, 282–5.

Tommerdahl M, Favorov OV, Whitsel BL (2010) Dynamic representations of the somatosensory cortex. *Neurosci Biobehav Rev* **34**, 160–70.

Tomycz ND, Deibert CP, Moossy JJ (2011) Cervicomedullary junction spinal cord stimulation for head and facial pain. *Headache* **51**, 418–25.

Tong DM, Zhou YT, Wang GS, *et al.* (2010) Hemorrhagic pure sensory strokes in the thalamus and striatocapsular area: causes, clinical features and long-term outcome. *Eur Neurol* **64**, 275–9.

Torvik A (1959) Sensory, motor and reflex changes in two cases of intractable pain after stereotactic mesencephalic tractotomy. *J Neurol Neurosurg Psychiatry* **22**, 299–305.

Toth S, Sólyom A, Toth Z (1984) One possible mechanism of central pain. Autokindling phenomenon on the phantom limb or sensory loss oriented patients. *Acta Neurochir (Wien)* Suppl **33**, 459–69.

Tourian AY (1987) Narcotic responsive "thalamic" pain treatment with propranolol and tricyclic antidepressants. *Pain Suppl* **4**, 411.

Tourian AY (1991) Deafferentation syndrome: medical treatment. In: Nashold BS, Ovelmen-Levitt J, eds., *Deafferentation Pain Syndromes. Pathophysiology and Treatment*. New York, NY: Raven Press, pp. 331–40.

Tracey I, Bushnell C (2009) How neuroimaging studies have challenged us to rethink: is chronic pain a disease? *J Pain* **10**, 1113–20.

Trappenberg TP (2010) *Fundamentals of Computational Neuroscience*, 2nd edn. Oxford: Oxford University Press.

Tremont-Lukats IW, Challapalli V, McNicol ED, Lau J, Carr DB (2005) Systemic administration of local anesthetics to relieve neuropathic pain: a systematic review and meta-analysis. *Anesth Analg* **101**, 1738–49.

Trentin L, Visentin M (2000) La predittività del test con lidocaina nel trattamento del dolore neuropatico. *Minerva Anestesiol* **66**, 157–61.

Triggs WJ, Beric A (1992) Sensory abnormalities and dysaesthesias in the anterior spinal artery syndrome. *Brain* **115**, 189–98.

Tronnier V, Rasche D (2009) Precentral stimulation for different neuropathic pain syndromes.clinical experience of 15 years. *Eur J Pain* **13**, S48, A138.

Tsai MD, Wang ADJ, Wei CP, Tsai MC (2010) Neuropathic pain following spinal cord trauma treated with cingulotomy: report of two cases. *Eur J Pain* 2010 suppl 4, 121 A428.

Tsai PS, Buerkle H, Huang LT, *et al.* (1998) Lidocaine concentrations in plasma and cerebrospinal fluid after systemic bolus administrations in humans. *Anesth Analg* **87**, 601–4.

Tseng SH (2000) Treatment of chronic pain by spinal cord stimulation. *J Formos Med Assoc* **99**, 267–71.

Tsubokawa T, Yamamoto T, Katayama T, Hirayama T, Sibuya H (1984) Thalamic relay nucleus stimulation for relief of intractable pain. Clinical results and beta-endorphin immunoreactivity in the cerebrospinal fluid. *Pain* **18**, 115–26.

Tsubokawa T, Katayama Y, Yamamoto T, Hirayama T (1985) Deafferentation pain and stimulation of the thalamic sensory relay nucleus: clinical and experimental study. *Appl Neurophysiol* **48**, 166–71.

Tsubokawa T, Katayama Y, Yamamoto T, Hirayama T, Koyama S (1991a) Treatment of thalamic pain by chronic motor cortex stimulation. *PACE Pacing Clin Electrophysiol* **14**, 131–4.

Tsubokawa T, Katayama Y, Yamamoto T, *et al.* (1991b) Chronic motor cortex stimulation for the treatment of central pain. *Acta Neurochirurgica Suppl* **52**, 137–9.

Tsubokawa T, Katayama Y, Yamamoto T, *et al.* (1993) Chronic motor cortex stimulation in patients with thalamic pain. *J Neurosurg* **78**, 393–401.

Tulgar M, McGlone F, Bowsher D, Miles JB (1991) Comparative effectiveness of different stimulation modes in relieving pain. Part II. A double-blind controlled long-term clinical trial. *Pain* **47**, 157–62.

Turk DC, Dworkin RH, McDermott MP, *et al.* (2008) Analyzing multiple endpoints in clinical trials of pain treatment: IMMPACT recommendations. *Pain* **139**, 485–93.

Turnbull IM (1972) Bilateral cingulumotomy combined with thalamotomy or mesencephalic tractotomy for pain. *Surg Gynecol Obstet* **134**, 958–62.

Turnbull IM (1984) Brain stimulation. In: Wall PD, Melzack R, eds., *Textbook of Pain*, Edinburgh: Churchill Livingstone, pp. 706–14.

Turner JA, Lee JS, Schandler SL, Cohen MJ (2003) An fMRI investigation of hand representation in paraplegic humans. *Neurorehab Neural Repair* **17**, 37–47.

Turton AJ, Butler SR (2001) Referred sensations following stroke. *Neurocase* **7**, 397–405.

Tuveson B, Leffler AS, Hansson P (2009) Influence of heterotopic noxious conditioning stimulation on spontaneous pain and dynamic mechanical allodynia in central post-stroke pain patients. *Pain* **143**, 84–91.

Uhlhaas PJ, Pipa G, Lima B, *et al.* (2009) Neural synchrony in cortical networks: history, concept and current status. *Front Integr Neurosci* **3**, art.17.

Uhle EI, Becker R, Gatscher S, Bertalanffy H (2000) Continuous intrathecal clonidine administration for the treatment of neuropathic pain. *Stereotact Funct Neurosurg* **75**, 167–75.

Umesaki A, Uno H, Niki H, *et al.* (2009) A case of cortical infarction with isolated sensory disturbance in the c8 nerve root area. *Eur Neurol* **62**, 124.

Urban BJ, Nashold BS (1978) Percutaneous epidural stimulation of the spinal cord for relief of pain. *J Neurosurg* **48**, 323–8.

Utsuki S, Oka H, Miyajima Y, Fujii K (2009) Usefulness of gamma knife pituitary surgery to control thalamic pain after treatment of thalamic malignant lymphoma and report of pathology of gamma knife lesions. *Neurol India* **57**, 185–7.

Van Bastelaere M, De Laat M (1999) Lamotrigine: a morphine-sparing drug for central pain. In: *9th World Congress on Pain, Book of Abstracts*. Seattle, WA: IASP Press, A211–P65.

Van de Kelft E, De La Porte C (1994) Long-term pain relief during spinal cord stimulation: the effect of patient selection. *Qual Life Res* **3**, 21–7.

Van der Bruggen MA, Huisman HB, Beckermann H, *et al.* (2001) Randomized trial of 4-aminopyridine in patients with chronic incomplete spinal cord injury. *J Neurol* **248**, 665–71.

Van Wagenen WP, Herren RY (1940) Surgical division of commissural pathways in the corpus callosum. *Arch Neurol Psychiatry* **44**, 740–59.

Vanzetta I, Slovin H (2010) A BOLD assumption. *Front Neuroenergetics* **2**, art. 24.

Vartiainen N, Kirveskari E, Kallio-Laine K, Kalso E, Forss N (2009) Cortical reorganization in primary somatosensory cortex in patients with unilateral chronic pain. *J Pain* **10**, 854–9.

Vedula SS, Bero L, Scherer RW, Dickersin K (2009) Outcome reporting in industry-sponsored trials of gabapentin for off-label use. *N Engl J Med* **361**, 1963–71.

Vega-Bermudez F, Johnson KO (2002) Spatial acuity after digit amputation. *Brain* **125**, 1256–64.

Velasco M, Brito F, Jimenez F, *et al.* (1998) Effect of fentanyl and naloxone on a thalamic induced painful response in intractable epileptic patients. *Stereotact Funct Neurosurg* **71**, 90–102.

Velasco M, Velasco F, Brito F, *et al.* (2002) Motor cortex stimulation in the treatment of deafferentation pain.

I. Localisation of the motor cortex. *Stereotact Funct Neurosurg* **79**, 146–67.

Velasco F, Arguelles C, Carrillo-Ruiz JD, *et al.* (2008) Efficacy of motor cortex stimulation in the treatment of neuropathic pain: a randomized double-blind trial. *J Neurosurg* **108**, 698–706.

Veldhuijzen DS, Greenspan JD, Kim JH, Lenz FA (2010) Altered pain and thermal sensation in subjects with isolated parietal and insular cortical lesions. *Eur J Pain* **14**, 535.e1–11.

Velik R (2010) From single neuron firing to consciousness: towards the true solution of the binding problem. *Neurosci Biobehav Rev* **34**, 993–1001.

Verdugo R, Ochoa JL (1991) High incidence of placebo responders among chronic neuropathic pain patients. *Ann Neurol* **30**, 229.

Verkhratsky A, Parpura V, Rodriguez JJ (2011) Where the thoughts dwell: the physiology of neuronal–glial "diffuse neural net". *Brain Res Rev* **66**, 133–51.

Veselis RA, Feshchenko VA, Reinsel RA, *et al.* (2004) Thiopental and propofol affect different regions of the brain at similar pharmacologic effects. *Anesth Analg* **99**, 399–408.

Vesper J (2010) Chronic motor cortex stimulation and predictive value of rTMS. *Eur J Pain Suppl* **4**, 135 A476.

Vestergaard K, Nielsen J, Andersen G, *et al.* (1995) Sensory abnormalities in consecutive, unselected patients with central post-stroke pain. *Pain* **61**, 177–86.

Vestergaard K, Andersen G, Jensen TS (1996) Treatment of central post-stroke pain with a selective serotonin reuptake inhibitor. *Eur J Neurol* **3** (Suppl 5), 169.

Vestergaard K, Andersen G, Gottrup H, Kristensen BT, Jensen TS (2001) Lamotrigine for central poststroke pain: a randomized controlled trial. *Neurology* **56**, 184–90.

Vick PG, Lamer TJ (2001) Treatment of central post-stroke pain with oral ketamine. *Pain* **92**, 311–13.

Vierck CJ (1973) Alterations of spatio-tactile discrimination after lesions of primate spinal cord. *Brain Res* **58**, 69–79.

Villemure C, Wassimi S, Bennett GJ, Shir Y, Bushnell MC (2006) Unpleasant odors increase pain processing in a patient with neuropathic pain: psychophysical and fMRI investigation. *Pain* **120**, 213–20.

Vogel HP, Heppner B, Humbs N, Schramm J, Wagner C (1986) Long term effects of spinal cord stimulation in chronic pain syndromes. *J Neurol* **233**, 16–18.

Von Hagen KO (1957) Chronic intolerable pain: discussion of its mechanism and report of eight cases treated with electroshock. *J Am Med Assoc* **165**, 773–7.

Vranken JH, Dijkgraaf MG, Kruis MR, van Dasselaar NT, van der Vegt MH (2005) Iontophoretic administration of S(+)-ketamine in patients with intractable central pain: a placebo-controlled trial. *Pain* **118**, 224–31.

Vranken JH, Dijkgraaf MGW, Kruis MR, *et al.* (2008) Pregabalin in patients with central neuropathic pain: a randomized, double-blind, placebo-controlled trial of a flexible-dose regimen. *Pain* **136**, 150–7.

Vranken JH, Hollmann MW, van der Vegt MH, *et al.* (2011) Duloxetine in patients with central neuropathic pain caused by spinal cord injury or stroke: a randomized, double-blind, placebo-controlled trial. *Pain* **152**, 267–73 .

Vuadens PH, Regli F, Dolivo M, Uske A (1994) Segmental pruritus and intramedullary vascular formation. *Schw Arch Neurol Psych* **145**, 13–16.

Vul E, Harris C, Winkielman P, Pashler H (2009) Puzzlingly high correlations in fMRI studies of emotion, personality, and social cognition. *Perspect Psychol Sci* **4**, 274–90.

Wade DT, Robson P, House H, Makela P, Aram J (2003) A preliminary controlled study to determine whether whole-plant cannabis extracts can improve intractable neurogenic symptoms. *Clin Rehabil* **17**, 21–9.

Wade DT, Makela P, Robson P, House H, Bateman C (2004) Do cannabis-based medicinal extracts have general or specific effects on symptoms in multiple sclerosis? A double-blind, randomized, placebo-controlled study on 160 patients. *Mult Scler* **10**, 434–41.

Waijima Z, Shitara T, Inoue T, Ogawa R (2000) Severe lightning pain after subarachnoid block in a patient with neuropathic pain of central origin: which drug is best to treat the pain? *Clin J Pain* **16**, 265–9.

Walker AE (1942a) Relief of pain by mesencephalic tractotomy. *Arch Neurol Psychiatry* **48**, 865–83.

Walker AE (1942b) Mesencephalic tractotomy. A method for the relief of unilateral intractable pain. *Arch Surg* **44**, 953–62.

Walker AE (1950) The neurosurgical treatment of intractable pain. *Lancet* **70**, 279–82.

Wall P (1988) Stability and instability of pain mechanisms. In: Dubner R, Gebhart GF, Bond MR, eds., *Proceedings of the 5th World Congress on Pain*. Amsterdam: Elsevier, pp. 13–24.

Wall PD (1995) Pain in the brain and lower parts of the anatomy. *Pain* **62**, 389–91.

Wallace MS, Charapata SG, Fisher R, *et al.* (2006) Intrathecal ziconotide in the treatment of chronic nonmalignant pain: a randomized, double-blind,placebo-controlled clinical trial. *Neuromodulation* **9**, 75–86.

Wallace MS, Rauck R, Fisher R, *et al.* (2008) Intrathecal ziconotide for severe chronic pain: safety and tolerability results of an open-label, long term trial. *Anesth Analg* **106**, 628–37.

Waltz TA, Ehni G (1966) The thalamic syndrome and its mechanisms. Report of two cases, one due to arteriovenous malformation in the thalamus. *J Neurosurg* **24**, 735–42.

Wang J, Zuo X, He Y (2010) Graph-based network analysis of resting-state functional MRI. *Front Systems Neurosci* **4**, 1–12.

Wang T, Collet JP, Shapiro S, Ware MA (2008) Adverse effects of medical cannabinoids: a systematic review. *CMAJ* **178**, 1669–78.

Wang X, Unui K, Kakigi R (2007) Early cortical activities evoked by noxious stimulation in humans. *Exp Brain Res* **180**, 481–9.

Warms CA, Turner JA, Marshall HM, Cardenas DD (2002) Treatments for chronic pain associated with spinal cord

injuries: many are tried, few are helpful. *Clin J Pain* **18**, 154–163.
Wasan AD, Artin K, Clark MR (2004) A case-matching study of the analgesic properties of electroconvulsive therapy. *Pain Med* **5**, 50–8.
Wasner G, Naleschinski D, Binder A, *et al.* (2008a) The effect of menthol on cold allodynia in patients with neuropathic pain. *Pain Med* **9**, 354–8.
Wasner G, Lee BB, Engel S, McLachlan E (2008b) Residual spinothalamic tract pathways predict development of central pain after spinal cord injury. *Brain* **131**, 2387–400.
Watt EE, Betts BA, Kotey FO, *et al.* (2008) Menthol shares general anesthetic activity and sites of action on the GABA(A) receptor with the intravenous agent, propofol. *Eur J Pharmacol* **590**, 120–6.
Waxman SG (2010) Channelopathic pain: a growing but still small list of model disorders. *Neuron* **66**, 622–4.
Weber H (1904) Ueber Anaesthesie durch Adrenalin. *Verh Dtsch Ges Inn Med* **21**, 616.
Webster LR, Fisher R, Charapata S, Wallace MS (2009) Long-term intrathecal ziconotide for chronic pain: an open-label study. *J Pain Symptom Manage* **37**, 363–72.
Weigel R, Krauss JK (2004) Center median-parafascicular complex and pain control. *Stereotact Funct Neurosurg* **82**, 115–26.
Weimar C, Kloke M, Schlott M, Katsarava Z, Diener HC (2002) Central poststroke pain in a consecutive cohort of stroke patients. *Cerebrovasc Dis* **14**, 261–3.
Werhagen L, Hultling C, Borg K (2010) Pain, especially neuropathic pain, in adults with spina bifida, and its relation to age, neurological level, completeness, gender and hydrocephalus. *J Rehabil Med* **42**, 374–6.
Werhahn KJ, Mortensen J, Kaelin-Lang A, Boroojerdi B, Cohen LG (2002) Cortical excitability changes induced by deafferentation of the contralateral hemisphere. *Brain* **125**, 1402–13.
Werner A (1961) Myélectomie dans un cas de paraplégie spastique douloureux. *Neurochirurgie* **7**, 140–5.
Wertheimer P, Mansuy L (1949) Reflexions sur la topectomie préfrontale. *Rev Neurol* **81**, 866–71.
Wessel K, Vieregge P, Kessler CH, Kömpf D (1994) Thalamic stroke: correlation of clinical symptoms, somatosensory evoked potentials, and CT findings. *Acta Neurol Scand* **90**, 167–73.
Wester K (1987) Dorsal column stimulation in pain treatment. *Acta Neurol Scand* **75**, 151–5.
Whitaker R (2010) *Anatomy of an Epidemic: Magic Bullets, Psychiatric Drugs, and the Astonishing Rise of Mental Illness in America*. New York, NY: Crown.
White JC (1963) Anterolateral chordotomy: its effectiveness in relieving pain of non-malignant disease. *Neurochirurgia (Stuttgart)* **6**, 83–102.
White JC, Sweet WH (1955) *Pain: Its Mechanisms and Neurosurgical Control*. Springfield, IL: Thomas.
White JC, Sweet WH (1969) *Pain and the Neurosurgeon: a Forty-Year Experience*. Springfield, IL: Thomas.
Widar M, Samuelsson L, Karlsson-Tivenius S, Ahlstroem G (2002) Long-term pain conditions after a stroke. *J Rehabil Med* **34**, 165–70.
Widar M, Ek AC, Ahlstroem G (2004) Coping with long-term pain after a stroke. *J Pain Symptom Manage* **27**, 215–25 (see also *J Clin Nurs* **13**, 497–505).
Widerström-Noga EG, Turk DC (2003) Types and effectiveness of treatments used by people with chronic pain associated with spinal cord injuries: influence of pain and psychosocial characteristics. *Spinal Cord* **41**, 600–9.
Widerström-Noga EG, Turk DC (2004) Exarcerbation of chronic pain following spinal cord injury. *J Neurotrauma* **21**, 1384–95.
Widerström-Noga EG, Felipe-Cuervo E, Yezierski RP (2001) Relationships among clinical characteristics of chronic pain after spinal cord injury. *Arch Phys Med Rehabil* **82**, 1191–7.
Widerström-Noga EG, Cruz-Almeida Y, Felix ER, Adcock JP (2009) Relationship between pain characteristics and pain adaptation type in persons with SCI. *J Rehabil Dev* **46**, 43–56.
Wiegand H, Winkelmuller W (1985) Behandlung des Deafferentierungsschmerzes durch Hochfrequenzläsion der Hinterwurzeleintrittszone. *Dtsch Med Wochenschr* **110**, 216–20.
Wiesner T, Leinweber B, Quasthoff S, *et al.* (2007) Itch, skin lesions – and a stiff neck. *Lancet* **370**, 290.
Wilke HJ (2008) Animal models for spinal research. *Eur Spine J* **17**, 1.
Willis WD (1991) Central neurogenic pain: possible mechanisms. *Adv Pain Res Ther* **19**, 81–102.
Willoch F, Schindler F, Wester HJ, *et al.* (2004) Central poststroke pain and reduced opioid receptor binding within pain processing circuitries: a [11C] diprenorphine PET study. *Pain* **108**, 213–20.
Wilsey B, Marcotte T, Tsodikov A, *et al.* (2008) A randomized, placebo-controlled, crossover trial of cannabis cigarettes in neuropathic pain. *J Pain* **9**, 506–21.
Wine WA, Ko GD, Tumarkin EJ (2007) Case series of multiple sclerosis patients with neuropathic pain improved with the oral cannabinoid nabilone. *Eur J Pain* **11** (Suppl 1), 139.
Winkelmuller M, Winkelmuller W (1996) Long-term effects of continuous intrathecal opioid treatment in chronic pain of nonmalignant etiology. *J Neurosurg* **85**, 458–67.
Wirth ED, Vierck CJ, Reier PJ, Fessler RG, Anderson DK (2002) Correlation of MRI findings with spinal cord injury pain following neural tissue grafting into patients with posttraumatic syringomyelia. *Progr Pain Res Manage* **23**, 313–30.
Wolksee PJ, Gracely RH, Greenberg RP, Dubner R, Lees D (1982) Comparison of effects of morphine and deep brain stimulation on chronic pain. *Am Pain Soc* Abst. 36.
Wongsarnpigoon A, Grill WM (2009) Optimization of parameter selection and electrical targeting. In: Canavero S, ed., *Textbook of Therapeutic Cortical Stimulation*. New York, NY: Nova Science, pp. 69–90.

Wood T, Sloan R (1997) Successful use of ketamine for central pain. *Palliat Med* **11**, 57.

Woolsey CN, Erickson TC, Gilson WE (1979) Localization in somatic sensory and motor areas of human cerebral cortex as determined by direct recording of evoked potentials and electrical stimulation. *J Neurosurg* **51**, 476–506.

Wright A (1870) Oil of peppermint as a local anaesthetic. *Lancet* **2464**, 726.

Wrigley PJ, Press SR, Gustin SM, *et al.* (2009) Neuropathic pain and primary somatosensory cortex reorganization following spinal cord injury. *Pain* **141**, 52–9.

Wu YT, Chiang SL, Lai MH, *et al.* (2010) Methylprednisolone worsening neuropathic pain in non-traumatic thoracic myelopathy. *J Clin Pharm Ther* **35**, 491–6.

Wycis HT, Spiegel EA (1962) Long-range results in the treatment of intractable pain by stereotaxic midbrain surgery. *J Neurosurg* **19**, 101–7.

Wydenkeller S, Maurizio S, Dietz V, Halder P (2009) Neuropathic pain in spinal cord injury: significance of clinical and electrophysiological measures. *Eur J Neurosci* **30**, 91–9.

Wyndaele M, Wyndaele JJ (2006) Incidence, prevalence and epidemiology of spinal cord injury: what learns a worldwide literature survey? *Spinal Cord* **44**, 523–9.

Yamamoto M, Yabuki S, Hayabara T, Otsuki S (1981) Paroxysmal itching in multiple sclerosis: a report of three cases. *J Neurol Neurosurg Psychiatry* **44**, 19–22.

Yamamoto T, Katayama Y, Hirayama T, Tsubokawa T (1997) Pharmacological classification of central post-stroke pain: comparison with the results of chronic motor cortex stimulation therapy. *Pain* **72**, 5–12.

Yamamoto T, Katayama Y, Fukaya C, *et al.* (2000) Thalamotomy caused by cardioversion in a patient treated with deep brain stimulation. *Stereotact Funct Neurosurg* **74**, 73–82.

Yamashiro K, Iwayama K, Karihara M, *et al.* (1991) Neurons with epileptiform discharge in the central nervous system and chronic pain. Experimental and clinical investigations. *Acta Neurochir (Wien) Suppl* **52**, 130–2.

Yanagida H, Arakawa K, Sakai K, Sadohara Y (2003) Intensity of central pain: analysis of pain scores in 18 patients. *Pain Pract* **3**, 117–19.

Yen HL, Chan W (2003) An East–West approach to the management of central post-stroke pain. *Cerebrovasc Dis* **16**, 27–30.

Yoshii N, Mizokami T, Ushikubo T, Kuramitsu T, Fukuda S (1980) Long-term follow-up study after pulvinotomy for intractable pain. *Appl Neurophysiol* **43**, 128–32.

Young CK, Eggermont JJ (2009) Coupling of mesoscopic brain oscillations: recent advances in analytical theoretical perspectives. *Progr Neurobiol* **89**, 61–78.

Young GB, Blume WT (1983) Painful epileptic seizures. *Brain* **106**, 537–54.

Young RF (1990) Clinical experience with radiofrequency and laser DREZ lesions. *J Neurosurg* **72**, 715–20.

Young RF (1995) Commentary. In: Schmideck HH, Sweet WH, eds., *Operative Neurosurgical Techniques. Indications, Methods and Results*, 3rd edn. Philadelphia, PA: WB Saunders, pp. 1399–401.

Young RF, Chambi I (1987) Pain relief by electrical stimulation of the periaqueductal and periventricular gray matter. Evidence for a non-opioid mechanism. *J Nerurosurg* **66**, 364–71.

Young RF, Goodman SJ (1979) Dorsal spinal cord stimulation in the treatment of multiple sclerosis. *Neurosurgery* **5**, 225–30.

Young RF, Rinaldi PC (1997) Brain stimulation. In: North RB, Levy RM, eds., *Neurosurgical Management of Pain*. New York, NY: Springer, pp. 283–301.

Young RF, Tronnier V, Rinaldi PC (1992) Chronic stimulation of the Kolliker-Fuse nucleus region for relief of intractable pain in humans. *J Neurosurg* **76**, 979–85.

Young RF, Vermeulen SS, Grimm P, *et al.* (1995) Gamma knife thalamotomy for the treatment of persistent pain. *Stereotact Funct Neurosurg* **64** (Suppl 1), 172–81.

Yun SP, Sun BC (2010) Apipuncture treatment for central post-stroke pain. *J Altern Complement Med* **16**, 223–4.

Zachariah SB, Borges EF, Varghese R, Cruz AR, Ross GS (1994) Positive response to oral divalproex sodium (Depakote) in patients with spasticity and pain. *Am J Med Sci* **308**, 38–40.

Zahs KR, Ashe KH (2010) "Too much good news" – are Alzheimer mouse models trying to tell us how to prevent, not cure, Alzheimer's disease? *Trends Neurosci* **33**, 381–9.

Zaki SA, Shenoy P, Shanbag P, Sundar U (2010) Thalamic pain syndrome due to cytomegalovirus vasculitis in an HIV-positive child. *Indian Pediatr* **47**, 621–3.

Zaletel M, Zvan B, Kobal J (2007) Influence of age on central post-stroke pain. *Eur J Pain* **11** (1 Suppl), 140.

Zhang SQ, Liu MY, Wan B, Zheng HM (2008) Contralateral body half hypalgesia in a patient with lateral medullary infarction: atypical Wallenberg syndrome. *Eur Neurol* **59**, 211–15.

Zhang X, Fan XN, Ding L, Zhang HT, Wu LZ, Wang HR (2010) [Acupuncture treatment of regulating spirit, activating blood and relieving pain for thalamic pain] *Zhongguo Zhen Jiu (Chinese Acupuncture)* **30**, 367–70.

Zuliani V, Rivara M, Fantini M, Costantino G (2010) Sodium channel blockers for neuropathic pain. *Expert Opin Ther Patents* **20**, 755–79.

Zvan B, Zaletel M (2010) Ageing and poststroke pain. *Eur J Pain Suppl* **4**, 107.

Zylicz Z (1997) Opioid responsive central pain of cerebrovascular origin: a case report. *Palliat Med* **11**, 495–6.

Index